RHINOPLASTY

RHINOPLASTY

A practical guide to functional and aesthetic surgery of the nose

Third enlarged edition

edited by G.J. Nolst Trenité

Kugler Publications / The Hague / The Netherlands

ISBN Book: 90 6299 206 4
ISBN DVD: 90 6299 207 2
ISBN Book and DVD: 90 6299 208 0

Distributors for USA and Canada:
Library Research Associates, Inc.
158 West Main Street, Suite 2
Walden, NY 12586
U.S.A.
Fax: (845) 778 1864
E-mail: lrainc@fronntiernet.net

For all other countries:
Kugler Publications
P.O. Box 97747
2509 CG The Hague
The Netherlands
Fax: +31.70.33 00 254
E-mail: info@kuglerpublications.com
website: www.kuglerpublications.com

Phototypeset by Palm Produkties, Nieuwerkerk aan den IJssel, The Netherlands
Printed by Koninklijke Drukkerij C.C. Callenbach b.v., Nijkerk, The Netherlands
Bound by Bindery Callenbach, Nijkerk The Netherlands

Kugler Publications is an imprint of SPB Academic Publishing bv, P.O. Box 97747, 2509 CG The Hague, The Netherlands

CONTENTS

CONTRIBUTORS

A.J.M. Balm, M.D., Ph.D.
Department of Head and Neck Oncology and Surgery, The Netherlands Cancer Institute – Anthonie van Leeuwenhoek Hospital, Plesmanlaan 121, 1060 CX Amsterdam, The Netherlands

M. Bönisch, M.D.
Department of Otorhinolaryngology, Diakonessen Krankenhaus Linz, Linz, Austria

T.R. Bull, F.R.C.S.
Consultant Surgeon, Royal National Throat, Nose and Ear Hospital & Charing Cross Hospital, and 107 Harley Street, London W1N 1DG, U.K.

R. Cobo, M.D.
Department of Otorhinolaryngology, Centro Medico Imbanaco, Carrera 38A# 5A-100 Cons 231 Rorre A, Cali, Colombia

W.J. Fokkens, M.D., Ph.D.
Department of Otorhinolaryngology, Academic Medical Centre of the University of Amsterdam, P.O. Box 22660, 1100 DD Amsterdam, The Netherlands

P.J.F.M. Lohuis, M.D., Ph.D.
Department of Otorhinolaryngology/Head and Neck Surgery, Academic Medical Centre of the University of Amsterdam, P.O. Box 22660, 1100 DD Amsterdam, The Netherlands

I.S. Mackay, F.R.C.S.
Consultant E.N.T. Surgeon, Royal Brompton Hospital and Charing Cross Hospital, London, U.K.

R. Meyer, M.D., Ph.D.
Centre de Chirurgie Plastique, 4 Avenue Marc-Dufour, CH 1007 Lausanne, Switzerland

M.J. Middelweerd, M.D., Ph.D.
Department of Otorhinolaryngology, Head and Neck Surgery, Free University Hospital Amsterdam, P.O. Box 7057, 1007 MB Amsterdam, The Netherlands

G.J. Nolst Trenité, M.D., Ph.D.
Department of Otorhinolaryngology/Head and Neck Surgery, Academic Medical Center, University Hospital of the University of Amsterdam, Meibergdreef 9, 1105 AZ Amsterdam Z.O., The Netherlands

F.W.A. Otten, M.D., Ph.D.
Department of Otorhinolaryngology, Diaconessenhuis, Houtlaan 55, 2334 CK Leiden, The Netherlands

R.M.L. Poublon, M.D., Ph.D.
Department of Otorhinolaryngology, Erasmus University Rotterdam, Dr. Molewaterplein 40, 3015 GD Rotterdam, The Netherlands

G. Rettinger, M.D., Ph.D.
Department of Otorhinolaryngology, Head and Neck Surgery, University of Ulm, Prittwitzstrasse 43, D-89075 Ulm/Donau, Germany

C.D.A. Verwoerd, M.D., Ph.D.
Department of Otorhinolaryngology, Erasmus University Rotterdam, Dr. Molewaterplein 40, 3015 GD Rotterdam, The Netherlands

H.L. Verwoerd-Verhoef, M.D., Ph.D.
Department of Otorhinolargyngology, Erasmus University Rotterdam, Dr. Molewaterplein 40, 3015 GD Rotterdam, The Netherlands

B.C. Vinayak F.R.C.S.
Department of Otorhinolaryngology, Radcliffe Infirmary, University of Oxford, Woodstock Road, Oxford, OX2 6HE, U.K.

H.D. Vuyk, M.D., Ph.D.
Department of Otorhinolaryngology, Ziekenhuis Gooi Noord, Rijksstraatweg 1, 1261 AN Blaricum, The Netherlands

C. Walter, M.D., Ph.D.
Department of Otorhinolaryngology and Facial Surgery, Klinik am Rosenberg, CH 9140 Heiden AR, Switzerland

T.D. Zijlker, M.D., Ph.D.
Department of Otorhinolaryngology, Ziekenhuis De Wever en Gregorius, Henri Dunantstraat 5, 6419 PC Heerlen, The Netherlands

FOREWORD

M. Eugene Tardy, Jr.

The pioneers of early rhinoplasty in the late nineteenth and early twentieth century would take pleasure in the fact that this complex operation still incorporates the fundamental principles identified by these visionary men. It is doubtful, however, that any among them could have foreseen the remarkable refinements rather routinely employed in the past decade.

Important developments have transformed aesthetic and reconstructive rhinoplasty from a procedure incorporating primarily *tissue reduction* and *sacrifice* to one of *tissue reorientation and reconstruction*. Time and experience combine to teach that the finest and most natural long-term outcomes are those in which *less* removal of nasal structures is effected, preserving natural form and function. Clearly the best rhinoplasty surgeons are those who think and plan long-term, tailoring the operation to the exact anatomy encountered, carrying out maneuvers designed to maintain control of the healing process. Cartilage grafting procedures, much more common now than in the past, lend unlimited possibilities to nasal contour sculpturing. Conservative preservation of the various components of the nasal framework and skin-subcutaneous tissue layer now reigns as a fundamental cardinal principle of modern rhinoplasty.

For the majority of our predecessors and teachers, the learning process for sophisticated rhinoplasty procedures was a long and arduous process, rooted in trial and error. The past two decades, stimulated by educators skilled in teaching techniques and aided by knowledge gained through anatomical studies and long-term follow-up of patients operated on by various techniques, have borne witness to a significant shortening of the otherwise steep and arduous learning curve to rhinoplasty excellence. Operative television brings the experience and techniques of experts from around the world to the eager learner at the flick of a video control button. The emergence of the open approach to certain difficult rhinoplasty anatomical problems allows the neophyte surgeon an unparalleled opportunity to witness exact relationships and variations in nasal anatomic components. Fresh cadaver dissection experience has clarified surgical concepts of value and disqualified those with questionable outcomes. A plethora of detailed textbooks on rhinoplasty has emerged in the past decade, providing surgical guidance based upon wide experience and careful patient follow-up.

To this veritable explosion of scholarly information, Nolst Trenité and his associate authors have added another valuable link to the puzzle of aesthetic and functional rhinoplasty.

In the expanded second edition of this successful text/atlas new chapters by surgeons of long experience and vision augment fundamental information from the first edition. A companion interactive CD-ROM vividly portrayed operative techniques discussed in the text. Emphasizing throughout the cardinal principles which apply in the overwhelming majority of rhinoplasty procedures, the authors present herein direct and compelling information for the neophyte and experienced surgeon alike. The clear language of the text is complemented by valuable illustrations designed to give the reader the understanding to apply rhinoplasty principles to a variety of anatomical variants encountered.

Throughout, the authors uniformly emphasize coordinated procedures to repair both functional as well as aesthetic deformities and disorders. Strong emphasis is placed on the significant advantages of cartilage autografts in the treatment of both primary and revision surgery, a philosophy that is generally shared by knowledgeable surgeons worldwide. Techniques which occasion less risk of sequelae or significant complication predominate throughout the volume.

This **third edition of Rhinoplasty**, edited by Gilbert Nolst Trenité and his contributory colleagues expands and enlarges the canons of nasal surgery elegantly demonstrated in the former editions. Six new chapters have been developed, including expanded and detailed discussions of septoplasty, ethnic rhinoplasty, refinements of the open approach, alar batten grafting and an enlarged section on nasal reconstructive techniques. Furthermore, a most valuable addition to the traditionally nicely illustrated written chapters incorporates an interactive DVD containing elements of live surgery, as well as instructive and vivid videoclips of surgical techniques.

Surgeons who share a deep interest and passion for the complex operation of rhinoplasty will enjoy the clear, precise and pragmatic approach incorporated herein. Professor Nolst Trenité and associates have produced what they sought to achieve – a vital and practical contemporary guide to rhinoplasty.

M. Eugene Tardy, Jr., M.D. F.A.C.S.
Professor of Clinical Otolaryngology – Head and Neck Surgery
Director, Division of Head and Neck Plastic Surgery
University of Illinois Medical Center at Chicago

INTRODUCTION

This book on rhinoplastic surgery was initiated by the Dutch ENT society because of the increasing interest of ENT surgeons not only in functional, but also in aesthetic surgery of the nose. This interest has been stimulated by a growing demand for aesthetic surgery.

In many cases there is a combined functional-aesthetic problem, which can be corrected in a one-stage operative procedure. The fast development of more atraumatic and refined operative techniques in the last decade, and the importance of good long-term results and dwindling mishaps in nasal surgery, emphasize the need for an up-to-date, step-by-step operative guide. Although there are many good books on the subject of rhinoplasty, there is a lack of practical guides covering surgical anatomy, pre- and postoperative management and basic techniques for septal-, tip- and osseocartilaginous vault surgery, especially for the less experienced rhinosurgeon.

This book is divided into three parts: the basic knowledge needed for rhinoplastic surgery (part I), the different operative techniques (part II), and capita selecta of special problems (part III), written by internationally renowned authorities on rhinoplasty.

We hope that this practical guide will be of use to many surgeons by helping them to perform one of the most challenging aspects of facial plastic surgery: rhinoplasty.

Gilbert J. Nolst Trenité

Second enlarged edition

It is with great pleasure that I present the second enlarged edition of *Rhinoplasty: A Practical Guide to Functional and Aesthetic Surgery of the Nose*.

The first edition was sold to all parts of the world, from Japan to Colombia in South America. The reviews in leading journals were overwhelmingly positive. Any small points of constructive criticism acted as a stimulus to improve the second edition. The book has been considerably extended and now contains 300, rather than 200, pages, not to mention about 200 extra full-color illustrations and three new chapters: 'External rhinoplasty, the benefits and the pitfalls', 'Nasal vestibular stenoses' and 'Guidelines for cadaver dissection'. The purpose of the last mentioned (a unicum in textbooks on rhinoplasty) is to stimulate neophyte rhinoplastic surgeons to start practising modern rhinoplasty techniques on cadaver specimens before proceeding to patients. A fourth new chapter, 'Surgical management of large septal perforations' by R. Meyer, on the very challenging treatment of septal perforations, replaces his earlier contribution 'Tip columella and ala'.

Moreover, a completely new teaching tool has been developed with the help of ETI (Expert Center of Taxonomic Identification) at the University of Amsterdam: An interactive CD-ROM with live-surgery video coverage of the different surgical procedures linked to the corresponding chapters, which enables the user to observe the surgery in combination with the techniques described.

I sincerely hope that this second enlarged edition, combined with its specific interactive CD-ROM, will contribute to shortening the learning process in one of the most difficult aspects of facial plastic surgery: that of rhinoplasty.

Gilbert J. Nolst Trenité

Third edition with interactive DVD

After the first edition, which was published in 1993, and the second edition with interactive CD ROM, published in 1998, this third edition is even more extensive, containing six new chapters: Septal surgery basic techniques; New concepts in reconstructive septoplasty; Developments in the open rhinoplasty approach; Ethnic rhinoplasty; Batten grafts for nasal valve collapse; and Nasal reconstruction.

Moreover, a sophisticated new interactive DVD has been developed in cooperation with the Audio Visual Center at the University of Amsterdam. Its goal is to provide a practical guide with the maximum impact on teaching. The DVD contains more than two and a half hours of live surgery and there are short video clips on specific surgical techniques to complement the various chapters.

The many positive reactions from all parts of the world regarding this practical guide to functional and aesthetic surgery of the nose, which has helped colleagues improve their surgical skills, have been a huge stimulus.

Once again, I sincerely hope that this third edition, with its interactive DVD that explicitly shows most of the modern techniques in rhinoplasty, will be of benefit to surgeons who wish to improve their skills in rhinoplasty, which today still remains the most challenging and difficult surgical procedure in plastic surgery of the face.

Gilbert J. Nolst Trenité

PART I: BASICS

1: ANATOMY

R.M.L. Poublon

Introduction

To gain access to the underlying structure of the nose, it is very important for the surgeon to have full knowledge of the anatomy of the nose, of its relationship with the remainder of the face and of the dynamic consequences of various surgical maneuvers on nasal integrity. In other words, when looking at the face, the attention should be drawn to the eyes when the nose is in harmony with the face. It should be realized that although the nose is in the center of the face, it is not in fact the focal point.

Modern facial analysis began in the Middle Ages with the work of Leonardo da Vinci and Albrecht Dürer. They were, however, more interested in the realistic depiction of faces than in defining an aesthetic ideal. In the last decades, this analysis has been intensified by orthodontists in their development of cephalometric measurements. However, certain simple proportions and rules have proven useful in analyzing the nose before surgery. Moreover, it should be borne in mind that we have to look through the skin and subcutaneous tissue to envisage the bony and cartilaginous framework. The terminology in describing anatomical relationships of nasal structures is illustrated in Figure 1.

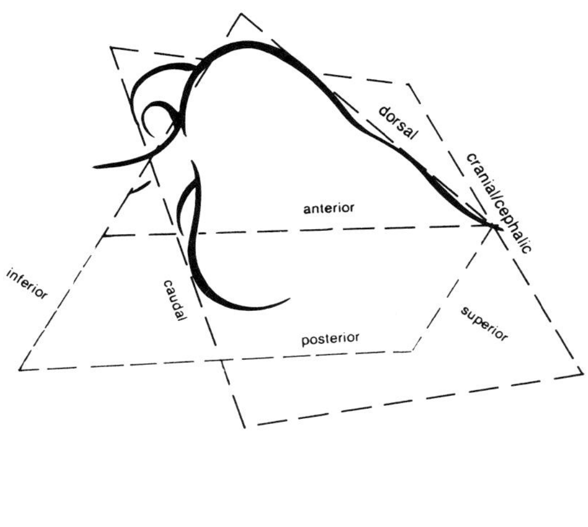

Fig. 1. Terminology and orientation.
Cranial means towards the head, dorsal means towards the dorsum of the nose, anterior means towards the front of the body.
Cranial (or cephalic) and caudal refer to opposite directions, as do inferior and superior, and anterior and posterior.

Bony pyramid

The deepest depression on the root of the nose in the midsagittal plane is the nasion. This is composed of the junction of the paired nasal bones with the nasal process of the frontal bone, thus forming the nasofrontal angle. The overlying soft tissue in this region is fairly thick and consists of skin, subcutaneous fat and the procerus muscle, which is in contrast with the thin layer of soft tissue at the caudal border of the nasal bones (Fig. 2).

Laterally, the nasal bones articulate with the frontal process of the maxillary bone: both constitute the bony nasal pyramid. This pyramid encapsules the nasal fossa, and contributes to the width of the bony nose in the upper third. It partially overrides the upper lateral cartilages, as with a rooftile. A thin layer of connective tissue between bone and cartilage is considered to be periosteum fused with perichondrium. The overlap tends to be more in the parasagittal than in the lateral plane. The inferior border of the pyramid up to the anterior nasal spine is called the piriform aperture. Mobilization of the bony pyramid is usually achieved with medial-oblique osteotomies in the nasal bones and with slightly curved lateral osteotomies in the frontal process of the maxilla, superior to the attachment of the inferior turbinate and just anterior to the lacrimal fossa.

Cartilaginous pyramid

The lower two-thirds of the nose is built up of cartilage. From early fetal life, the cartilaginous framework consists of a T-bar-shaped bilateral vault fused in the midline to the septum. Whereas in early childhood this cartilage extends from the

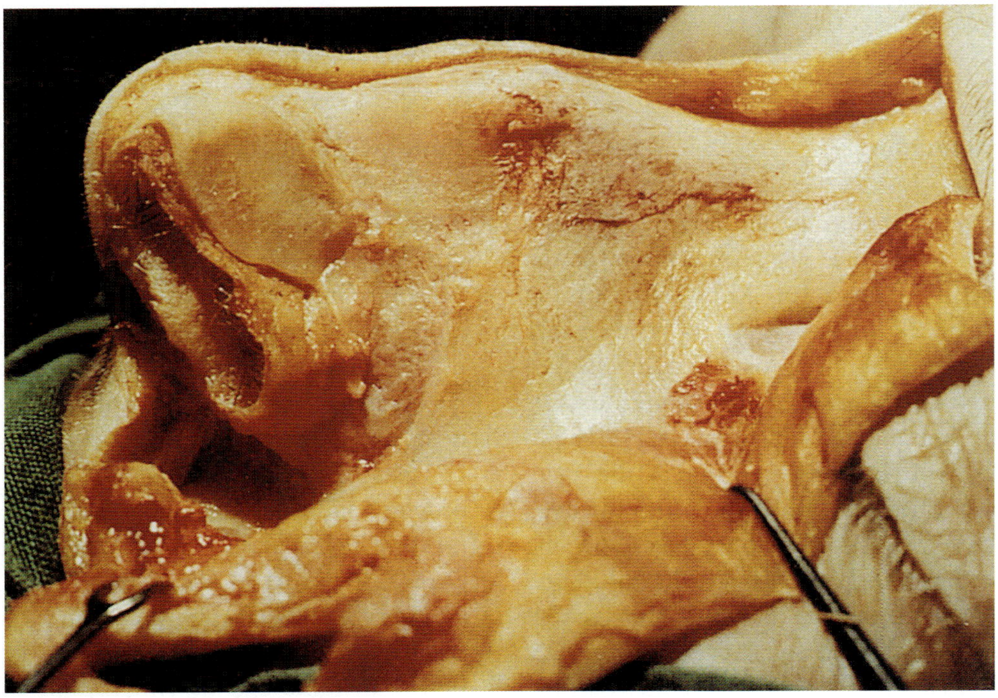

Fig. 2. Lateral view of the nasal pyramid in relation to the overlying subcutaneous tissue and skin.

tip of the nose into the still cartilaginous skullbase, during further growth the cranial parts of the upper lateral cartilages regress, ultimately giving them the triangular shape of adulthood (Fig. 3a,b). Therefore, nasal septal cartilage and upper lateral cartilages form one cartilaginous complex. Surgery on the nasal dorsum will therefore impose the medial aspect of the upper lateral cartilages as well as the cartilaginous nasal septum.

Cranially, the upper laterals are overlapped by the nasal bones and frontal process of the maxilla, and caudally, by the cephalic border of the lower lateral cartilages. A thin layer of connective tissue between bone and cartilage is considered as periosteum fused with perichondrium. Laterally, the upper laterals are attached and supported to the piriform aperture with dense connective tissue. This firm attachment can be damaged after surgery or trauma, which will give rise to functional as well as aesthetic complaints. The region of overlap with and attachment to the lower laterals is called the scroll region and forms the first major support mechanism to the nasal tip. Three different forms of overlap between upper and lower lateral cartilage can be found. A true rooftile overlap is most frequently seen in which the cephalic margin of the lower lateral covers the free caudal margin of the upper lateral. In the second form of overlap the cephalic margin of the lower lateral covers a reverse curled free caudal margin of the upper lateral cartilage. This variation can be identified when the vestibulum is inspected in the valve area. Sometimes a true overlap between lower and upper lateral cartilage is missing mostly due to the aging process. An intercartilaginous incision, to undermine the nasal dorsum, will loosen this prominent support mechanism which could result in tip ptosis.

The relationship between the upper laterals and the nasal septum is of extreme clinical importance at its caudal end and this region is called the nasal valve area. This region is the functional unit which includes the nasal septum medially, the caudal end of the upper

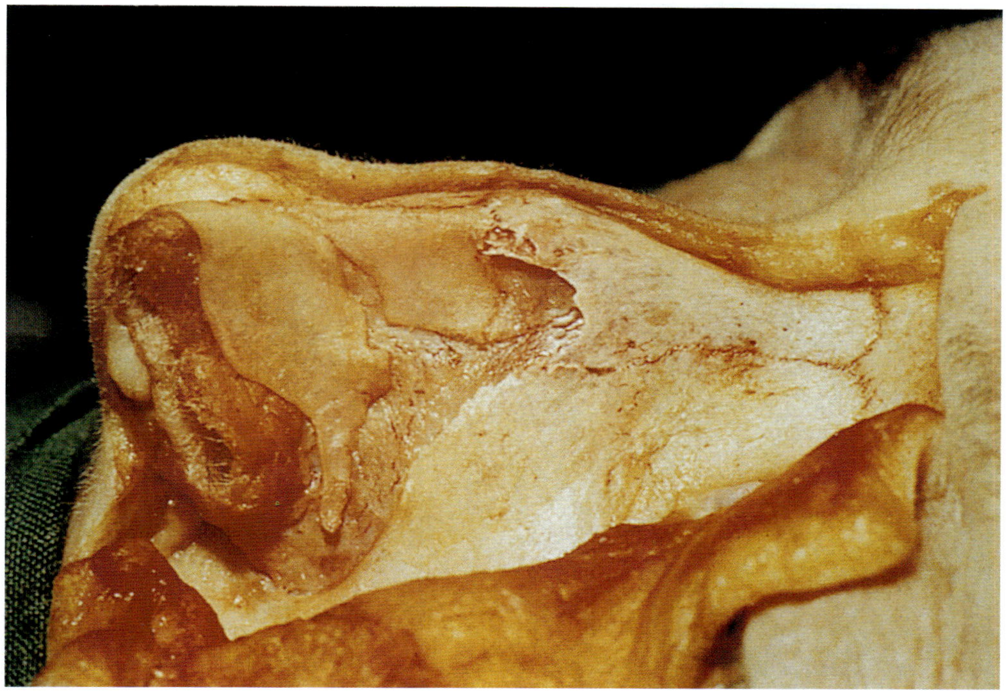

Fig. 3a. Lateral view of the nasal pyramid with special interest to the relationship between upper lateral cartilage and the bony pyramid.

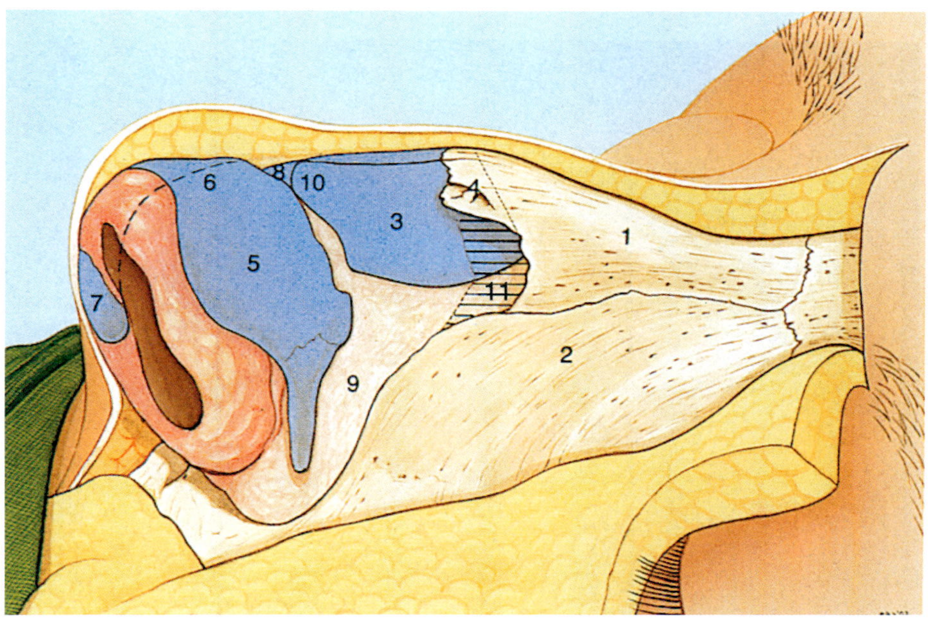

Fig. 3b. 1. nasal bone 2. frontal process of the maxillary bone 3. upper lateral cartilage 4. area of overlap (nasal bone-upper lateral) 5. lateral crus of lower lateral cartilage 6. dome area with tip defining point 7. medial crus of lower lateral cartilage 8. quadrangular (septal) cartilage 9. connective tissue 10. scroll region 11. shaded part of removed nasal bone.

laterals and the piriform aperture laterally, the floor of the nose and the head of the inferior turbinates posteriorly. The nasal valve is that specific triangular slit-like portion of the nose between the caudal end of the upper lateral cartilage and its relationship to the nasal septum. Normally it ranges between 10 and 15 degrees. The epithelial lining of the nasal vestibule changes here from keratinizing squamous epithelium into nasal mucosa.

Lobule

The tip is the most forward projecting part of the lobule. The part immediately

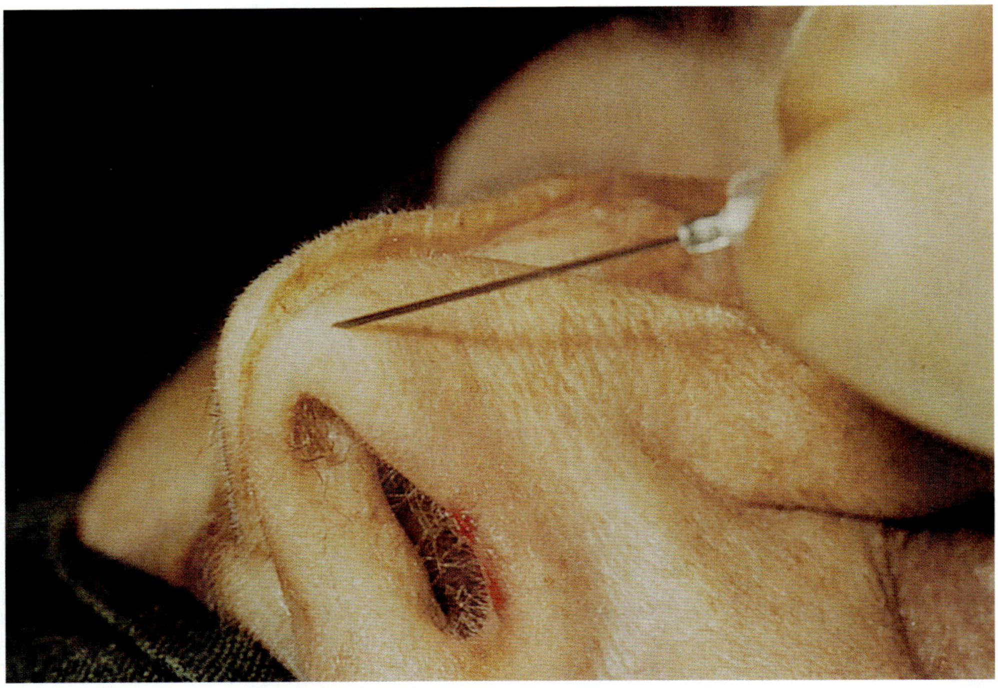

Fig. 4. Oblique view of the lobule. The inferior border of the lower lateral cartilage is indicated on the skin leaving a small triangular area where cartilage is lacking (soft triangle of Converse).

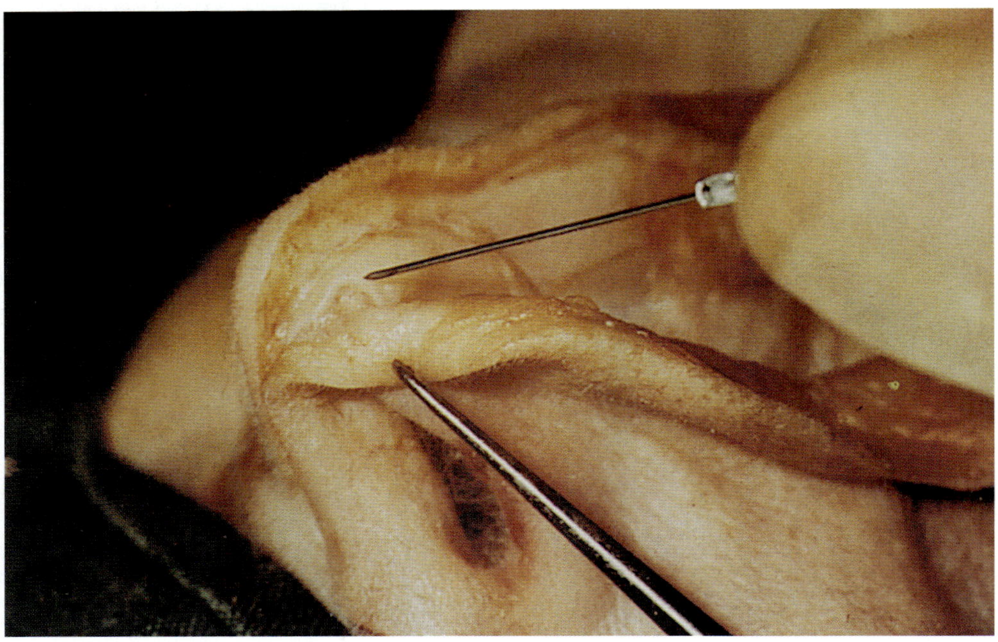

Fig. 5. Oblique view of the lobule. The inferior border of the lower lateral cartilage is indicated where the medial crus diverges into the lateral crus (angle).

above the tip is called the supratip and the part below the intratip. The lower lateral cartilages encompass the nostrils, leaving a small triangular area between the medial and lateral crus (soft triangle of Converse) (Figs. 4 and 5). The medial component or medial crus forms the columella and the lateral component or lateral crus provides the cartilaginous framework of the ala.

The medial footplate attachment to the caudal border of the septal cartilage forms the second major tip support mechanism. The junction of the columella and the

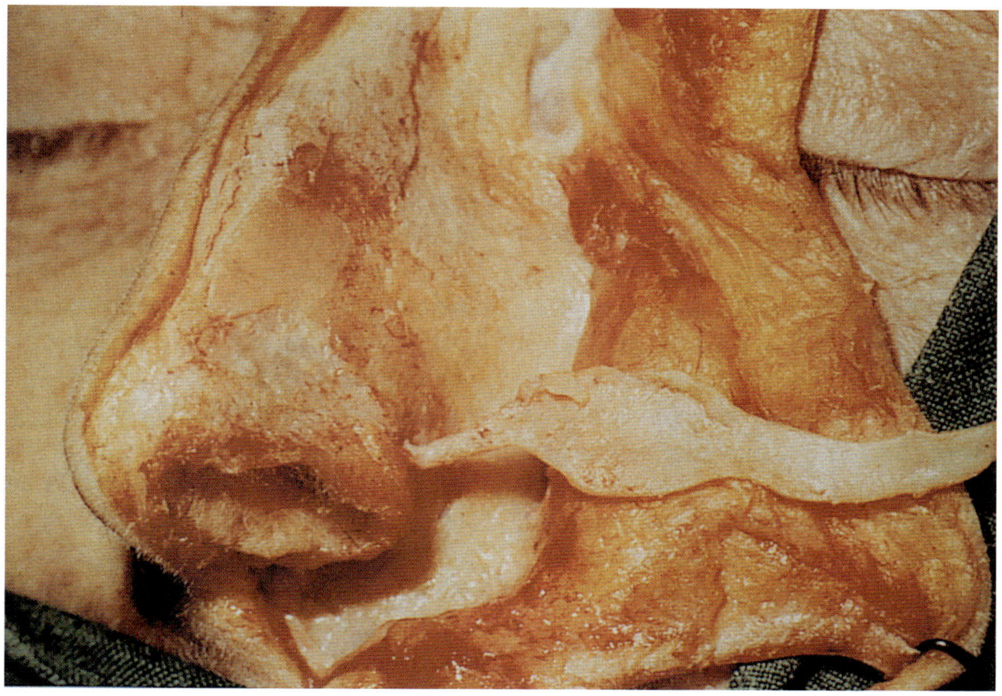

Fig. 6. Oblique view of the lobule. The lower lateral cartilage is rolled aside leaving the vestibular skin in its original position. Note the hinge area with the sesamoid cartilage.

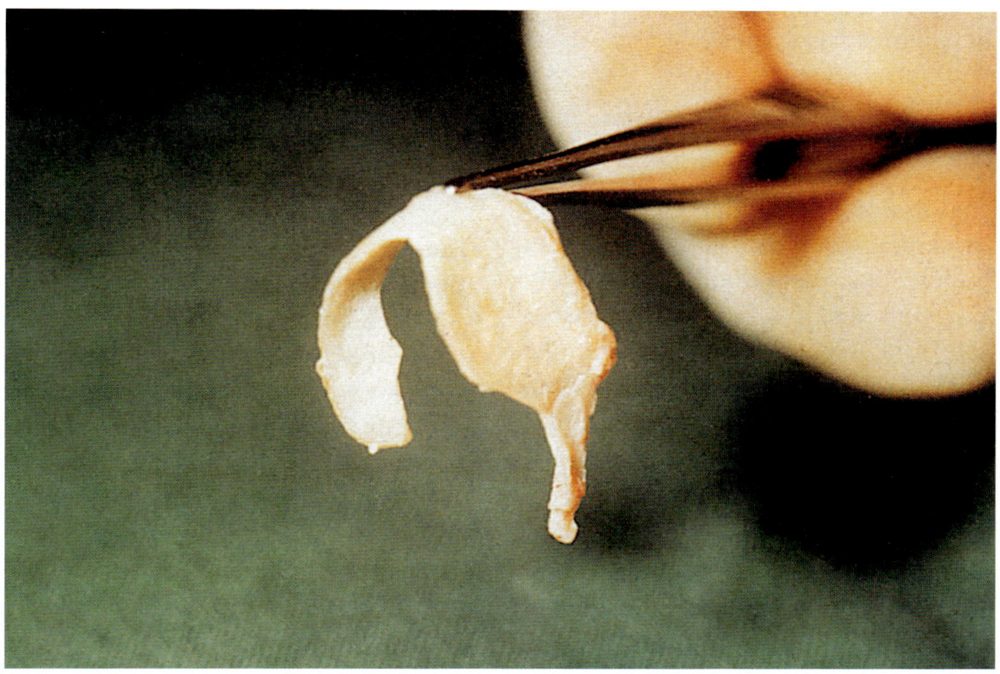

Fig. 7. Oblique view of the lower lateral cartilage. Medial crus beginning at its footplate, the transition into the lateral crus and the tail of the lower lateral cartilage with the sesamoid cartilage. Note the resilience of the cartilage giving strength to the nostril.

upper lip forms the nasolabial angle. Changes of this angle can give the illusion of rotation of the tip. A blunt angle results in an upward rotation, *e.g.*, a prominent anterior nasal spine or overdevelopment of the septal cartilage. A sharp angle results in a downward rotation, *e.g.*, underdevelopment of the septal cartilage or excessive resection of cartilage ('retracted columella'). The lateral crura diverge in the supratip area into the ala, leaving a small triangular area between them which contains the septal angle (weak triangle of Converse). Laterally, the oval-shaped cartilage is connected with dense fibro-fatty tissue to the piriform aperture. This area is called the hinge area. Small segments of cartilage (sesamoid cartilages) can be found in this region (Fig. 6).

The tip-defining point (highest projecting point) is usually associated with the transition of the medial and lateral crus (or angle). Size, shape and resilience of the medial as well as the lateral crus form the third major support mechanism of the nasal tip (Fig. 7). Other minor supporting factors are:

- the strong ligamentous attachment of the skin to the interdomal region;
- the cartilaginous and membranous nasal septum;
- the sesamoid complex extending the support of the lateral crura to the piriform aperture (hinge area);
- the anterior nasal spine.

Nasal septum

The nasal septum is composed of a bony and a cartilaginous part (Figs. 8a, b). In early childhood, the septum is completely cartilaginous and ossifies during further growth from a center just posterior to the crista galli in a ventro-caudal direction. This ossification is partly intramembranous in the first years of childhood and partly endochondral, up until puberty.

The bony part consists of the perpendicular plate of the ethmoid and the vomer as well as the crest of the premaxilla and palatine. The perpendicular plate forms the upper and anterior part of the bony septum. It is continuous cranially with the crista galli and the cribriform plate. The vomer extends from the rostrum of the sphenoid, articulates anterior to the perpendicular plate superiorly and with the quadrangular cartilage inferiorly. The posterior margin is free, separating the posterior nasal apertures or choanae.

The quadrangular cartilage is the medial part of the T-bar-shaped cartilaginous framework of the mobile nose. In early childhood, this cartilage reaches the sphenoidal rostrum and the paired nasal bones. During further growth, the extension of cartilage diminishes due to ossification, sometimes leaving a sphenoidal process between the perpendicular plate and vomer. This may give rise to spur formation.

The superoposterior margin of the septal cartilage is connected to the inferior border of the internasal suture. In an anterior direction, the septal cartilage ends in the supratip area just above the level of the lower lateral cartilages. Caudally, the septum reaches the medial crura of the lower lateral cartilages, divided from them by a thin strip of membranous septum, and meets the anterior septal spine antero-inferiorly. In this region, fibers of the perichondrium and periosteum interchange, resulting in a firm attachment of the septal cartilage to the spine. Inferiorly, the septal cartilage sits in the groove of the maxillary crest with the same confluence of perichondrial and periosteal fibers.

The T-bar-shaped cartilaginous framework of septum and upper laterals gives the growing nasal cartilage enough strength for it to be capable of exerting pressure on the overlying and neighboring bony parts of the skull. Resection or destruction of cartilage due to trauma or surgery result in underdevelopment of the nose or even in a saddle-shaped deformity. A cartilaginous connection is seldom created after interruption of the continuity of the cartilage, due to inadequate wound healing. This will ultimately result in deviations and duplications.

Fig. 8a. Lateral view of the nasal septum covered with mucosa (1), hard and soft palate (2), anterior skull base (3) with frontal sinus (4) cribriform plate (5) crista Galli (6) sphenoid sinus (7) and pituitary fossa (8), posterior skull base (9) separated from the nasopharynx (10) by the clivus (11).

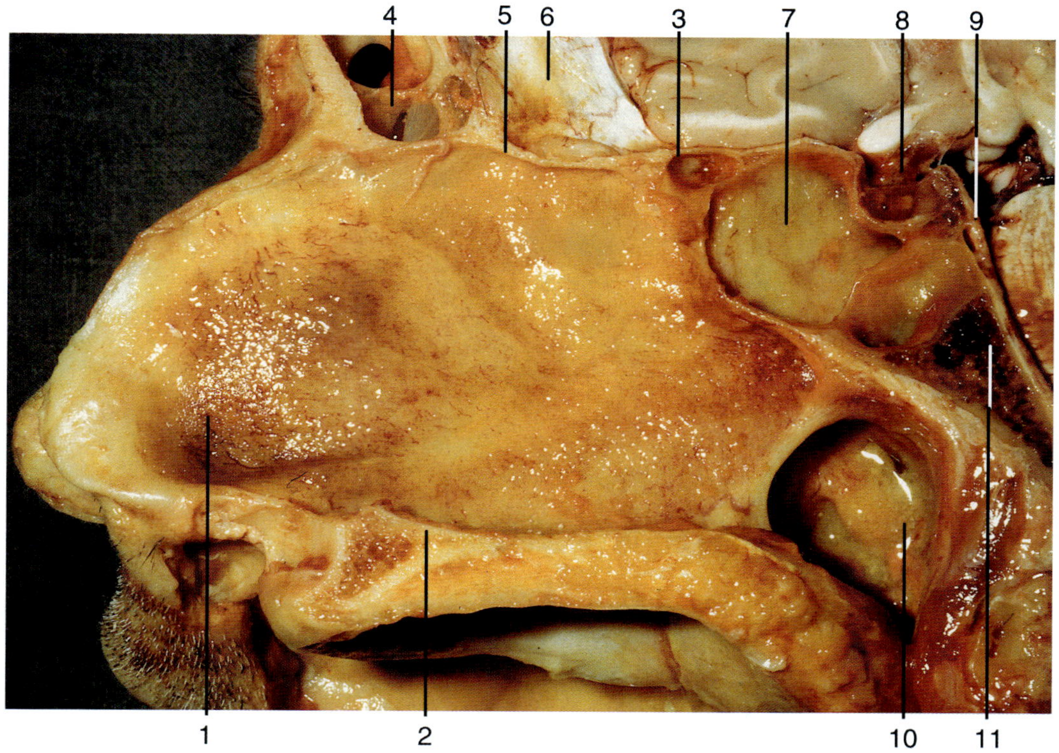

Fig. 8b. Lateral view of the nasal septum, consisting of septal cartilage (1), sphenoid tail of septal cartilage (2), perpendicular plate (3), vomer (4), palatine process of maxillary bone (5). It should be noted that the septal cartilage extends more than 10 mm under the nasal bone in this already 58-year-old specimen. A slight convexity of the septal cartilage can be observed just superior to the anterior nasal spine. Posterior to the anterior nasal spine, the incisival canal be identified.

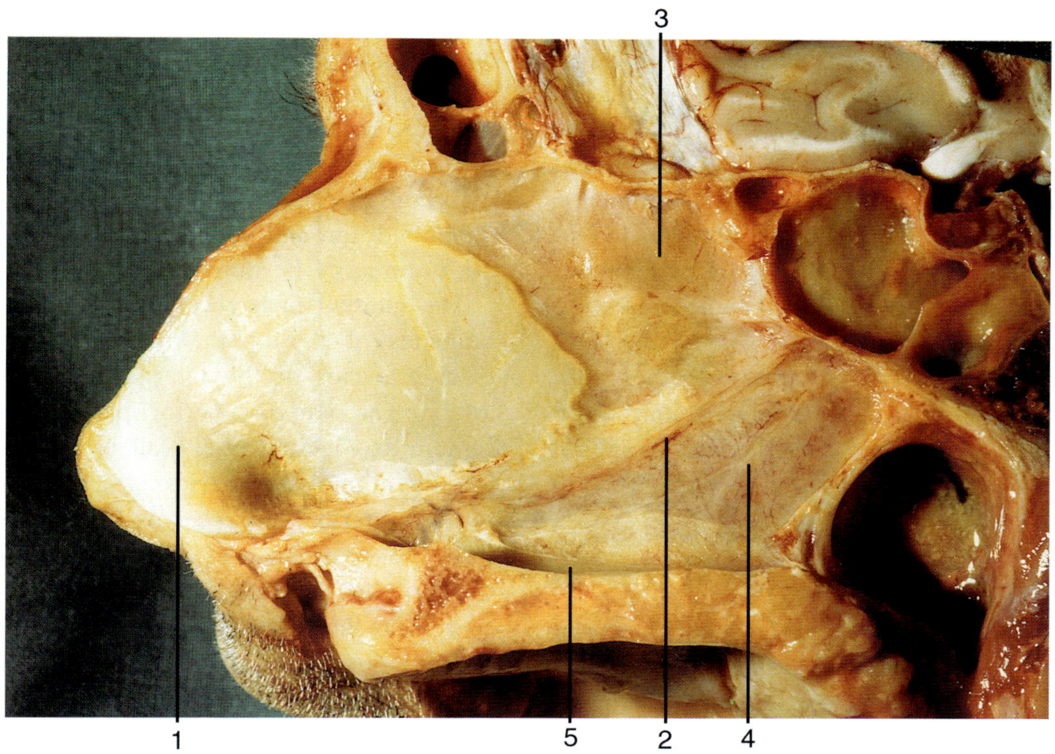

Skin

The thickness of the nasal skin differs from person to person, due to the amount of subcutaneous fat, sebaceous glands and nasal musculature. The skin over the dorsum and sides of the nose is usually thin and loosely connected to the osseous and cartilaginous framework. It is much thicker and more firmly adherent over the

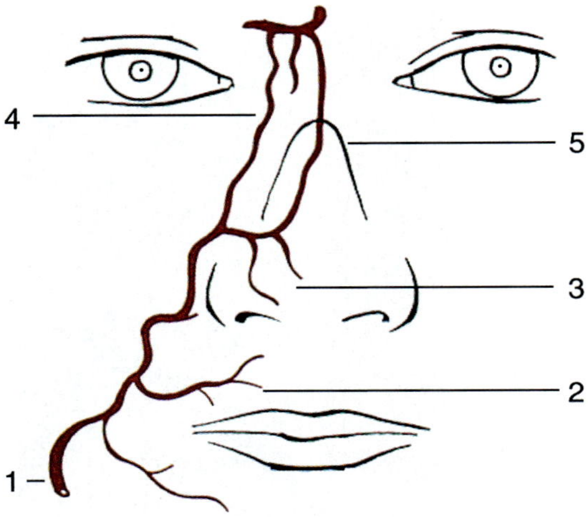

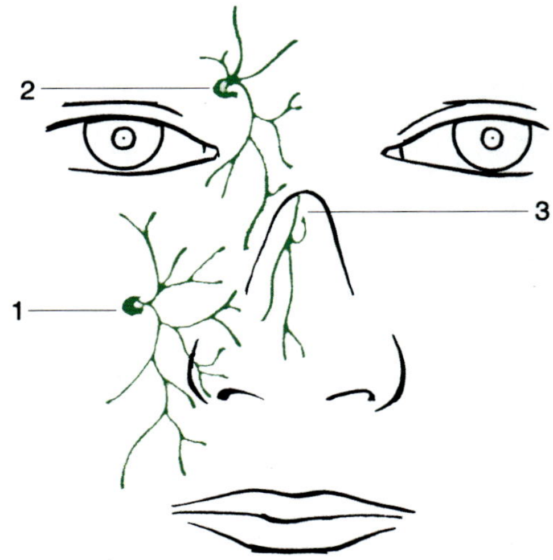

Fig. 9. Arterial nasal blood supply in frontal view.

Facial artery (1), superior labial artery (2), superior and inferior alar artery (3), angular artery (4), dorsal branch of the ophthalmic artery (5).

Fig. 10. Sensory nerve supply to the external nose in frontal view.

(Infraorbital branch of the maxillary nerve (1), infratrochlear branch of the ophthalmic nerve (2), external branches of the ethmoidal nerve (3)).

nasofrontal junctions and lower laterals. Pores of sebaceous glands are often quite prominent in the tip.

Assessment of skin texture and thickness should play a significant role in surgical planning. A too superficial undermining in refinement procedures to the nasal tip and correction of the nasal skeleton can lead to scar formation with areas of contraction and retraction. This can reveal palpable cartilage and bony remnants. Sometimes discoloration occurs, due to damage to the overlying skin. Extreme caution must be taken when creating pockets sufficiently deep into the subcutaneous tissue to avoid further skin damage. Alar rim retraction may even result from the over-reduction of lateral crura and needless sacrifice of underlying vestibular skin.

Blood supply

The arterial blood supply to the external nose is achieved by branches of the facial artery, as well as the ophthalmic artery. At the alar base, the facial artery divides into the labial, alar and angular arteries (Fig. 9). The superior labial artery supplies the upper lip and columella. The superior and inferior alar arteries run along the caudal and cephalic margin of the lower lateral cartilage. These supply the lobule. The angular artery runs upward along the lateral nasal wall and supplies the dorsum. It communicates with the dorsal nasal branch of the ophthalmic artery close to the medial orbital angle. All these larger vessels run laterally along the cartilaginous and bony framework and, working in close proximity with the perichondrium and periosteum, they need not necessarily be damaged.

The internal nose receives blood from branches of the ophthalmic artery and from branches of the internal maxillary artery. The antero-superior part of the septum and lateral nasal wall is supplied by the ethmoidal arteries, whereas the postero-inferior part receives blood from the sphenopalatine and descending palatine arteries. The greater palatine artery serves the antero-inferior portion of the nose, running through the incisive canal. It communicates with branches of the sphenopalatine artery. The network of vessels on the anterior septum, just posterior to the vestibular skin, contributes to Kiesselbach's plexus. This area is the most common site for epistaxis.

The mucosa on the inferior and middle

Fig. 11. Muscles of the nose. M. procerus (1), M. dilatator (2), M. levator labii superior (3), M. depressor septi (4), M. nasalis (5).

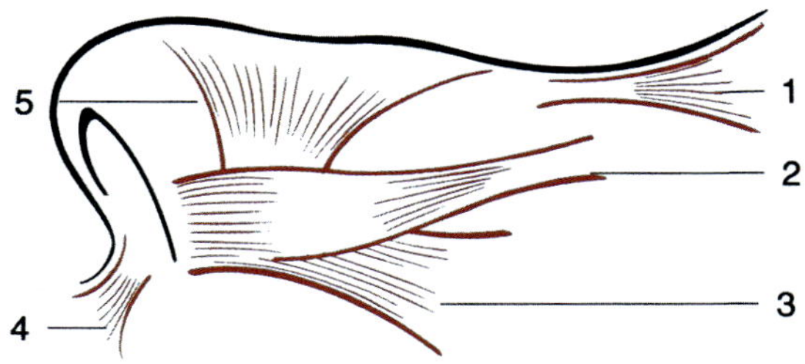

turbinates has a prolific vascular (cavernous) structure. The venous system drains posteriorly via the sphenopalatine vessels into the pterygoid plexus, occasionally intracranially to the cavernous sinus.

Nerve supply

The nerves of the external nose can be divided into sensory and motor nerves. The sensation in the skin of the middle third of the face (cheek, ala and upper lip) is derived from the infraorbital branch of the maxillary nerve (Fig. 10). The infratrochlear branch of the ophthalmic nerve supplies the upper third of the nose and the medial orbital angle. The middle third of the nasal dorsum and tip of the nose get their nerve supply from the external branches of the ethmoidal nerve. The motor nerve supply to the facial musculature is derived from the facial nerve.

The antero-superior part of the internal nose (lateral nasal wall and septum) is supplied by the ethmoidal nerve, while branches of the maxillary nerve and pterygopalatine ganglion supply the posterior part. It is noteworthy that the sensation in the antero-inferior part of the septum and lateral nasal wall is derived from branches of the alveolar nerve and superior dental plexus. Damage to this region (*e.g.*, inferior meatus antrostomy, inferior septal tunnelling) may give rise to numbness of the upper teeth.

Musculature

The muscles of the nose are primarily elevators, which shorten the nose and dilate the nostrils. One of these is the *M. procerus*, which can be regarded as a continuation of the frontal muscle and is inserted on the aponeurotic layer of the nasal dorsum (Fig. 11). This layer can be found on the lower aspect of the nasal bones and the upper part of the upper lateral cartilages.

The *M. Dilator* (*pars alaris musculi nasalis*) opens the nostrils and originates from the nasomaxillary suture and fibro-fatty tissue which support the lower laterals with the piriform aperture. Its insertion is at the skin of the nasolabial groove. The *M. levator labii superior* dilates the nares and originates in the frontal process of the maxillary bone. It is attached to the perichondrial layer of the lower lateral cartilage. The *M. depressor septi* lowers the nasal tip and opens the nostrils in deep inspiration. It forms part of the orbicularis muscle of the upper lip and inserts in the columella. The only muscle to effect compression of the nose, lengthen the nose and contract the nostrils is the *M. nasalis* (*pars transversa musculi nasalis*). Therefore, it antagonizes the *M. procerus*. It originates immediately lateral to the piriform aperture and inserts in the aponeurotic layer on the nasal dorsum.

All this muscular tissue should be protected during rhinoplasty, since its injury can cause a rigid appearance and immovability of the nose. A tension nose can be regarded as an exception to this rule. Surgical division of the *M. depressor septi* to release the pull at the nasal tip can then be advocated.

2: AESTHETICS

G.J. Nolst Trenité

Introduction

Before analyzing the nasal deformity and planning the operative procedure, it is necessary to see the face as a whole and be aware of the fact that, in addition to the *nose*, there are four other major aesthetic components in the facial complex: *forehead, eyes, lips and chin*. Changing the proportions and angles of the nose interferes directly with the other aesthetic parts. When these components are balanced in harmony, this creates beauty. Therefore knowledge of facial proportions is essential for every rhinoplastic surgeon.

Facial proportions

There is no absolute standard for the aesthetic proportions of the face. This differs depending on *sex*, *age*, *body type* and *facial characteristics*. The female nose is relatively smaller, the dorsum and lobule narrower, than that of the male. In profile, the female dorsum may show a slight concavity while, in the male dorsum, a slight convexity is acceptable. The naso-labial angle should be less acute in females (more tip rotation) than in males.

The aging nose tends to become elongated due to loss of elasticity of the skin, resulting in drooping of the tip. Degenerative changes in the alveolar process of the maxilla give the nose a more prominent appearance.

The nose should be in harmony with the body type. A short person can have a smaller nose with more tip rotation than a tall individual. The shape of the nose will also be determined by the shape of the face. A characteristically long or oval face requires a longer and narrower nose, whereas a round or square face will be more harmonious with a shorter, broader nose. Moreover, facial familial features should be considered in the preoperative assessment of an individual patient.

Frontal view (Fig. 1)

To evaluate the proportions, the face is roughly divided into three equal horizontal planes (hairline-glabella-subnasal-menton). With regard to the nose, the intercanthal distance should be more or less equal to the width of the alar base, which is more or less equal to the width of the eyes. The nasal width is aesthetically about 70% of the nasal length NT (nasion-tip). In its midfacial proportions, the nose should make a gentle curve (unbroken line) from the supra orbital ridge to the tip-defining point on the same side. The upper rim of the nares should resemble the wings of a seagull in flight. The columella is slightly lower with the nares just visible.

Lateral view (Figs. 2a,b and c)

In the lateral view, the Frankfort plane (the line between the superior border of the external auditory canal and the inferior border of the infra-orbital rim) should be horizontal. Similarly to the frontal view, the face is divided into three equal parts to evaluate the proportions.

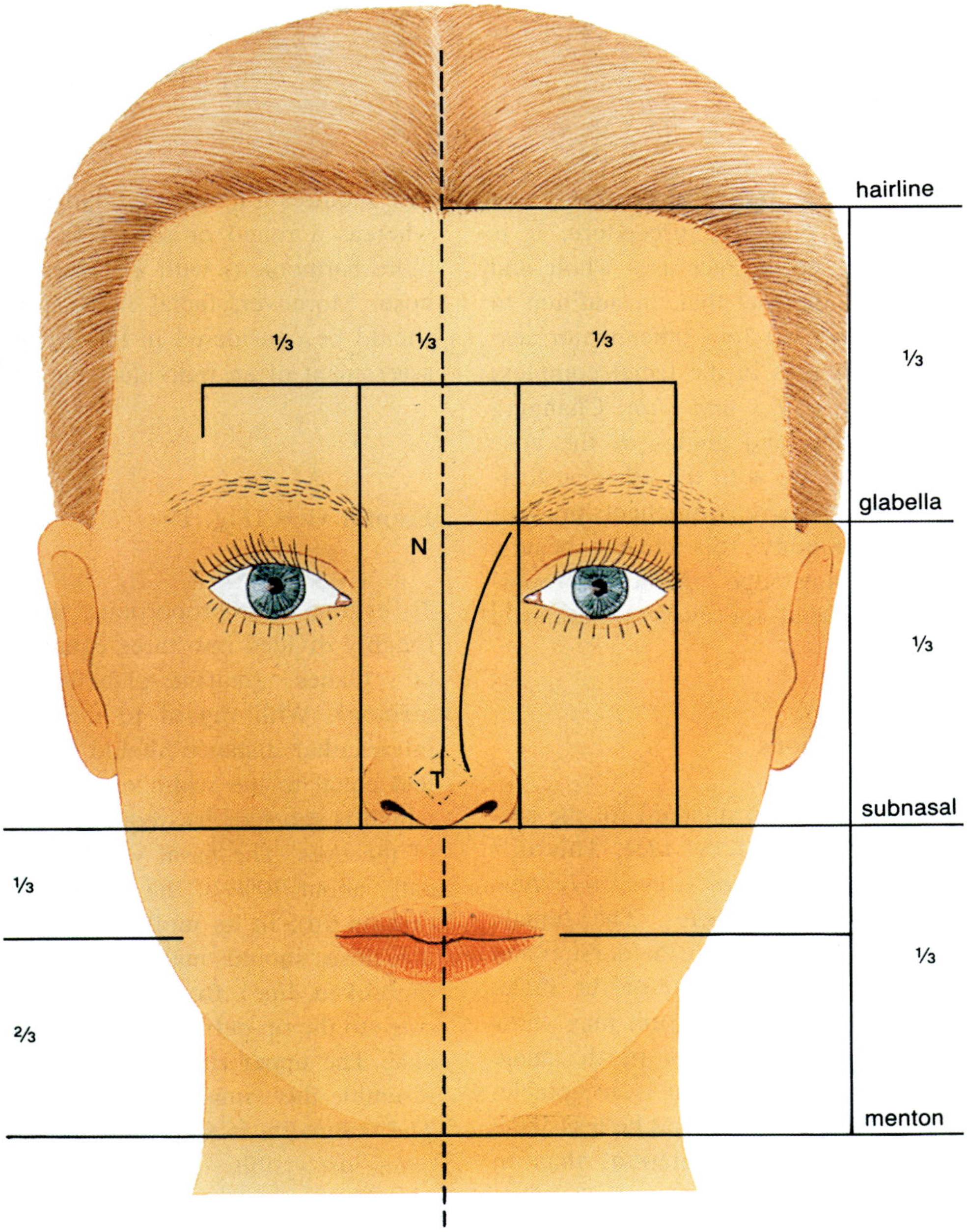

Fig. 1. Frontal view of the face divided into aesthetic proportions (equal thirds) with a gently curving unbroken line from the supra-orbital ridge along the lateral border of the dorsum to the tip-defining point on the same side.

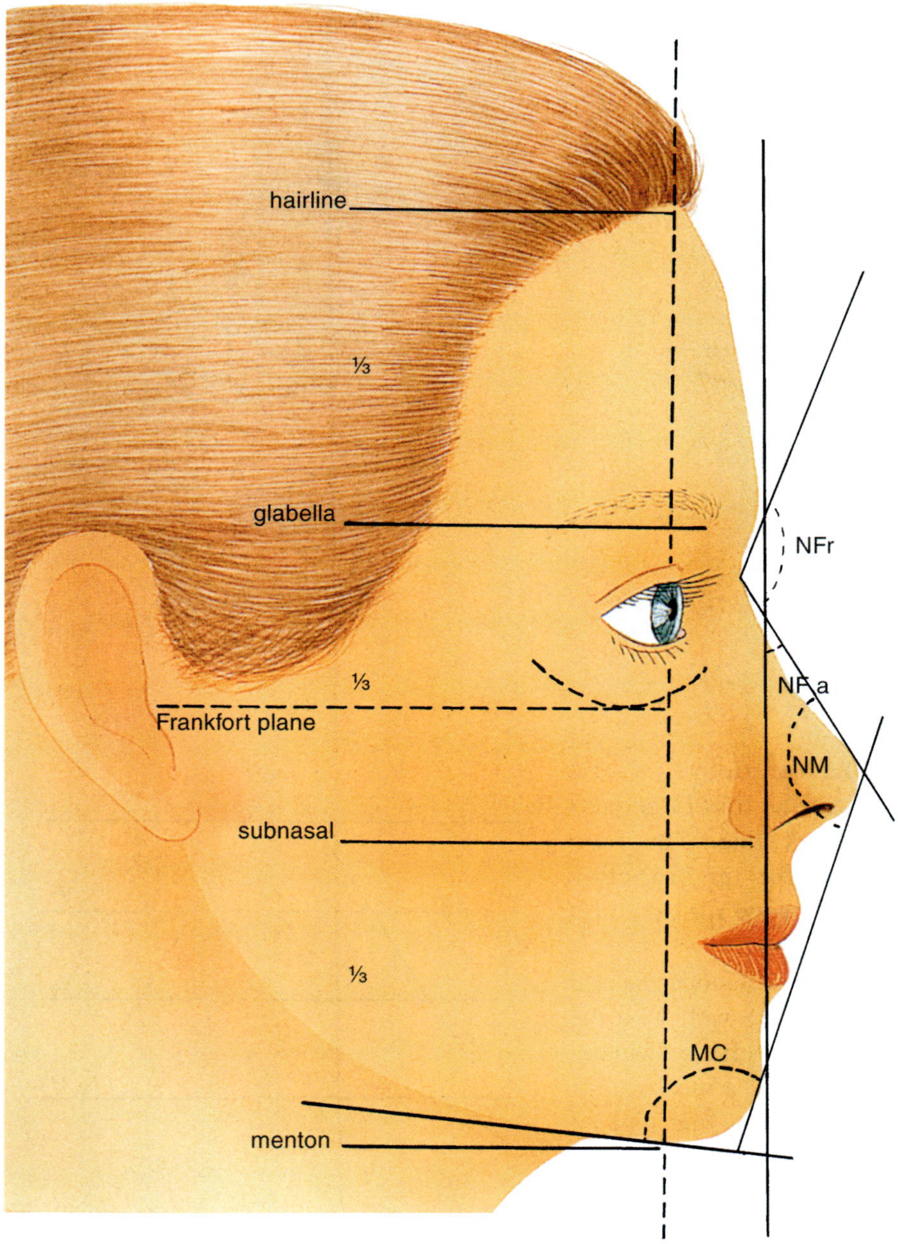

Fig. 2a. Lateral view of the face with the horizontal Frankfort plane, divided into three equal aesthetic proportions. Soft tissue angles and lines relate the major aesthetic components (aesthetic triangle of Powell and Humphreys).

In the case of the lateral view, it is important to assess:
- projection of the tip
- tip-rotation
- tip-columella-lip complex
- alar-lobular complex
- supra-tip break
- columella double break

Powell and Humphreys have come up with a new concept: the aesthetic triangle to analyze facial proportions. In the lateral view, this aesthetic triangle relates the major aesthetic components of the face by soft tissue angles and lines (Fig. 2a). The normal ranges for the various angles are:
- nasofrontal (NFr) 115–130 degrees
- nasofacial (NFa) 30–40 degrees
- nasomental (NM) 120–132 degrees
- mentocervical (MC) 80–95 degrees

Projection of the tip can easily be assessed by the method of Goode. Using this method, a vertical line is drawn from

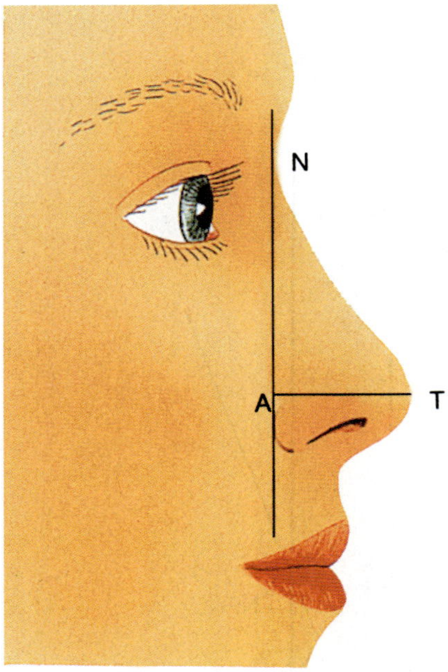

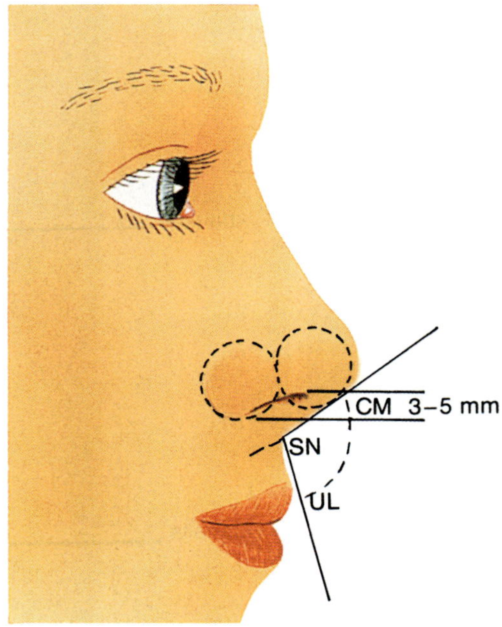

Fig. 2b. The ratio TA/TN as a measure for tip projection.

Fig. 2c. The nasolabial angle (CM-SN-UL), the ratio between ala and lobule and extension of the columella below the nares (3– 5 mm).

the nasion (N) to the alar groove (A) and a horizontal line from the tip (T) perpendicular to the vertical line. The ratio TA/TN is a measure for tip projection (Fig. 2b). The normal range for this ratio is 0.55–0.60.

The normal range of the Goode method for tip projection correlates well with the nasofacial angle of the aesthetic triangle. The nasolabial angle (NL), a measure for tip rotation, is defined by a line tangent to the most anterior part of the columella (CM) to the subnasale (SN) and a line intersecting the SN and the mucocutaneous border of the upper lip (UL) with a normal range of 90–120 degrees (female 105–120 degrees, male 90–105 degrees). The columella should extend 3–5 mm below the nares. The lateral relationship between ala and lobule is approximately 1:1 (Fig. 2c). A slight overgrowth of the lobule is aesthetically acceptable, whereas that of the alar part is not. Just cephalic to the tip, there should be a slight depression known as the supratip break. The columella double break has an anterior lobular part and a posterior columellar part.

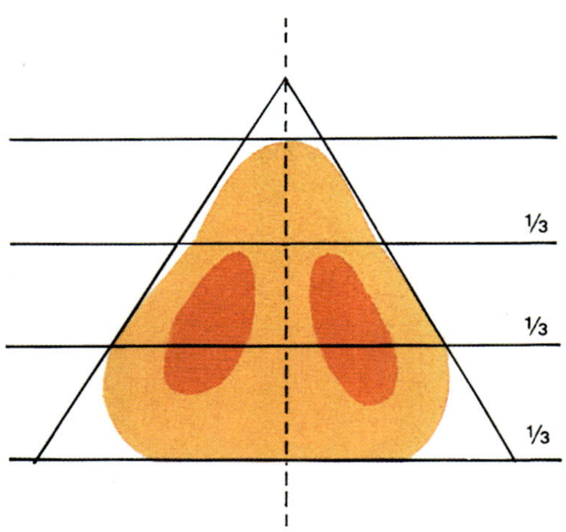

Fig. 3. Basal view of the nose which should have approximately the form of an equilateral triangle with the lobular, intermediate and basal part of the columella as three equal segments.

Basal view (Fig. 3)

The base of the nose has approximately the form of an equilateral triangle with the nostrils comprising two-thirds of the height. The columella can be divided into three equal segments, the anterior lobular, a narrower intermediate and a wider basal segment. In the adult Caucasian nose, the nares should be oval and in a slightly oblique position.

Oblique view (Fig. 4)

The oblique view is an underestimated projection. It gives an overall impression of the contours of the lateral nasal wall. The oblique projection is therefore especially important in assessing asymmetries and irregularities of the bony cartilaginous vault. There should be a smoothly curving line from the dome over the dorsum and radix into the supraorbital ridge.

With these general aesthetic guidelines in mind, the surgeon should apply the criteria mentioned above to each individual case.

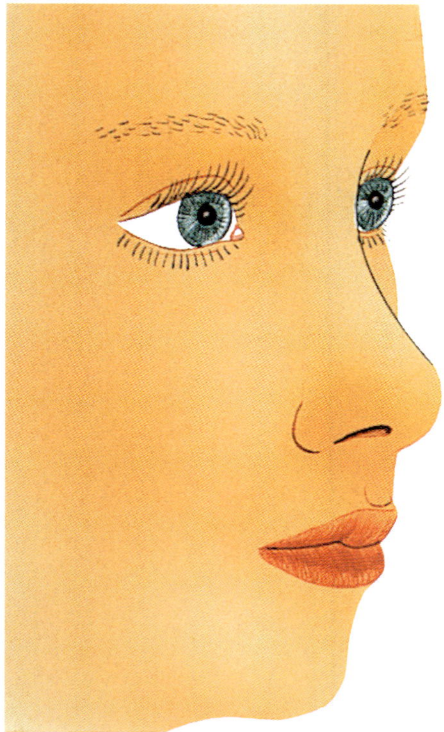

Fig. 4. Oblique view with a smoothly curving line from the dome over the dorsum and radix into the supraorbital ridge.

3: PREOPERATIVE MANAGEMENT

G.J. Nolst Trenité

Introduction

Successful rhinoplasty depends not only on a good operative result, but also on fulfillment of the patient's expectations. To achieve this goal, an extensive preoperative assessment is very important. During the first consultation, the psychological eligibility of the candidate for rhinoplasty should be considered and only after a thorough anatomical evaluation, and taking into account the medical history, should assessment of the possibilities and limitations of the operation be made.

Consultation

Interview

It is important to take *enough time* to listen carefully to the functional and aesthetic complaints of the patient. The surgeon should evaluate the motivations, expectations and mental health of the patient wanting to undergo rhinoplasty. Care should be taken not to select patients with weak motivations and unrealistic expectations. Written information for the patient on the operation, and what to expect from anesthesia, duration, possible complications, postoperative period (pain, swelling, bandages), stay in hospital, removal of stitches, etc., and a medical history questionnaire, are helpful and time saving.

Special medical history data should be emphasized when dealing with the rhinoplasty patient:

- tendency for bleeding
- family bleeding disorders
- hypertension
- cardiac disorders
- allergic disorders
- medication (aspirin)
- keloid formation
- previous septo-rhinoplasty
- nasal trauma
- nasal and sinus diseases
- psychological problems
- psychiatric history

Physical examination

Although a short look at the nose of the patient may reveal the aesthetic problem, a thorough external and internal examination of the nose, by inspection and palpation, is essential in order to establish what changes are possible and which operative technique should be used.

External inspection: Before concentrating on the problems of the nose, evaluation of "the balance of the nose with the other facial components" and establishment of possible asymmetries is important. Ethnic and family characteristics should be taken into account. Facial asymmetries are often not noticed by the patient. The patient's attention should be drawn to possible asymmetries, to prevent later complaints about the postoperative result.

The quality of the skin (thickness, elasticity, pathological condition) plays an important role in assessment of the surgical possibilities. The thinner the skin the more chance there is of visible postoperative irregularities in the skeleton of the nose. Therefore, a thin skin demands an extremely careful surgical approach. However, the advantage is that subtle corrective refinements can be carried out better in these patients than in patients with

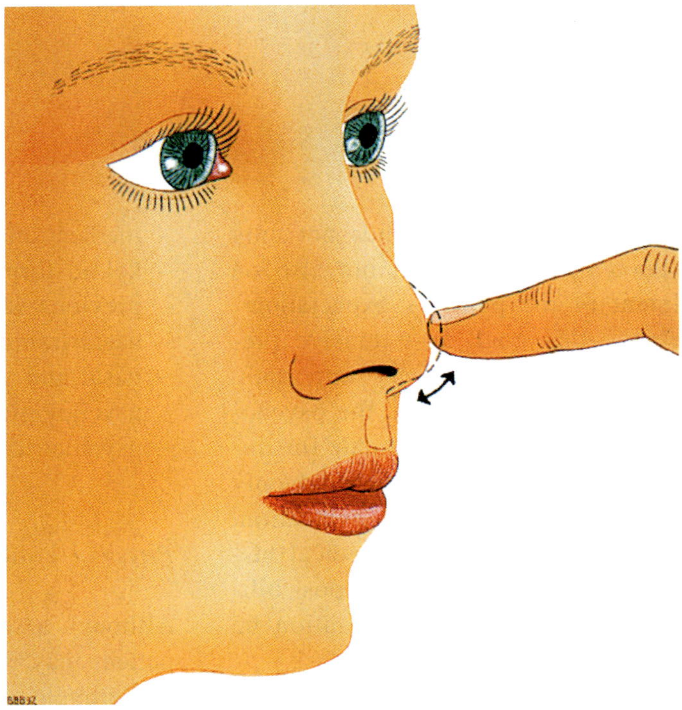

Fig. 1. Tip recoil.

thick skins. A very thick skin with an abundance of subcutaneous adipose tissue considerably limits the possibilities of correction. The tendency for an inexperienced surgeon in particular to carry out an overcorrection in these cases by extensive resection of the cartilaginous nose skeleton, produces the possibility of postoperative scar retraction and, consequently, of undesirable deformities.

The more specific abnormalities in the shape of the nose that should be inspected are:

- length and projection
- shape of the tip of the nose
- columella
- lip-tip-columella base complex
- cartilaginous and bony dorsum
- radix nasi

External palpation: Palpation of the nose gives important additional information on the skin and skeleton of the nose. The skin is palpated with two fingers to define the elasticity and 'size of skin sleeve'. In an extensive nose reduction, contractility of the skin is especially important. The bridge of the nose is palpated to diagnose any irregularities and to define the length of the ossa nasalia. In nasal tip surgery, it is important to have an idea of the 'tip support'. The degree of 'tip support' contributes to the choice of incisions, surgical approach and operative techniques. A way of testing this 'tip support' is by pushing down and then immediately releasing the tip of the nose – tip recoil (Fig. 1). By palpating the alar cartilages, information is collected about shape, size and elasticity. In case of insufficient elasticity of the alar cartilages, caution is required with regard to an extensive resection of the cartilage.

Internal inspection: Before inspecting the internal nose with a speculum, assessment of a possible 'alar collapse' during gentle inhalation is advisable. 'Alar collapse' is not only determined by the weakness of the nostrils but also by the functioning of the ostium internum. Stenosis in the area of the valve causes a stronger underpres-

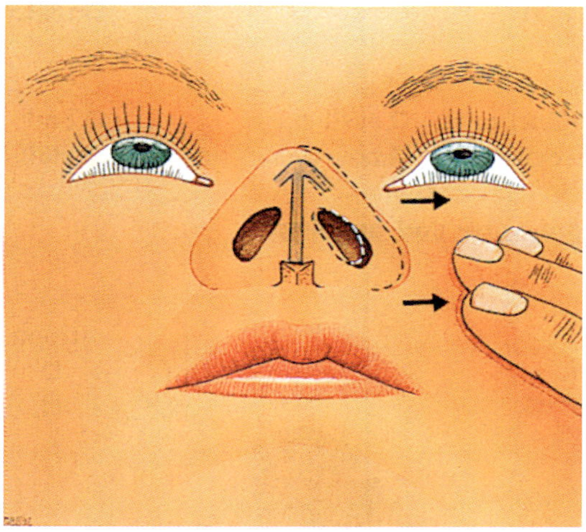

Fig. 2. Cottle test.

sure on inhalation and consequently a more powerful inhalation. Correct diagnosis is of vital importance in the choice of surgery (alar grafts, internal valve surgery or upward rotation of the lateral crus). After inspection of the vestibulum for, for example, pathology of the skin and protrusion of the lateral crura, the ostium internum is assessed. The angle between upper lateral cartilage and septum is normally 10 to 15 degrees. Stenosis due to septum deviations, deviating anatomy of the upper lateral (ballooning) or scarring due to trauma or 'previous surgery', may result in inhalation problems.

Further internal inspection should follow in order to assess possible mucosa pathology (*e.g.*, atrophy, edema, polyps, septal deviations or concha hypertrophy).

Internal palpation: Palpation of the vestibulum provides relevant information on overgrowth of the caudal septum deviations which may interfere with a possibly planned tip rotation, on septal deviations and on the size of the medial crus and size and position of the anterior nasal spine. With the aid of an instrument, palpation of the more proximal part of the septum is important in the evaluation of any septal cartilage present which can serve as a support and, if necessary, be taken and used as 'craft material'. A simple test to detect any limitation in inhalation at the level of the ostium internum is to pull the cheek lateral-wise during gentle inhalation through the nose, the so-called Cottle test (Fig. 2). The sign is positive when inhalation noticeably improves with this maneuver.

Aesthetic evaluation

According to the aesthetic standards (see Chapter 2 on aesthetics), the nose is assessed in relation to the remaining facial features. In planned shape changes, as well as considering the patient's wishes, age, sex, body type and familial features should be taken into account. The nose is assessed in a frontal, lateral, oblique and basal way, whereby a distinction is made between the radix, dorsum and tip of the nose (see chapter on aesthetics).

With regard to the remaining features, the naso-frontal and naso-labial angles as well as the nose-chin relation are assessed.

Communication

Based on the examination, the surgical possibilities, wishes and limitations are discussed with the patient. A mirror and preoperative photographs are of practical value for this purpose. Surgical risks, postoperative complications, such as subsequent bleeding and infections, and also possible dissatisfaction with the postoperative result, should be discussed in detail with the patient. From a 'medico-legal' point of view, it is wise to have the patient sign a document of 'informed consent'. Pre- and postoperative instruction forms can contribute to communication and are time-saving as well.

SEPTO-RHINOPLASTY ASSESSMENT FORM

Name ... born ... ☐ male ☐ female
pat. reg. No. .....

Septo-rhinoplasty: ☐ functional ☐ aesthetic ☐ both
Type: ☐ primary ☐ revision ☐ non-caucasion ☐ cleft lip

Septum, valve and turbinates

Septum pathol.

☐ deviation
area 1 2 3 4 5 L
area 1 2 3 4 5 R
☐ perforation
diam. ... cm.
☐ cartilage loss
area 1 2 3 4 5
☐ other

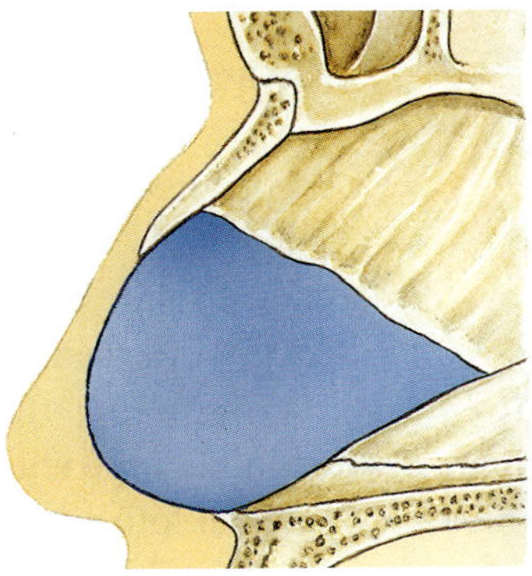

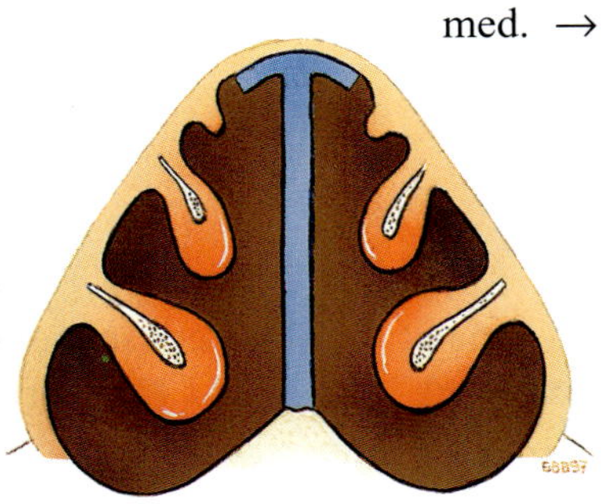

Turbinate pathol.

	atroph.	hypertr.	other
inf. →	☐	☐	☐
med. →	☐	☐	☐

Valve pathol.

☐ too narrow
☐ too wide
☐ other

Tip columella, vestibulum and ala

Tip pathol.

☐ bulbous
☐ bifid
☐ asym.
☐ overproj.
☐ underproj.

Tip recoil

weak →1→2→3→4→5 strong

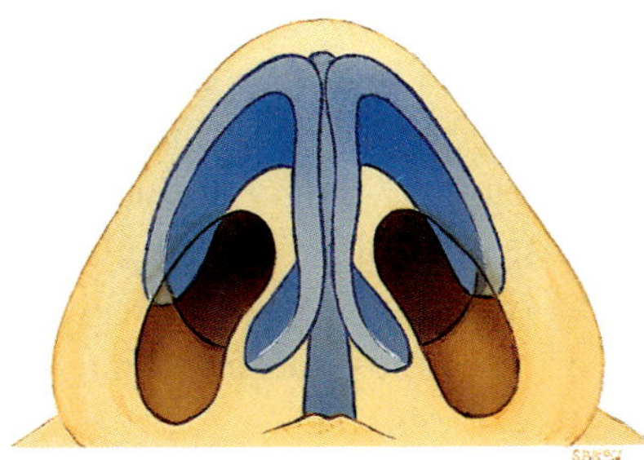

Columella pathol.

☐ retracted
☐ deviated
☐ broadened
☐ other

Vestibulum pathol.

☐ stenosis
☐ other

Alar pathol.

☐ insuff. ☐ flaring ☐ other

Osseo-cartilaginous vault

Skin qual.

thin →1→2→3→4→5 thick

Vault pathol.

☐ deviated
☐ cartil. ☐ bony ☐ both
☐ irregular
☐ cartil. ☐ bony ☐ both
☐ saddle
☐ cartil. ☐ bony ☐ both
☐ hump
☐ tension nose

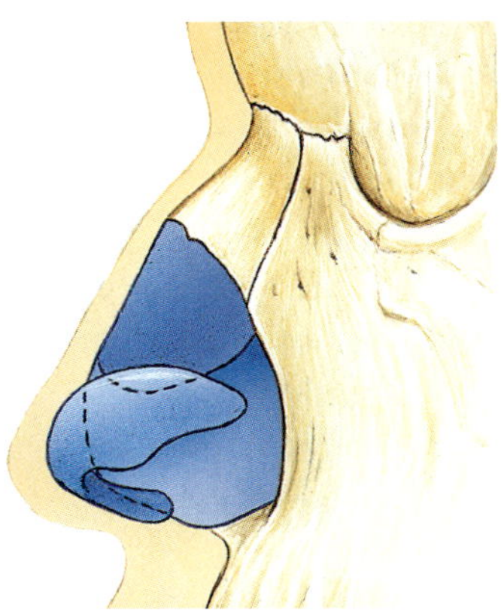

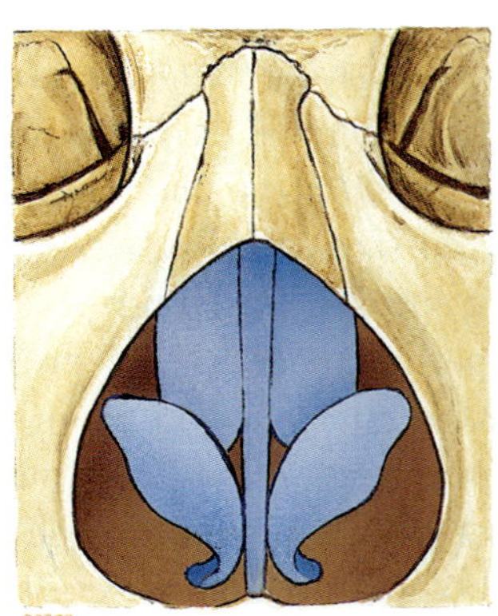

Rhinometry

☐ acoustic
☐ mano

Photography

☐ standard
☐ other

Anesthesia: ☐ local
☐ iv analgesia
☐ general

☐ day care
☐ hospitalization

☐ pre-assessment

Expected operation time ..... Operation date ....

Fig. 3a.

SEPTO-RHINOPLASTY OPERATION FORM

Name ... born ... □ male □ female
pat. reg. nr. .....
operating date .... anaesthesia: □ local □ i.v. □ general

Approach

□ endonasal
□ delivery
□ open

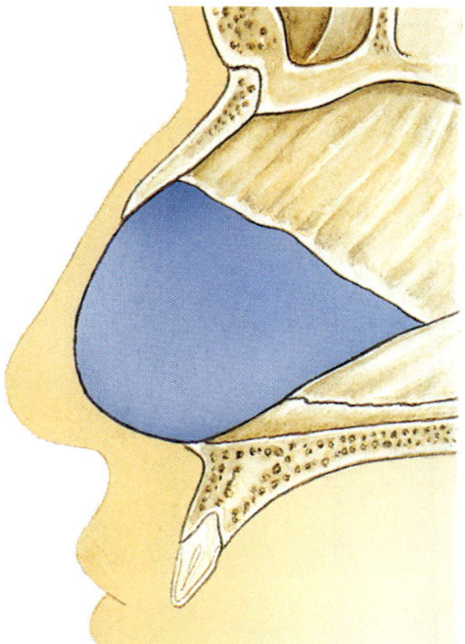

Incisions

□ hemitransf.
□ Killian
□ part. transf.
□ compl. transf.
□ marginal
□ rim
□ intercartil.
□ transcartil.
□ V-Y procedure
□ Z-plasty
□ broken columella

Type of grafts

□ autog. septal
□ autog. ear
□ autog. rib
□ composite ear
□ allogeneic
□ xenograft
□ alloplast
□ skin

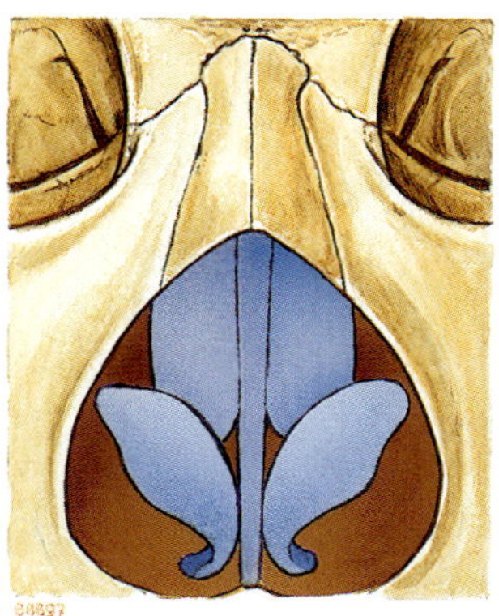

Graft site

□ spreader
□ columella strut
□ shield
□ tip onlay
□ dorsal onlay
□ dorsal lat.
□ alar batton
□ maxillary
□ naso-front.
□ naso-lab.

Technique

Septoplasty

Cart. septal work
□ basal strip
□ post. chondrotomy
□ scoring
□ splinting
□ resection

Bony septal work
□ ant. spine red.
□ ant. spine realignm.
□ perpend. plate
□ vomer
□ grafting

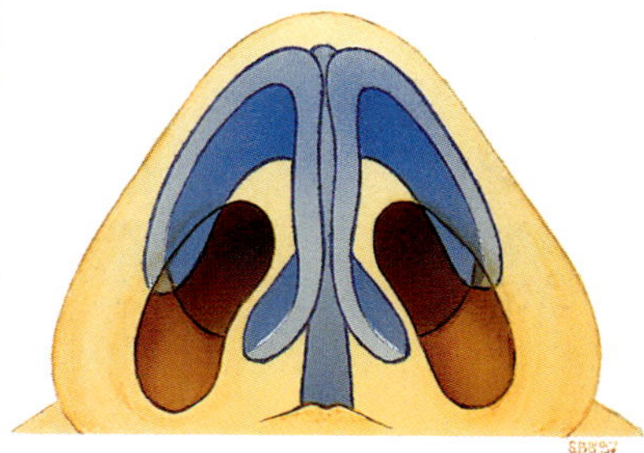

Turbinate reduct.
□ inf. □ L □ R
□ med. □ L □ R

Tip surgery

□ cephalic resection
□ complete strip
□ incomplete strip
□ suturing
□ interdomal
□ transdomal
□ lat. crural steal

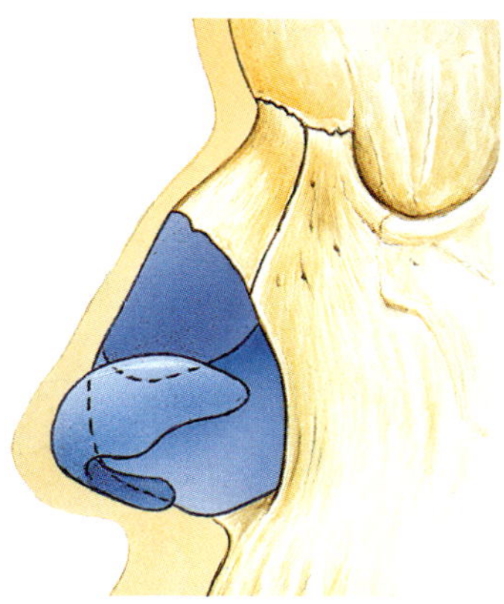

Bony cart. vault surg.
□ hump resection
□ upper lateral
□ augmentation

Osteotomies
□ medial-oblique
□ intermediate
□ lateral (intranasal)
□ lateral (percutaneous)
□ infraction
□ outfraction
□ realignment

Alar base surgery

□ V-shape wedge
□ invert. V-shape wedge
□ rectang. shape wedge

Direct postoperative care

□ packing removal . . . days p.o.
□ dressing removal . . . days p.o.
□ sutures removal . . . days p.o.
post op. consultation date . . . . . .

□ daycare
□ hospitalization
□ antibiotics
□ other med.

Fig. 3b.

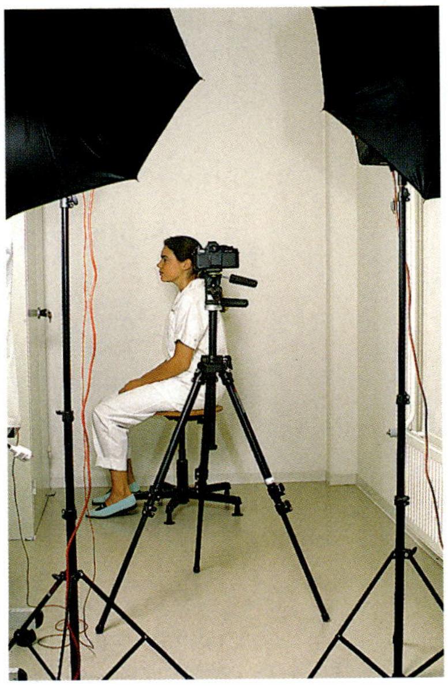

Fig. 4. A standard set-up for photographic documentation.

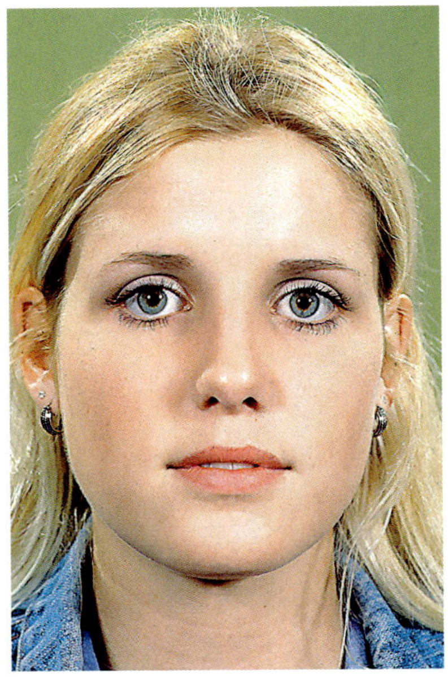

a

Fig. 5a. Frontal view.

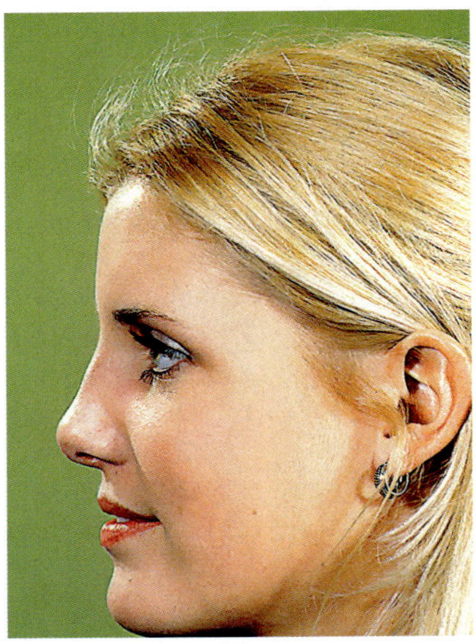

b

Fig. 5b. Lateral view (right side not shown).

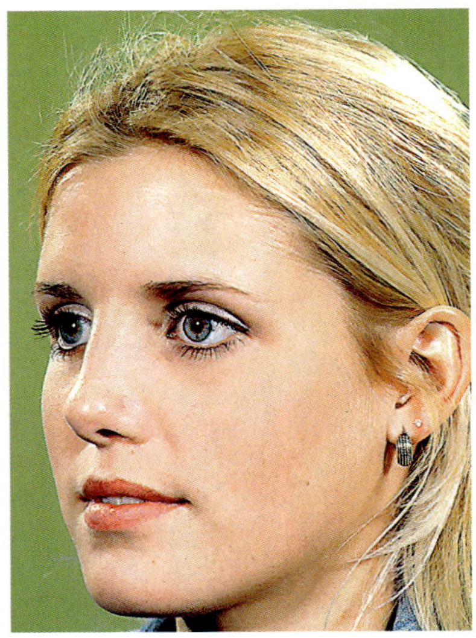

c

Fig. 5c. Oblique view (right side not shown).

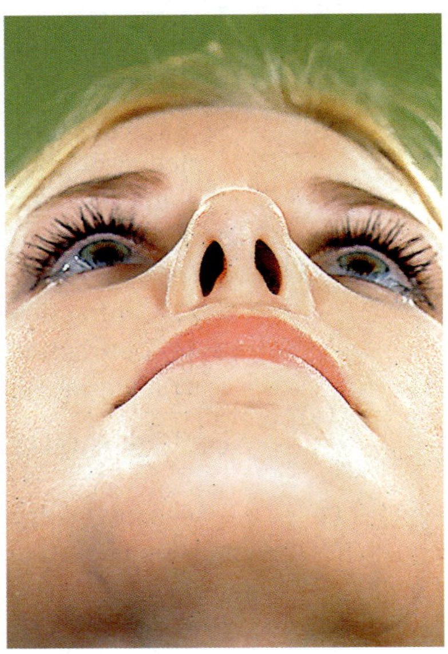

d

Fig. 5d. Basal view.

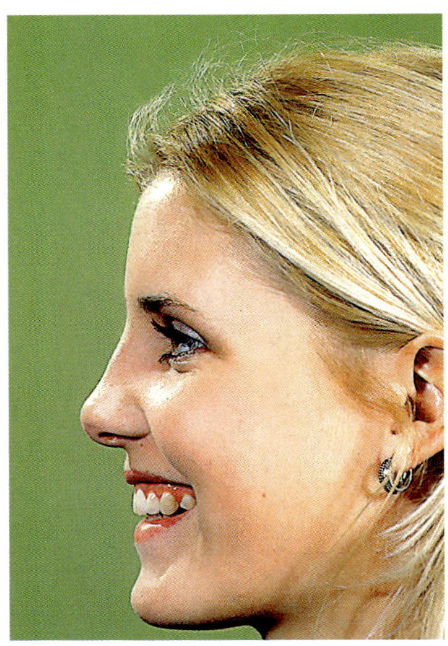

e

Fig. 5e. Smiling lateral view.

Documentation

For the treatment, and from a 'medico-legal' point of view, a complete medical record with carefully documented preoperative findings (see Fig. 3a) is of great importance. As rhinoplasty is an elective operation, an extensive medical history with the aid of a questionnaire is indicated in order to exclude any surgical or anesthetic risks.

The extent of preoperative laboratory and X-ray examinations (X-sinus, X-thorax) depends on the patient's state of health. A surgical plan (possibly on a standard form) (see Fig. 3b) with proposed changes, incisions, approaches, and techniques, is a helpful reminder, especially when considerable time elapses between consultation and operation and, moreover, it forces the surgeon to make a well-considered plan.

Photography

Both pre- and postoperative photographic documentation is necessary for:

- consultation with the patient
- preoperative planning
- reference during operation
- assessment of results
- 'medico-legal' purposes

For useful photographic documentation, standardization of the photographs is necessary. A standard set-up of permanent equipment in a studio would be most suitable. The equipment should consist of a reflex camera with a 100 to 135 mm lens with a 100 ASA 35 mm film (or slides). For a correct soft exposure, two flash lights with an umbrella on either side of the camera would be sufficient. In addition, a neutral background is important (Fig. 4).

For adequate documentation, at least six photographs are needed (Figs. 5a–e):

- *A frontal view* with the patient looking straight into the camera with a horizontal eyeline.
- *A lateral view* (on both sides). The ear should be visible for determination of the Frankfort plane which must be horizontal.
- *An oblique view* (on both sides) at an angle of 45 degrees, is important for assessment of the nose contour and for any asymmetries.
- *A basal view* with the tip of the nose in a more or less vertical position to make pre- and postoperative comparison possible.
- *A smiling lateral view* to document the dynamics of the nasal tip.

For photographic documentation during the operation, a 105 mm macro-lens with ring flash is most suitable.

4: ANESTHESIA AND PREOPERATIVE MEDICATION

G.J. Nolst Trenité

Introduction

Rhinoplasty can be carried out under either local or general anesthesia. The goals for appropriate anesthesia are: amnesia, analgesia, sedation and a 'dry' operation field. The advantages of a general anesthetic are complete amnesia, analgesia and sedation, but a disadvantage is the often far from bloodless operation field. Therefore, the use of complementary topical and local infiltration anesthetics are necessary to acquire a more or less 'dry' operation field. With the use of new inhalation anesthetic agents (enflurane), the use of local anesthetics is less restricted, as was the case with halothane. Nevertheless, local anesthesia (topical in combination with infiltration) is still the best choice for ambulant nasal surgery, because of its low risks and more or less bloodless operation field. The bloodlessness of the operation field depends to a large extent on the technique of administration of the anesthetic solution. In combination with intravenous analgesia and sedation, with close monitoring of vital signs, it moreover ensures a relaxed, cooperative patient. In children and when the operation procedure is estimated to be of long duration (more than two hours), the preference is for general anesthesia.

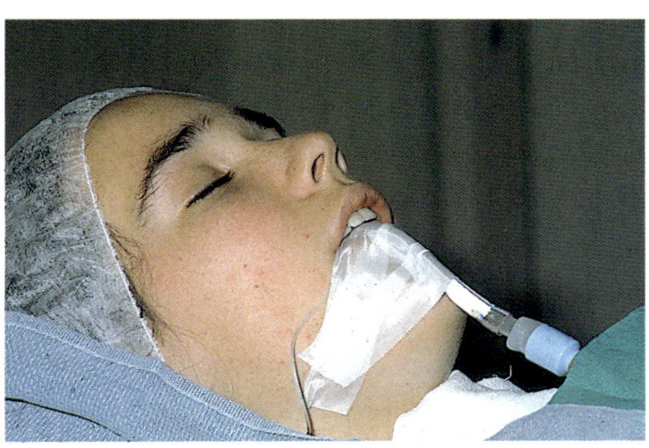

Fig. 1. Reverse Trendelenburg position with the endotracheal tube in a caudal direction.

Preoperative care and medication

Preoperative evaluation with regard to medical history, physical examination and laboratory tests, should not only be carried out in cases of general anesthesia, but also when local anesthesia is planned. Oral tranquilizers (benzodiazepines) taken the night before and two hours before surgery, and a clear explanation of the anesthetic procedures, are very helpful for the patient's relaxed state when entering the operating room.

Position

The patient should be put into a slight reverse Trendelenburg position to facilitate venous drainage. In general anesthesia, the oral endotracheal tube should be pointed in a caudal direction in order not to disturb the relaxed state of the upper lip and nasal base (Fig. 1).

Intravenous analgesia and sedation

The anesthesiologist establishes an intravenous route for the controlled administration of short-acting analgesia (alfentanyl) and sedatives (propofol), and will take care of monitoring vital signs:
- electrocardiogram
- blood pressure
- pulse oximeter

Local anesthetics

Cocaine-HC1 is an excellent anesthetic and vasoconstrictive agent for topical use in the nose. A concentration of 5% is appropriate. Care should be taken not to

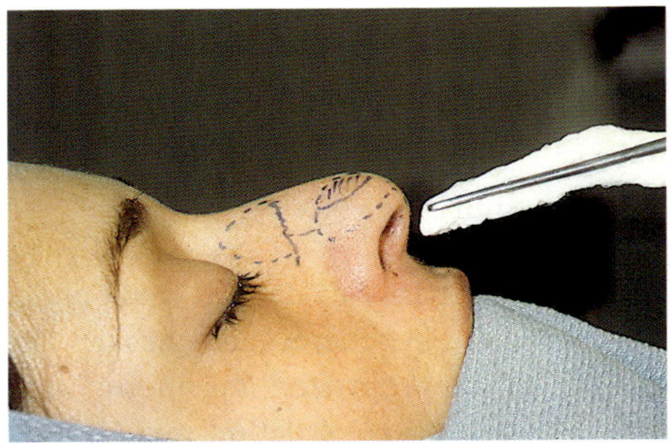

Fig. 2. Application of cotton strips with topical anesthetic agent.

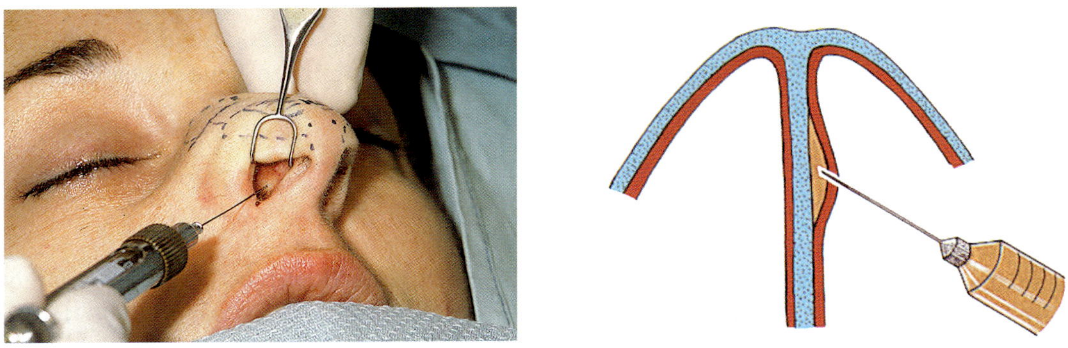

Fig. 3a,b. Infiltration of the local anesthetic in the septum, submucoperichondrial.

use more than 200 mg (4 ml of 5% solution) to prevent a toxic reaction. Combination with epinephrine should not be used, in order to prevent cardiac disrhythm. Lidocaine (1% or 2%) in combination with 1:100,000 epinephrine are the most commonly used injectable agents for infiltration anesthesia (toxic dose of lidocaine in combination with epinephrine in the range of 500 mg) in nasal surgery. Nevertheless, there is an increasing popularity for bupivacaine 0.25-0.5% which has a considerably increased length of anesthetic action, but in higher concentrations (0.5%) the chance of tissue damage.

Local anesthesia technique

Local anesthesia of the nose starts with the application of a topical agent (cocaine 5% 2-3 ml) on cotton strips in each nasal fossa, giving adequate vasoconstriction and anesthesia (Fig. 2). The next step is the infiltration of lidocaine 1% or 2% in combination with epinephrine 1:100,000. For complete analgesia and vasoconstriction, no more than 6 ml of the solution is needed. A 27-gauge long needle is very useful for deposition of the anesthetic agent in the surgical dissection planes. There is no need for specific nerve blockage. As the infiltration is uncomfortable for the patient, deeper intravenous sedation is advisable during this short period. Distortion of the nose caused by improper deposition and an overdose of the local anesthetic should be prevented.

Infiltration sequence

Septum

When submucoperichondrial tunnelling of the septum is indicated for reconstruction or graft harvesting, it is helpful to infil-

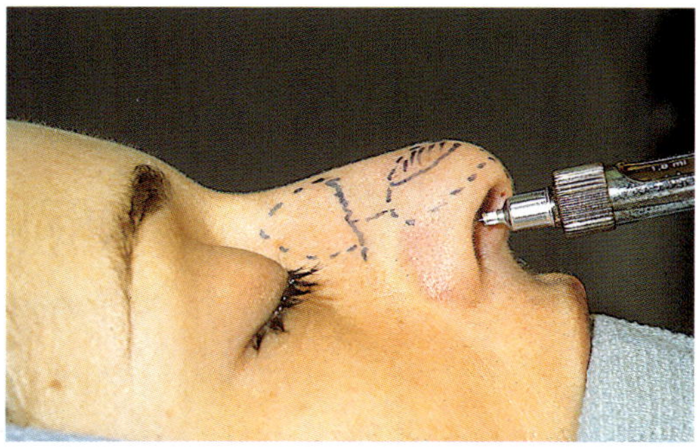
a

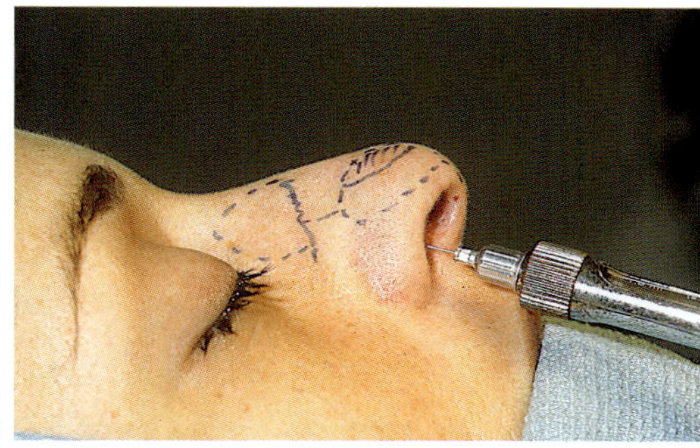
b

Fig. 4a,b. Deposition of the anesthetic solution laterally and medially in the surgical dissection plane of the dorsum.

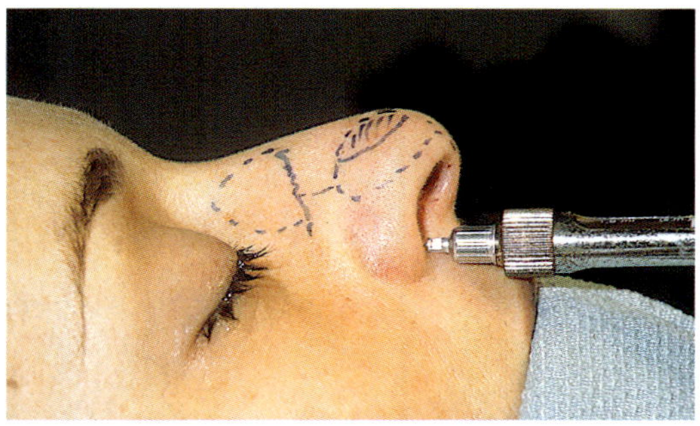

Fig. 5. Deposition of the local anesthetic along the intended course of the lateral osteotomy.

trate the septum submucoperichondrially, resulting in a hydraulic dissection, which facilitates further dissection in the proper plane (Fig. 3a,b).

Dorsum

Using the intercartilaginous approach, the 27-gauge needle penetrates the epithelium. The needle is advanced along the dorsum in the dissection plane, close to the perichondrium and periosteum (Fig. 4a). Deposition of a small amount of anesthetic solution is done while retracting the needle up to the point of penetration, then advancing it again in a more medial or lateral position (Fig. 4b). Deposition again takes place while retracting the needle until the complete area of dissection is covered. This procedure is then repeated on the opposite side. With a total amount of anesthetic of up to 2 ml, there should be no distortion of the nose when the deposition takes place in the proper planes.

Lateral wall

The solution is deposited along the intended course of the lateral osteotomies, starting at the margin of the pyriform aperture medial and lateral to the ascending process of the maxilla, while retracting the needle (Fig. 5). This procedure, combined with the use of micro-osteotomes (leaving the periosteum attached), will give a considerable reduction of postoperative ecchymosis.

Columella and nasal base

The needle penetrates the columella base in the epithelium of the nostril floor and then advances just lateral to the alar base at the opposite side, while deposition takes place during withdrawal of the needle (Fig. 6a,b). Using the same penetration site, a deposit is placed into the columella (Fig. 7). The needle is rotated 180° and advanced up to the point just lateral of the alar base at the opposite side, followed by deposition of the anesthetic during withdrawal. In the case of an external approach, an extra injection through the skin of the nasal tip between the domes to the anterior columella is necessary, leaving a small deposit, during withdrawal followed by rotation of the needle into the supratip areas for an extra deposit of the local anesthetic.

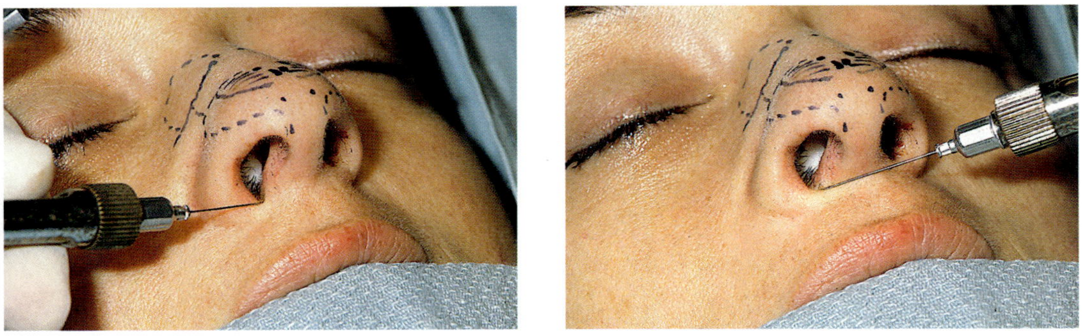

a b

Fig. 6a,b. Infiltration of the anesthetic solution into the nasal base through one penetration site.

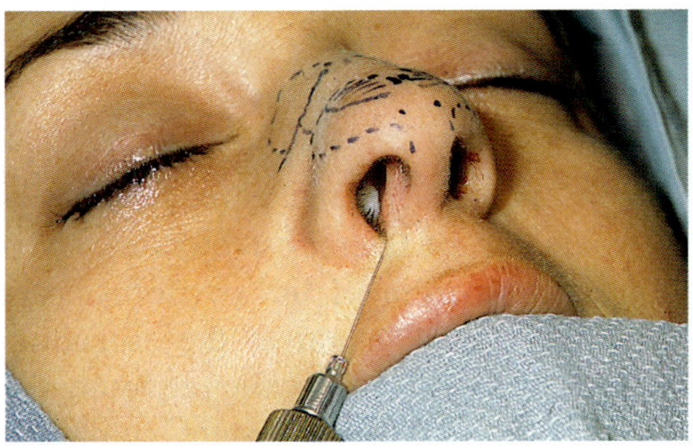

Fig. 7. Deposition of the local anesthetic in the columella using the same penetration site as for the nasal base.

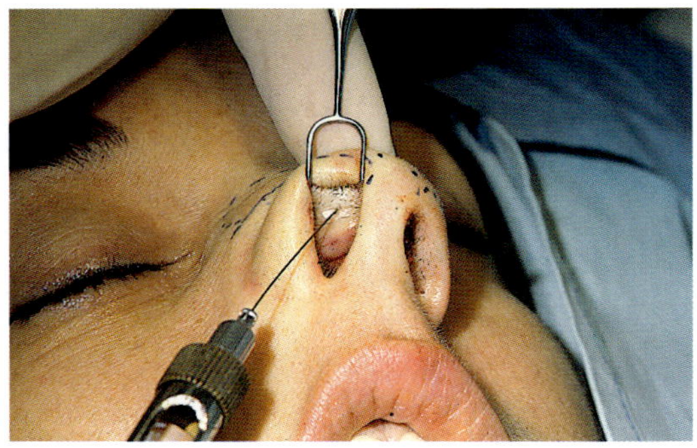

Fig. 8. Subperichondrial deposition of the anesthetic solution along the intended course of the transcartilaginous incision.

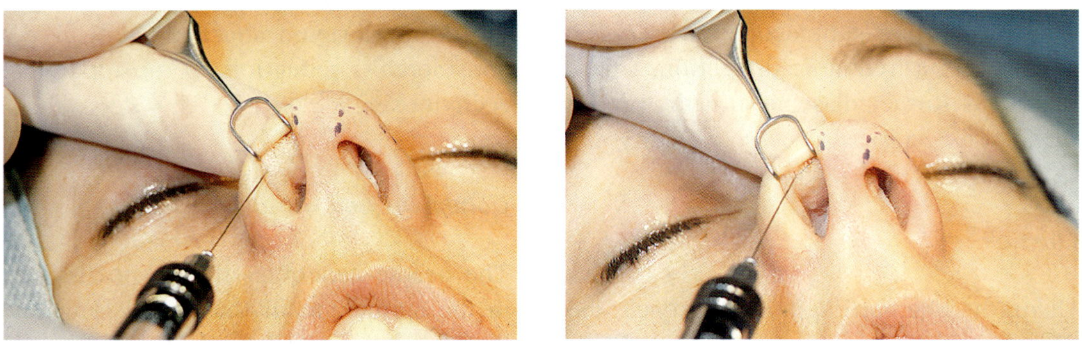

a b

Fig. 9a,b. Small multiple deposits of the local anesthetic along the caudal margin of the lateral crus.

Tip

Local infiltration of the nasal tip should be attuned to the specific approach. In the case of a non-delivery approach using a transcartilaginous incision, the local anesthetic should be deposited subperichondrially along the incision line, which facilitates the dissection (Fig. 8). When a marginal incision is planned in the case of a delivery or external approach, small multiple deposits of the local anesthetic solution are placed along the caudal edge of the lateral crus extending to the anterior side (Fig. 9a,b). In the case of the alar rotation technique (with total delivery of the lateral crus), there are also deposits subperichondrially at the vestibular side of the lateral crus.

Alar base

Planning a wedge resection of the alar base, local anesthetic is infiltrated into the alar lobule, leaving a small deposit without disturbing the original contour.

5: POSTOPERATIVE CARE AND COMPLICATIONS

G.J. Nolst Trenité

Introduction

Postoperative care starts with the application of an adequate internal and external nose dressing. The follow-up does not end with removal of the nose dressing. In order to become a good nose surgeon, follow-up of at least one year (postoperatively) is necessary to follow the dynamics of the healing process, thereafter at five to ten years. Early or late complications, if any, should be prevented as far as possible and should be treated adequately. However, careful oral and written instructions prevent unnecessary postoperative complications.

Packing and Dressing

Packing

The goal of the nose packing (internal nose dressing) is:
- to ensure good tissue approximation
- to prevent hematomas, swelling and bleeding
- to prevent synechia
- to prevent displacement by splinting

It would be wrong to suppose that, in case of an inadequate postoperative result, the packing can permanently influence the position of the septum or the shape of the nose. Such temporary modelling hardly influences the final postoperative result. The packing can generally be removed after 24 hours, unless an extensive reconstruction of the septum has been performed.

Packing applied too tightly and for too long disrupts adequate venous and lymphatic drainage. Septal suturing to prevent subperichondral hematomas further reduces the necessity of lengthy packing (Fig. 1). Material such as impregnated gauze strips or telfa gauze (Fig. 2a), which do not adhere to the mucous membrane and as such can be removed without pain or damage, has proved to be most suitable for packing.

Dressing

The goal of the external nose dressing is:
- to fix the skin on the under-layer, thereby reducing dead space
- to prevent hematomas and swelling
- to prevent displacement by outside trauma
- to prevent widening of the lateral walls by intranasal edema

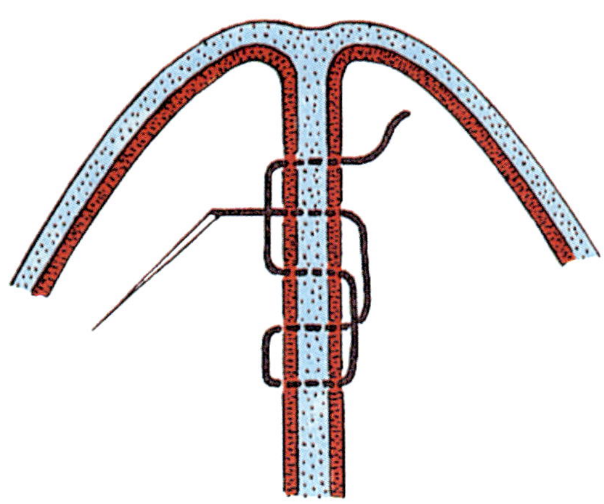

Fig. 1. Septal mattress sutures to prevent subperichondrial hematomas.

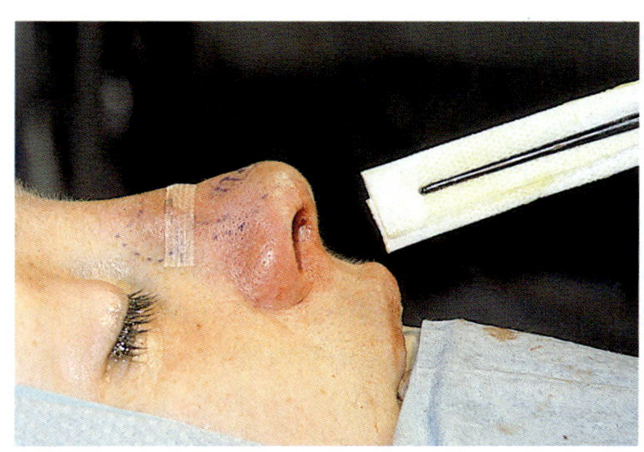

a

Fig. 2a. Packing of the nose with telfa gauze.

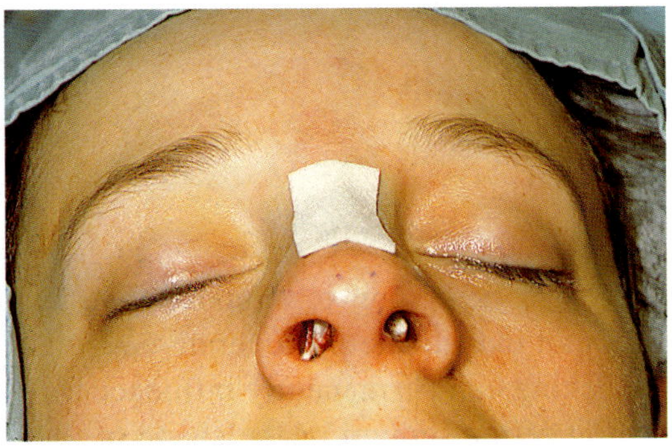
b

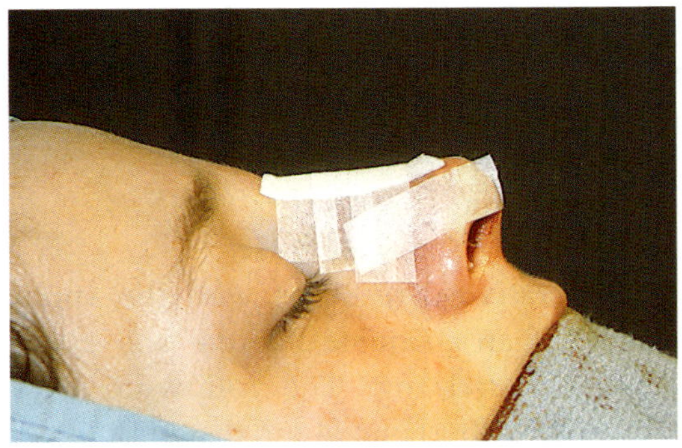
c

Fig. 2b. Gel foam to prevent extraction of the skin while removing the external nose dressing.

Fig. 2c. Overlapping strips of hypo-allergenic paper-tape and a sling of paper-tape to enclose the lobule.

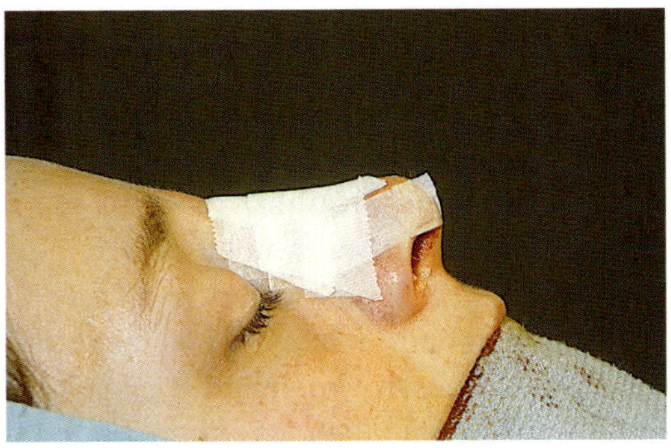
d

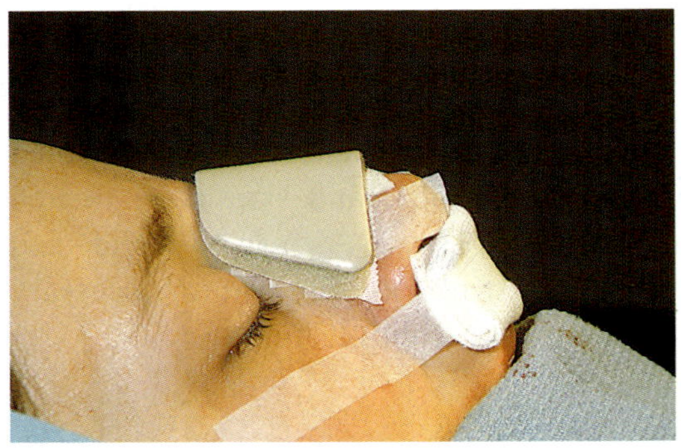
e

Fig. 2d. Second layer of cloth-tape.

Fig. 2e. A two-piece Denver® splint.

Only in specific operative techniques, such as wedge excisions with pushdown of the bony pyramid, does the external nose dressing also aim to fix and shape the bony pyramid. Inadequately fractured nasal bones cannot be fixed permanently by the external nose dressing. The external nose dressing consists of three layers: hypo-allergenic paper-tape, adhesive cloth-tape and splint.

Before applying the external dressing, operative edema, if any, is reduced by massage of the nasal covering. Thereafter, the skin of the nose is rubbed with Tinctura Benzoin or Mastisol followed by the application of a piece of gel foam, (which prevents extraction of the skin from the underlying nasal skeleton while removing external nose dressing) (Fig. 2b) after which overlapping strips of paper-tape are applied, right across the bridge of the nose, including the supratip area. A sling of paper-tape is then applied, not extending below the nostril apexes, to enclose the lobule (Fig. 2c).

Then a layer of adhesive cloth-tape is applied over the paper-tape (Fig. 2d).

As a splint, various materials, such as aluminium, plastic or plaster of Paris, can be used. The splint only covers the bridge of the nose (Fig. 2e). Lateral and frontal extensions allow the possibility of distortion due to movements of the facial musculature. A splint applied too tightly may result in ischemia of the skin. This also applies to the adhesive tape, especially in dorsum and tip implantations which put the skin under pressure. The dressing procedure is finished by a ‘moustache dressing’ to catch any nasal discharge (Fig. 2e). External nose dressings are generally removed after one week.

Early postoperative period (up to six weeks)

Oral and written instructions are of great importance to the patient in order to les-

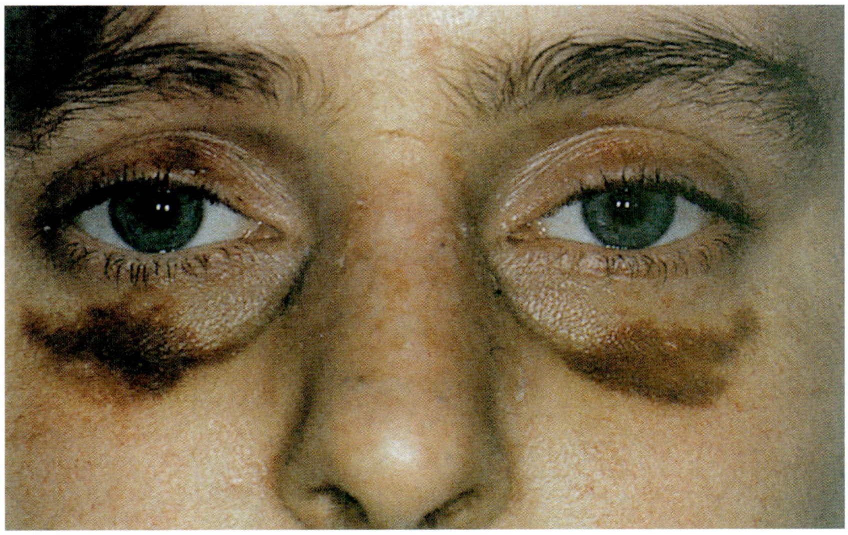

Fig. 3. Extended ecchymosis and an allergic reaction of the nasal skin due to cloth-tape.

sen the possibility of complications in the postoperative period.

Postoperative instructions for the patient:
- raise the head of the bed when resting or sleeping;
- apply cold compresses regularly during the first day after operation;
- prevent blowing the nose fiercely and when sneezing occurs, sneeze through the mouth;
- do not use any agents containing salicyl during the first ten days;
- avoid any intensive physical activity or traumatizing sports for six weeks;
- do not wear spectacles resting on an operated nose bridge until six weeks after operation;
- do not drink alcohol or smoke during the first weeks after operation.

It is also important to give oral and written information about the postoperative period, such as:
- postoperative follow-ups
- changing the dressings
- the moment of removing the stitches
- nose-toilet
- dry mouth
- complaints of nasal congestion due to reactive mucosa swelling
- temporary subfebrile temperature
- possible complications

In order to prevent complications, a knowledge of them is necessary. We can distinguish between early and late complications.

Early complications

- extensive edema and ecchymosis
- allergic skin reactions to cloth-tape
- hematomas
- infections
- skin ischemia and necrosis

Edema and ecchymosis were more or less normal phenomena in the old operative techniques for bony pyramid. As a precaution, the eyelids were taped with plaster. With modern techniques (micro- osteotomies), there is in general minimal edema and ecchymosis so that taping of the eyelids is no longer necessary. The use of hypo-allergenic paper-tape has greatly reduced *allergic skin reactions* to plaster (Fig. 3).

Hematomas mostly arise from careless preparation outside the surgical planes and from unfavorable conditions during anesthesia (CO_2 accumulation, high BP and coagulation disorders). Upper lip hematoma generally provides little chance of infection and often recovers spontaneously. In paranasal hematomas

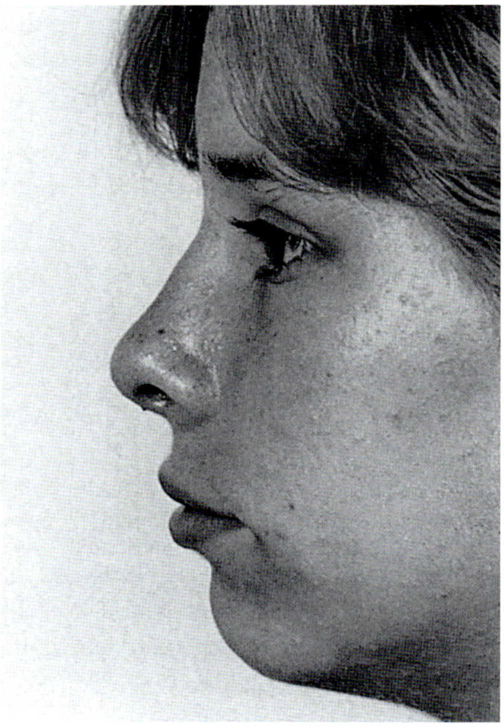
a

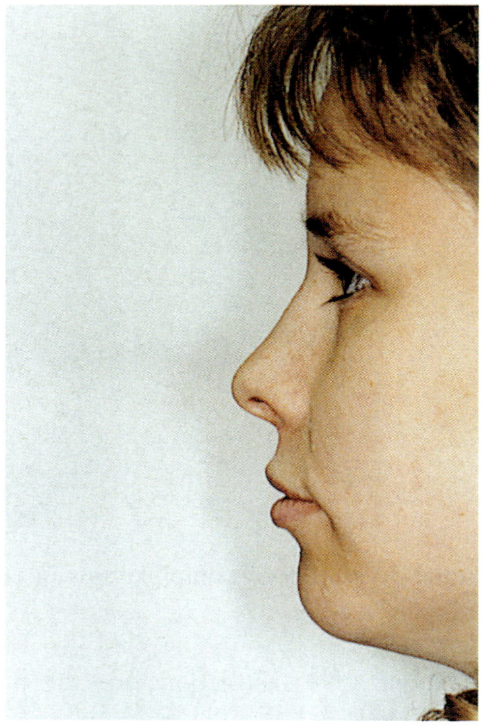
b

Fig. 4a. Lateral view of a 14-year-old girl four weeks after immediate reconstruction (with autogenous rib cartilage) of a completely destroyed cartilaginous nasal septum, due to an abscess.

Fig. 4b. Lateral view of the same girl (after puberty) at the age of 19 years with adequate outgrowth of nose and upper jaw.

(subperiostal), due to lateral osteotomies, there is a chance of infection via the paranasal sinuses. Treatment consists of drainage of the hematoma followed by a local compression dressing and antibiotics. Dorsum hematomas are treated in the same way as paranasal hematomas. Inadequate treatment may result in necrosis of the triangular cartilages.

Septum hematomas occur most frequently. If subperichondral on both sides, they will result in necrosis of the septum cartilage. This can be prevented by loosening the perichondrium wherever possible on one side only and, after septum correction, by fixing the perichondrium blades around the septal cartilage again with the aid of matrass sutures. Septum hematomas can also be prevented by careful pledgeting of the nose for 24 hours. Drainage, repledgeting and antibiotics are the treatment of choice.

Infections: superficial pustulae of the skin caused by covering plasters usually disappear quickly after removal of the dressing. Recovery can be speeded up by antibiotics and corticosteroid creams. Paranasal abscesses are treated in the same way as hematomas, provided that the drain for the removal of pus is left in place slightly longer.

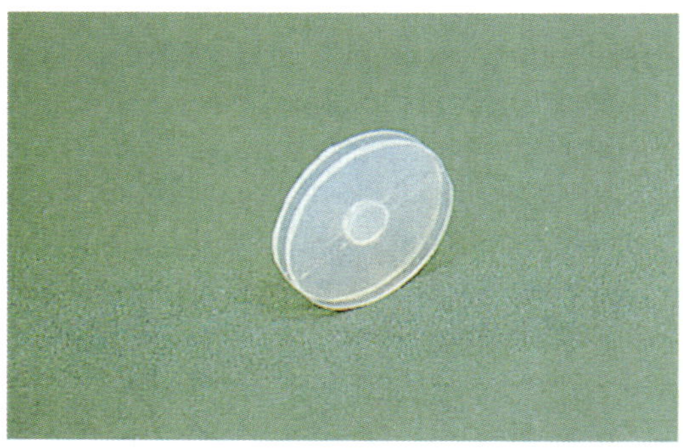

Fig. 5. Silastic septal button for non-surgical closure of a septal perforation.

Dorsum and septum abscesses are serious complications because of the chance of lasting damage to the cartilaginous skeleton of the nose. In dorsum hematomas, it is necessary for synthetic implants to be removed at once, whereas allogeneic (homologous) cartilage or bone

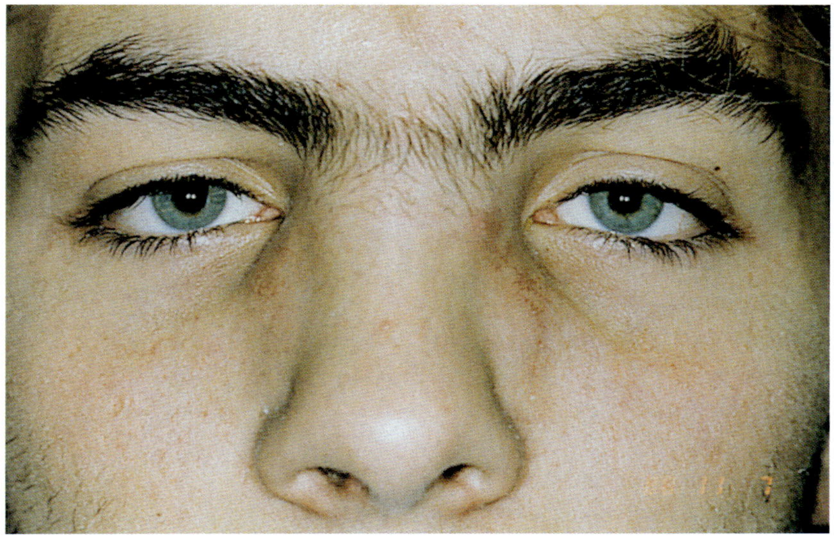

Fig. 6. Paranasal callus after (very low) lateral osteotomies.

implants can initially remain. In septum abscesses, the cartilaginous septum often disappears to a large extent due to *necrosis*.

Direct reconstruction of the septum with autogeneic or allogeneic cartilage (auricle or rib) after drainage of the abscess often gives a satisfactory recovery, despite the infectious area in which the graft is inserted. In this way, the nose bridge will be prevented from sinking in. In children therefore, the morphogenetic function of the cartilaginous septum can recover, resulting in prevention of growth inhibition of the nose and upper jaw (Fig. 4a, b).

Skin ischemia and necrosis is a serious complication. In earlier days, the combination of a too tight nasal packing and dressing (leaving the nasal tip free) could disturb the blood supply to the free skin of the nasal tip. Nowadays the use of septal suturing, short stay and loose packing (telfa) diminishes stagnation of the blood supply to the tip. Other causes are too aggressive subdermal thinning of the skin and too tightly fitting nasal implants, and these should be prevented. Any sign of tissue ischemia should be treated immediately by removing a tight dressing, application of local ice bags and, if necessary, reoperation to change or resculpture a too large implant. If there is any sign of an infection, high doses of broad spectrum antibiotics should be prescribed.

The late postoperative period (six weeks to one year)

A satisfactory postoperative result is no guarantee of the final result. Particularly after extensive changes to the nose skeleton, it is difficult to predict the final result. Inadequate operative techniques and/or wrong application can lead to unsatisfactory results and complications which often do not materialize until the late postoperative period. Therefore, a long-term follow-up is important to gain experience which can lead to adjusting and refining operative techniques. Photographic documentation at regular intervals, pre- and postoperatively, is of great importance here.

A postoperative follow-up scheme (after the first six weeks) at three, six, nine, and 12 months, and thereafter, if possible, every second year, would be adequate. In order to prevent complications, knowledge as well as observation of each patient is important.

Late complications

- nose passage disorders
- septal perforation
- deviation and irregularities of the dorsum
- paranasal callus
- saddle nose
- pollybeak deformity
- tip distortion
- tip ptosis
- columella retraction

Late complications often arise from undesired scarring due to mistakes in operative techniques and as a result of early complications such as hematomas and infections.

Nose passage disorders due to redeviation of the septum after correction of a deviated nasal septum occur in about 20% of cases. Stenoses of the ostium internum are less frequent but more difficult to treat. Firstly, recorrection of the septum is needed. Stenosis of the ostium internum often requires complicated surgical reconstruction with z-plasties and/or spreader grafts.

Septal perforation due to extensive cartilage resection and/or a corresponding lesion on either side of the mucoperichondrium which has not been carefully sutured, or which remains after a septum abscess, may give rise to recurring epistaxis, crustation, an unpleasant whistle (in a small perforation) and loss of support of the cartilaginous dorsum in a large perforation. For minor perforations, the treatment is surgical. In the case of major perforations (larger than 3 cm), there is less chance of success with surgical closure. In a number of cases, a Silastic septal button may be the solution (Fig. 5).

Deviations and irregularities of the dorsum often arise from a careless operative technique in combination with scar retraction. Frequent causes of these dorsum deviations are insufficient mobilization of the ossa nasalia or strong septum deviation being left untreated. After some time has elapsed, careless smoothing of the bony and cartilaginous dorsum can result in visible irregularities, especially in thin-skinned patients. The subcutaneous implantation of cartilage in the dorsum after hump resection is a common procedure. However, when crushed septal cartilage is used, it may lead to resorption and/or growth of new cartilage and consequently to visible irregularities. This cartilage growth occurs especially in young adults in whom growth of the nose is not yet complete.

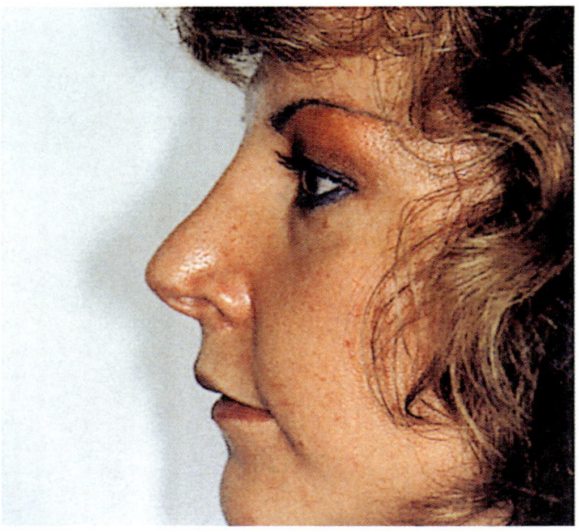

Fig. 7a. A soft-tissue pollybeak deformity.

Paranasal callus may arise after a paranasal hematoma and left-over crushed bone or splinters. In most cases the callus disappears spontaneously (Fig. 6).

Pollybeak deformities are frequently occurring complications of rhinoplasty. We can distinguish between soft-tissue and cartilaginous pollybeaks (Fig. 7a,b). Revision surgery is needed in both cases. Careful preparation directly at the cartilaginous dorsum prevents lesions of the nose musculature and soft tissue, which can result in scar retraction and consequently in a soft-tissue pollybeak. Ade-

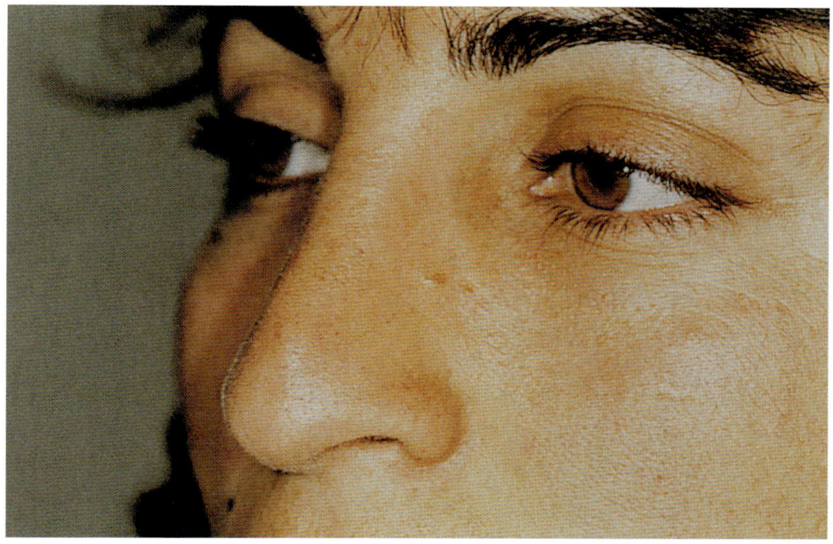

Fig. 7b. A cartilaginous pollybeak.

quate resection of the cartilaginous dorsum and avoidance of too much loss of tip support prevents a cartilaginous pollybeak.

Tip distortion arises from undesired scarring often in combination with disturbance of the continuity of the alar cartilages. Therefore, careful consideration should be given to an interrupted strip technique for the tip of the nose.

Tip ptosis arises to a slight degree when the tissues lose their elasticity in the aging process. However, this increases when the support structures have been over-sacrificed in early tip surgery. Therefore, knowledge of the tip support mechanisms is essential in order to prevent these complications.

Columella retraction is most frequently caused by overzealous resection of the caudal part of the septum. Skin scarring due to careless making and/or closing of columella incisions in the 'external approach' may also lead to disfiguring columella retractions.

PART II: OPERATIVE TECHNIQUES

6: SEPTOPLASTY AND TURBINATE SURGERY

M.J. Middelweerd

Septoplasty

'So the septum goes, so goes the nose', is an ancient but very true statement (see Fig. 11a-d). In the case of a saddle-nose deformity, a retracted columella, and especially in the crooked nose, the importance of the shape and condition of the septum is illustrated. In most rhinoplasty cases, at least minor septal surgery is indicated and this procedure may vary from mere cartilage graft harvesting to entirely reshaping or rebuilding the septum. In this chapter, various nasal septal deformities and the surgical approaches for their correction are described.

Anatomy

The septum consists of the perpendicular plate of the ethmoid, the vomer, the premaxilla and the quadrangular cartilage (Fig. 1). The quadrangular cartilage is connected to the perpendicular plate with a firm syndesmosis.

The bony parts of the septum are covered with periosteum and the cartilaginous part with perichondrium. Strong connective tissue fibers which cross from one side of the septum to the other (Fig. 2), connecting the perichondrium with the periosteum, attach the cartilaginous septum to the vomer and premaxilla. Directly continuous with the quadrangular cartilage are the triangular or upper lateral cartilages, establishing the cartilaginous dorsum of the nose. Caudally located at the caudal end of the quadrangular cartilage is the membranous septum, connecting the cartilaginous septum with the columella. In the membranous septum, the feet of the medial crura of the alar cartilages connect with the caudal border of the quadrangular cartilage, providing support for the nasal tip (Fig. 3).

Part of the cartilaginous nasal septum has a supportive function for the nose. The supportive part is demonstrated when drawing a vertical line from the anterior-most part of the nasal bone (keystone area) in a midsagittal plane of the nose (Fig. 1). Caudo-anteriorly from this line, resections should be carried out very conservatively. The mucosal lining of the septum is of the respiratory ciliary

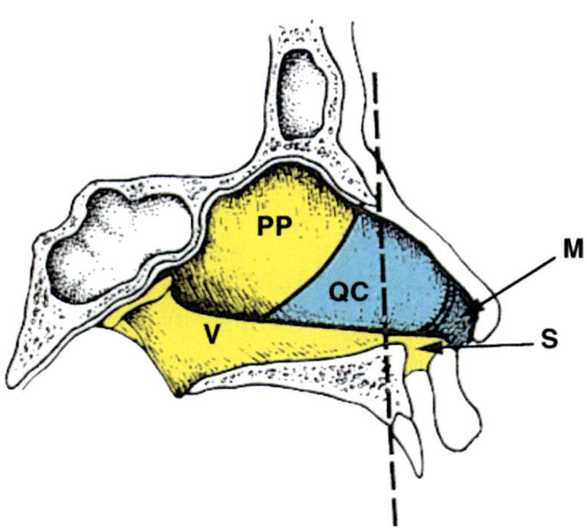

Fig. 1. The nasal septum in components. QC, quadrangular cartilage; PP, perpendicular plate; V, vomer; S, spina nasalis anterior; M, membranous septum. The dashed vertical line represents a plane, ventrally from which resections should be carried out very conservatively.

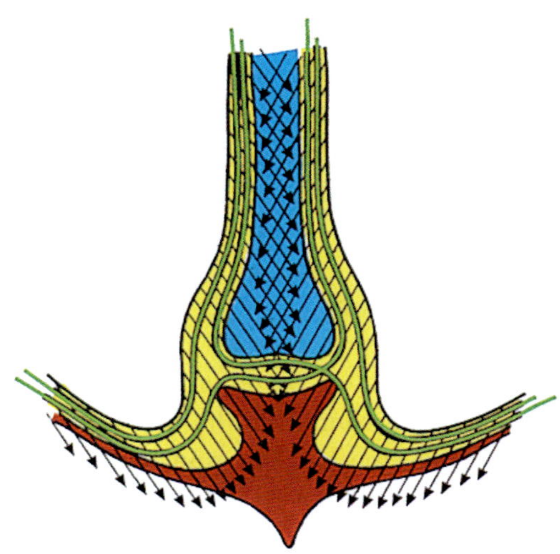

Fig. 2. Coronal section of the vomer (red) on top of which the cartilaginous septum (blue) is attached. The arrows indicate the strong connective tissue fibers which connect the mucoperichondrium and the mucoperiosteum to the base of the septal skeleton. Actual crossing of fibers from left to right and vice versa is indicated by the green lines.

epithelial type and its blood supply plays a vital role in the oxygen supply to the cartilaginous septum.

Classification of septal deformities

Septal deviations can be located in the bony part or the cartilaginous part, but mostly they are a combination of both. In general, cartilaginous deviations have the severest impact on the nasal airway. Deformities of the cartilaginous septum can be caused by intrinsic and extrinsic factors.

Intrinsic factors

Trauma to the cartilaginous septum may give rise to dislocation or fracturing. The earliest dislocating trauma may occur during the process of natural birth. Moreover, Cottle has even described neonatal septal dislocations in newborns delivered by Caesarian section, suggesting that intrauterine pressure trauma to the nose caused the deformity.

Fracturing of the cartilaginous septum brings about the loss of interlocked stress (Fry) within the septum. The fracture line may be directed horizontally or vertically. Due to the loss of interlocked stress, the fractured elements tend to override and block the nasal airway unilaterally. Fractures may also cause partial resorption of the cartilaginous septum, due to hematoma. Saddle formation and/or columellar retraction may be the result.

Extrinsic factors

These are factors originating from the structures surrounding the cartilaginous septum, causing its deviation without any intrinsic deformity in the cartilaginous septum itself. A deviated perpendicular plate will give rise to a deviated cartilaginous septum, because of their tightly connected syndesmosis and the limited space available in the nose. An abnormally large premaxillary spine may dislodge the caudal septal border. Dislocation of the vomer-maxilla junction gives lateral displacement of the cartilaginous septum, showing a normal connection between the vomer and the cartilaginous septum. Primary correction of these surrounding structures will cause secondary straightening of the cartilaginous septum. Additional reduction of the cartilaginous septum is often necessary to create a sufficient airway.

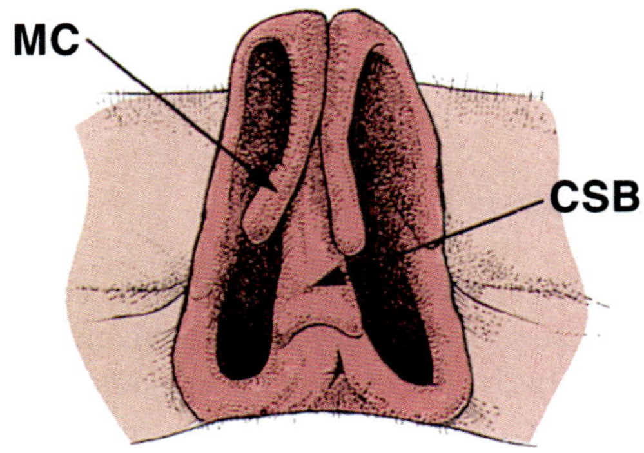

Fig. 3. Caudal view of the nasal septum, showing the attachment of the medial crura (MC) of the alar cartilages to the caudal septal border (CSB). This connection is situated in the plane of the membranous septum.

Approach

Four different approaches for surgical access to the septum are possible, each with its own indications and merits. All the incisions have the goal of providing an entrance to the submucoperichondrial/subperiosteal plane of the septum.

1. Killian incision

A vertical incision in the septal mucoperichondrium, 1.5 cm cranially from the caudal septal border. The mucoperichondrium is relatively easily elevated from this part of the septum and the incision gives good access to all parts of the septum, except for the caudal-most cartilaginous portion. This is a very suitable incision for cartilage harvesting purposes and correction of perpendicular plate deviations.

2. Total transfixion incision

A vertical vestibular skin incision, caudally from the caudal septal margin through the membranous septum. This incision gives good access to all parts of the septum and, in combination with intercartilaginous incisions, provides superb exposure of the valve area and the rest of the nasal dorsum. It is particularly useful if the dorsum has to be lowered. When a complete total transfixion is made, the attachments of the medial crura to the caudal septum are sacrificed, which will reduce tip projection and may cause retraction of the columella. If deprojection of the tip is not desired, a modified total transfixion incision is applied, remaining superior to the medial crural attachments with the septum.

3. Rethi incision

This horizontal mid-columellar incision can be utilized for the septum when an external approach has been selected for performing the rhinoplasty. After elevating the skin from the nasal tip and dorsum, the medial crura of the alar cartilages are divided and, after subsequently dividing the membranous septum, the caudal septal border is exposed. In cases where a large part of the caudal septal border is absent, this direct midline approach can facilitate the separation of the adhering mucoperichondrial flaps without tearing, because of the absence of an angle between the instruments and the tissue, as is present in total or hemitransfixion. In such a case, the Rethi incision may even be the method of preference in septoplasty without further rhinoplasty.

4. Hemitransfixion incision

A vertical vestibular skin incision is made at the level of the caudal septal edge, as described by Cottle *et al.*, preserving the integrity of the membranous septum. This gives good access to the entire septum, including the premaxilla.

Creating tunnels

Cartilaginous septum

A choice can be made between elevating the perichondrium from the cartilaginous septum unilaterally or bilaterally. Although elevating unilaterally may in theory leave a better blood supply to the cartilaginous septum, bilateral elevation of the mucoperichondrium gives better access to more severe deviations. If bilateral mucosal tearing is avoided, this proves to be a safe method.

Vomer

Spurs are usually removed after bilateral mucoperiosteal flap elevation, whereas ridges of the vomer are usually removed after unilateral tunnelling.

Perpendicular plate

When correction of perpendicular plate deviation is necessary, the mucoperiosteum is always elevated bilaterally to provide adequate exposure.

A distinction is made between superior and inferior tunnelling. The superior tunnel is defined as reaching as far inferiorly as the firm cross-fiber attachment of the cartilaginous septum to the vomer. The inferior tunnel is made subperiostally, starting at the premaxilla along the floor of the nose, close to its junction with the vomer. The inferior tunnel is advocated in cases of very inferiorly-located ridges blocking the nasal airway; joining the inferior and superior tunnels by dissecting the crossing fibers, gives good exposure in these cases. However, after elevating the periosteum from the perpendicular plate, the crossing fibers may be relatively easily dissected reversely, returning posteriorly to the caudal septum. With this technique, the relatively traumatizing inferior tunnel may be avoided in the great majority of cases.

Correction technique for septal deformities

Basic septoplasty

After elevating the mucoperichondrium and the mucoperiosteum uni- or bilaterally, a basal cartilaginous incision, separating the cartilaginous septum from the vomer, is made and the perpendicular plate is separated from the cartilage by means of a posterior chondrotomy. A horizontal strip or a boomerang-shaped piece of cartilage is removed, leaving the caudal-most cartilaginous part attached to the nasal spine. A 'swinging door' is created in this way. The deviated part of the bony septum can now be exposed by swinging the cartilaginous septum laterally. The deviated part of the bony septum is removed with forceps or an osteotome.

Fragments of the removed cartilage are repositioned between the mucoperichondrial layers, to prevent their direct adherence and thus the risk of septal perforation. The bone fragments removed are also partly replaced. With this basic technique, the majority of septal deviations may be corrected successfully (Fig. 4).

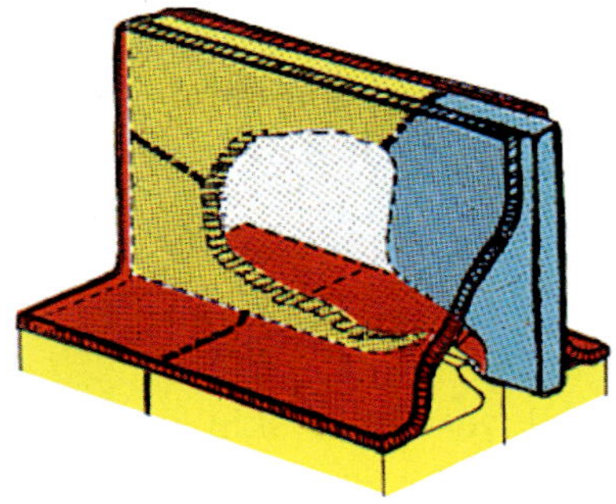

Fig. 4. Schematic representation of the nasal septum after a basic septoplasty. A basal cartilaginous strip and part of the perpendicular plate have been removed. Parts of the removed bone and cartilage fragments have to be replaced in the indicated defect to prevent adherence of the two mucosal layers.

Moderate cartilaginous bending despite the basic technique

Bending of the cartilage in a vertical plane requires vertical scoring incisions on the concave side of the deviated part. Horizontal bending is corrected with horizontal scoring incisions on the concave side of the deviated part (Fig. 5).

The severely deflected caudal cartilaginous septal margin

This deformity may be the cause of severe airway blocking and deviation of the cartilaginous nasal dorsum. After elevating the perichondrium bilaterally, the cartilaginous septum is detached from the premaxilla.

There are two ways to correct this deflection by breaking the spring of the cartilage:

1. multiple vertical partial thickness (at least 50%) cuts on the concave side;
2. vertical wedge resection on the convex side.

These two techniques are often combined. Fixation of the corrected cartilage is performed with mattress sutures through both layers of mucoperichondrium, tying the knot on the former convex side. The caudal septum end may be secured to the nasal spine with an additional suture (Fig. 6).

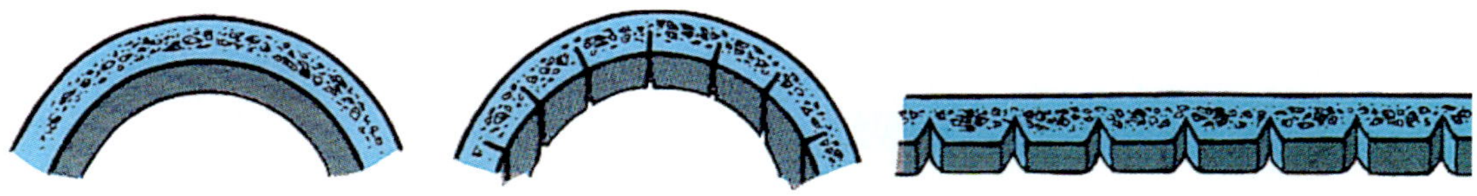

Fig. 5. Schematic representation of a curved piece of cartilage. Scoring incisions of at least 50% thickness on the concave side allows straightening of the cartilage.

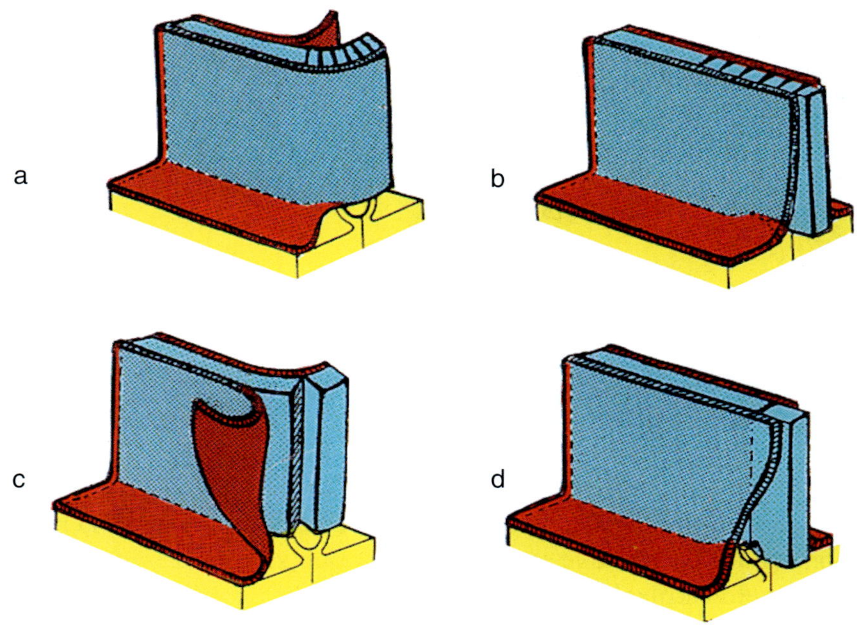

Fig. 6. Schematic representation of correcting a seriously vertically deflected cartilaginous septum. *a,b.* Vertical scoring incisions on the concave side. *c,d.* Vertical wedge excision on the convex side.

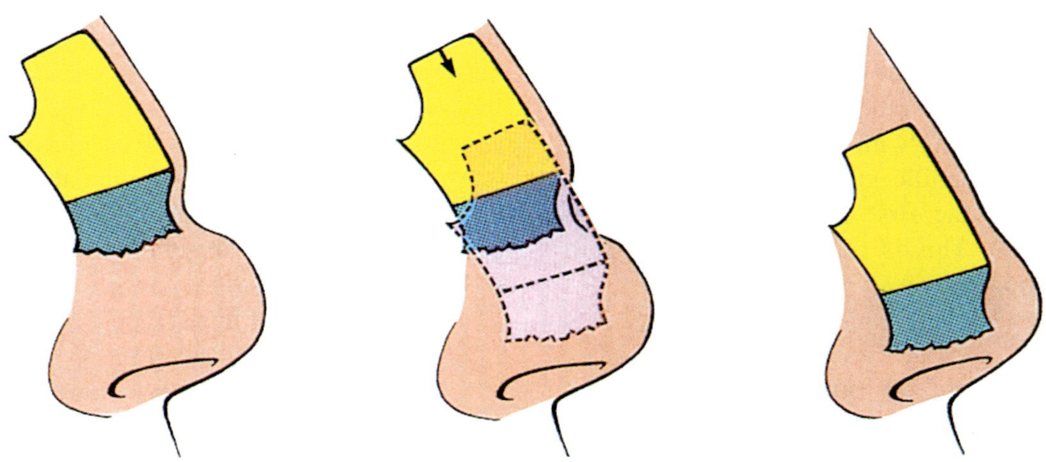

Fig. 7. Schematic representation of the advancement of a bony/cartilaginous septal complex to correct sagging of the nasal dorsum after overresection of the septum in the keystone area.

Cartilaginous sagging of the dorsum

This deformity is caused by loss of support from the cartilaginous septum in the keystone area, mostly after severe trauma or previous septal surgery. After elevating the mucoperichondrium from the cartilaginous remnants, the perpendicular plate may be taken out and reshaped to be shifted more caudally, providing new support in the keystone area (Fig. 7). If too little perpendicular plate is left, a cartilaginous autograft from the auricle may be inserted, with both good functional and aesthetic results (Fig. 8a,b).

Splinting and packing

In general, absorbable mattress sutures, fixating the bilateral mucoperichondrial layers upon the cartilaginous septum,

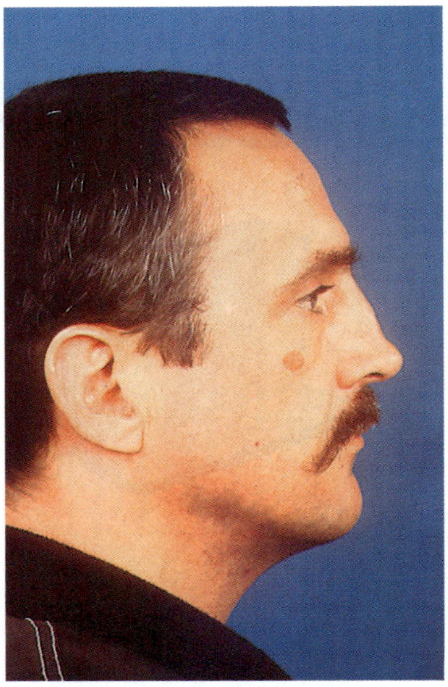
a

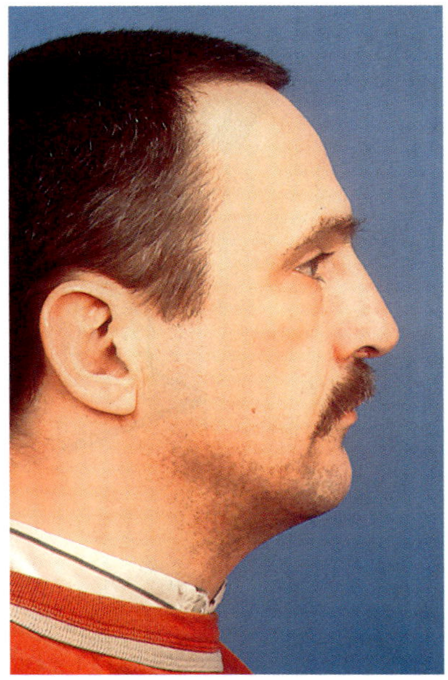
b

Fig. 8a,b. Pre- and postoperative views of a patient with supratip impression due to loss of dorsal support after triple septoplasty, Dorsal correction with implantation of autogenous auricular cartilage.

provide enough protection against the development of postoperative septal hematoma. In severe cartilaginous septal deviations, postoperative splinting of the septum may be of help for temporary support. The splints can be removed seven to ten days postoperatively. Light (if any) bilateral packing with strips of telfa or a strip of hydrophilic gauze, is enough for collecting the first sanguinolent nasal discharge. This is removed 12 to 48 hours postoperatively.

Surgery of the turbinates

The inferior turbinate plays the most important role in nasal airway patency, in comparison to the medial and superior turbinate. Surgery of the medial turbinates will therefore not be discussed in this chapter.

Surgical reduction of the volume of the inferior turbinates is indicated in cases of hyper-reactivity of the nasal mucosa, responding insufficiently to medical therapy. Especially in reduction rhinoplasty, a sufficient nasal airway may be secured by inferior turbinate reduction. The turbinate consists of a bony skeleton enveloped by richly vascularized nasal mucosa.

Airway obstruction may be caused by the bony component or by the mucosal component of the turbinate. Distinction between these components can be made by assessing the increase of airway diameter after decongesting the nasal mucosa.

There are several procedures to enhance the airway in the inferior nasal meatus:

- submucous electrocoagulation
- lateral outfraction of the lower turbinate
- partial resection of hypertrophic mucosa of the inferior turbinate (Fig. 9)
- submucous resection of the os turbinale
- partial resection of both the bone and the mucosa of the inferior turbinate. Mucosal cryosurgery and ectrocautery show only temporary effect in our hands.

Surgical technique

Inferior turbinate surgery can be performed quite well under local anesthesia. The mucosa of the inferior turbinate is infiltrated along its entire length with xylocaine 1% and adrenalin 1 in 100,000.

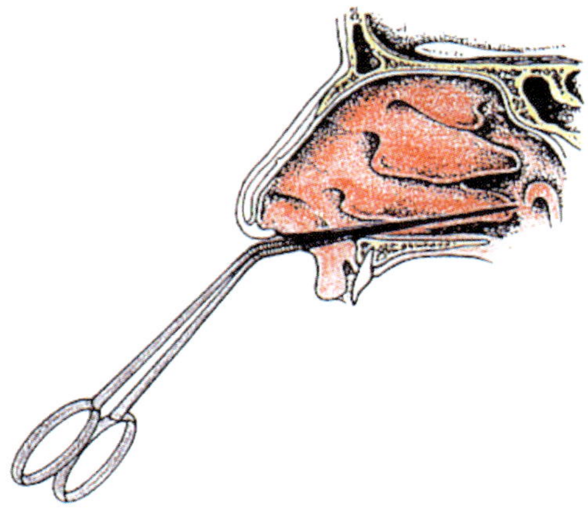

Fig. 9. Resection of a strip hypertrophied mucosa of the inferior turbinate with a pair of Fomon's scissors.

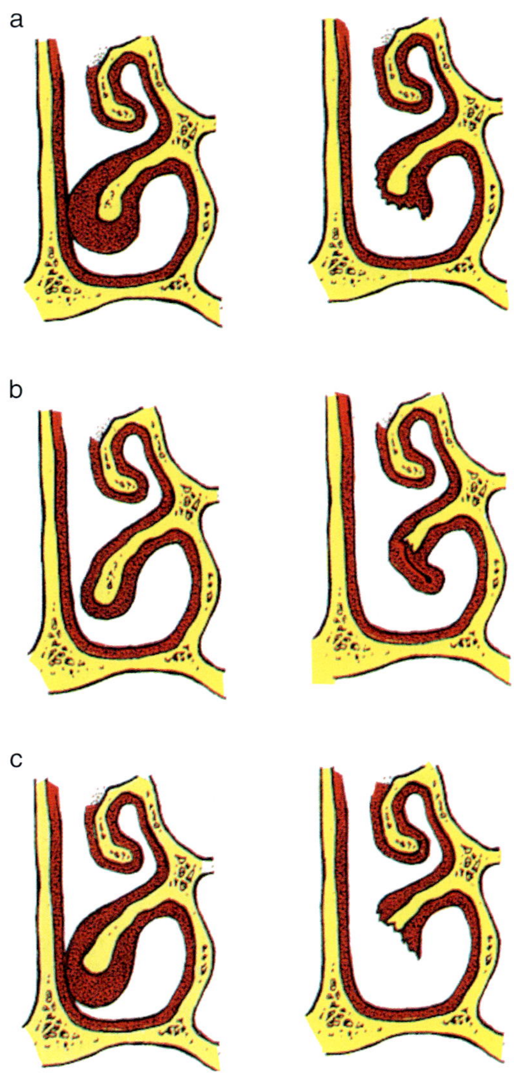

Fig. 10. Reduction surgery of the inferior turbinate. *a.* Isolated mucosal hypertrophy; mucosal resection alone. *b.* Isolated enlargement of the os turbinale; submucous bone resection alone. *c.* Combination of *a* and *b*; combined resection of bone and mucosa.

Furthermore the nasal mucosa is anesthesized with cocaine crystals or a 5–10% solution applied on surgical patties.

Mucosal resection of the inferior turbinate (Fig. 10a)
Starting from the most anterior portion of the inferior turbinate, a strip of mucosa and submucous tissue from the inferior part of the turbinate is resected with a pair of Fomon's or Heymann's scissors (Fig. 9). The posterior extent of the resection is determined by the individual anatomy; the mucosal hypertrophy may be located in the anterior part or posterior part of the turbinate or may concern its total length.

Submucous resection of the os turbinale (Fig. 10b)
A vertical incision is made in the mucosa covering the most anterior part of the inferior turbinate. A submucoperiosteal plane is developed with, *e.g.*, a Freers' elevatorium. The os turbinale can be cut to the desired proportions with a pair of bone cutting scissors or an osteotome. The incision is sutured with absorbable material. This procedure is only indicated in case of a predominantly bony 'hypertrophy' of the inferior turbinate.

Combined resection of inferior turbinate mucosa and bone (Fig. 10c)
This procedure is performed essentially in the same way as the mucosal resection. Part of the turbinate bone, however, is removed together with the mucosa to create a sufficient airway. Again, the anterio-posterior extent of the resection is individually determined. This procedure is indicated in cases with combined bony and mucosal turbinate hypertrophy.

Postoperative care
The nose is packed for 48 hours postoperatively. Nasal crusting and sanguinolent discharge will occur during the first two weeks. Sodium hydrocarbonate 1.4% nasal washouts are advised in this period.

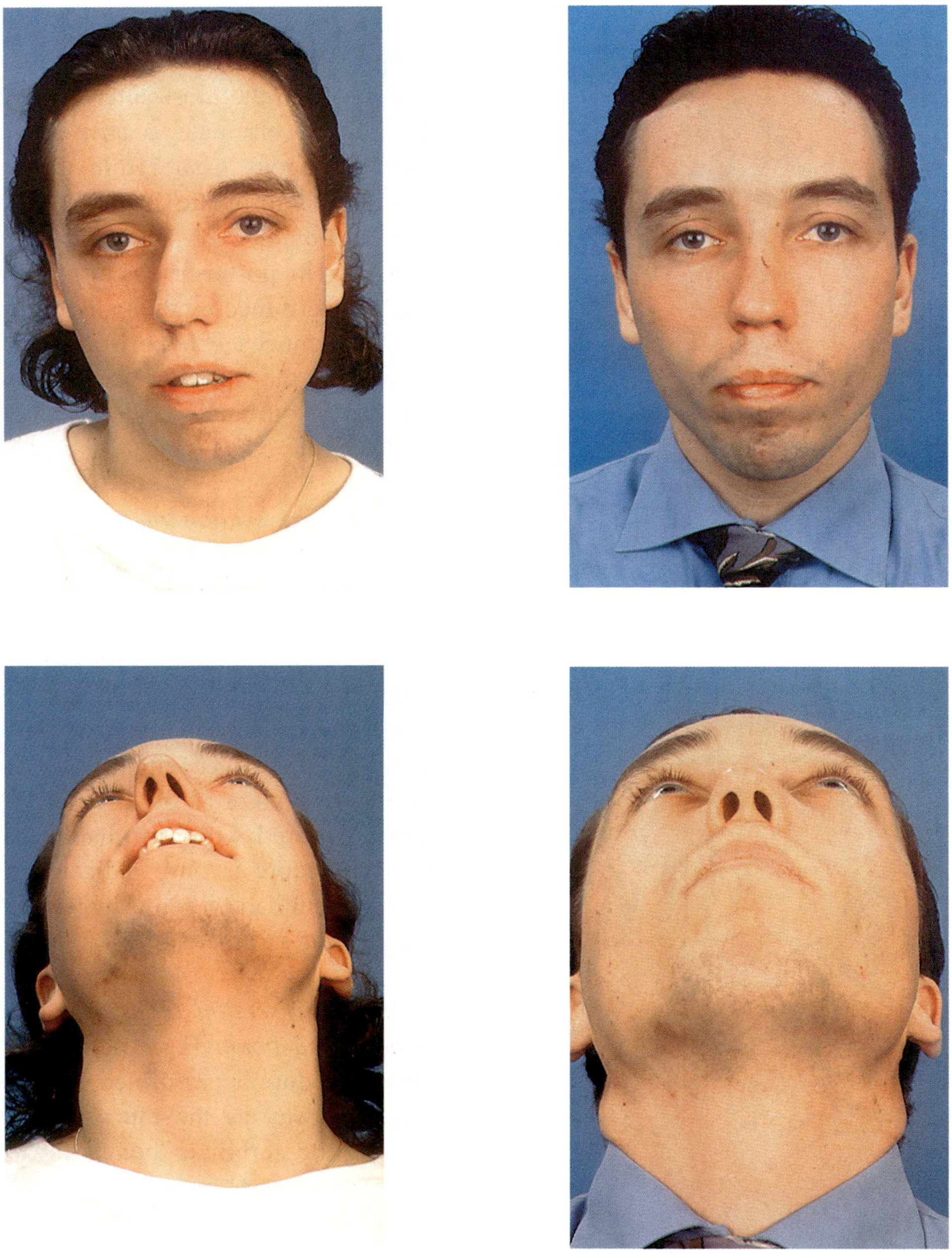

Fig. 11 a-d. Pre and postoperative views of a patient with congenital deviation of the nose mainly due to septal deformity. Septo-rhinoplasty was performed.

Complications

The most important complication after turbinate resection is the risk of severe postoperative bleeding in less than 1% of cases. The occurrence of synechiae should be prevented by adequate postoperative packing and by avoiding a raw area between the inferior turbinate and the septum. Ozena (intranasal crusting and foetor) is predominately a theoretical complication. In large numbers of patients reported by Courtiss and Goldwyn, it was only found extremely rarely. Extensive resections in the middle nasal meatus are much more likely to have this effect and should be avoided.

7: GRAFTS IN NASAL SURGERY

G.J. Nolst Trenité

Introduction

In the last century all kinds of biological and non-biological materials were used for augmentation of the nasal dorsum and to correct tip deformities. Non- biological implants have a high risk of local infection and extrusion of the implant, compared to biological grafts. Although the common use of new biocompatible synthetic materials (teflon, mersilene, goretex, etc.) give very good results in other parts of the body, this is not so for the nose due to its vulnerability for trauma, inducing an antigenic reaction in the tissue surrounding the implant. Allogeneic (homologous) and xenogeneic (heterologous) materials still have some extended resorption of the graft. Up until now, autogenous (autogeneic, autologous) material has always been regarded as the graft material of choice in nasal surgery, despite the additional harvesting procedure. In most cases there is a preference for autogenous cartilage over bone, because of the lack of flexibility of bone and its tendency to be resorbed.

Autogenous graft material

As autogenous graft material for the nose, we can use single or composite grafts:

Single grafts	*Composite grafts*
– cartilage	– double layer graft (skin, cartilage)
– bone	– triple layer graft (skin, cartilage, skin)
– skin	

Donor sites

Most donor sites for autogenous grafts are easily accessible during nasal surgery. There are, however, two exceptions: costal cartilage and iliac crest bone.

The most frequently used donor sites are:
for cartilage (Fig. 1a,b,c):
– the septum
– the auricle
– costal cartilage
for bone (Fig. 2):
– iliac crest or cranium
for full skin and composite grafts (Fig. 3):
– the auricle

Recipient sites

The recipient site for bone is usually confined to the dorsum. Single full skin grafts have a tendency to retract and are therefore only suitable for small skin defects over the cartilaginous and bony nasal skeleton. Double and triple layer composite grafts are indicated for defects with tissue loss of the tip, ala or columella. Autogenous cartilage is generally used in most recipient sites.

The main recipient sites for grafts in nasal surgery are:
– radix
– septum
– dorsum
– nasal side wall
– tip
– ala
– columella
– naso-labial groove

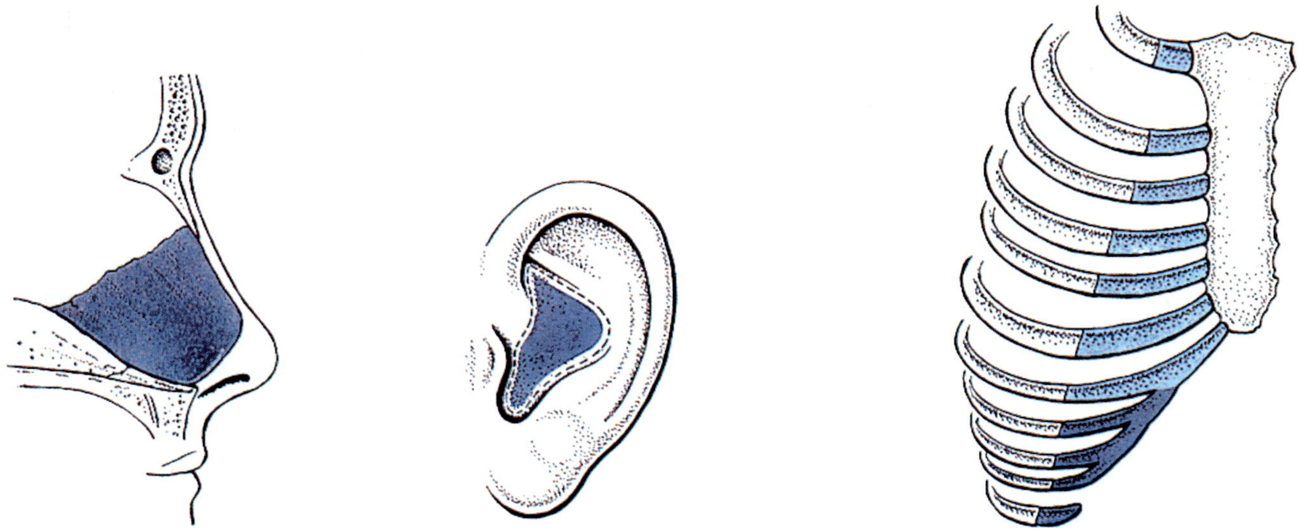

a b c

Fig. 1a,b,c. Donor sites for autogenous cartilage grafts – dark blue areas.

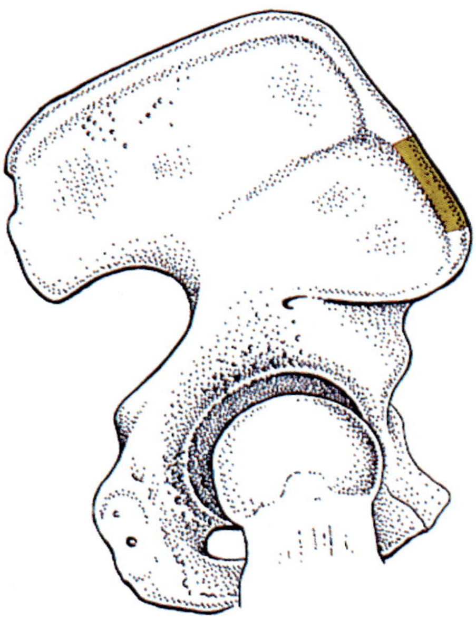

Fig. 2. Iliac crest with brown area as donor site for bone.

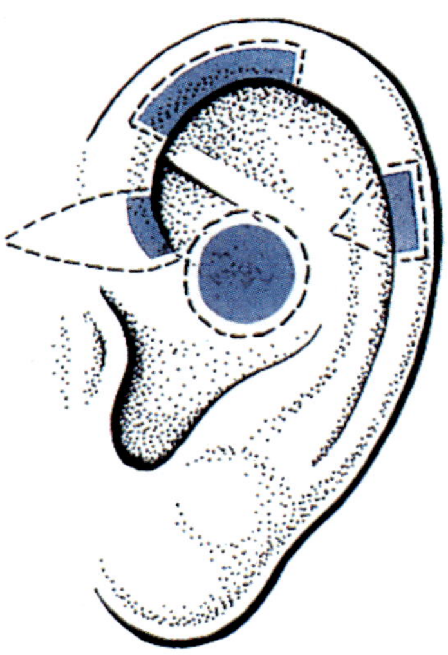

Fig. 3. Different areas of the auricle for harvesting composite grafts.

Indications

Radix

By changing the horizontal and vertical position of the deepest depression of the root of the nose, using a small cartilaginous graft, this will result in lengthening of the nose and diminishing an apparent over-projection of the nasal tip (Fig. 4a,b).

Septum

The choice of a graft for augmentation of the nasal dorsum depends on the etiology and extent of the correction needed. Postoperative sagging of the cartilaginous dorsum after septal surgery is best treated with rebuilding or repositioning of the cartilaginous septum (Fig. 5a,b). For rebuilding the septum autogenous cartilage from the posterior portion of the septum (if still available), conchal cartilage or costal cartilage (less accessible) is suitable. In case of a septal abscess with excessive loss of septal cartilage, immediate rebuilding with autogenous costal cartilage or allogeneic 'bank' cartilage is indicated, to prevent saddling and, if it concerns a growing child, additional midfacial growth disturbances.

Dorsum

In a saddle nose caused by a too low cartilaginous dorsum with normal tip support, a cartilaginous septal or conchal graft is appropriate (Fig. 6a,b). A nose with severe saddling involving the whole osseocartilaginous vault could be a good candidate for a bone graft (Fig. 7a,b). Due to the tendency of iliac crest bone to be resorbed, cranial bone or costal cartilage grafts are now more popular. When this severe saddling is combined with loss of tip support, a (two piece) costal cartilage graft is very suitable (Fig. 8a,b).

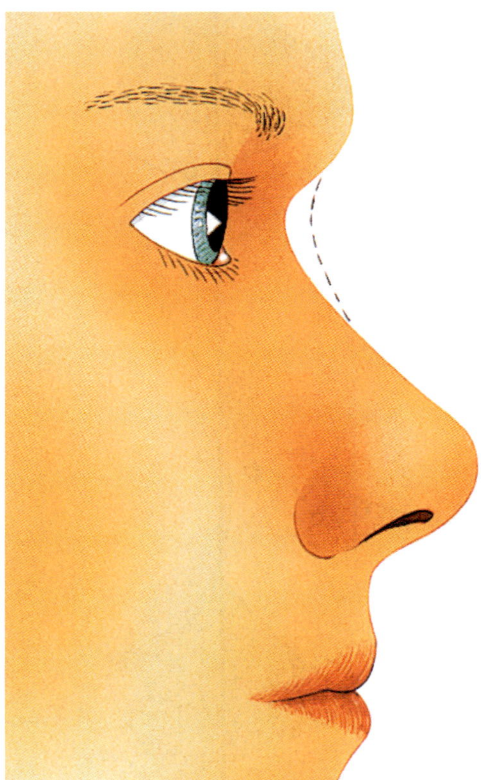
a

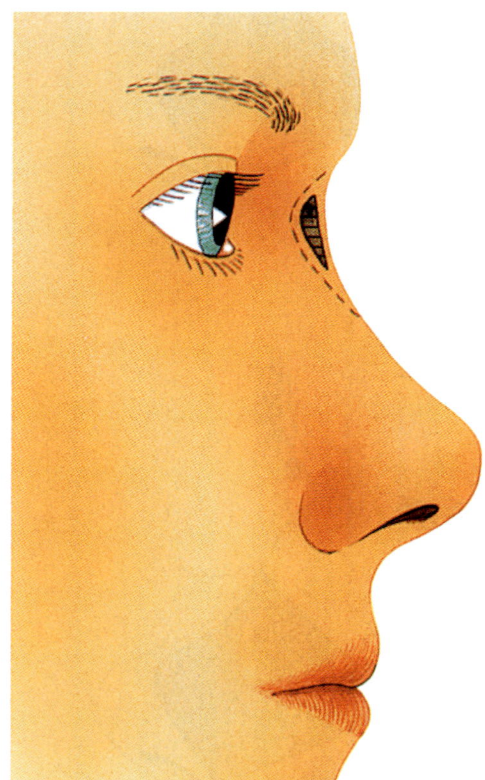
b

Fig. 4a. A too deep nasofrontal groove resulting in an apparent overprojection of the nose.

Fig. 4b. Autogenous cartilage graft (blue striped area) to lengthen the nose and to correct the apparent overprojection.

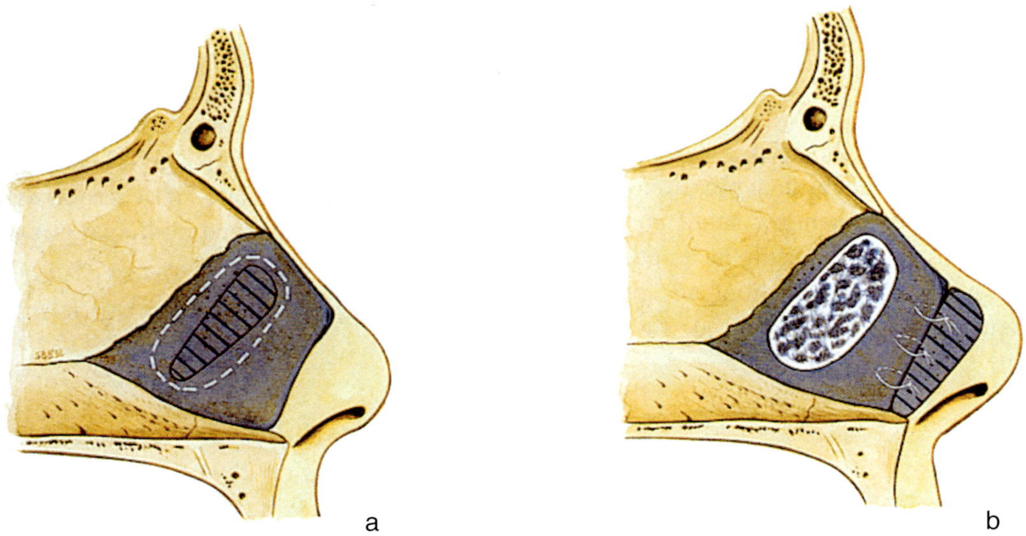

a b

Fig. 5a. Sagging of the cartilaginous dorsum, diminished tip support and retraction of the columella due to overresection of the caudal part of the septum.

Fig. 5b. Rebuilding the septum with autogenous septal cartilage (blue striped area). Reimplantation of crushed left-over cartilage in the donor site to prevent a septal perforation.

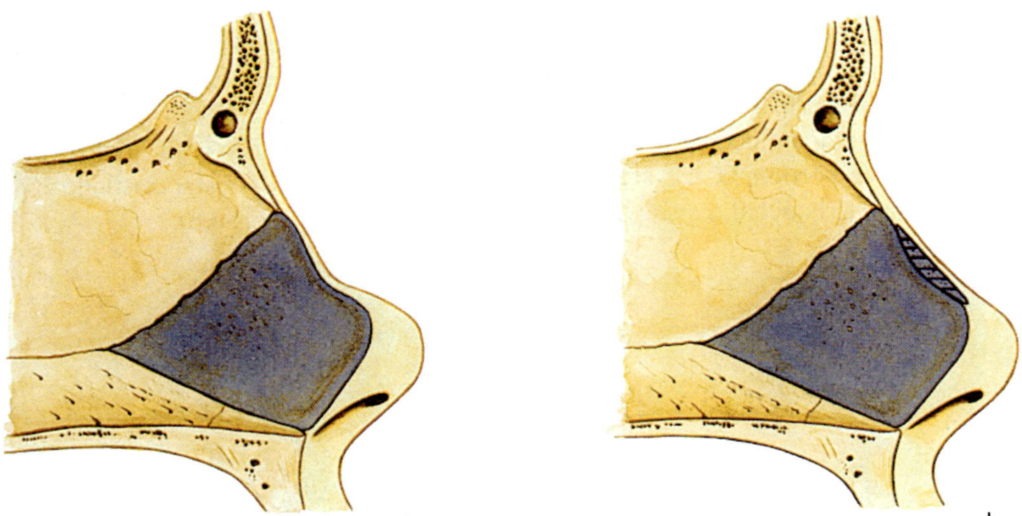

a b

Fig. 6a. Saddle nose caused by a too low cartilaginous dorsum with normal tip support.

Fig. 6b. Autogenous septal or conchal cartilage (blue striped area) to rebuild a sagging cartilaginous dorsum.

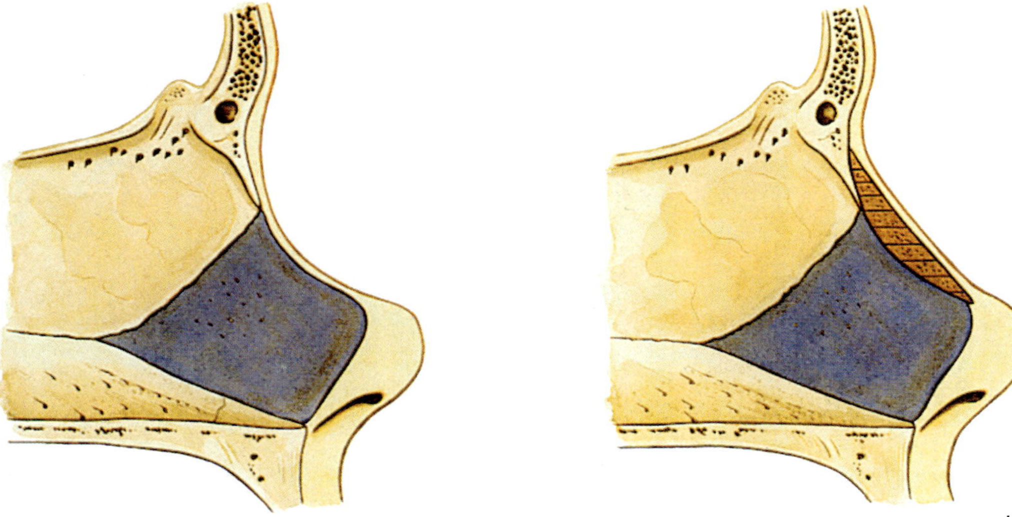

a b

Fig. 7a. Severe saddling involving the whole osseocartilaginous vault.

Fig. 7b. Autogenous bone graft – brown striped area – to augment the nasal (bony and cartilaginous) dorsum.

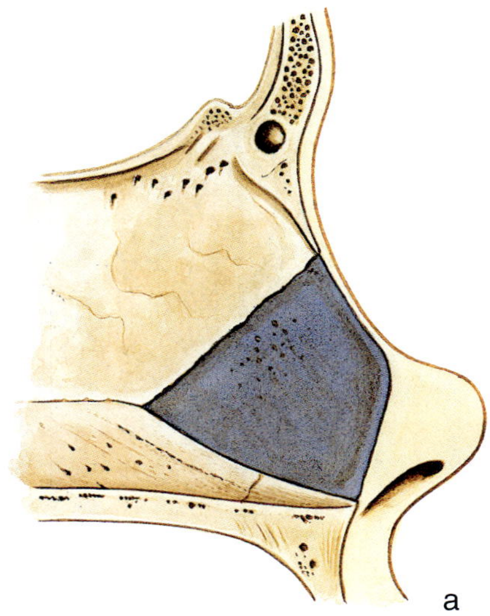
a

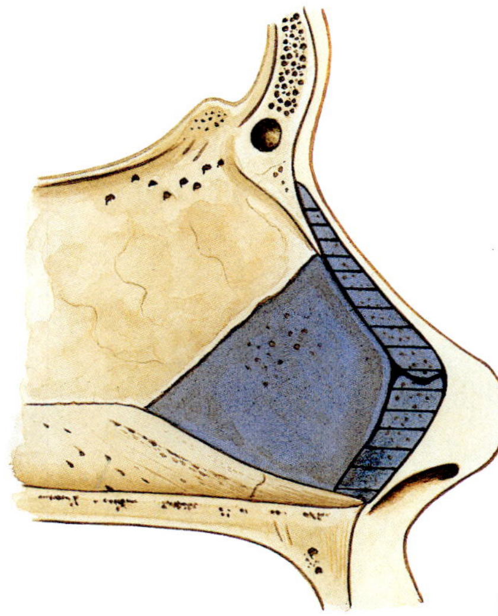
b

Fig. 8a. A combination of severe saddling and diminished tip support.

Fig. 8b. A two piece autogenous costal cartilage graft (blue striped areas) to reconstruct the normal projection of the nose.

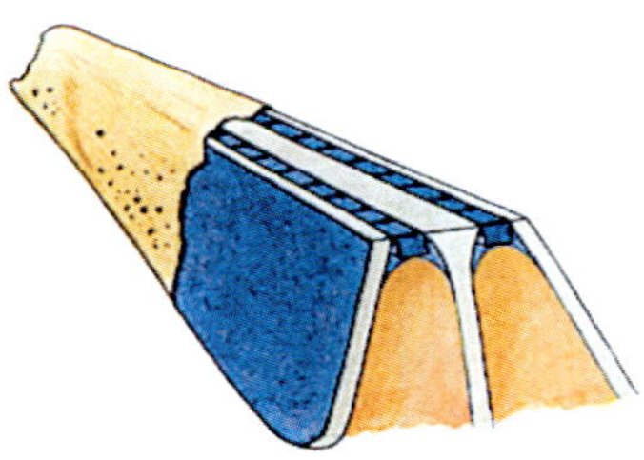
a

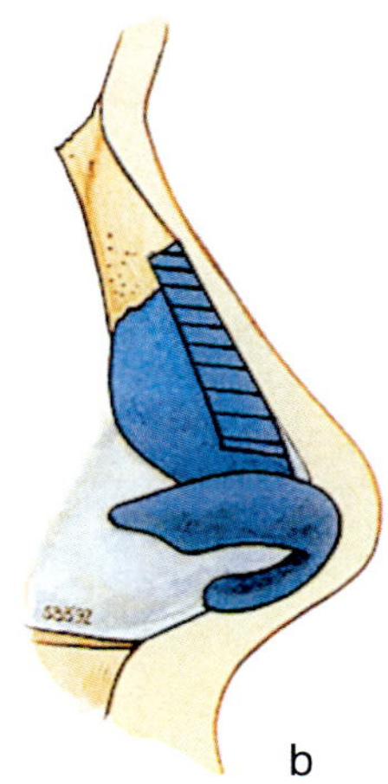
b

Fig. 9a. Spreader grafts of autogenous septal cartilage (blue striped areas) to restore a too narrow nasal valve and an aesthetically too narrow midnose.

Fig. 9b. Autogenous septal onlay graft (blue striped area) to camouflage avulsion of the upper lateral from the nasal bone.

Nasal side wall

Mid-nose collapse due to excessive resection of the upper lateral or avulsion of the upper lateral from the nasal bone (K-area) can be treated with a septal cartilage graft (Fig. 9a,b).

Tip, ala and columella

For tip augmentation, cartilaginous grafts from the concha, septum, or a combination of these, can be used depending on the operative technique and extent of the correction. Conchal cartilage is very suitable as an onlay tip graft because of its natural bending properties (Fig. 10). Septal cartilage is the material of choice for a columella strut for extra tip support, and for a shield-type tip graft for extra tip definition and projection (Fig. 11a,b). In certain cases of alar rim defects, resulting in alar collapse, a conchal cartilage graft with its concave side towards the vestibulum can be very effective. When there are not very large alar, tip or columellar defects with cartilage and soft tissue loss, and in cases of vestibular stenosis, composite grafts are indicated.

Naso-labial angle

To correct an acute naso-labial angle, due to some retraction of the columellar

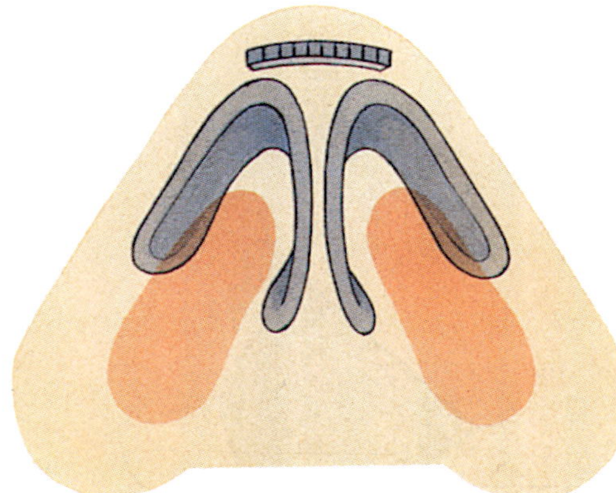

Fig. 10. Onlay tip graft of autogenous cartilage of the concha, which is very suitable due to its natural bending.

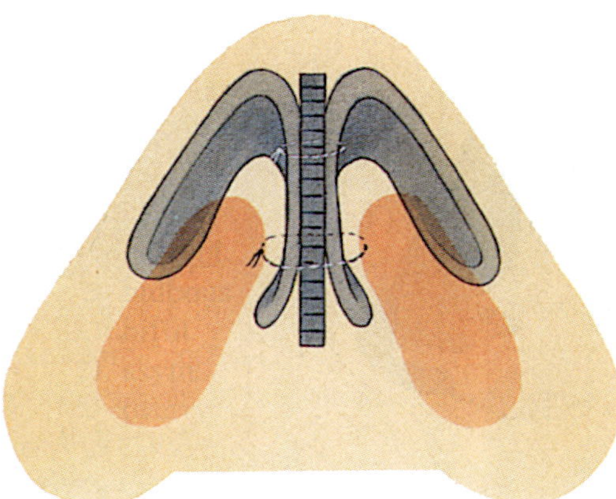

a

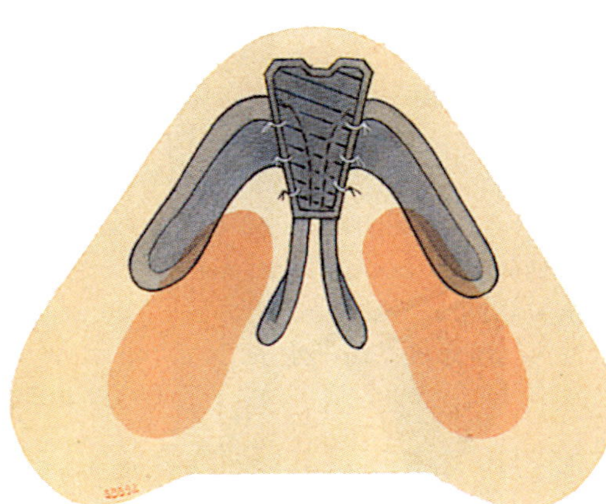

b

Fig. 11a. Columella strut of autogenous septal cartilage for extra tip support fixed by mattress sutures to the medial crura.

Fig. 11b. Shield-type tip graft sculptured from autogenous septal cartilage to gain extra tip projection and definition.

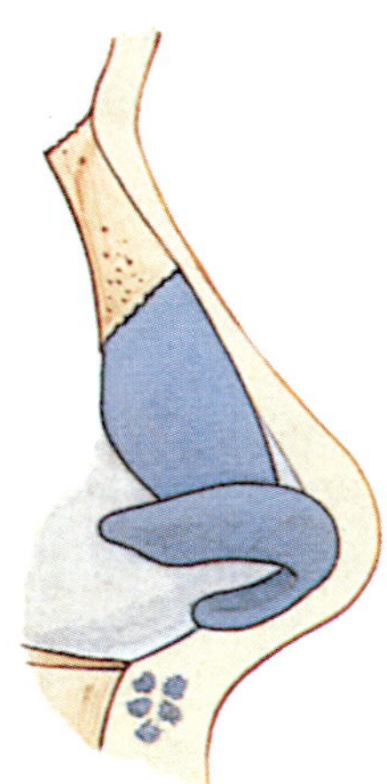

Fig. 12. Small pieces of autogenous cartilage to correct an acute nasal-labial angle.

base, small pieces of available septal or conchal cartilage in a subcutaneous pocket are appropriate (Fig. 12).

Harvesting technique

The harvesting technique described in this chapter is restricted to only the most frequently used autogenous grafts in nasal surgery.

Septal cartilage

When there is no indication for correction of a deviated septum, the hemi- transfixion incision should be replaced by a Killian incision (blade No. 15), so as not to disturb the septo-columellar junction (Fig. 13b). The initial incision through the mucoperichondrium can be made at either side of the septum. With a sharp, pointed, curved pair of scissors, dissection is started in the subperichondrial plane and continued with a Cottle or Joseph elevator to free the mucoperichondrium over the area of septal cartilage to be resected (Fig. 13b). Previous hydraulic dissection with a local anesthetic will facilitate this procedure (Fig. 13a). After incising the cartilage, a subperichondrial tunnel should be made over the corresponding area at the opposite side (Fig. 13c). Care should be taken not to damage the mucoperichondrium, to prevent perforation of the septum. After additional horizontal and vertical chondrotomies with a beaver knife, the planned amount of septal cartilage can be harvested. In choosing the cartilage harvesting area, care should be taken not to disturb the continuity of that part of the quadrangular cartilage anteriorly to the imaginary line between the most caudal point of the nasal bones (rhinion) and the anterior nasal spine, to prevent sagging of the cartilaginous nasal dorsum (Fig. 14ab). A blunt forceps should be used to remove the graft material in order not to damage the cartilage. After the sculpturing procedure, the left-over cartilage should be used as a crushed implant in the area of previously resected cartilage, to prevent the mucoperichondrium blades from sticking together. This procedure diminishes the chance of a

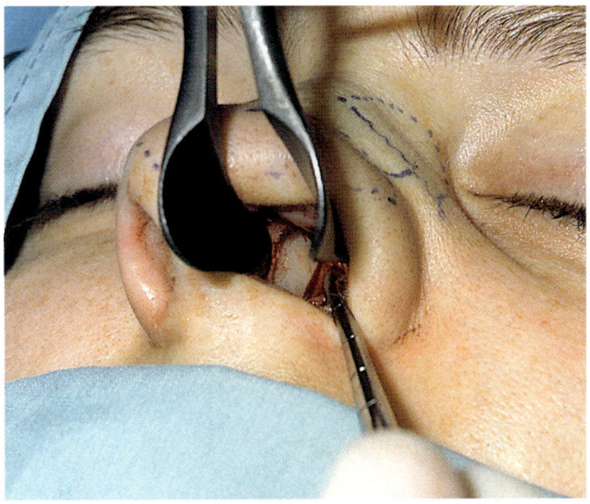
b

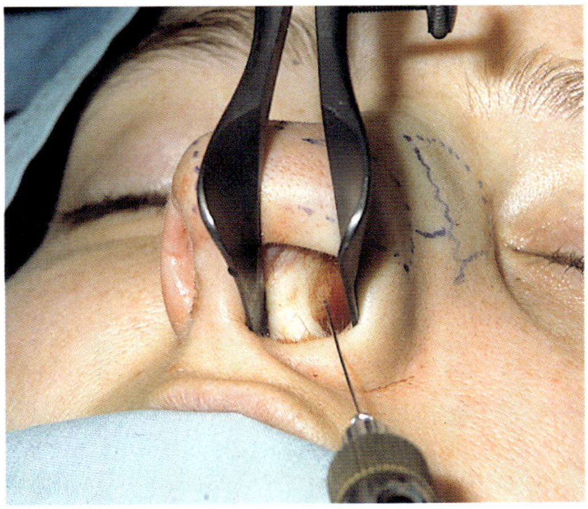
a

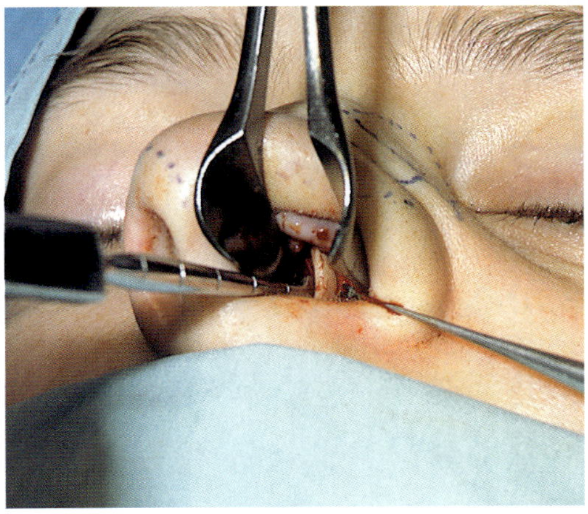
c

Fig. 13a. Hydraulic dissection with local anesthetic.

Fig. 13b. Freeing the mucoperichondrium from the septal cartilage after a Killian incision.

Fig. 13c. Vertical transcartilaginous incision followed by freeing the mucoperichondrium at the opposite side.

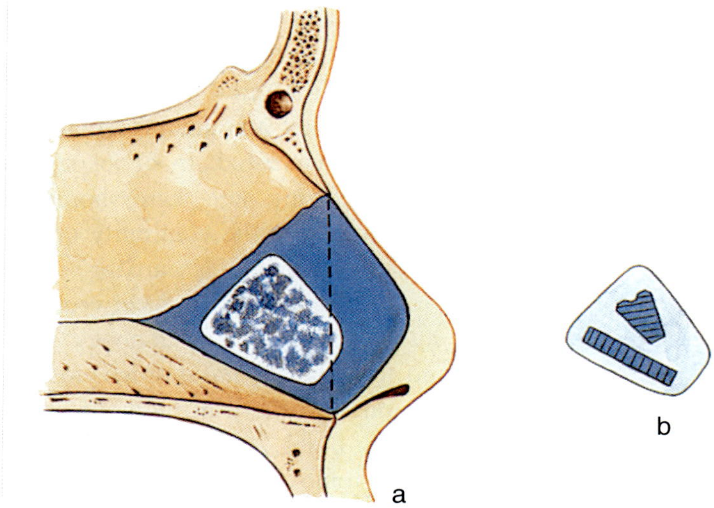

Fig. 14a. Donor site of septal cartilage, posterior to the dotted line to guarantee septal support of the nasal dorsum with reimplantation of crushed cartilage.

Fig. 14b. Harvested septal cartilage for sculpturing columella strut and shield tip graft.

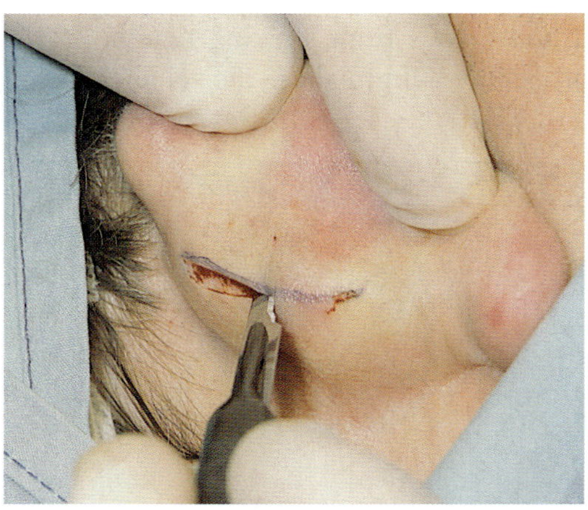

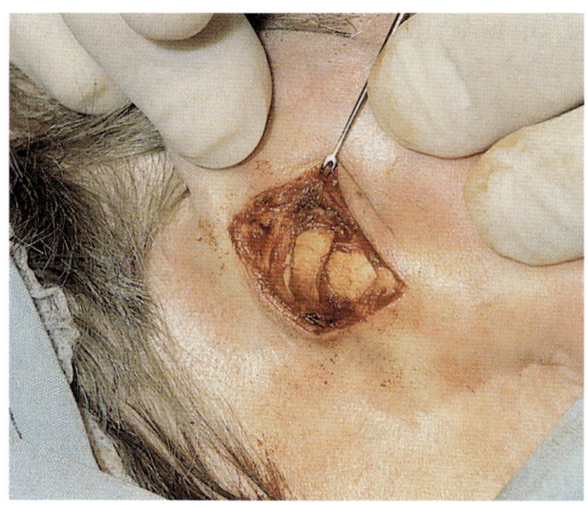

Fig. 15. Retro-auricular skin incision.
Fig. 16. Two parallel incisions through cartilage and 'post-auricular' perichondrium.

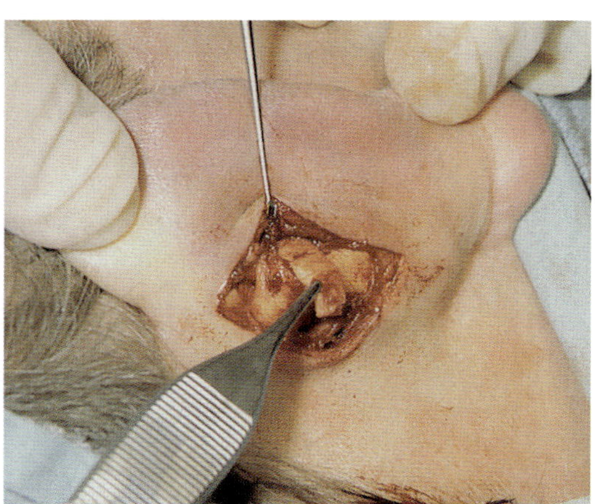

Fig. 17. Resection of the first onlay tip graft.

Fig. *18a.* Harvesting a second graft.

a 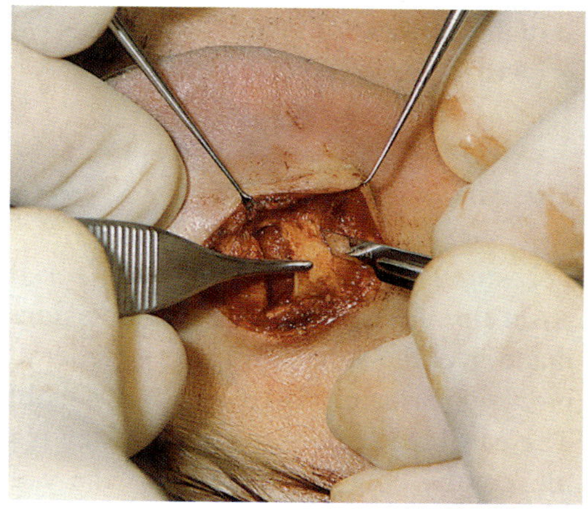

b 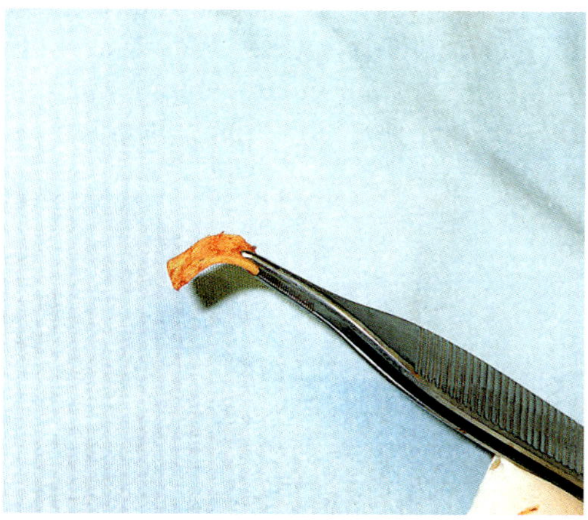

c 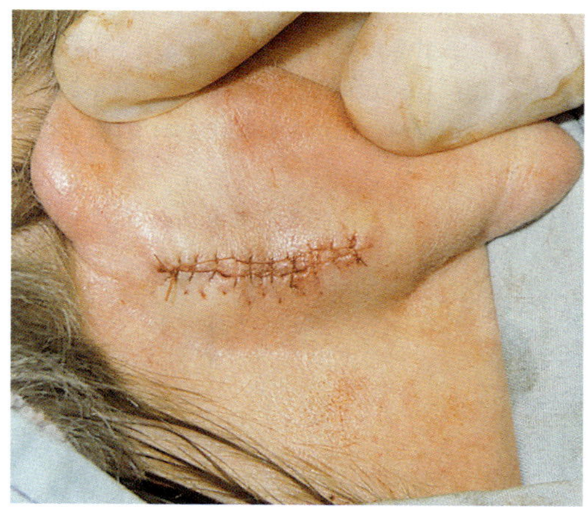

Fig. 18b. Natural bending of the conchal cartilage graft.

Fig. 18c. Skin closure with 5/0 atraumatic nylon 'running' suture.

a 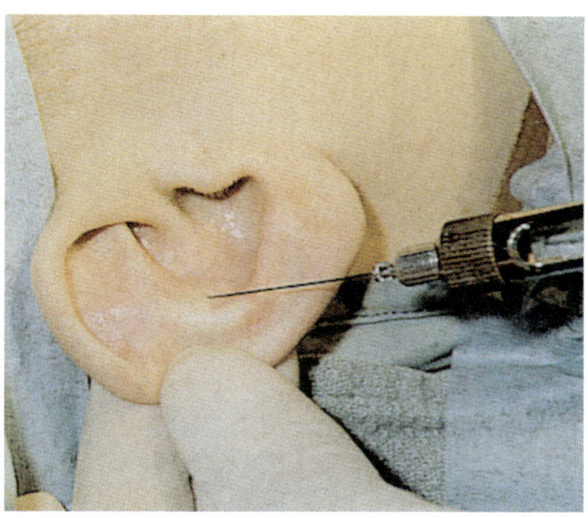

b 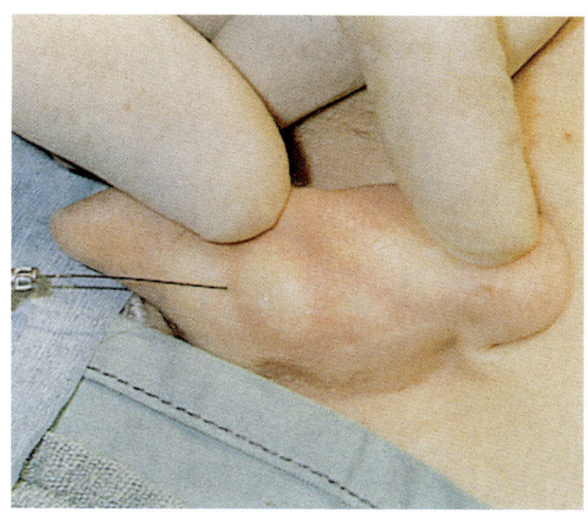

Fig. 19. Application of local anesthesia. *a.* Anterior side in subperichondrial plane. *b.* Posterior side in supraperichondrial plane.

septal perforation and stimulates the growth of new septal cartilage.

Ear cartilage

For small cartilage onlay grafts for the nasal tip, a retro-auricular skin incision is made over the concha (Fig. 15). Generally, pieces measuring 5–10 mm are suitable. The cartilage grafts can be harvested from the cymba conchae (cranial to the radix helices) or cavum conchae (caudal to the radix helicis), depending on the appropriate degree of bending which is needed. After freeing the soft tissue by blunt dissection over the area to be resected, two transcartilaginous incisions (No. 15 blade) are made through the cartilage and 'post-auricular' perichondrium (Fig. 16), followed by subperichondrial dissection on the pre-auricular side with a sharp, pointed, curved pair of scissors, and finally by resection of the cartilage graft (Fig. 17). If necessary this can be followed by harvesting of a second piece of conchal cartilage (Fig. 18a,b). The skin can easily be closed with a 5/0 atraumatic nylon 'running' suture (Fig. 18c). To harvest a large piece of conchal cartilage, the pre-auricular approach is technically easier than the postauricular approach, but is less elegant as it leaves a pre-auricular scar.

After infiltration of a local anesthetic solution (2% lidocaine with 1:100,000 epinephrine) at the anterior side of the concha into the subperichondrial surgical plane, to facilitate the dissection, the posterior side is infiltrated, but now in the supraperichondrial plane (Fig. 19a,b). To outline the postauricular semicircular skin and cartilage incision, three needles are

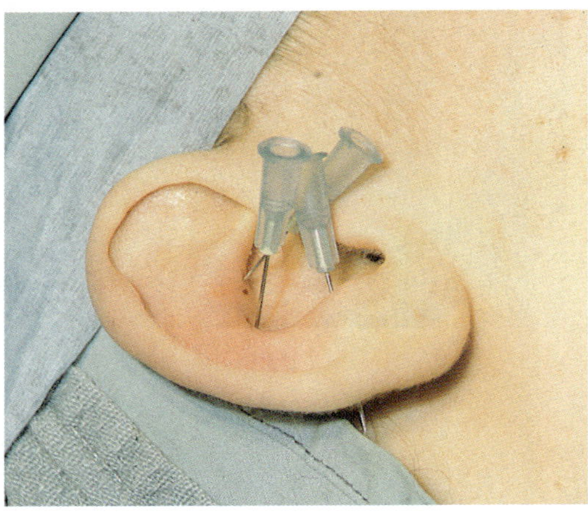

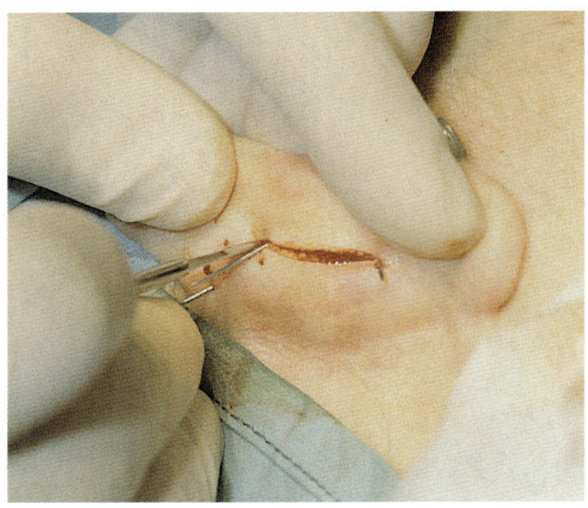

Fig. 20. Three through-and-through needles to mark the post-auricular skin and cartilage incisions.

Fig. 21. Skin incision along the landmark of the needles.

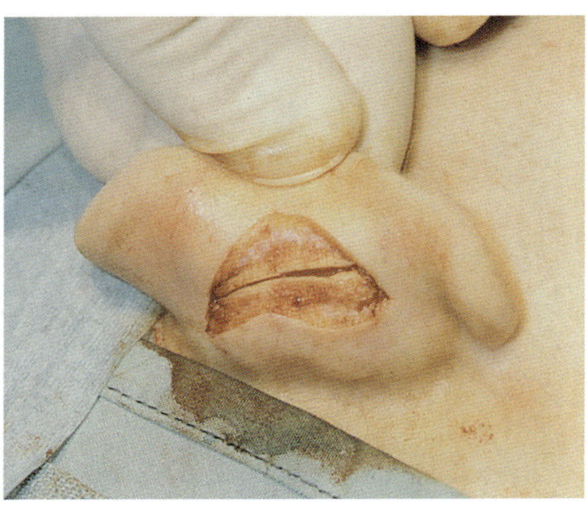

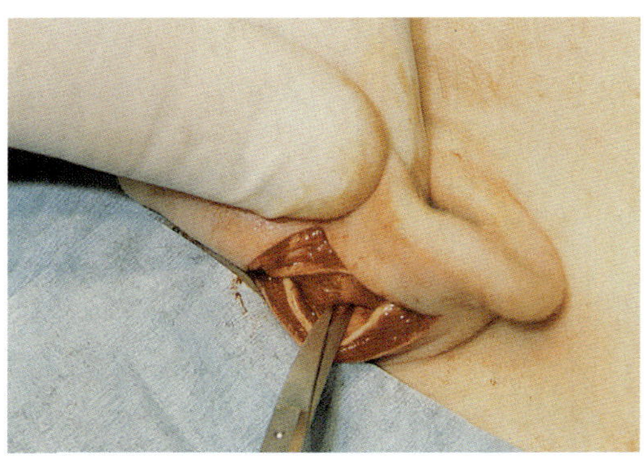

Fig. 22. Transcartilaginous incision leaving the pre-auricular perichondrium intact.

Fig. 23. Subperichondrial tunnelling over the cavum and cymba conchae.

used, stabbed through the auricle from the anterior side just medial to the antihelix, following the lateral border of the cavum and cymba conchae (Fig. 20).

After incising the skin along the line indicated by the needles (Fig. 21), the postauricular perichondrium and conchal cartilage are incised, leaving the perichondrium intact on the anterior side (Fig. 22). With a sharp, pointed, curved pair of scissors, subperichondrial tunnelling is then carried out over the cavum and cymba conchae (Fig. 23). The next step is to free the cartilage at the posterior side by blunt dissection in a supraperichondrial plane (Fig. 24). The cartilage is now incised just lateral of the ear canal, leaving the radix helicis intact for structural support and finally resected (Fig. 25a,b). After meticulous hemostasis, the skin incision is closed with a 5/0 atraumatic running suture. Carefully applied conchal packing, secured with through-and-through mattress sutures (Fig. 26), and a light compression ear bandage will prevent the formation of hematoma.

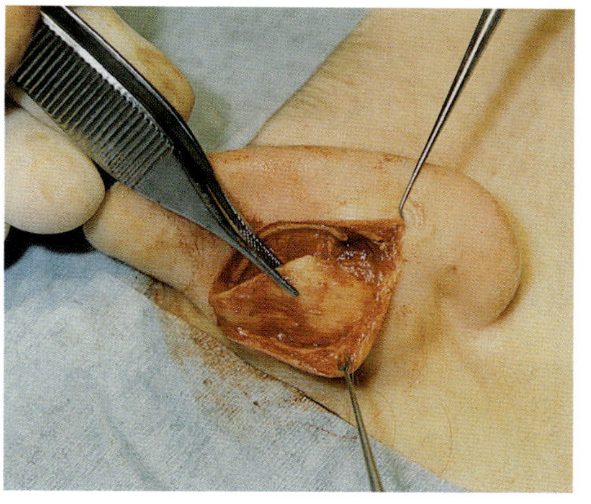

Fig. 24. Supra-perichondrial dissection at the posterior side.

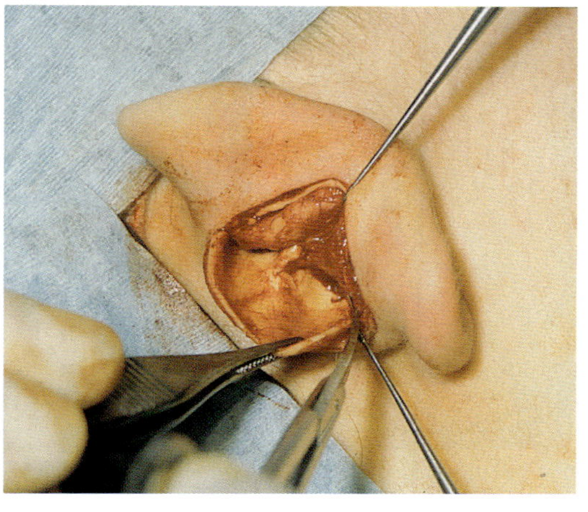

a

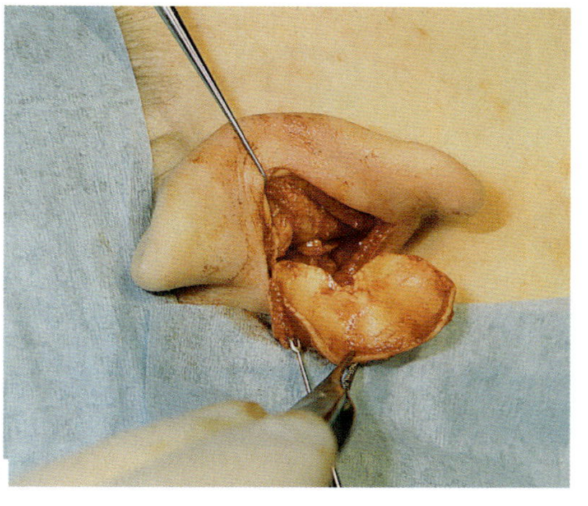

b

Fig. 25a,b,c. Resection of the cartilage graft leaving the radix helicis intact.

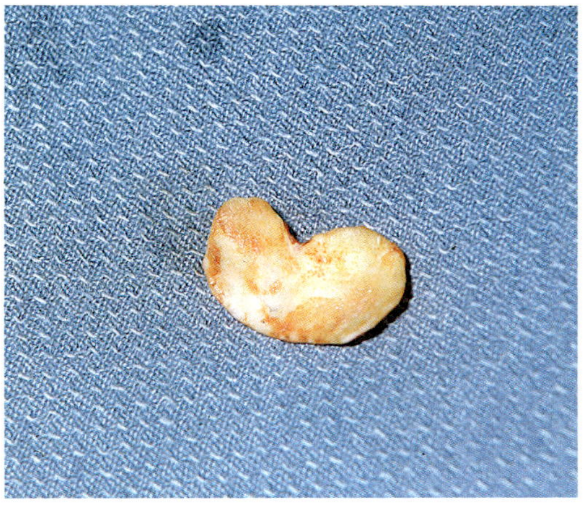

c

Fig. 25c.

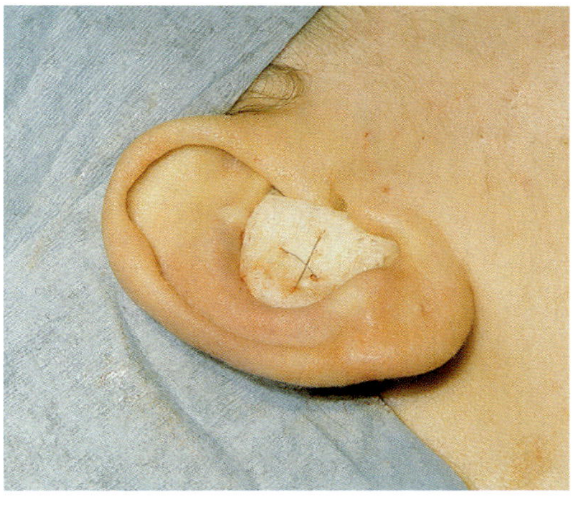

Fig. 26. Conchal packing fixed with through-and-through mattress sutures.

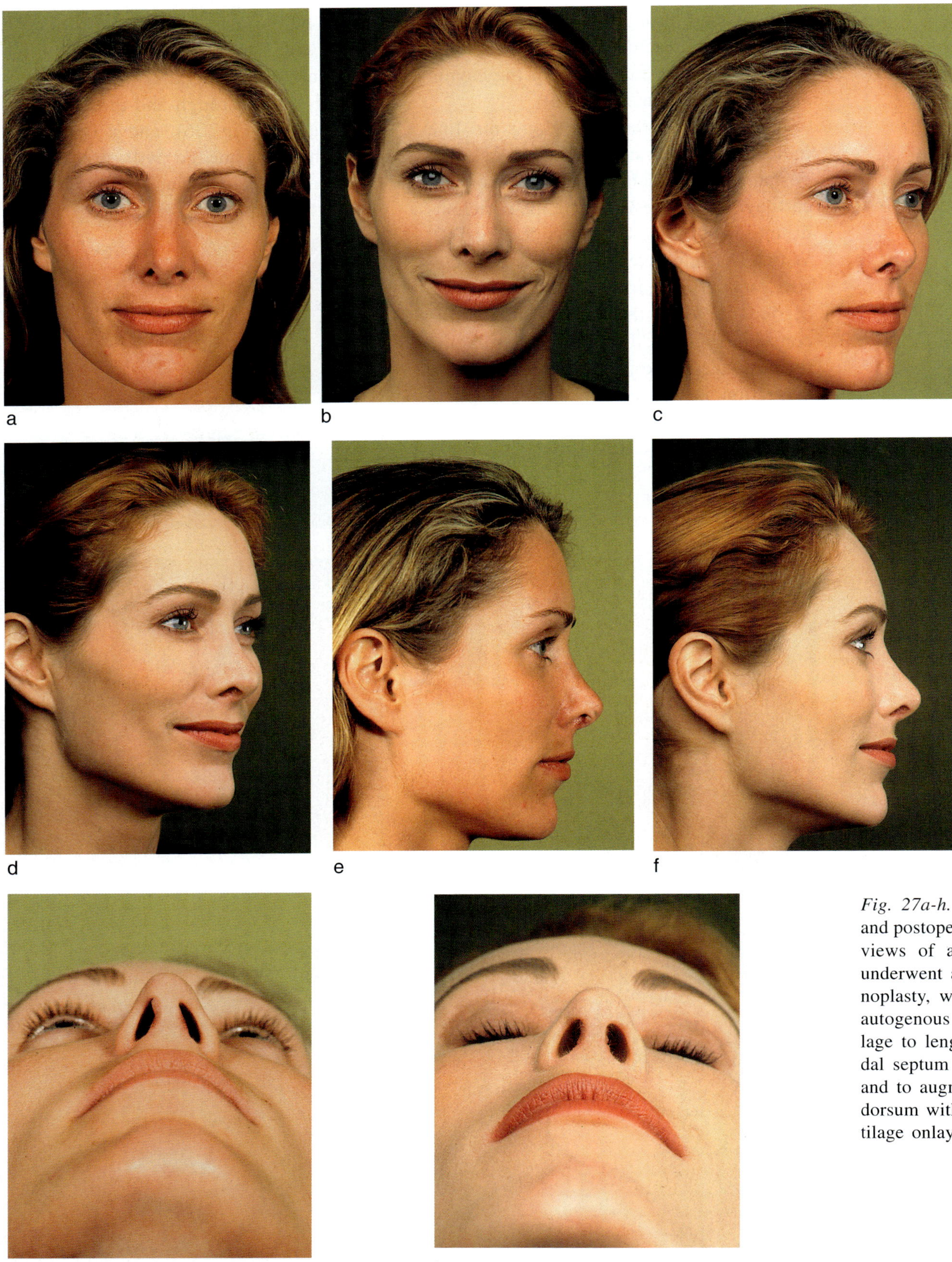

Fig. 27a-h. Pre- (*a,c,e,g*) and postoperative (*b,d,f,h*) views of a patient who underwent a revision rhinoplasty, with the use of autogenous septal cartilage to lengthen the caudal septum with a batton and to augment the nasal dorsum with a septal cartilage onlay graft.

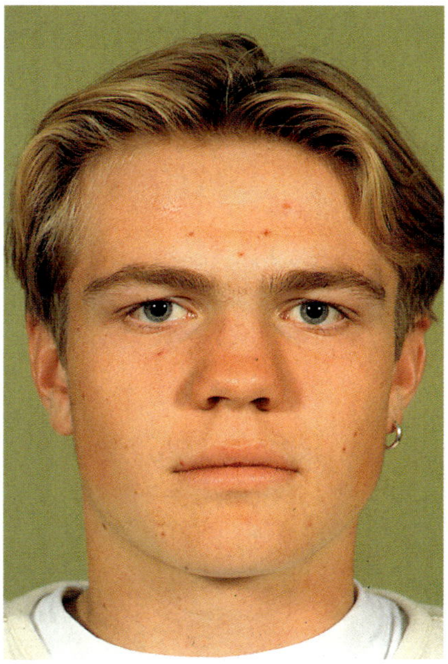
a

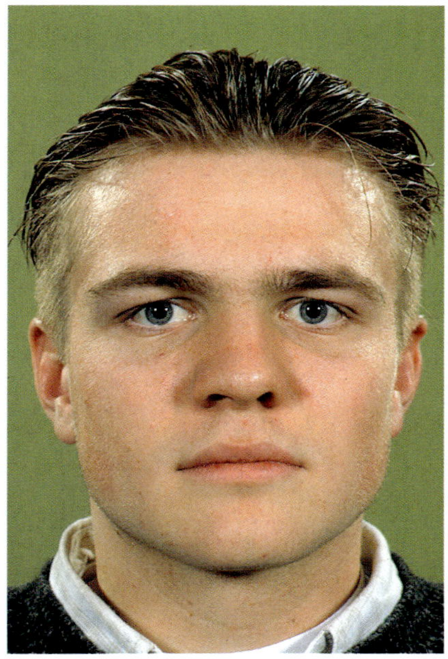
b

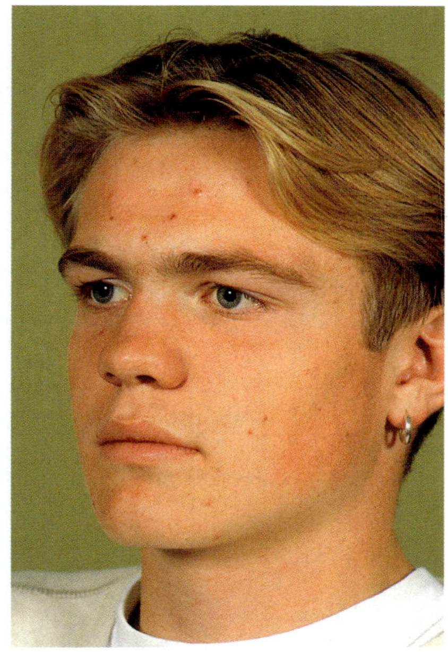
c

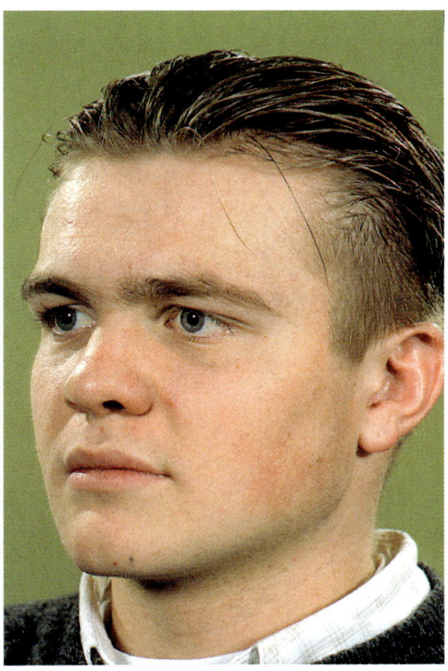
d

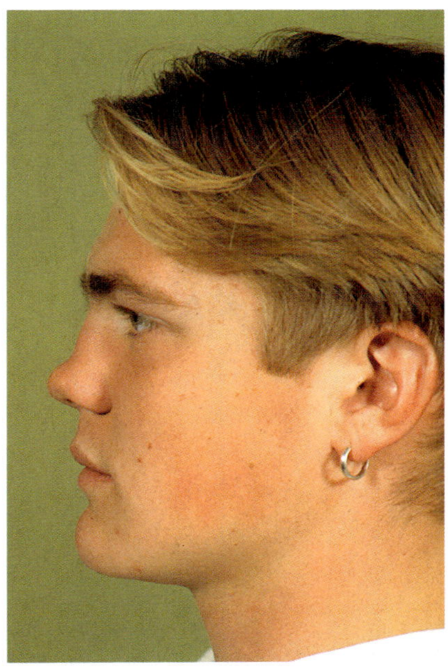
e

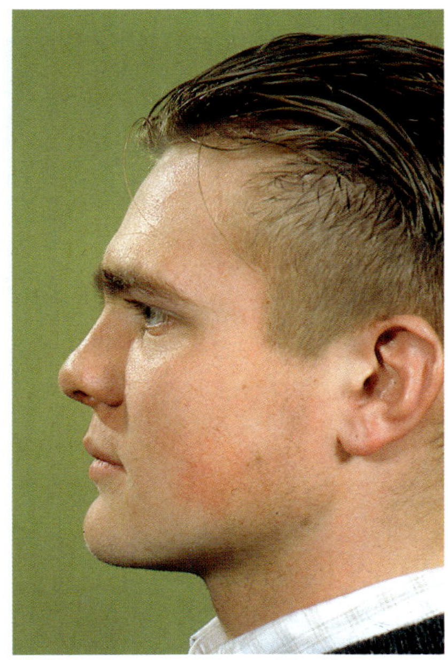
f

Fig. 28a-f. Pre- (*a,c,e*) and postoperative (*b,d,f*) views of a rhinoplasty in case of severe trauma. Through an external approach the fractured septum was rebuilt which, in combination with a dorsal conchal cartilage onlay graft, resulted in a normal profile.

In Figures 27-31 pre- and postoperative views are shown of patients who underwent a rhinoplasty with autogenous cartilage grafting procedures. Figures 32a-k show the preoperative harvesting procedure of rib cartilage and the reconstruction of the nasal framework.

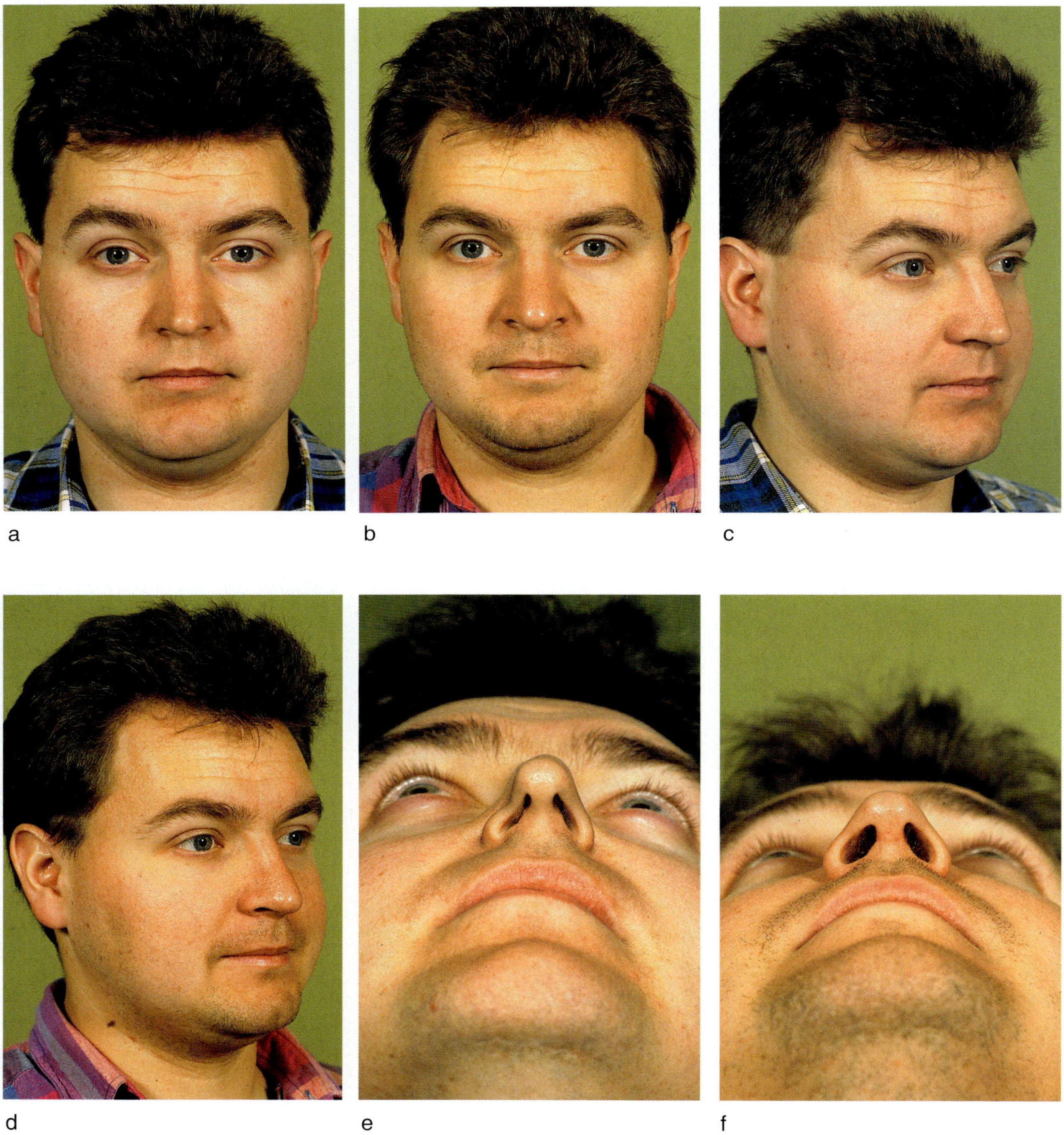

Fig. 29a-f. Pre- (*a,c,e*) and postoperative (*b,d,f*) views of a patient with functional problems due to a too narrow nasal valve (right more than left), who underwent an external rhinoplasty. After a moderate reduction of the dorsal height, spreader grafts were harvested from the cartilaginous septum and placed between septum and upper laterals through an external approach. Due to widening of the nasal valve area forced inspiration did not result in alar collapse anymore.

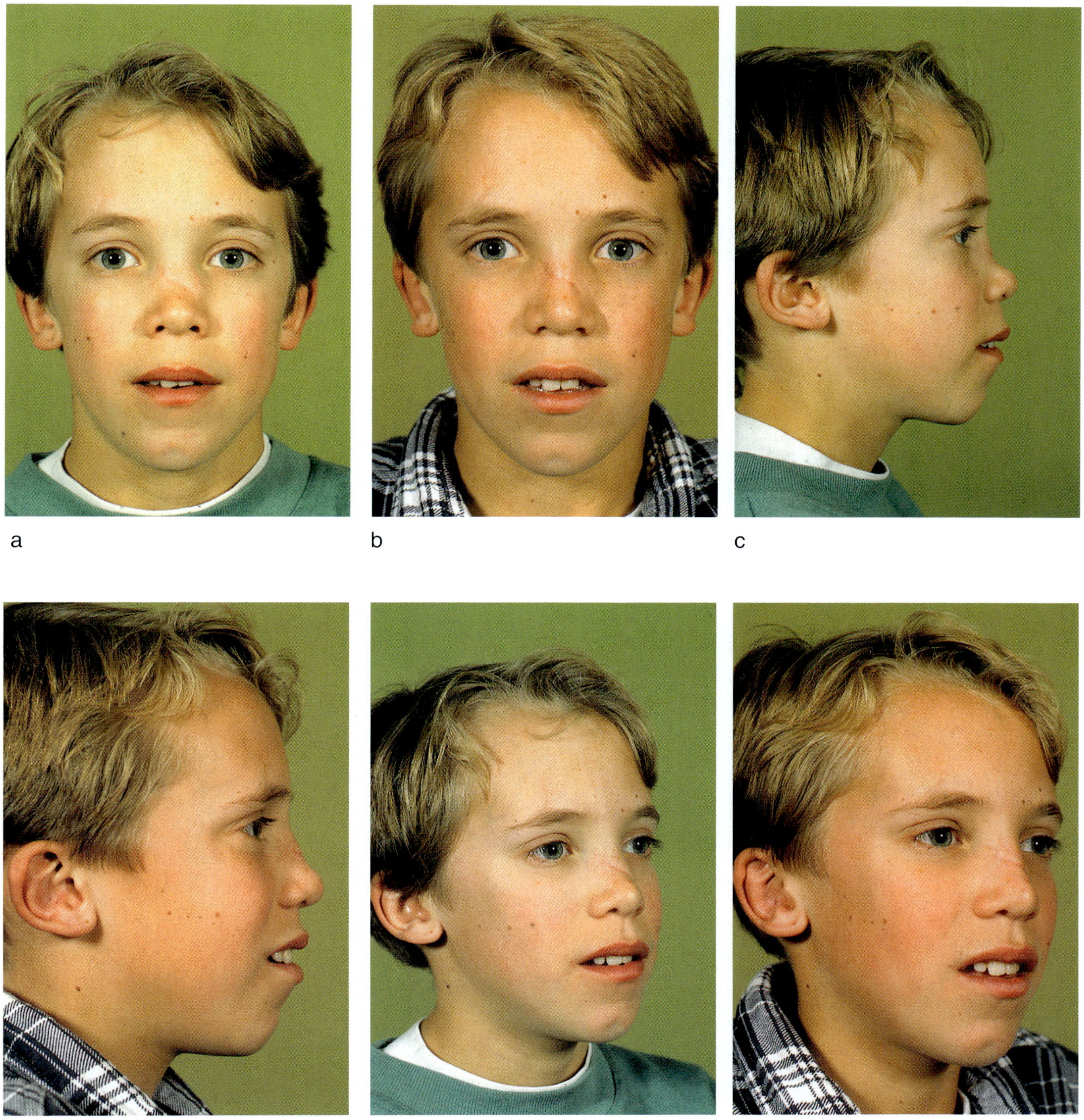

a b c

d e f

Fig. 30a-f. Pre- (*a,c,e*) and postoperative (*b,d,f*) views of an 11-year-old boy with severe psychological problems with his facial appearance, due to a severe nasal trauma resulting in a saddle deformity. He underwent an endonasal septorhinoplasty to straighten the deformed septum, to narrow the bony pyramid with micro-osteotomies and to augment the nasal dorsum with a conchal cartilage onlay graft. – In case of rhinoplasty in children, the surgeon should be aware that performing a rhinoplasty on a growing nose can interfere with midfacial growth even with the use of new atraumatic operative techniques. See Chapter 20 (Verwoerd and Verwoerd-Verhoef).

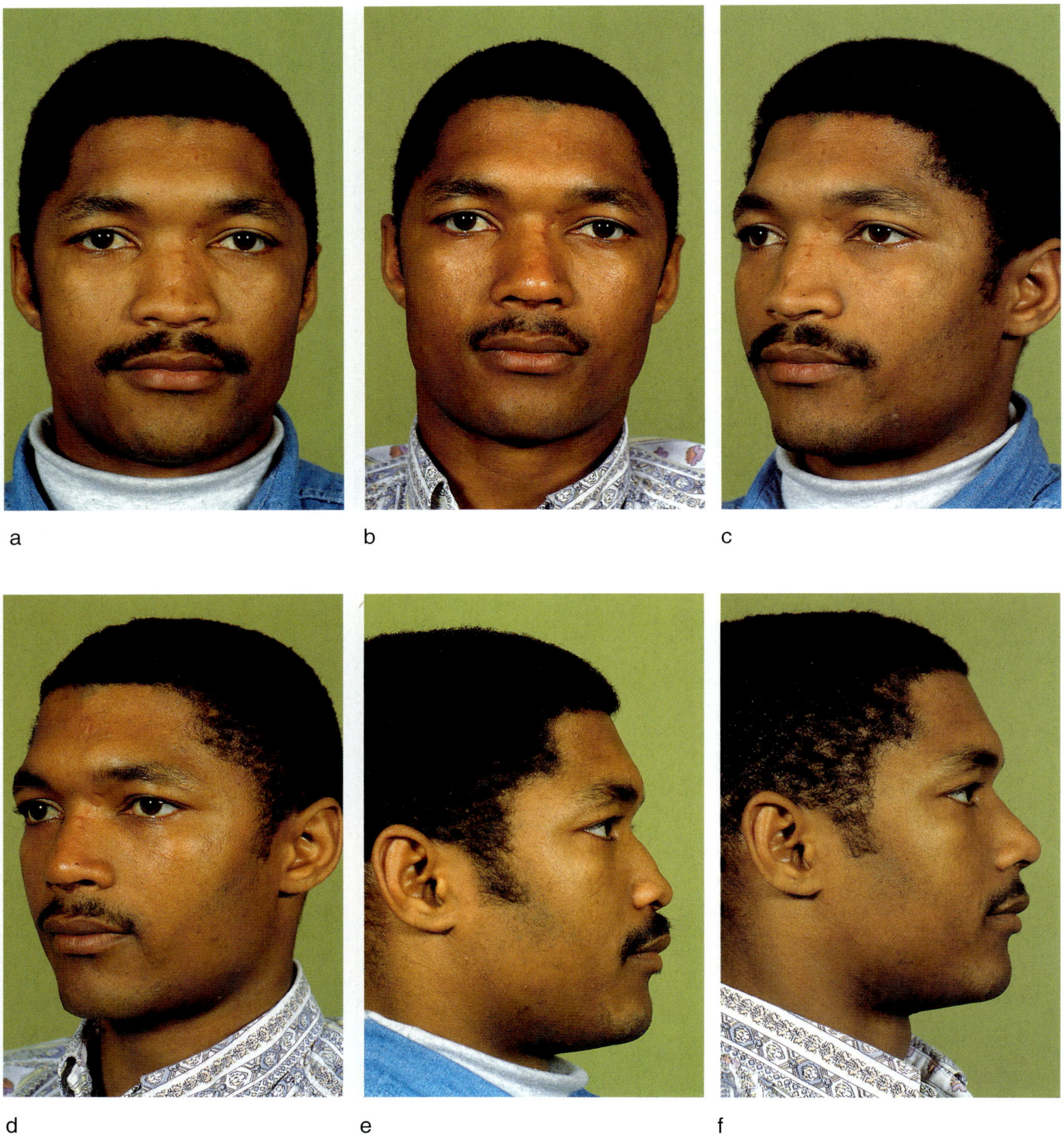

Fig. 31a-h. Pre- (*a,c,e,g*) and postoperative (*b,d,f,h*) views of a patient after multiple nasal traumata with loss of most of his cartilaginous framework. An external rhinoplasty was performed. Instead of a broken columella incision a V-incision was made at the base of the columella to perform a V-Y procedure to lengthen the columella. To rebuild the nose, autogenous rib cartilage was used.

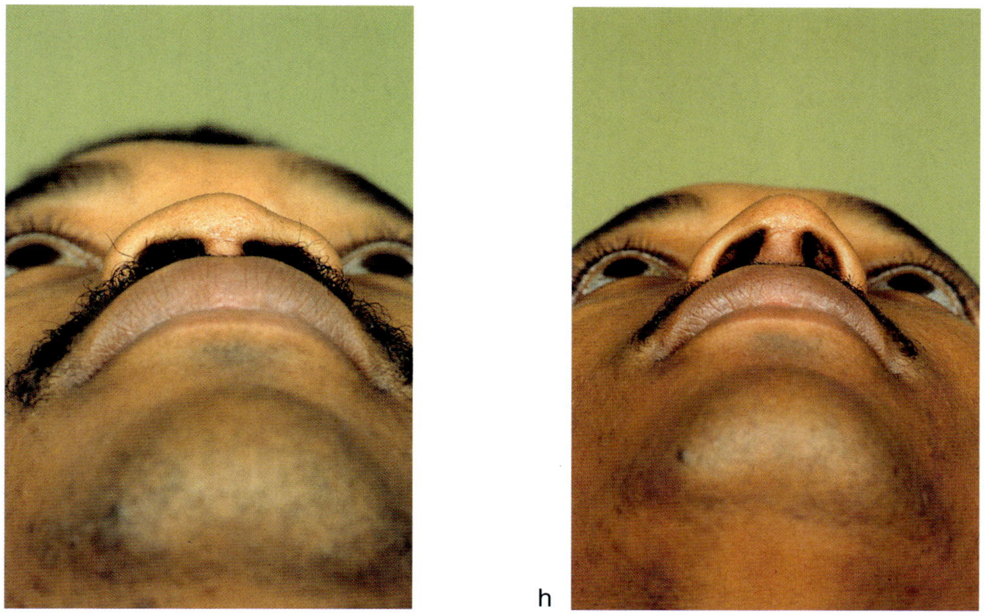

Fig. 31g-h.

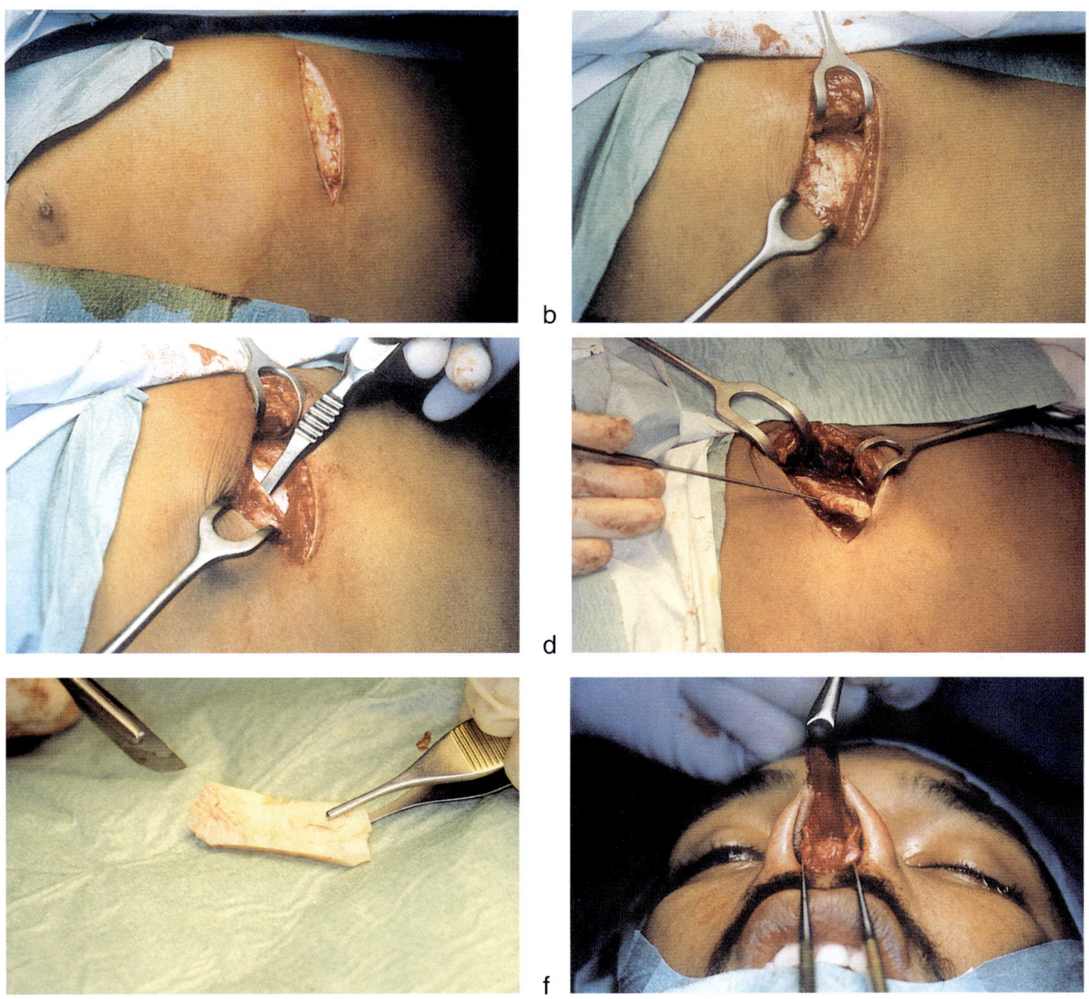

Fig. 32a-k. Surgical procedure for the harvesting of cartilage from the eighth rib which was sculptured in two pieces, a columella strut and a dorsal onlay graft. To prevent warping the superficial part of the rib cartilage was removed. Through an external approach, airway and dorsal profile were restored by a two-piece reconstruction in combination with a tip onlay graft to restore tip definition.

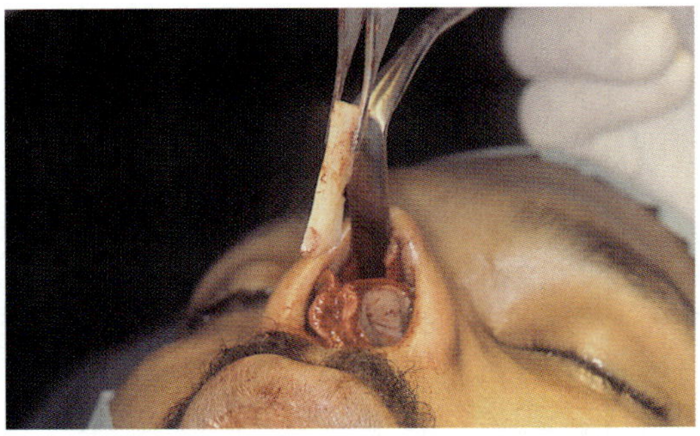

g

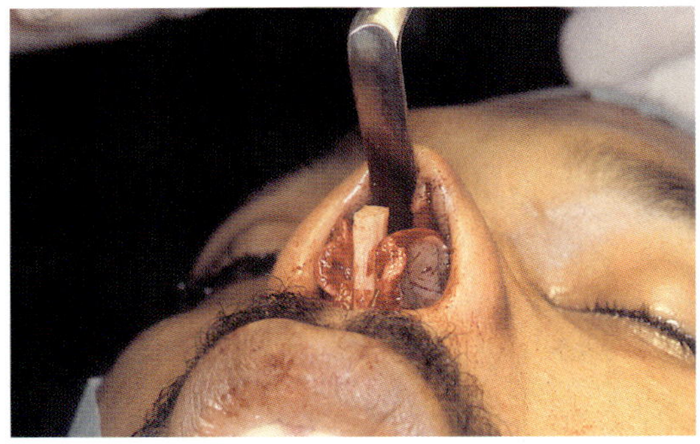

h

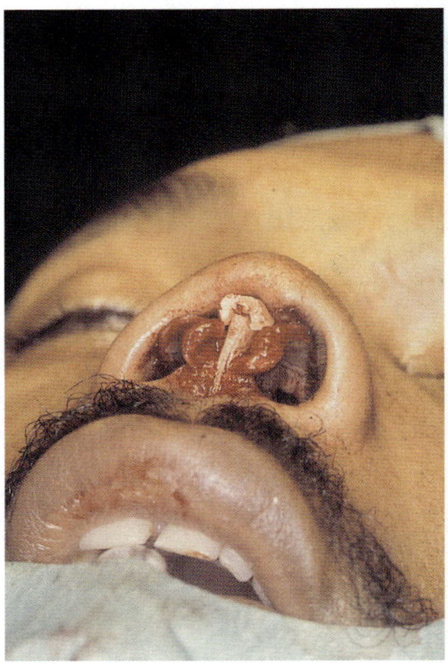

i

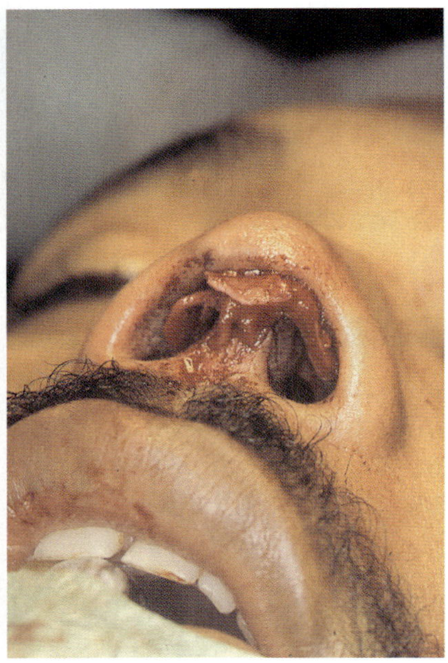

j

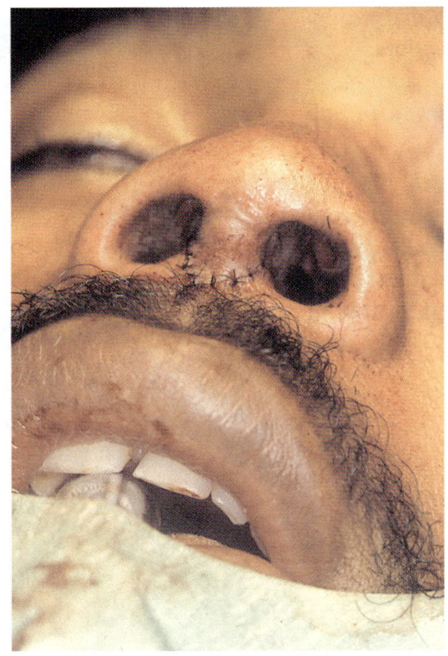

k

Fig. 32g-k.

8: ALAR INSUFFICIENCY SURGERY (alar collapse)

G.J. Nolst Trenité

Introduction

An insufficient ala will collapse due to the negative pressure built up in the nose even by quiet inspiration. Alar collapse resulting in impaired nasal inspiration is easily overlooked when inspecting the nose with a speculum. Examination of the nasal vestibular often reveals a protruding lateral crus in cases of alar insufficiency (Fig. 1).

The higher the negative pressure, the easier it is for the insufficient ala to collapse. Not only forceful inspiration through the nose, but also pathophysiological findings in the nasal valve area, resulting in an extra negative pressure build up, will influence the grade of alar collapse. Therefore, thorough examination of the nasal valve area (caudal end of the upper lateral, septum, head of the inferior turbinate and piriform aperture) is important for determining the appropriate surgical procedure to improve nasal breathing. Care should be taken not to disturb the relationship between caudal end of the upper lateral to the septum with a spectulum while examining the valve area. There are several reasons for insufficient alar resistance:

- specific nasal anatomy with a malpositioned lower lateral;
- loss of elasticity of the soft tissue between the upper and lower laterals in the process of aging;
- tissue damage and scar formation after trauma (surgical and non-surgical).

As insufficient alar resistance is a common cause of impaired nasal breathing in very old patients, surgical intervention can be restricted by health. In these cases, a vestibulum device (Fig. 2) worn in bed is a good choice for ensuring nasal breathing during the period of sleep. In nearly all other cases, surgical intervention is indicated. There are two basic principles in surgical repair:

1. improvement of alar resistance with graft material
2. reallocation of the lateral crus

The use of autogenous cartilage is especially indicated when the lack of alar resistance is caused by the overzealous resection of upper and lower lateral cartilages in rhinoplasty. Conchal cartilage to rebuild lower lateral and septal cartilage to reconstruct the middle third of the lateral nasal wall, are the best choice. In the case of a malpositioned lateral crus, surgical reallocation is indicated.

In this chapter, the reallocation of the alar cartilage by upward rotation of the lateral crus will be emphasized.

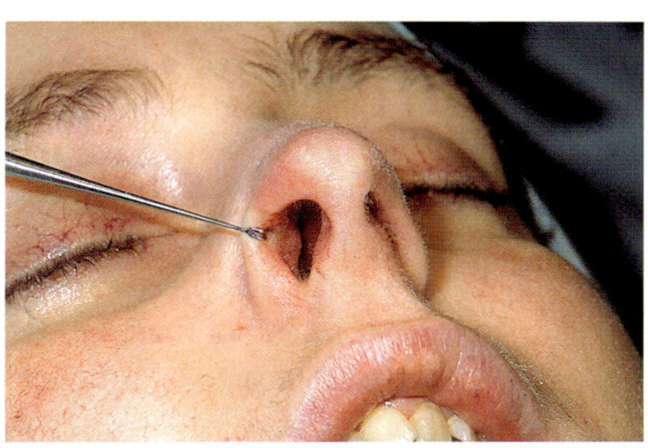

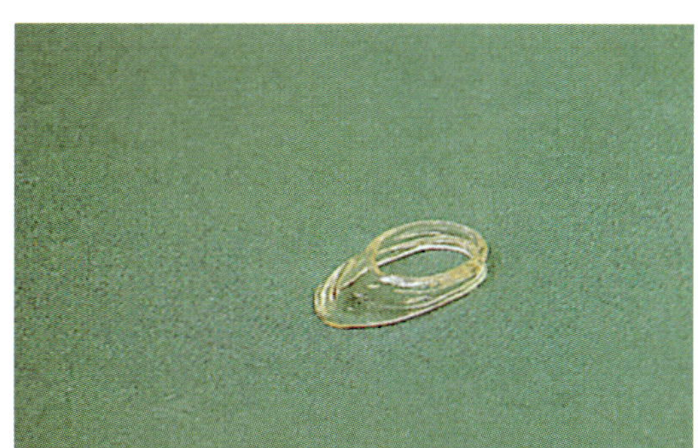

Fig. 1. A protruding lateral crus in the vestibulum.

Fig. 2. A vestibulum device ('nose shoe') to prevent alar collapse.

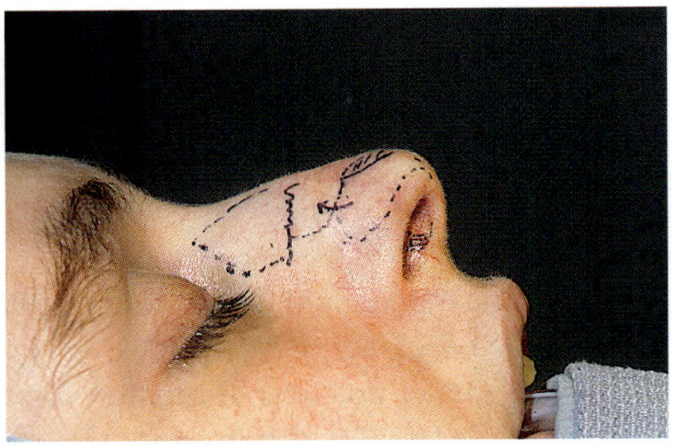

Fig. 3. Landmarks outlined on the nasal skin with marking of the new position of the lateral crus (arrow) and partial resection of the cephalic part of the lateral crus (striped area).

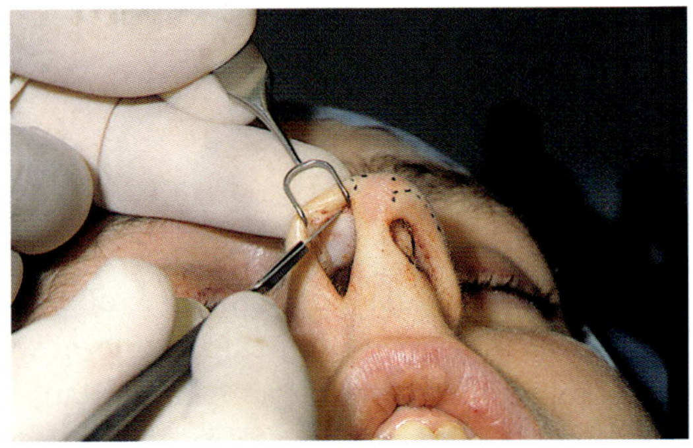

Fig. 4. Marginal incision along the caudal border of the lower lateral.

Experimental work by Rettinger and Masing showed that by changing the plane of the lateral crus (upward rotation), the distance between the medial and lateral crus will increase and at the same time build up more intrinsic tension in the cartilage. This improves the alar resistance to the negative pressure during inspiration. Rotation of the alar cartilage in collapsed alae, as described by the above-mentioned authors, is relatively easy to perform in a limited time (about one hour for both sides) under local anesthesia via the endonasal approach, with a low chance of complications.

Operative techniques

The surgical procedure for the insufficient ala can be differentiated as follows:
- rotation of the lateral crus (pure functional surgery);
- rotation of the lateral crus combined with resection of a cephalic part of it (combination of functional and aesthetic surgery);
- narrowing of a broad columella (adjunctive technique to widen the nasal vestibule).

Rotation of the lateral crus

The first step is to outline the landmarks of the nasal skeleton on the skin. Then, the lateral crus is determined and marked

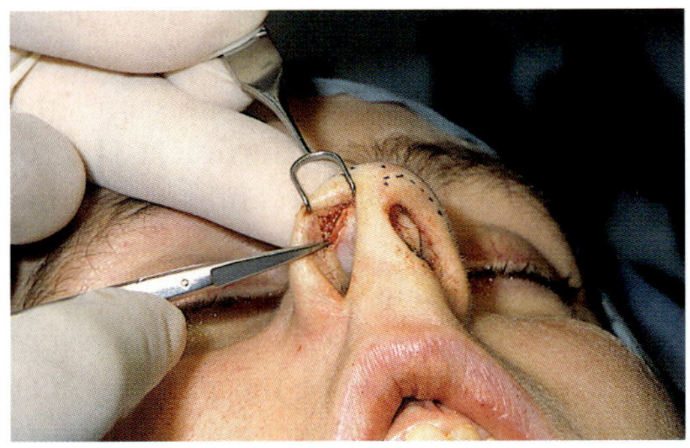

Fig. 5. Subperichondrial dissection at the vestibular side of the lateral crus with a pair of curved sharp pointed scissors.

(Fig. 3). Local anesthesia (combined with intravenous or general anesthesia) is used to ensure a dry operation field and to facilitate the subperichondrial dissection at the vestibular side of the lateral crus and should be performed approximately 15 minutes before the dissection is started. A standard marginal incision (No. 15 blade) is made along the caudal border of the lower lateral, including the dome area (Fig. 4). With a pair of curved sharp pointed scissors, the vestibular skin, including the underlying perichondrium, is freed from the lateral crus (Fig. 5). When starting the dissection, it is easier to begin just lateral of the dome, instead of far lateral where the right surgical plane is more difficult to find. After freeing the vestibular side of the lateral crus around the dome up to the medial crus, the non-vestibular side is dissected free from the overlying soft tissue in a supraperichondrial plane (Fig. 6a,b). The lateral crus

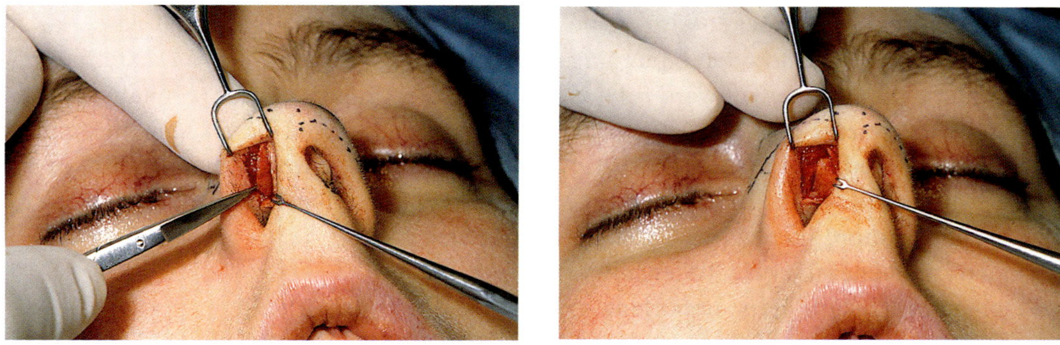

a b

Fig. 6a,b. Supraperichondrial dissection of the lateral crus at the non-vestibular side.

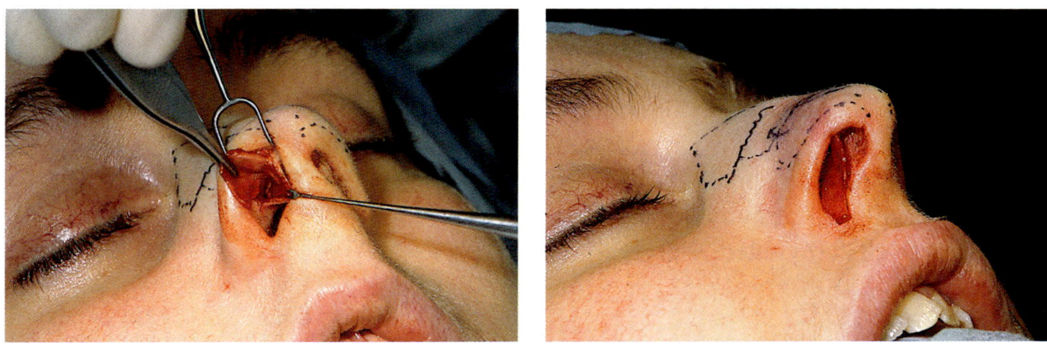

a b

Fig. 7a,b. Delivery of the lateral crus.

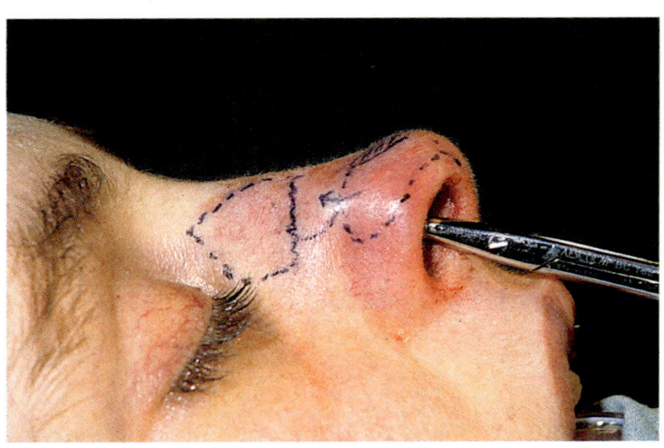

Fig. 8. The making of a pocket to fit the upwardly rotated lateral crus.

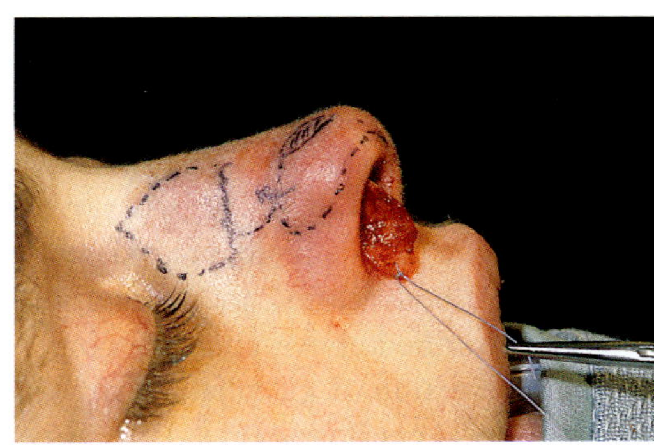

Fig. 9. Absorbable guiding suture placed through the distal end of the lateral crus.

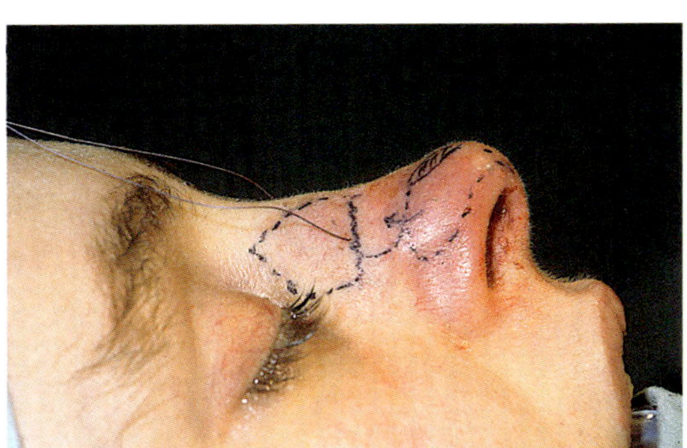

Fig. 10. Leading thread through the nasal skin to rotate and fixate the upper lateral in the new upward position.

can easily be delivered now (Fig. 7a,b). After the delivering procedure, a not-too-large pocket is made extraperichondrially to the upper lateral in the area already indicated, either by sharp or blunt dissection (Fig. 8).

An (absorbable) guiding suture (*e.g.*, 4/0 Vicryl with a straight needle is very appropriate) is placed through the distal end of the lateral crus (Fig. 9).

This leading thread with straight needle

is now brought into the pocket with a fine needle holder or mosquito clamp, piercing the skin at the planned new upward rotated position of the lateral crus (Fig. 10). The thread can be fixed with a small steristrip on the skin (Fig. 14). In the normal anatomical situation, there is just a slight overlap of the lateral crus. To ensure a good operative result, it is important to overcorrect the position of the lateral crus in a more cephalic position. Adjuvant fixation of the lateral crus with fibrin glue, or with through-and-through mattress sutures, should be done in case of large pockets, or when there is a considerable cartilage spring, to prevent postoperative caudal rotation.

The marginal incision should be closed meticulously with 5/0 atraumatic absorbable sutures (*e.g.*, 5/0 coated Vicryl).

Rotation of the lateral crus combined with resection of a cephalic part of it

The alar cartilage rotation technique is very appropriate for purely functional purposes. From an aesthetic point of view, the new upwardly rotated lateral crus can give a somewhat bulky tip or will give more expression to an already pre-existent bulky tip. In both cases, the operative procedure described above could be combined with resection of a cephalic strip of the lower lateral cartilages (Fig. 11). Care should be taken not to weaken the cartilage spring too much. If osseocartilaginous vault surgery is necessary, the same marginal incision can be used as long as the lateral crus has not yet been fixed in place (Fig. 12a,b). In special cases, as in cleft-lip patients, when an external approach is indicated, the cephalic rotated lateral crus should be fixed with non-absorbable 6/0 sutures (*e.g.*, Goretex) in the planned position to the upper lateral cartilage.

Narrowing of a broad columella

Widening the nasal vestibule by narrowing a broad columella in cases of alar insufficiency is helpful in improving nasal breathing. Narrowing of the broad columella can be accomplished by resecting a redundancy of intercrural soft tissue followed by one or two mattress sutures. When the medial crural footplates are the main reason for the broad columella, a partial distal cartilage resection of medial crura should be done. To obtain access to the crural footplate, a small vertical incision (No. 15 blade) over the crural footplate is the easiest way. With a pair of curved pointed scissors, the footplate is freed from the surrounding soft tissue and delivered with a single hook (Fig. 13). After the appropriate resection of cartilage, the skin is sutured with a 6/0 nylon suture (Fig. 14), and if necessary followed by one or two mattress sutures for extra narrowing.

In Figures 15 and 16 pre- and postoperative views of patients who underwent rhinoplasty with upper rotation of the lateral crura to correct alar collapse are presented.

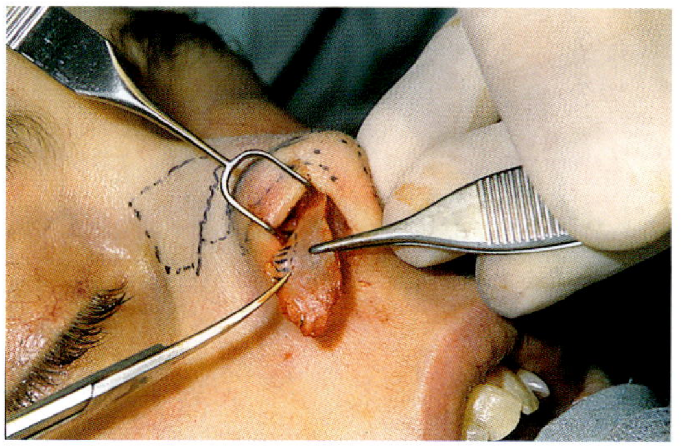

Fig. 11. Resection of the marked cephalic part of the lateral crus.

a
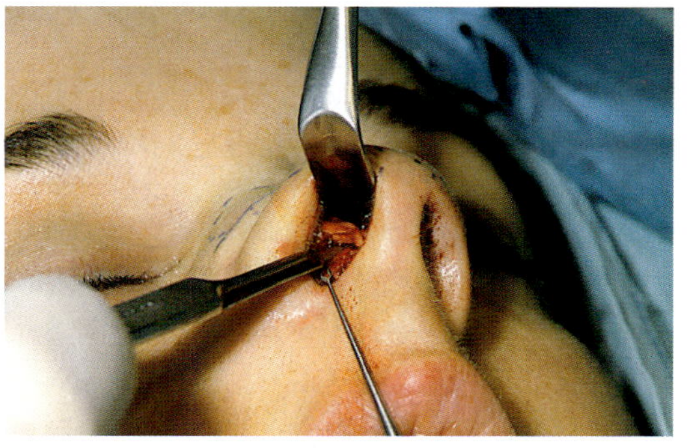
b
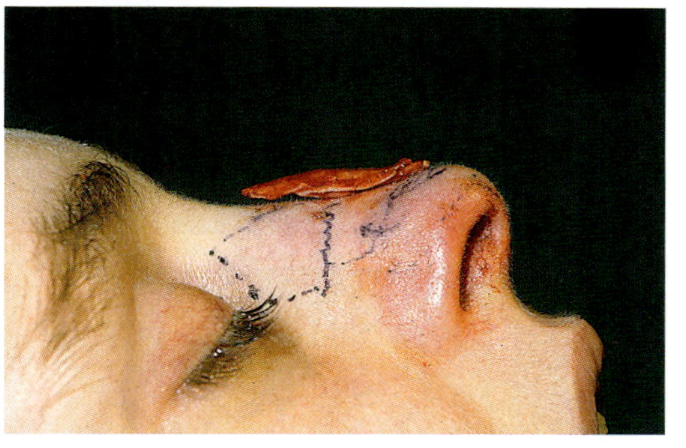

Fig. 12a,b. Resection of a cartilaginous and bony hump.

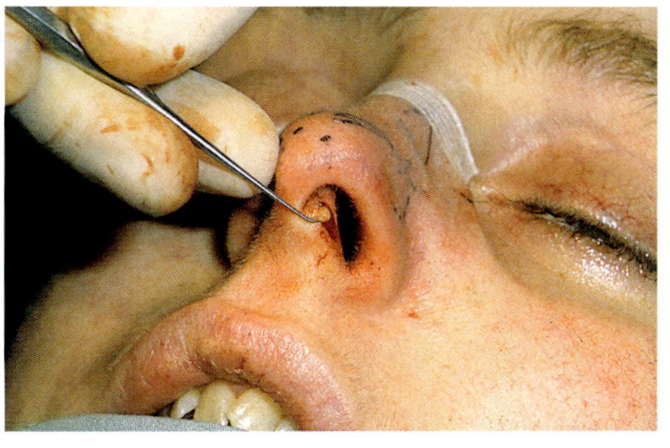

Fig. 13. Delivery of the medical crural footplate.

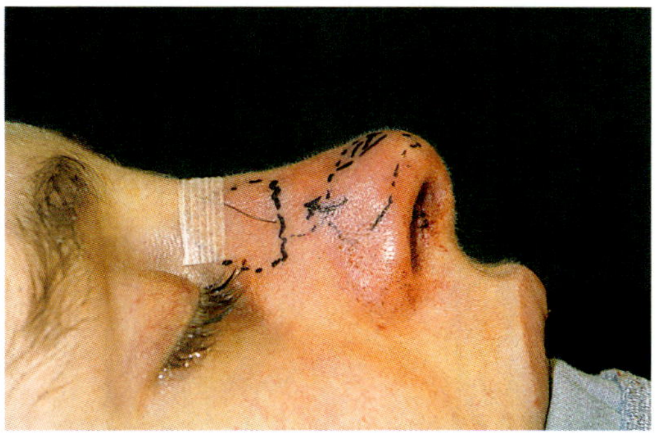

Fig. 14. Lateral view of the nose after upward rotation of the lateral crura, hump resection, median oblique and lateral micro-osteotomies, partial resection of the distal end of the medial crura and suturing of the skin incisions.

a
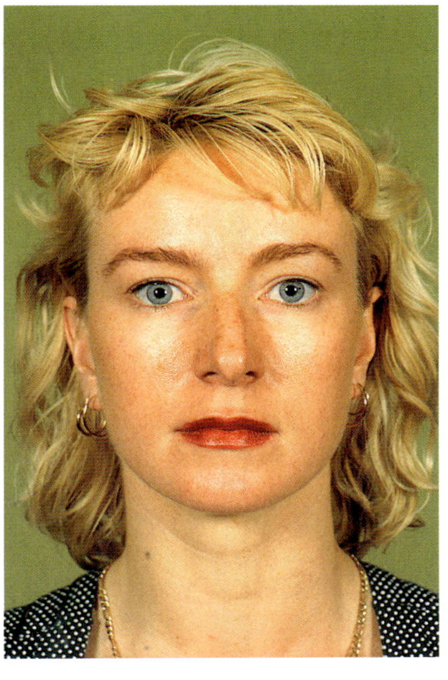
b
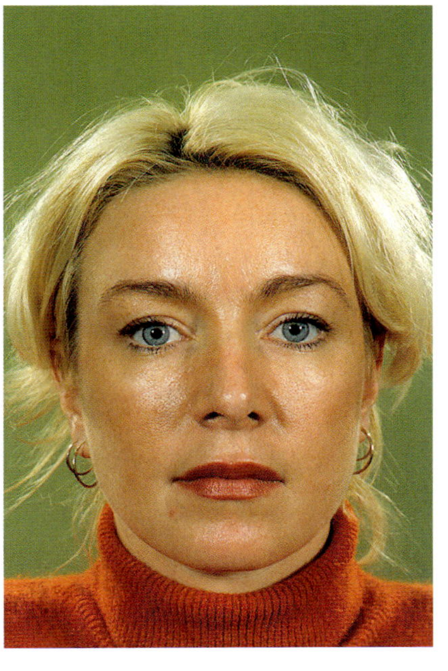

Fig. 15a-b. Legend, see next page.

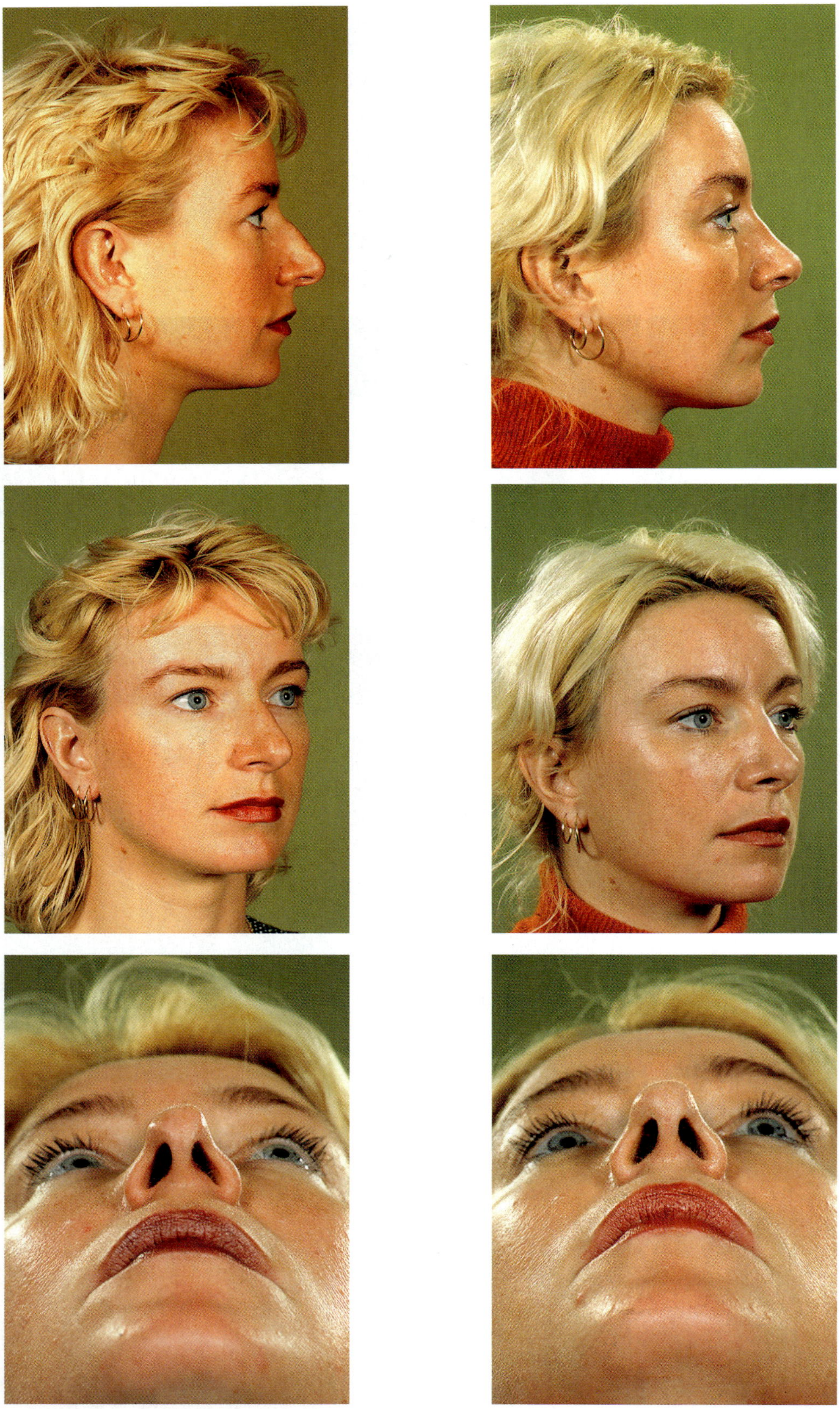

Fig. 15a-h. Pre- and post-operative views of a patient with alar collapse due to a malposition of the lateral crura. Furthermore, there is a bony cartilaginous hump with a slight deviation of the dorsum to the left and slight asymmetry of the nasal tip. Through marginal incisions the lateral crura were delivered (up to the dome), bilateral cephalic resection and at the left side a scoring procedure in the dome area to correct tip asymmetry were performed. Through the marginal incision the overlying soft tissue was dissected from the osseocartilaginous vault followed by hump resection, medial oblique micro-osteotomies and repositioning of the lateral crura with a guiding suture into a prepared pocket in a more cephalic position. Finally, lateral micro-osteotomies were performed, followed by realignment and infraction of the dorsum.

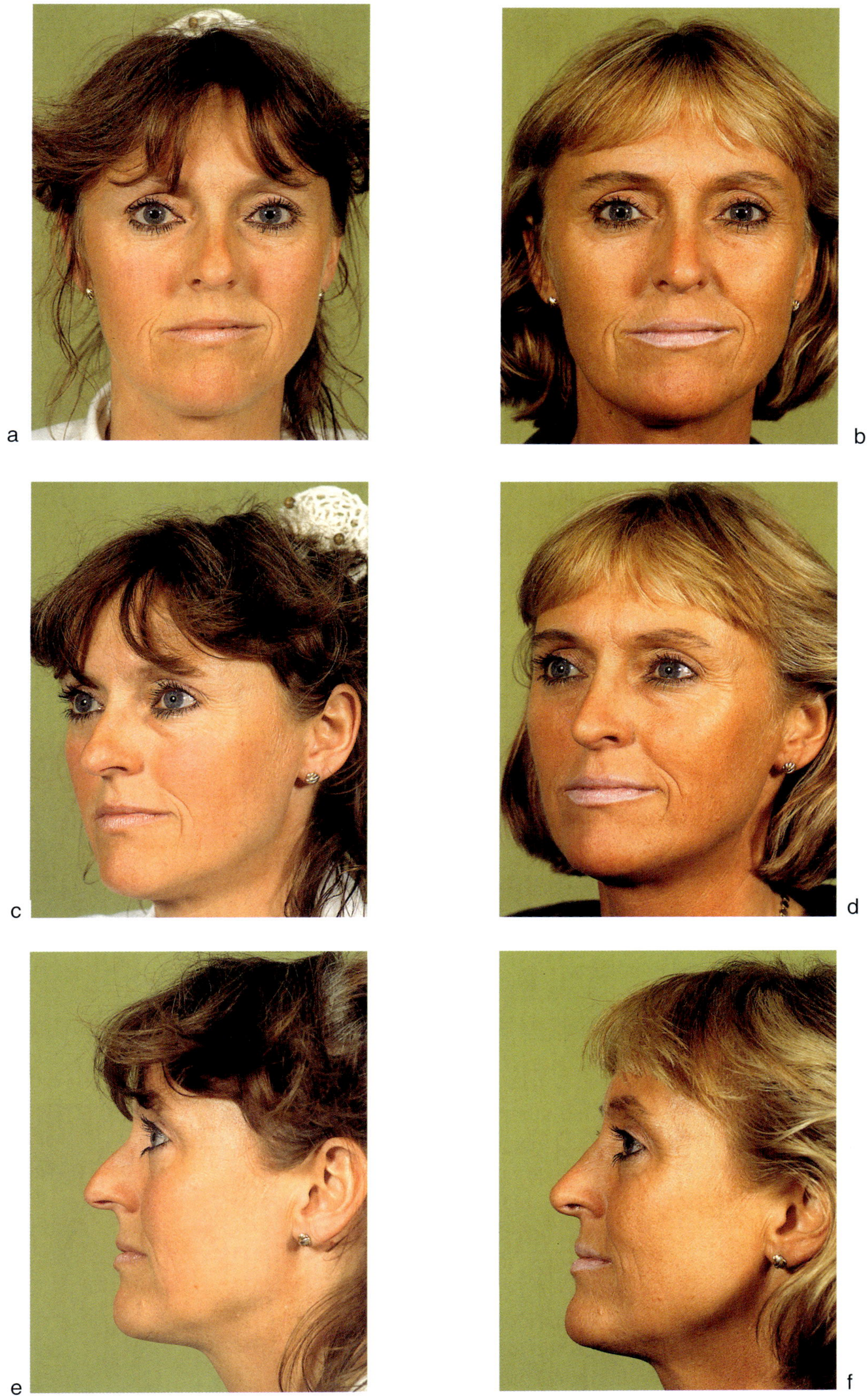

Fig. 16a-h. Pre- and postoperative views of a patient with alar collapse due to malposition of the lateral crura in combination with an overdeveloped cartilaginous vault. Through a marginal incision the lateral crura were delivered followed by bilateral cephalic resection to prevent bulbosity. To create more upward rotation of the nasal tip a small caudal septal cartilage strip was resected through hemitransfixion incision. The marginal incision was also used to approach, denude and lower the cartilaginous vault. Finally the lateral crura were repositioned more cephalically with a guiding suture.

g 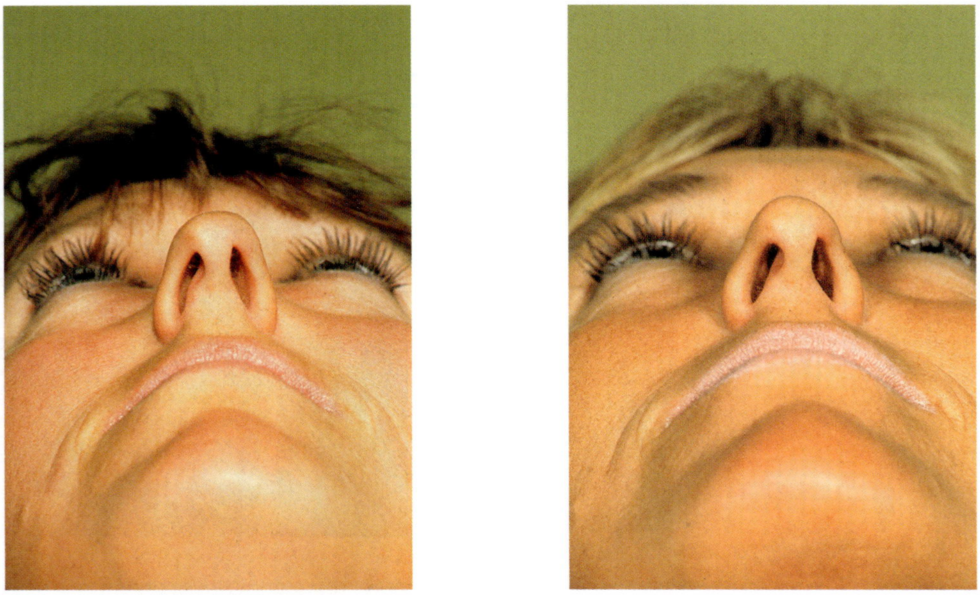 h

Fig. 16g-h.

9A: NASAL VALVE SURGERY
A modified Z-plasty

G.J. Nolst Trenité

General introduction

The nasal valve is of utmost importance in nasal breathing. It is the narrowest part of the nasal airway and plays an active regulating role in nasal airflow. The nasal valve area is composed of different interrelated structures, the pathology of one or more of which can disturb normal nasal breathing. The different structures comprise:

- upper lateral cartilage
- septum
- piriform aperture
- head of the inferior turbinate
- alar muscles

In the case of nasal airway obstruction, internal inspection of the nose emphasizing the nasal valve area should be done without a speculum, which could distort the valve angle (normally 10–15° in a leptorrhine nose) and thereby prevent differentiation between alar collapse and nasal valve obstruction (Fig. 1).

A combination of pathology of the different structures of the nasal valve area can exist. Most frequently, septal deviations in the valve area and medial displacement or overzealous resection of the upper lateral cartilage after rhinoplasty, cause nasal valve problems. If these skeletal abnormalities are the reason for the nasal airway obstruction, reallocation and/or grafting has to be carried out. Valve problems due to septal deviations in the valve area should be corrected with standard septoplasty techniques (see Chapter 6).

In mild cases of medial displacement of the upper lateral cartilage, resulting in a too narrow nasal valve, *a modified Z-plasty*, in which a medial based composite skin-cartilage flap from the cephalic part of the lower lateral is rotated in a surgically created space between the septum and upper lateral, is an appropriate technique to restore normal function.

In the case of severe narrowing of the middle third of the nose, due to medial displacement or loss of cartilage, resulting in functional and aesthetic problems, spreader grafts to widen the nasal valve and to augment the lateral nasal wall are indicated.

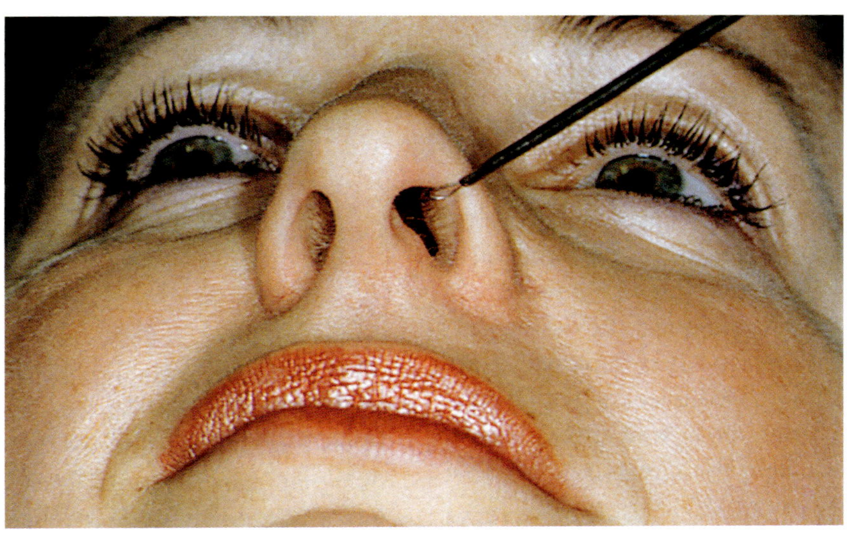

Fig. 1. Inspection of the vestibulum and the nasal valve area.

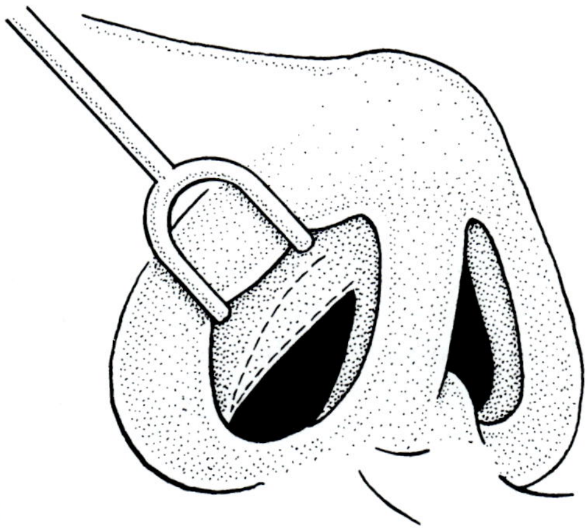
a

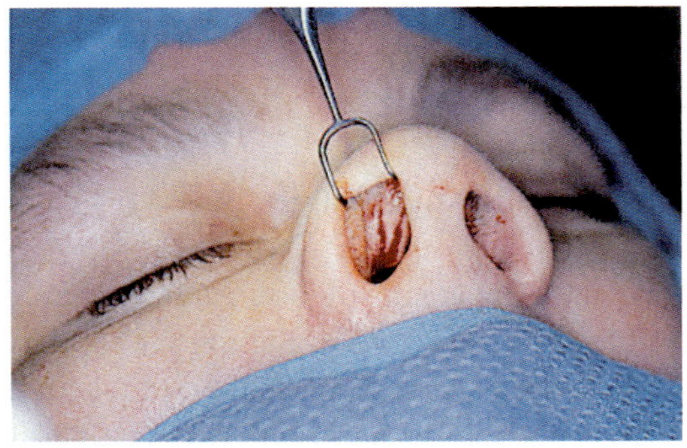
b

Fig. 2a,b. Transcartilaginous and intercartilaginous incision (*a.* schematically depicted, *b.* peroperative view).

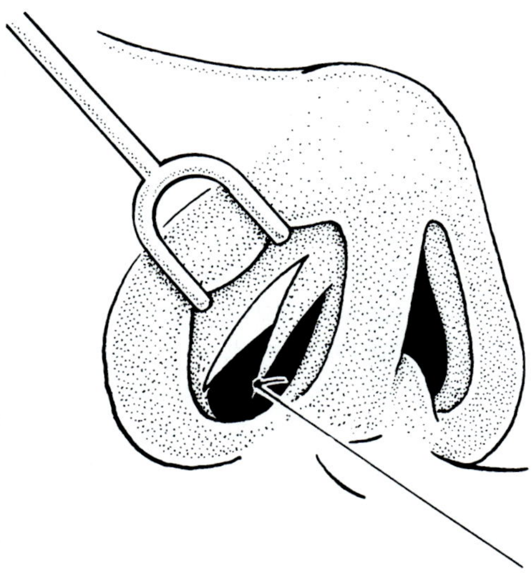
c

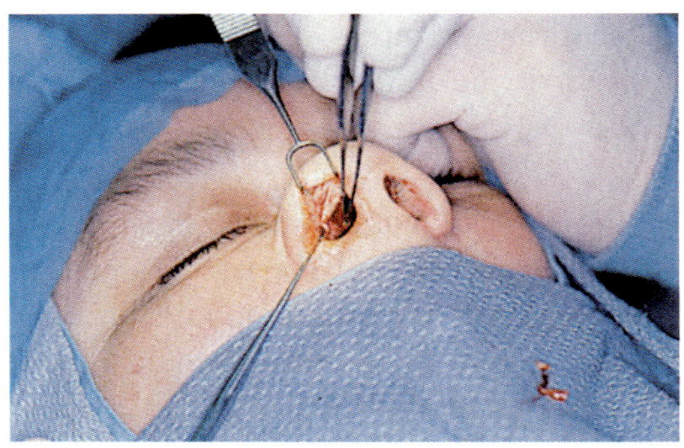
d

Fig. 2c,d. Medial based skin-cartilage flap from the cephalic part of the lateral crus (*c.* schematically depicted, *d.* peroperative view).

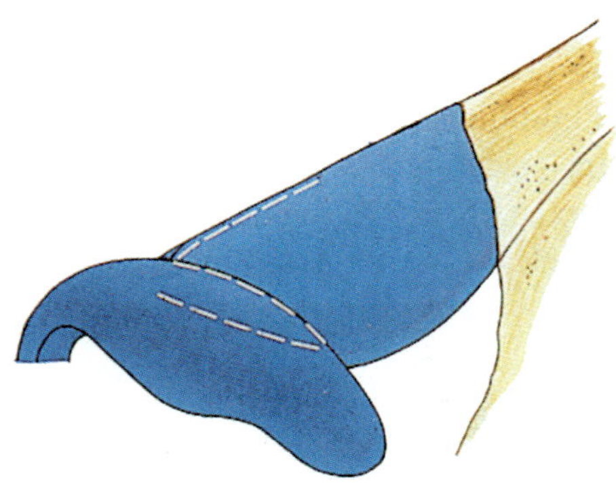

Fig. 3. Asymmetric Z-incision (transcartilaginous – intercartilaginous – transcartilaginous).

Modified Z-plasty to widen the nasal valve angle

Introduction

The use of a medial-based skin-cartilage flap from the cephalic part of the lateral crus as a surgical treatment for nasal valve obstruction was introduced by Walter. In principle, this technique follows the definition of a Z-plasty: two flaps which are raised and interposed over each other such that the tissue is borrowed from areas of excess and interposed on areas of deficiency.

Operative technique

After trimming the vibrissae and appropriate local anesthesia has been applied, a transcartilaginous incision (No. 15 blade) is made, starting approximately 3–4 mm lateral of the midline (quadrangular cartilage) and then proceeding laterally, separating a cephalic strip of

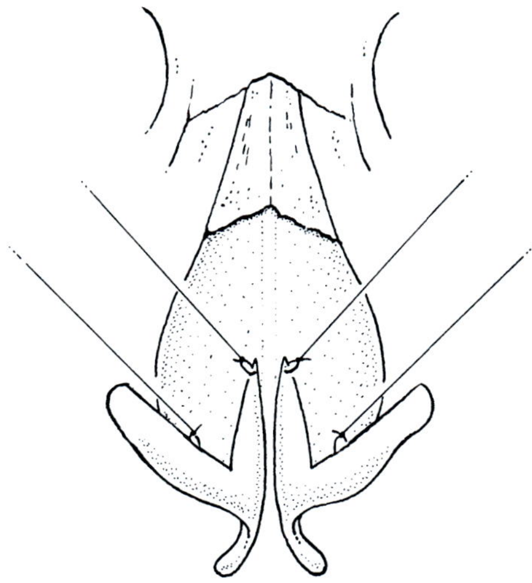

a

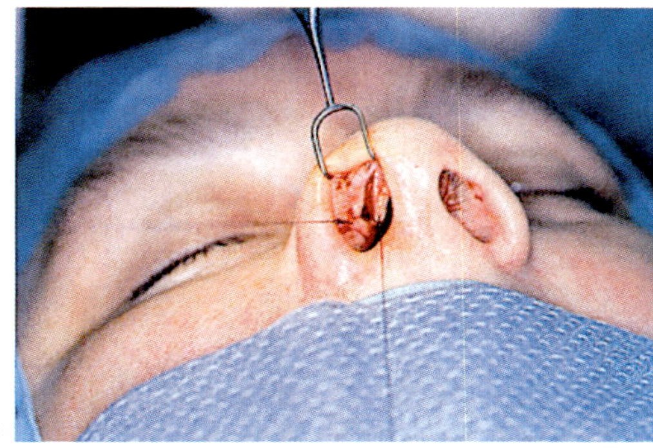

b

Fig. 4a,b. Guiding sutures through the lateral end of the skin-cartilage flap and the caudal rim of the upper lateral (*a.* schematically depicted, *b.* peroperative view).

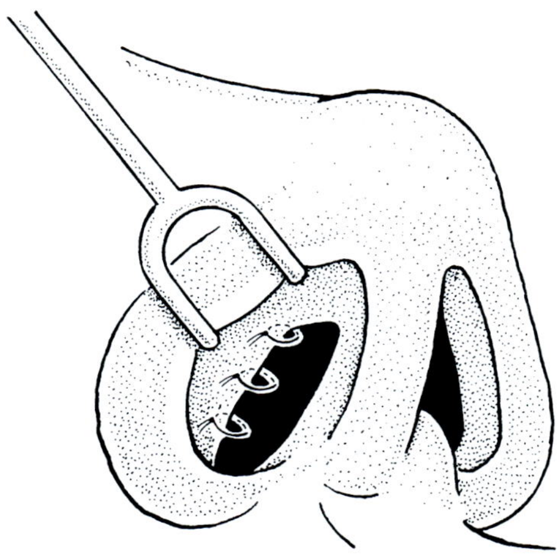

a

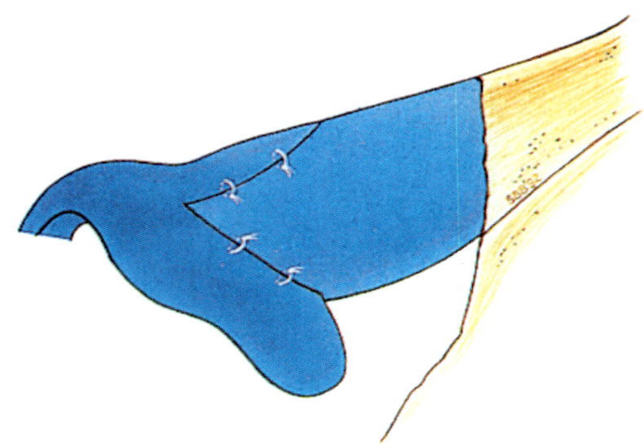

b

Fig. 5a. Suturing of the displaced caudal end of the upper lateral to the new cephalic border of the lower lateral crus. *b.* Suturing of the cranially-rotated skin-cartilage flap to the laterally displaced and fixated upper lateral.

cartilage 3–4 mm from the lower lateral (gradually diminishing) over a length of approximately 10–15 mm up to the cephalic border of the lower lateral. At this point, an intercartilaginous incision (central limb of the asymmetric Z) is made up to the nasal valve angle (Fig. 2a,b,c,d), followed by a second transcartilaginous incision along the quadrangular cartilage, separating it from the upper lateral (Fig. 3).

After this asymmetric Z-incision, the medial-based skin-cartilage flap after being dissected free can be interposed between the upper lateral and the quadrangular cartilage, with a guiding suture through the nasal skin (Fig. 4a,b). The upper lateral 'flap' is deplaced laterally with another guiding suture and fixed with 5/0 coated Vicryl sutures to the (new) cephalic border of the lateral crus (Fig. 5a,b). Suturing of the medial rotated flap is difficult and not always necessary. Good fixation can often be established with the guiding suture fixed with tape on the nasal skin for five days, combined with nasal packing.

9B: NASAL VALVE SURGERY
Spreader grafts

Lateral augmentation of the middle third of the nose with spreader grafts

T.D. Zijlker and H.D. Vuyk

Introduction

Reconstruction of the middle third of the nose may be necessary in certain functional and/or aesthetic problems. This hidden area is relatively unknown, probably because of its lack of surgical exposure in the traditional closed endonasal approach in rhinoplasty. Overly aggressive resection of cartilage and/or bone without adequate reconstruction, may cause functional and aesthetic sequelae. The open approach enables the surgeon to analyze the pathology and to restore shape and function with the help of cartilage inlay grafts in a more sophisticated, secure and practical way.

Anatomy

The middle nasal vault is composed of the upper lateral cartilages, which are firmly connected to the overlying bony nasal bridge at the so-called 'K-area' and in the midline they are fused with the cartilaginous septum, thus forming a T-shaped construction, which supports the nasal dorsum and defines the contour of the nose (Fig. 1). The angle between the septum and the upper lateral cartilages increases from caudal to cranial (Fig. 2a-c).

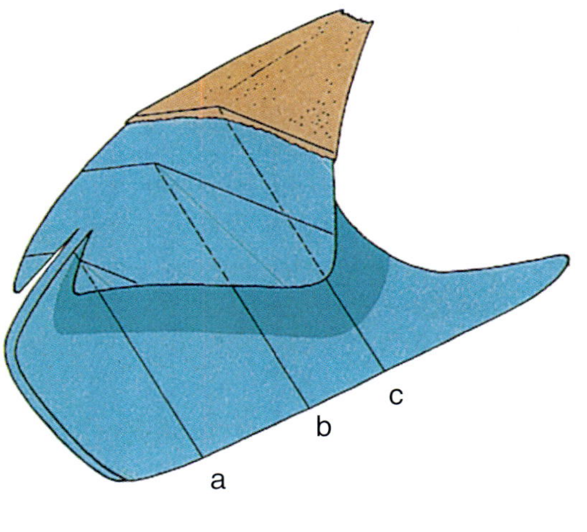

Fig. 1. Upper lateral cartilages fuse end to end with the cartilaginous septum and side to side with the nasal bones.

Physiology

The region between the caudal end of the septum and the upper lateral cartilages represents the narrowest part of the entire airway and is called the nasal valve area. Inward displacement towards the septum of the caudal edge of the upper lateral cartilages on inspiration and the reverse action on expiration should be considered a physiological phenomenon (Fig. 3a,b). The capacity of the involved structures to withstand inward sucking, preventing a partial or total collapse of the nasal valve region, is of utmost importance for normal nasal breathing.

Aesthetics

The middle nasal vault plays an important role in the aesthetics of the external nose. It should be a natural flowing, non-distracting connecting area between the cartilaginous lower third and the bony upper third of the nose.

Pathology

Functional and/or aesthetic pathology may be due to either congenital or iatrogenic causes. The latter should be prevented by all means. Profound knowledge of the surgical anatomy and physiology of the nose, delicate tissue handing, and

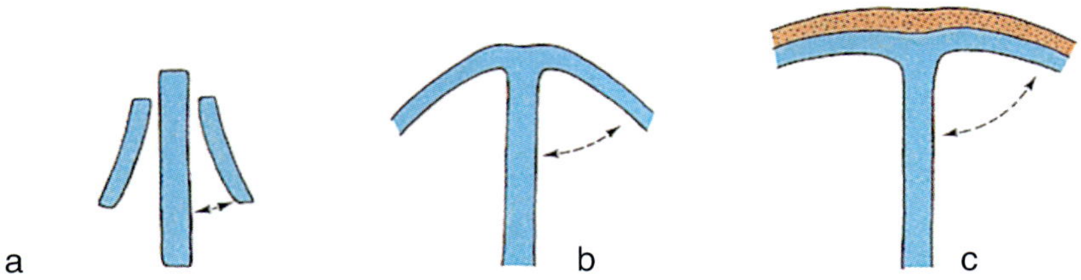

Fig. 2a-c. Schematically drawn cross-sections through the nose. The angle between the septum and the upper lateral cartilages increases from caudal to cranial.

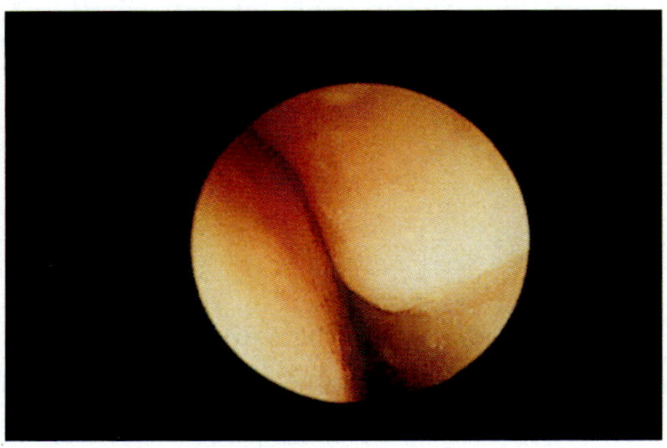

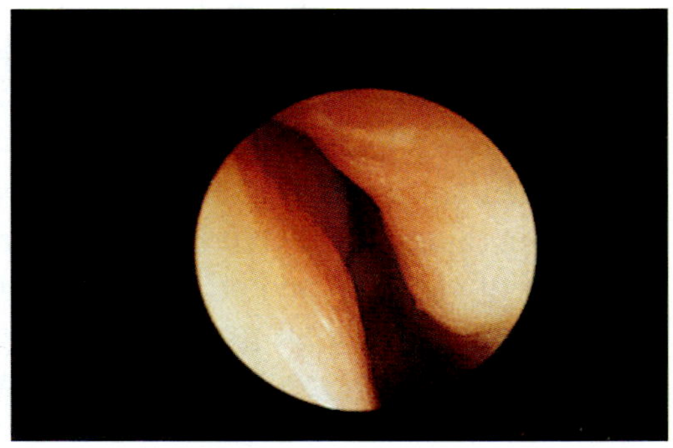

Fig. 3a. Nasal valve area during inspiration. *b.* Nasal valve area during expiration.

the use of non-aggressive techniques for correction of the preoperatively well-defined problems, are prerequisites in this respect.

Which patients are prone to these unwanted sequelae, and how can we recognize the potential danger at an early stage? How can we prevent and treat them adequately?

A patient with a high bony-cartilaginous dorsum who seeks rhinoplasty may be a complication-prone patient. The upper lateral cartilages mostly add more to the hump than the bony part of the nose. Correction demands hump reduction with special attention being paid to reconstruction of the created open roof, not only by using infraction of the nasal bones, but also sometimes by using spreadergrafts. Danger signs are short nasal bones, long flaccid and weak upper lateral cartilages, sometimes even with an almost parallel plane to the septum, and a nasal valve angle of less than the normal range of 10°–15°, and thin overlying skin. In the classic 'tension nose', one or more of these features can be seen. Functional problems may also arise because of the qualitative aspects of the tissue, such as relative weakening of the tissues as seen in aging noses.

The result of not appreciating these potential problems may produce a nose with a collapsed middle third with an unnatural, operated-on appearance, and nasal obstruction due to nasal valve collapse.

Treatment

Surgical treatment of the insufficient nasal valve by means of lateral augmentation is a relatively unknown but simple concept. Lateral augmentation means uni- or bilateral insertion of autogenous single (or double) cartilaginous grafts paramedially to the septum (Fig. 4).

These grafts spread the upper lateral cartilages away from the septum. This increases the diameter of the nasal valve and decreases its tendency to collapse. Moreover, from an aesthetic point of view spreader grafts restore the width of the nose by its mass.

As already discussed in this chapter, nasal physiology depends strongly on the condition of the nasal valve area.

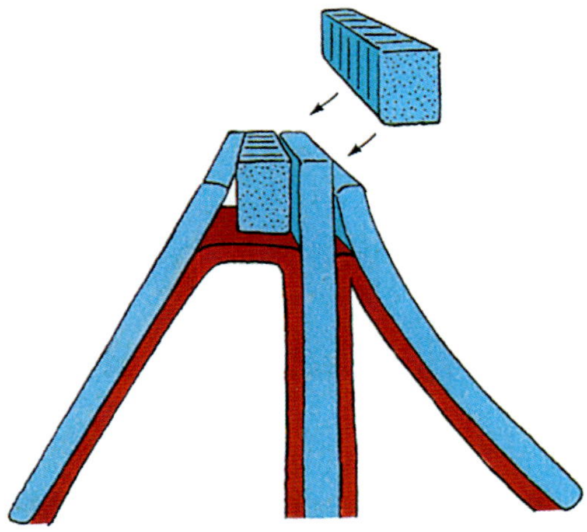

Fig. 4. Lateral augmentation with spreader grafts.

Grafting means repositioning, widening and strengthening of the various structures. Concurrent problems, such as caudal septal deviation, scar tissue formation, or anterior turbinate pathology, should not be overlooked and corrected in one stage.

Early publications on the use of spreader grafts in the reconstruction of the middle nasal vault advocate the closed endonasal technique for insertion. However, precise placement and fixation are almost impossible.

The open approach has greatly facilitated the placement of grafts. The use of grafts made of autogenous cartilage, derived from the nasal septum, tip, ear or costal, has proved to be versatile.

Technique

Harvesting

In the preoperative planning, grafting must be considered. Cartilage is preferably taken from the nasal septum (Fig. 5). Auricular cartilage is second choice, because of the relative weakness and curvature. If requested, resected cartilaginous hump remnants, cephalic portions of the lower lateral cartilages or costal cartilage may serve as donor material. Thus, large exposure of the surgical field, including the ear(s) or chest, may be required. If no septal pathology exists, the cartilage is harvested separately by a posterior 'Killian' incision. If the remaining cartilage strut is at least 10–15 mm in width in the caudal and dorsal region, no unwanted late effects, such as loss of tip projection or saddle nose deformity, need be expected.

Manufacturing

A stick-shaped graft is carved with a No. 11 blade, of an average size of 15 × 1 × 3 mm (Fig. 6). Some cases may require longer or broader grafts. Single or double grafts can be used if there is enough material available. It is easier to fix the various parts together in advance. Absorbable suture material or tissue glue can be used. The use of Histoacryl glue in experienced hands may be useful and time saving, but this is not entirely without dispute because of the potential histotoxicity and damage in well-vascularized tissues.

Surgical exposure

The open or external approach is used. Bilateral marginal incisions are connected with a notched V-shaped midcolumellar skin incision, after which the columellar flap is developed and the overlying skin elevated in the epiperichondrial, avascular plane, as extended as necessary (Figs. 7–10).

After exposure of the caudal end of the cartilaginous septum, the superior submucoperichondrial tunnels are developed on both sides, with an extension underneath the upper lateral cartilages, taking care not to tear the flaps. The caudal ends of the upper lateral cartilage are identified and saved (Fig. 11a,b).

With Converse scissors, the upper lateral cartilages are sharply dissected from the dorsal edge of the septum (Fig. 12). The length of the grafts is measured and the adapted graft will be placed on one

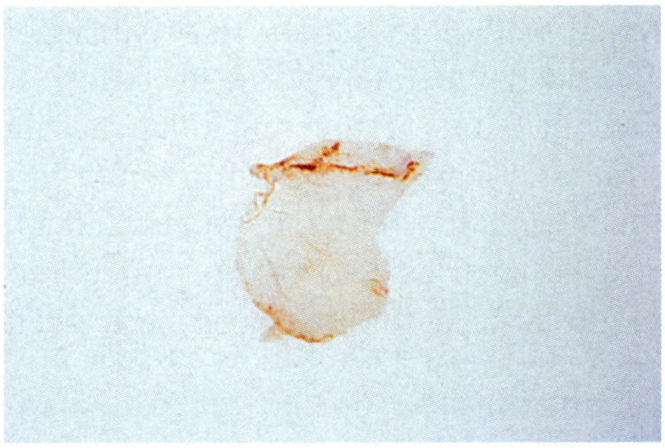

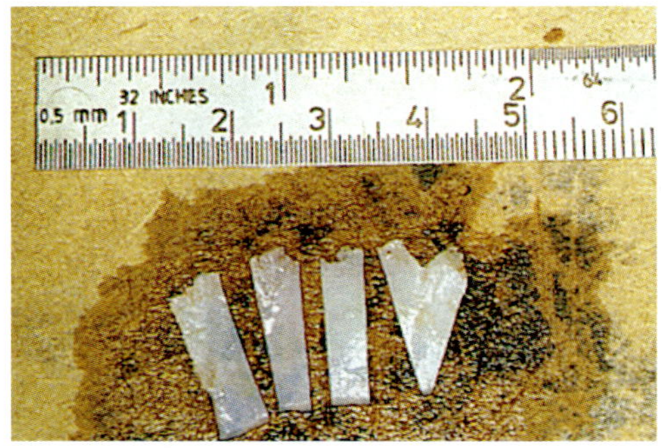

Fig. 5. Harvested cartilage.

Fig. 6. Different types of grafts used in open rhinoplasty: from left to right; columellar strut, bilateral spreader grafts, tip graft.

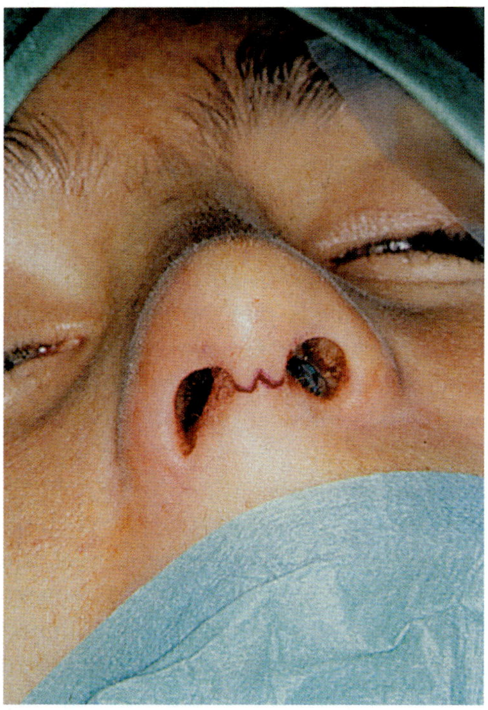

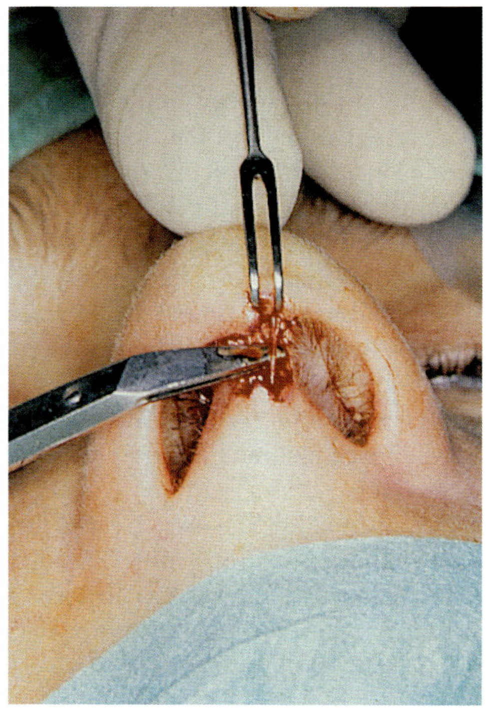

Fig. 7. Notched transcolumellar incision at the level of the midportion of the medial crura.

Fig. 8. Dissection of the flap from the medial crura. After exposure, the columellar artery is cauterized.

side, between the dorsal edge of the septum and the medial border of the upper lateral cartilages (Figs. 13 and 14). A 5/0 Vicryl suture is used to fixate these three layers together in the desired position, parallel to the septum, with a mattress suture technique (Fig. 15a,b). The same procedure is followed for the contralateral side.

The final dorsal refinement may take place at the end of the operation. All other rhinoplastic maneuvers can be carried out before insertion of these particular grafts.

The septum is closed with a running hemostatic suture, mattress suture or splints. The supratip dead space is closed with 4/0 catgut on a straight needle, to prevent a soft tissue polly-beak' formation (Fig. 16). The skin is redraped and meticulously closed in one layer with 6/0 nylon sutures (Fig. 17a,b). The marginal incisions are closed with 5/0 fast absorbing Vicryl sutures. After compression of the nasal dorsum and the tip, to diminish the chance of hematoma, a double layer of papertape is administered to the nose followed by the application of a cast. Perioperative antibiotic prophylaxis is given, as well as an antibiotic containing nasal ointment. No further packing is used.

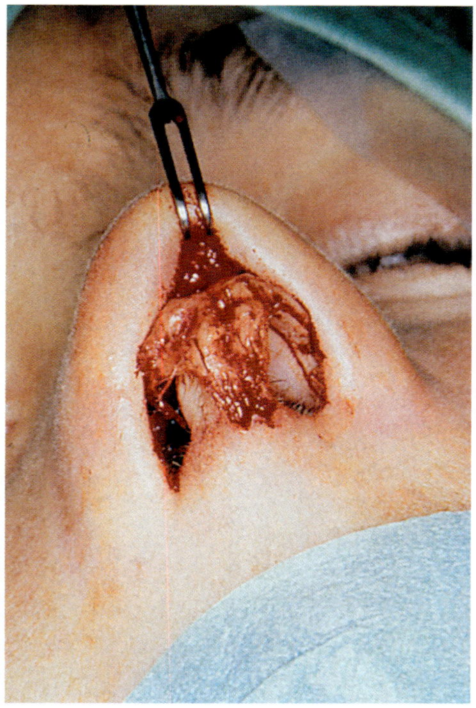

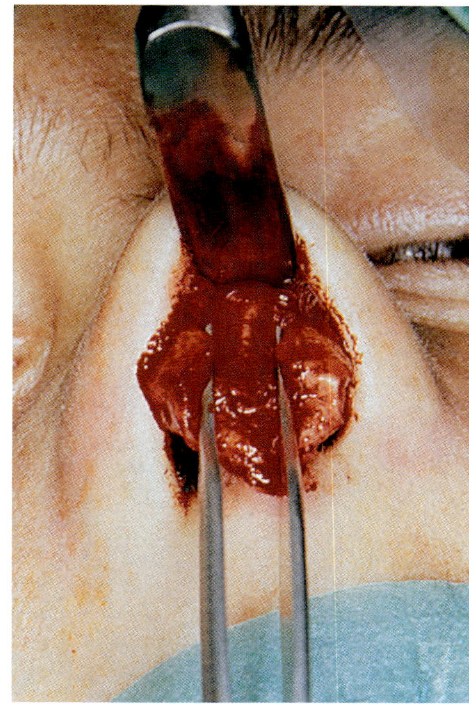

Fig. 9. The lower lateral cartilages in their mutual relationship. Note the asymmetry at the level of the domal region.

Fig. 10. The interdomal ligament is divided. An avascular plane is found and blunt and sharp dissection is used to expose the nasal dorsum.

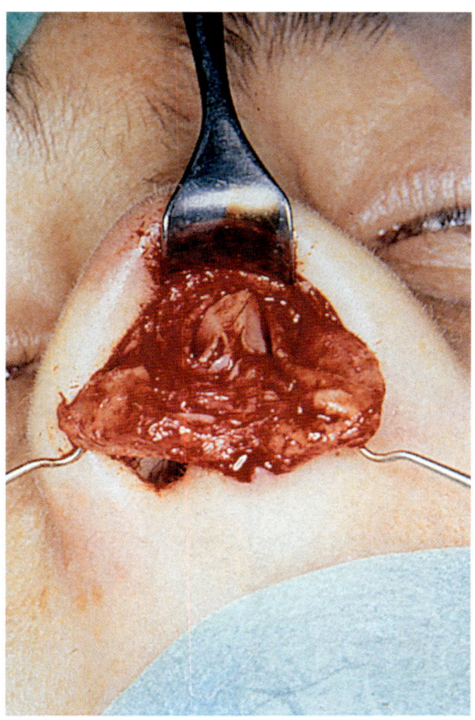

a

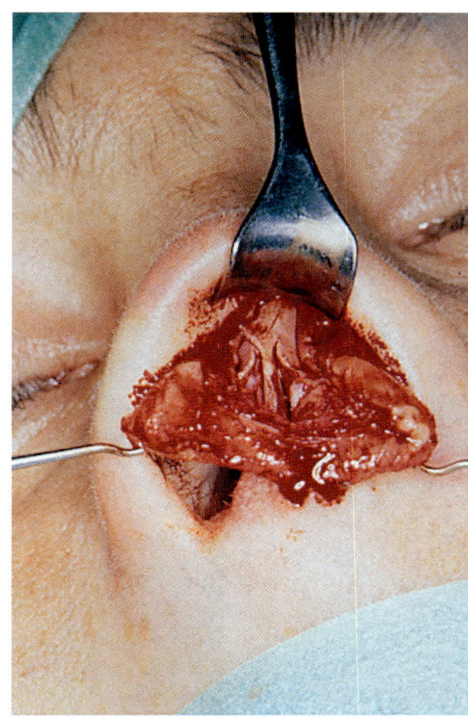

b

Fig. 11. The cartilaginous vault. *a.* Dissection of the perichondrial sheet covering the upper lateral cartilage. *b.* Elevation of bilateral mucoperichondrial septal flaps.

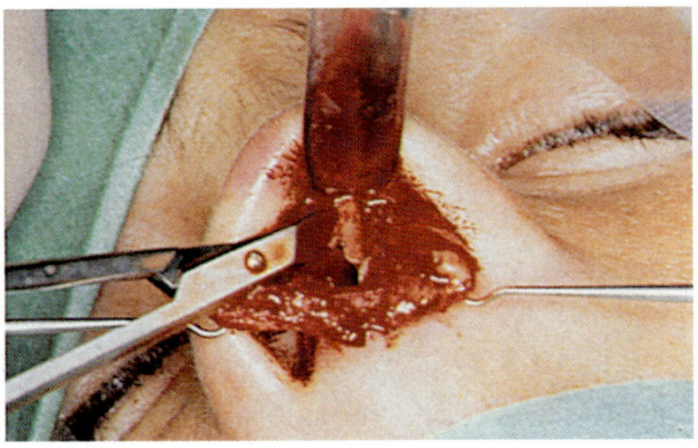

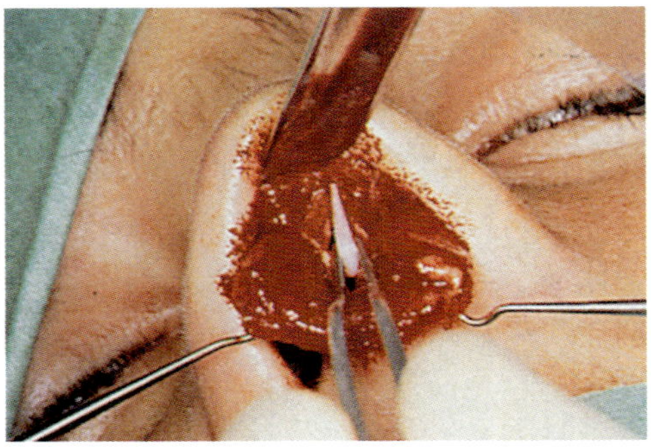

Fig. 12. Converse scissors are used to separate the upper lateral cartilage from the cartilaginous septum.

Fig. 13. Spreader graft inserted on the left side.

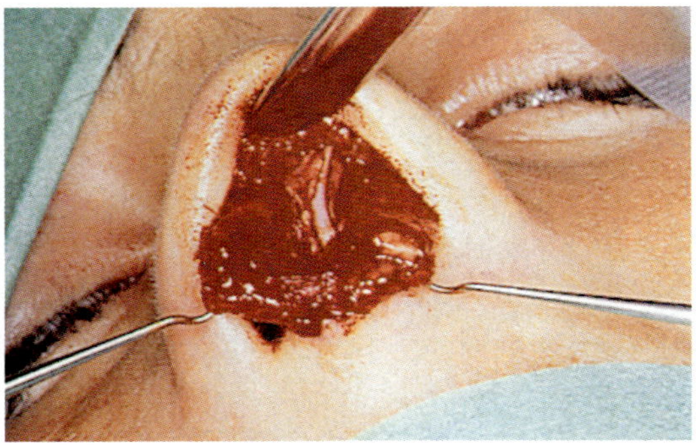

Fig. 14. A slight curvature to the left of the graft after cross hatching the graft. The medial border of the upper lateral cartilage is pushed in a lateral direction.

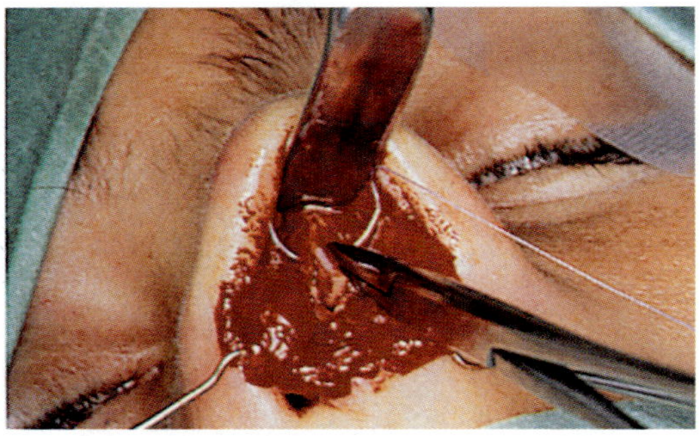

a

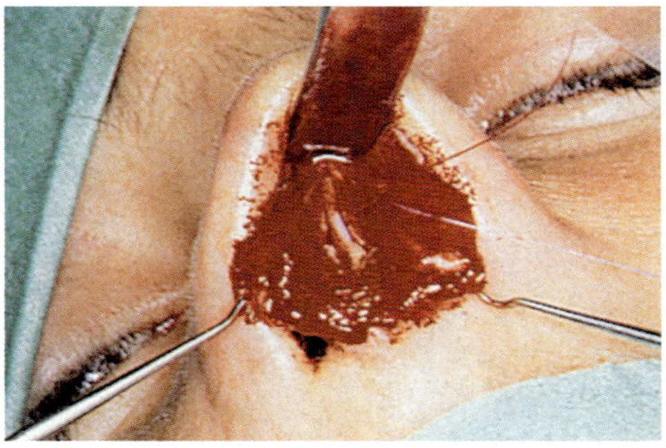

b

Fig. 15a,b. The graft is sutured in place, using mattress suture technique. A final dorsal refinement remains possible.

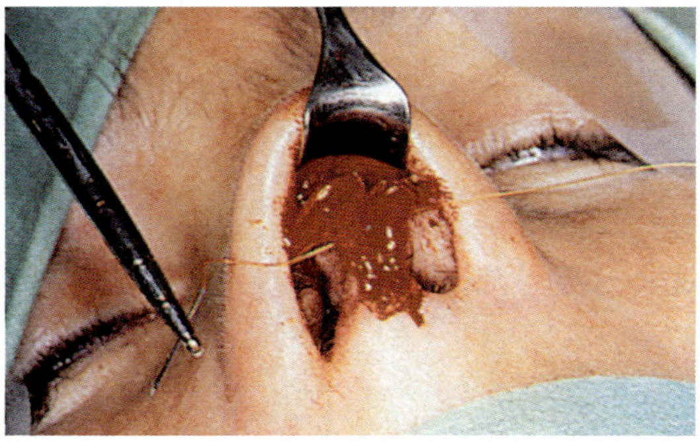

Fig. 16. The supra tip dead space is closed with an interdomal apposition mattress suture.

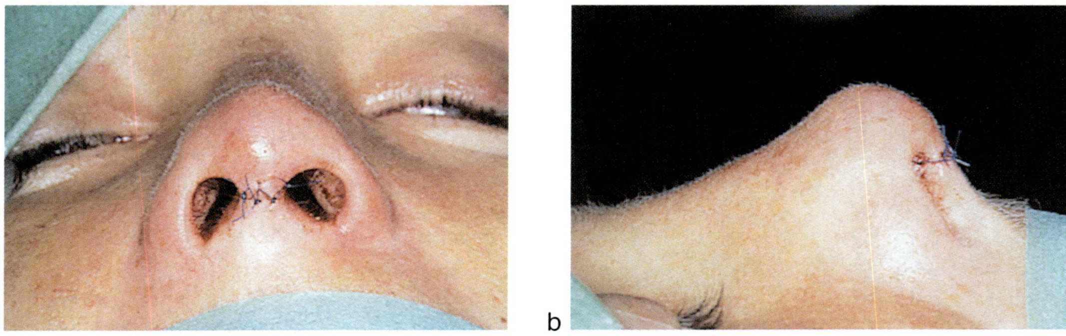

Fig. 17a,b. The midcolumellar incision is closed.

10: BASIC APPROACHES AND TECHNIQUES IN NASAL TIP SURGERY

G.J. Nolst Trenité

Introduction

The variety of procedures for nasal tip surgery and the individual differences in tip anatomy are complicated by the confusing terminology in the international literature. It was Tardy who advocated a systematic rational approach to the nasal tip. With this framework in mind, the inexperienced nasal surgeon can use the appropriate incisions, approaches and techniques more easily. The basic philosophy is to operate as atraumatically as possible and to preserve tip support, which is very important in getting good long-term postoperative results. There are three basic surgical approaches to the tip of the nose:

1. the non-delivery approach
   - cartilage-splitting
   - retrograde eversion
2. the delivery approach
3. the external approach

Indications for each of these approaches depend on the specific anatomy of the nose and the proposed changes:
- volume reduction
- reconstruction
- rotation
- change of projection

Surgical Procedures

The non-delivery approach is very appropriate for:
- small volume reduction of the lateral crus
- slight cephalic rotation of the tip

Volume reduction can easily be done using a transcartilaginous incision, in which only slight surgical trauma occurs.

The operative procedure for the cartilage splitting non-delivery approach is as follows: after drawing the skeletal landmarks and boundaries on the skin of the nose, the most cephalic part of the lateral crus to be resected is outlined with a marking pen on the external skin (Fig. 1). It is helpful to indicate on the vestibular skin where the transcartilaginous incision should be made. This can be done either by a through-and-through needle from the outside or, more elegantly, by using the inprint of a surgical instrument on the vestibular skin (Fig. 2a,b).

Care should be taken to preserve at least 5 mm of uninterrupted cartilage (in a vertical dimension) of the lateral crus. Although many surgeons make their incisions through the vestibular skin and cartilage at once, it facilitates the dissection of the vestibular skin to do this in two stages. A vestibular skin incision with a

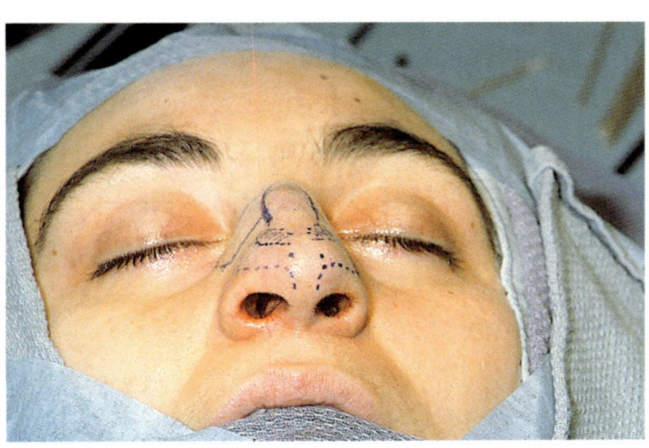

Fig. 1. Drawing of the skeletal landmarks and the planned resection on the skin.

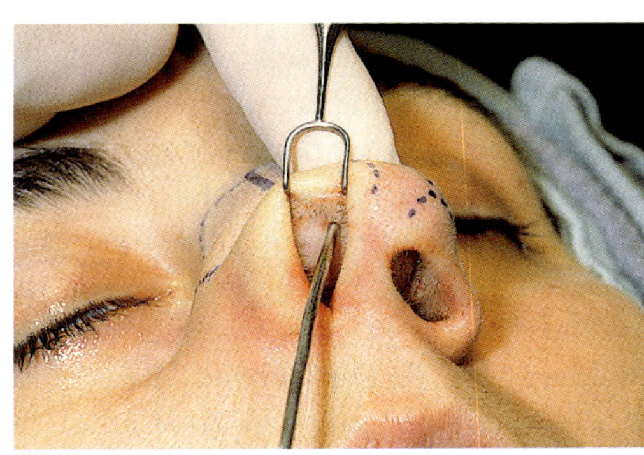

a

Fig. 2a. Inprint of the vestibular skin with a suction tube to mark the planned site of the transcartilaginous incision.

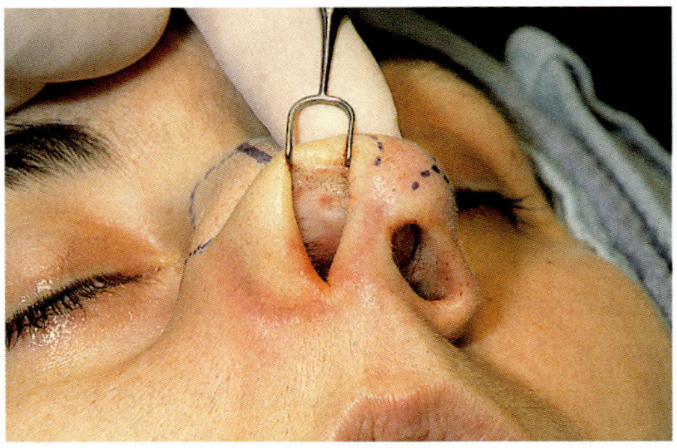

b

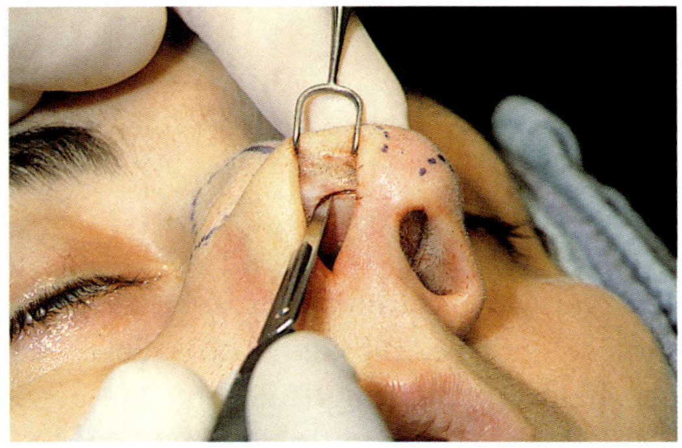

Fig. 2b. Suction tube inprint of the vestibular skin.

Fig. 3. Vestibular skin incision.

a

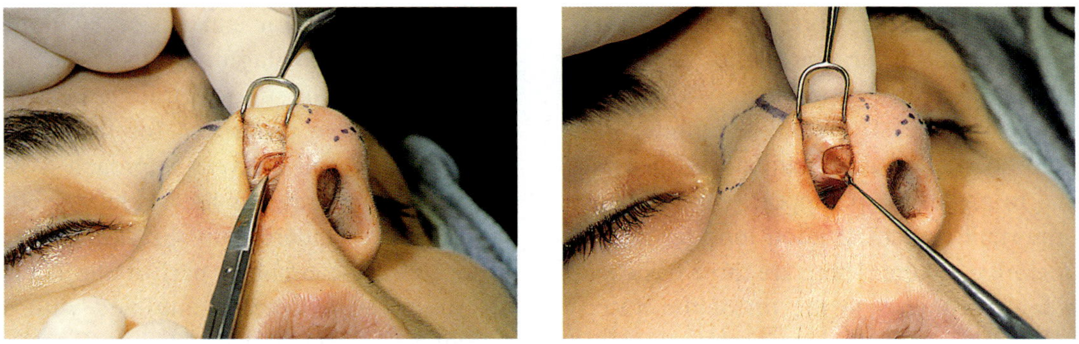

b

Fig. 4a,b. The vestibular skin is dissected free from the cephalic part of the lateral crus to be resected.

a

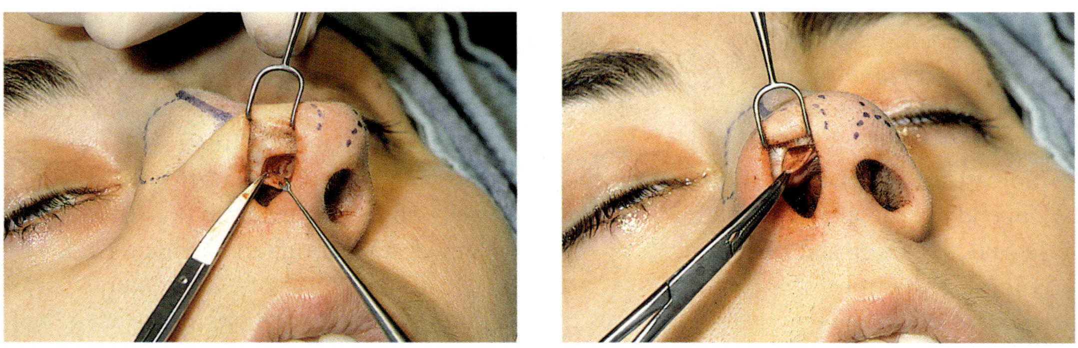

b

Fig. 5a,b. Dissection at the nonvestibular site after splitting the cartilage.

No. 15 blade (Fig. 3) is followed by dissecting the vestibular skin free from the proposed resection of the cephalic part of the lower lateral cartilage with a pair of sharp pointed curved scissors (Fig. 4a,b). After splitting the cartilage (No. 15 blade), the non-vestibular side of the cephalic part to be resected is dissected free from the overlying soft tissue and removed (Fig. 5a,b,c,d). Pressure of the middle finger of the operator's hand (holding the double-hooked ala retractor) on the lateral crus will give excellent exposure and control during surgery. After sufficient and symmetric volume reduction, the vestibular skin should be sutured carefully with 5/0 atraumatic absorbable suture material. This simple tip refinement procedure gives minimal surgical trauma, leaving the integrity of the lower lateral intact ensuring the best chances for uncomplicated healing process.

Nowadays, *the retrogade-eversion approach* is performed less often. Instead of a transcartilaginous incision, an *inter-*

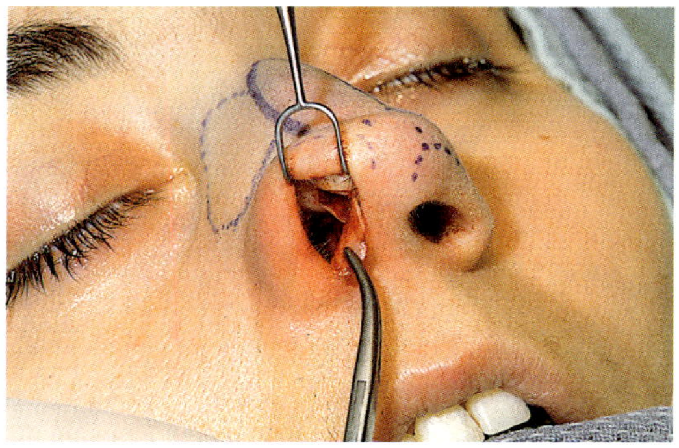
c

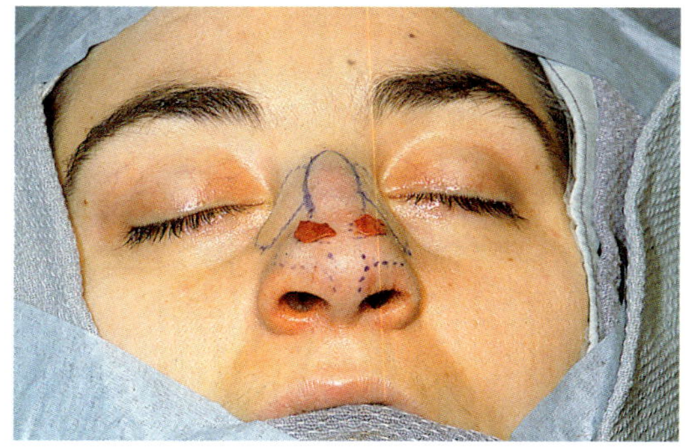
d

Fig. 5c,d. Resection of the cephalic parts of the lateral crura.

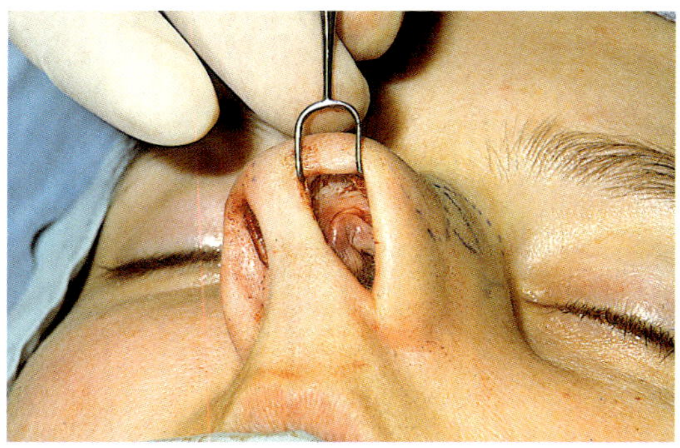

Fig. 6. Intercartilaginous incision caudal to the valve area and around the anterior septal angle.

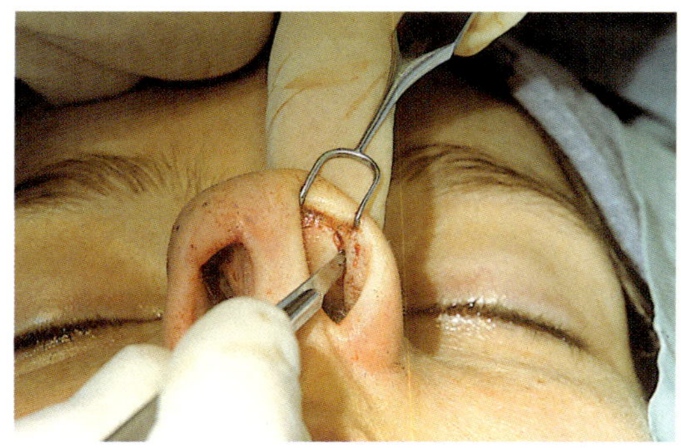

Fig. 7. Marginal incision.

cartilaginous incision is made followed by retrograde dissection over the lateral crus at the non-vestibular side, eversion of the lateral crus and resection of the planned cephalic portion of the cartilage.

The delivery approach, although more traumatic, is indicated when the planned changes to the nasal tip are more than just a small volume reduction. The indications for this approach are:

- asymmetry
- bifidity
- extra cephalic tip rotation
- diminishing of the tip projection

With this approach, it is possible to modify the alar cartilages under direct vision up to the dome and interdomal area. Different operative techniques can be applied:

- precise excision of cartilage to achieve good symmetry
- remodelling the alar cartilages by scoring and morselization
- interdomal suturing to correct bifidity
- interruption of the continuity of the alar cartilage to reduce an extremely overprojected tip ('pinocchio' nose) or to enhance cephalic tip rotation.

The surgical procedure to deliver the alar cartilages starts with an *intercartilaginous incision* with a No. 15 blade. It is important to make this incision caudally to the valve area to prevent unnecessary scarring in the valve area. This intercartilaginous incision should be carried well around the anterior septal angle (Fig. 6). If not, delivery could be stagnated.

The next step is to make a *marginal incision* (No. 15 blade), hugging the caudal edge of the lower lateral to prevent surgical damage to 'the soft triangle'. The incision starts at the upper part of the caudal edge of the medial crus, then goes around the dome and follows the caudal edge of the lateral crus as far as necessary (Fig. 7). After these two incisions, the non-vestibular side of the lateral crus is freed from the soft tissue by dissection with a pair of sharp pointed curved

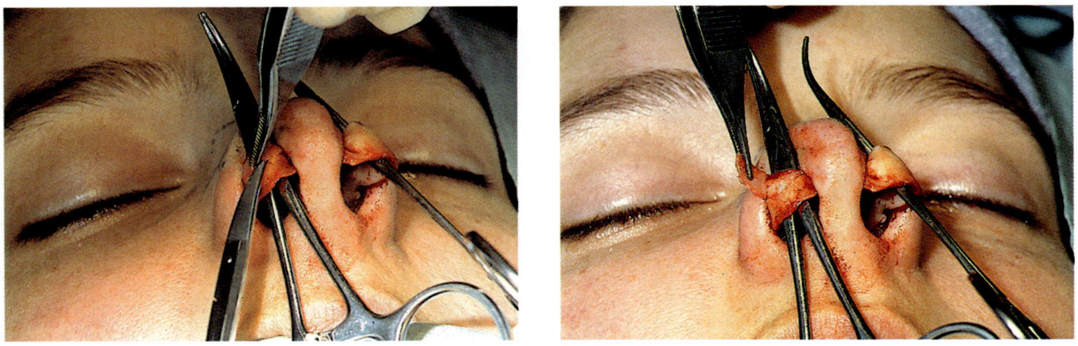

a b

Fig. 8a,b. Precise dissection and excision of a cephalic portion of the lateral crus.

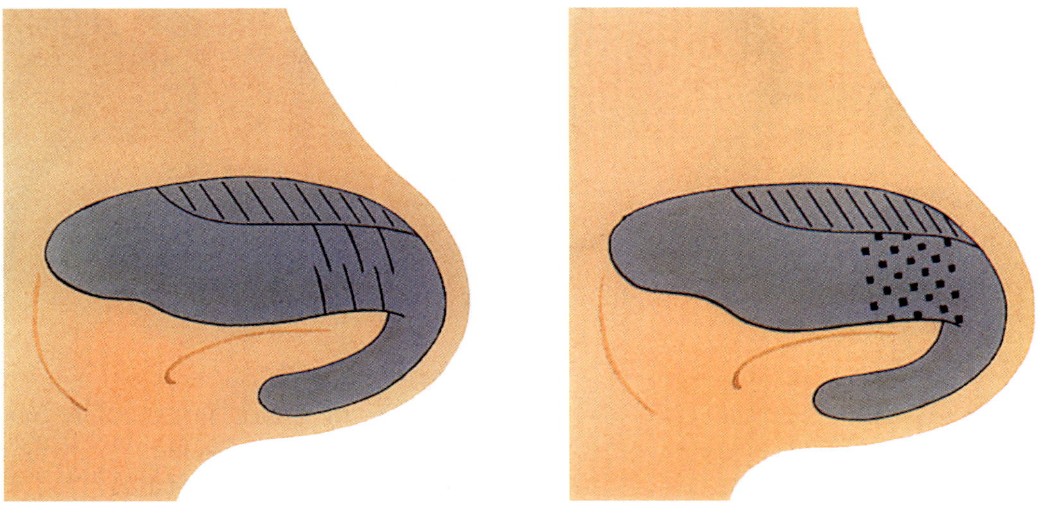

a b

Fig. 9. Weakening procedure of the lateral crus: *a.* scoring, *b.* morselization.

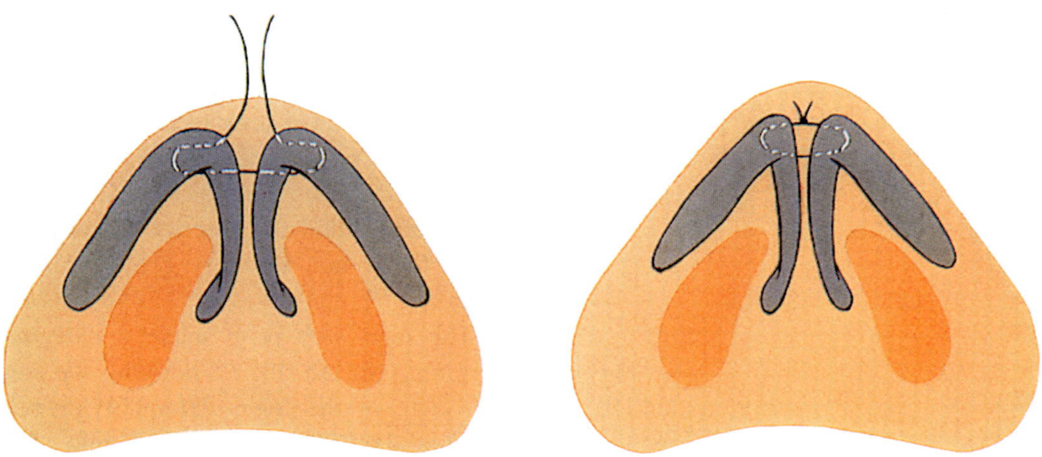

a b

Fig. 10a,b. Horizontal mattress suture technique to correct bifidity of the tip.

scissors. To deliver the bipedicle chondrocutaneous flaps, small hemostats are very handy. Precise excision of cartilage is now possible under direct vision (Fig. 8a,b). In the case of bulging of the lateral crus, the weakening procedure (scoring or morselization) is performed, if indicated in combination with resection of a cephalic portion of the lateral crus (Fig. 9a,b).

The delivery approach is also appropriate in the case of bifidity of the nasal tip, in which the horizontal mattress suture technique can be performed to

Fig. 10c,d. Mattress suture with 6/0 Goretex of left lower lateral followed by transportation of the needle with a mosquito clamp to the right side for the same procedure.

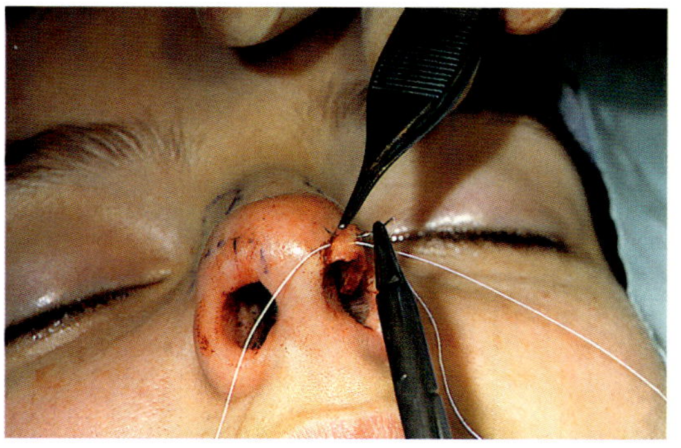
c

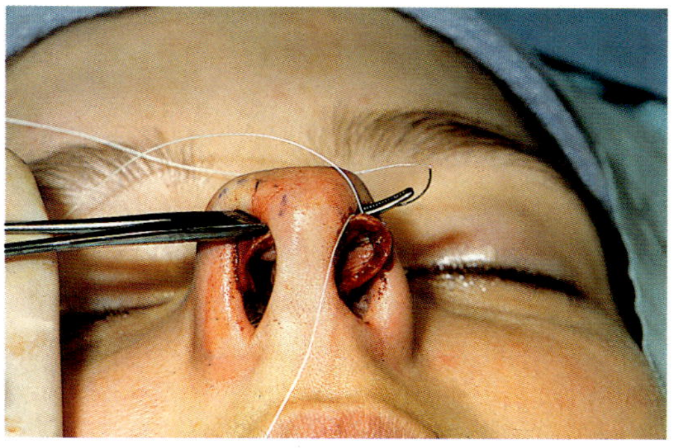
d

Fig. 10e. Direct postoperative result after advancing the domes with horizontal mattress suture technique.

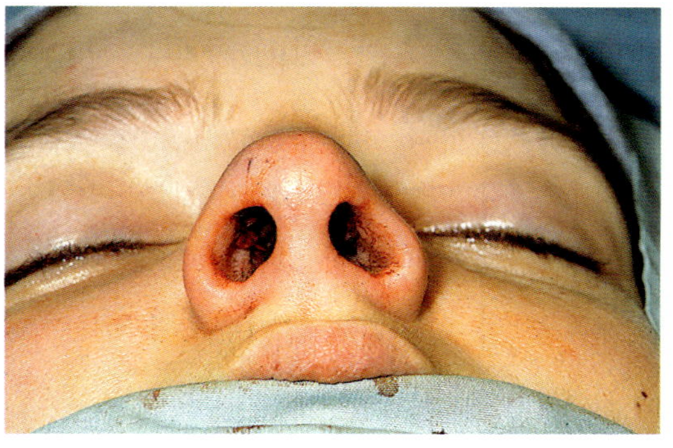
e

advance the domes with a non-absorbable (goretex) or a slow absorbable (PDS) atraumatic suture (Fig. 10a,b,c,d,e).

Interrupting the continuity of the alar cartilage can give some unpredictable scarring, especially visible in thin-skinned noses. In the case of dome amputation to reduce a 'pinocchio' nose, an onlay tip graft will hide possible irregularities in the healing process (Fig. 11a,b).

To reduce tip projection and to obtain sufficient cephalic tip rotation, as is indicated in correcting a tension nose, the continuity of the alar cartilage is interrupted by transection of the lateral crus at the junction of its middle and lateral third, followed by resection of the cartilage segment of the lateral third and cephalic part (Fig. 12a,b). A supplementary procedure to enhance tip rotation is resection of a caudal strip of cartilage in the septum. The surgeon should be aware that the healing process is less predictable, with more chance of postoperative asymmetries, with the delivery approach than with the non-delivery approach.

The external approach, although even more traumatic and time consuming, gives the best exposure of the three approaches. This approach enables the surgeon to perform bimanual surgery, and it makes judgment of the specific deformities much easier. Therefore, it is especially indicated in the case of:

- congenital deformities such as the cleft-lip nose

Fig. 11a. Dome amputation.

Fig. 11b. Sutured lower laterals with an onlay tip graft to hide possible postoperative irregularities.

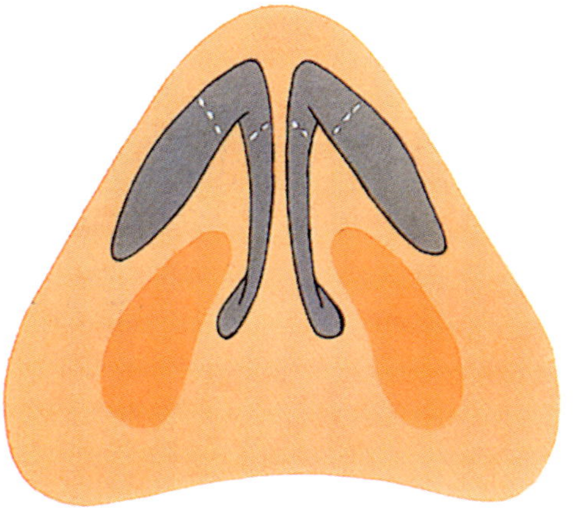
a

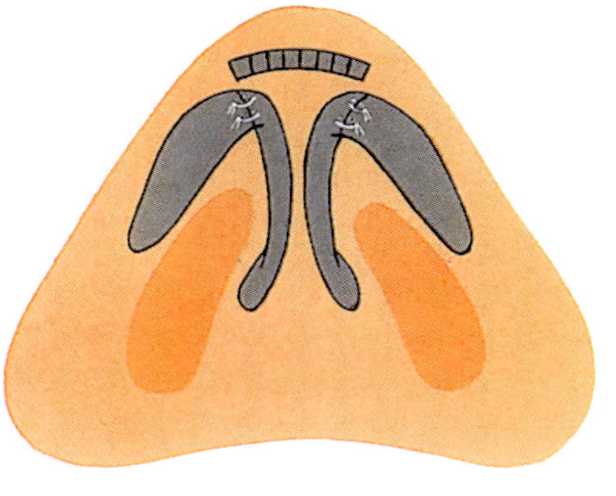
b

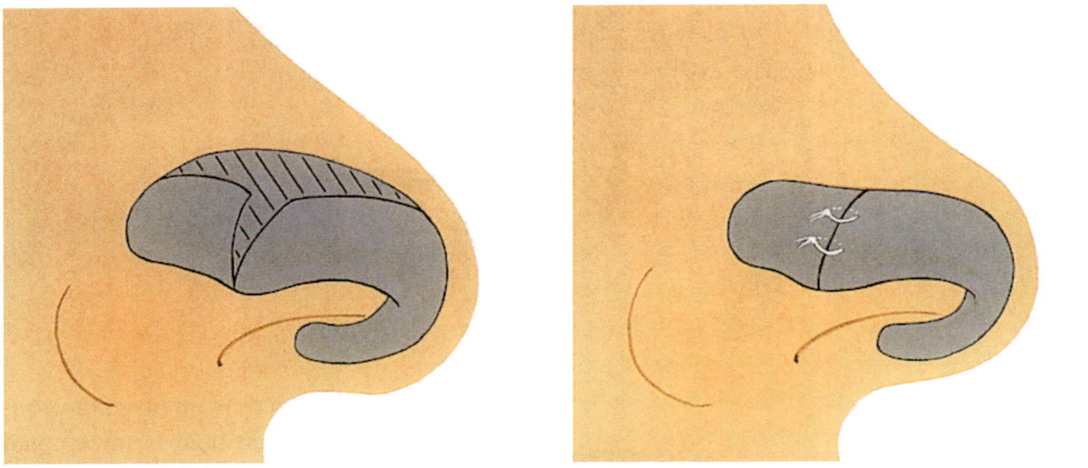

a b

Fig. 12a,b. Interrupted strip technique to obtain adequate cephalic tip rotation in case of a tension nose.

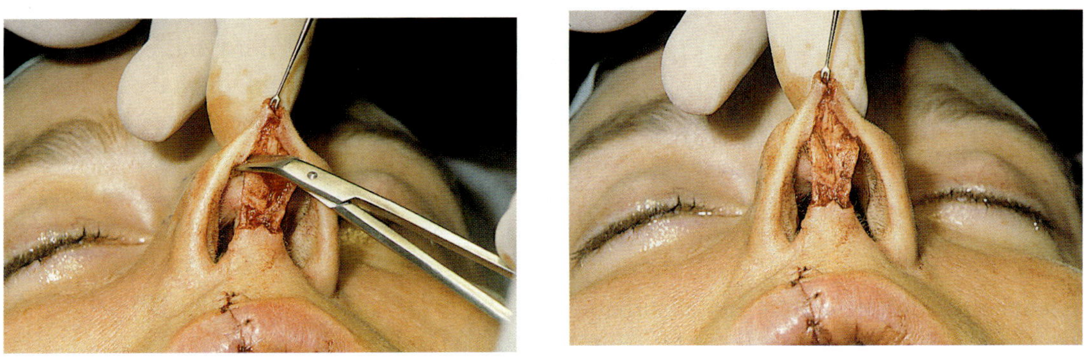

a b

Fig. 13a,b. External approach after careful preparation of the columella skin flap avoiding injury to the underlying cartilage of the medial crura.

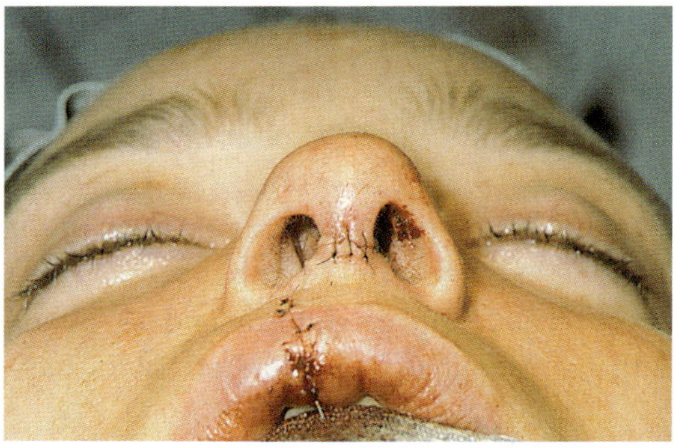

Fig. 14. Meticulous suturing of the midcolumellar incision with 6/0 nylon.

- extensive revision surgery
- severe nasal trauma
- elaborate reduction and augmentation procedures

Nevertheless, there is a tendency to use the external approach routinely, especially by less experienced nasal surgeons. This is justified as long as the surgeon weighs the surgical trauma of the chosen approach against the possibilities of a satisfying postoperative result in each individual case.

Careful preparation of the columella skin flap (Fig. 13a,b), without disturbing the underlying cartilage of the medial crura, and meticulous suturing of the midcolumellar skin incision (Fig. 14), to prevent skin necrosis and visible scarring, are prerequisites. The operative technique will be described in a step-by-step fashion in Chapter 12.

In Figures 15-18 clinical cases of a non-delivery, a delivery and an external approach are shown.

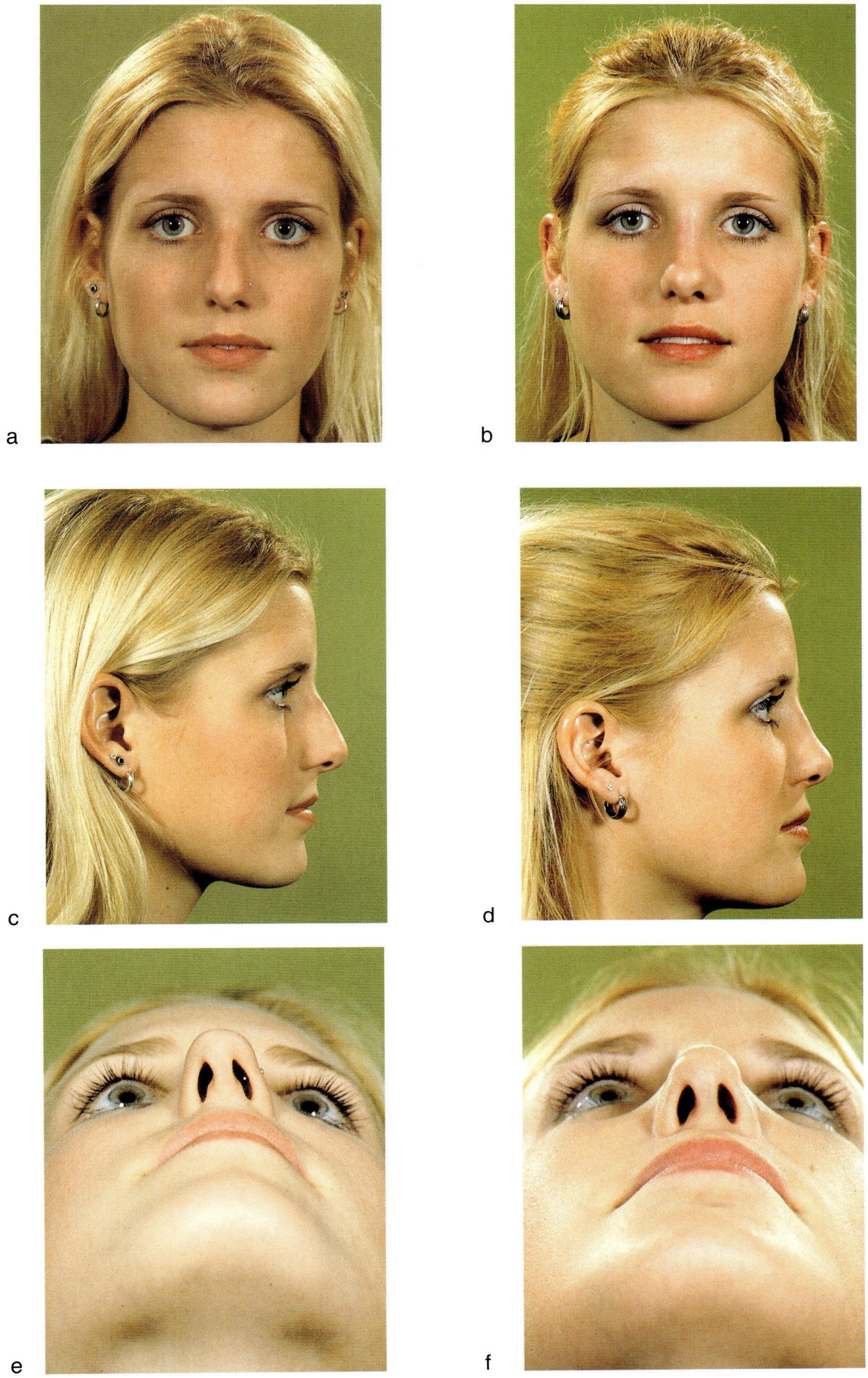

Fig. 15a-f. Pre- and postoperative views of a patient who underwent a rhinoplasty by the non-delivery approach. First a septoplasty was performed to correct a caudal septal deviation to the left followed by a cephalic resection of the lower laterals. Furthermore, a cartilaginous bony hump was removed followed by medial oblique, lateral micro-osteotomies and infraction of the nasal bones.

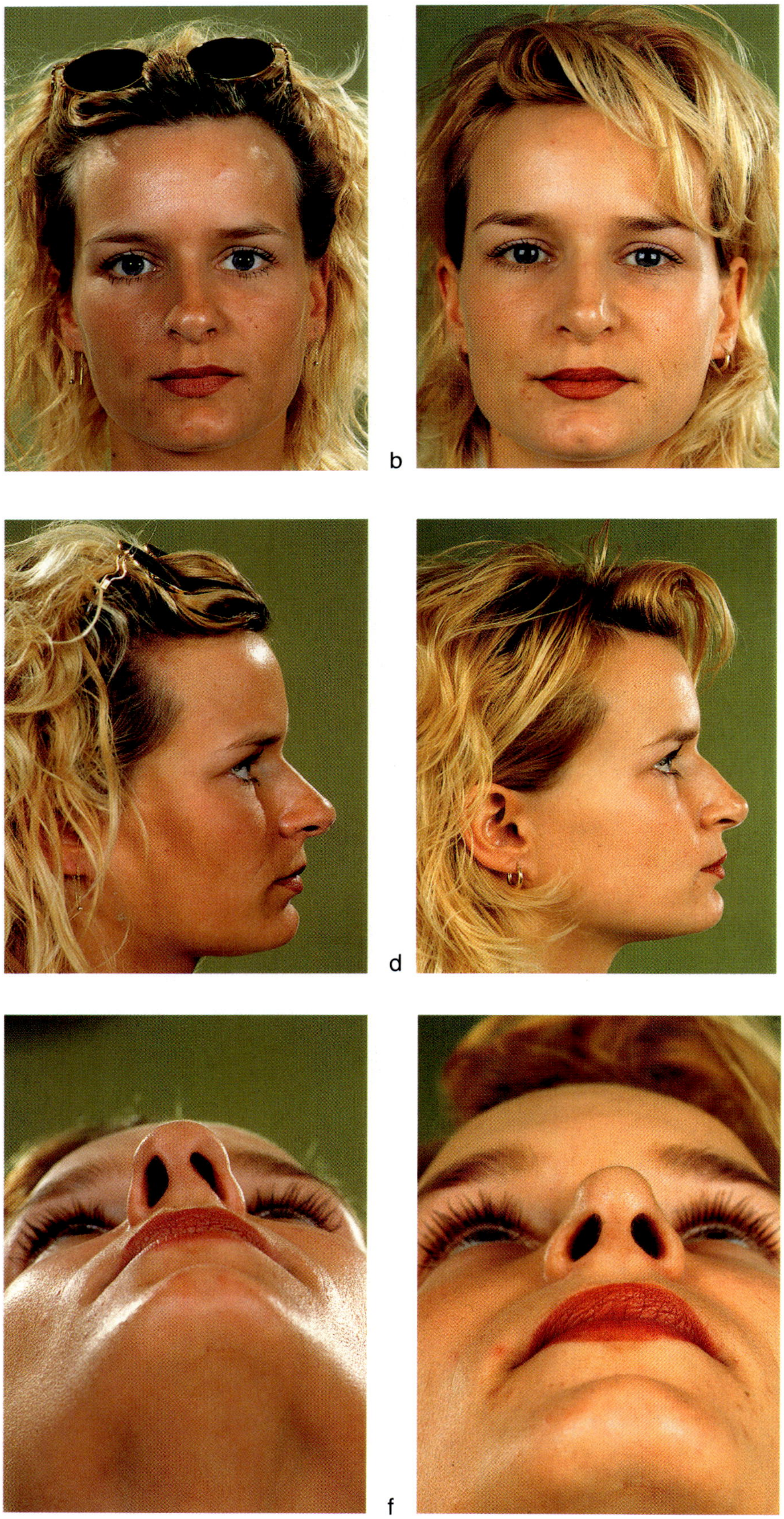

Fig. 16a-f. Pre- and postoperative views of a rhinoplasty by the delivery approach, to narrow the broad trapezoid tip with transdomal and interdomal suturing followed by a bilateral cephalic resection of the lower laterals and a small resection of the cartilaginous dorsum. The assymetry of the nostrils due to a caudal septal deviation to the left was corrected by a septoplasty through a hemitransfixion incision.

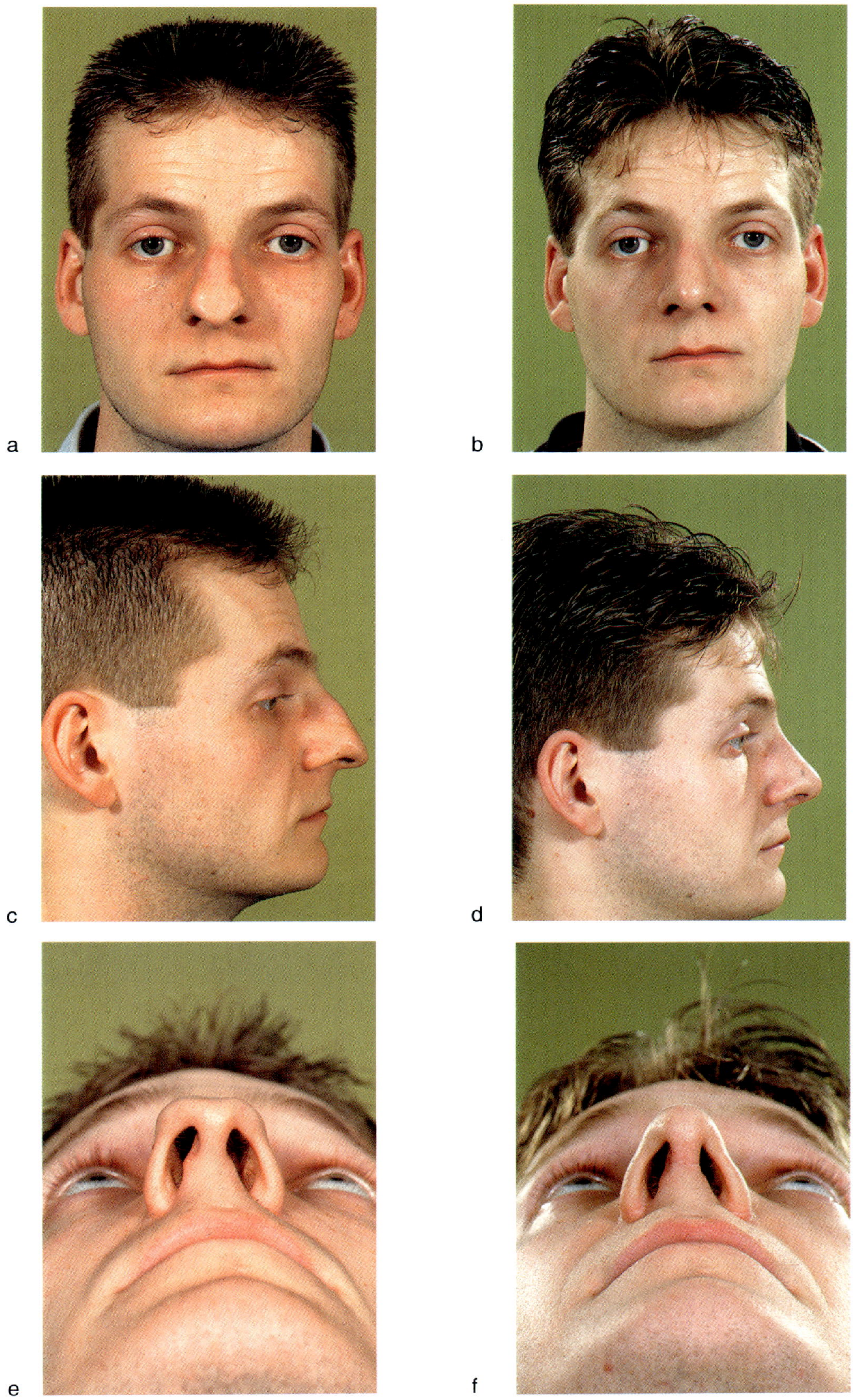

Fig. 17a-f. Pre- and postoperative views of a patient with a congenital deformity of the nose with agenesis of the nasal bones, overdevelopment of the cartilaginous vault and an extreme trapezoid deformity of the nasal tip. Narrowing of the tip with inter- and transdomal suturing and adequate cephalic tip rotation was performed with an interrupted strip technique through an external approach. Finally alar base wedge resections were performed to correct alar flaring.

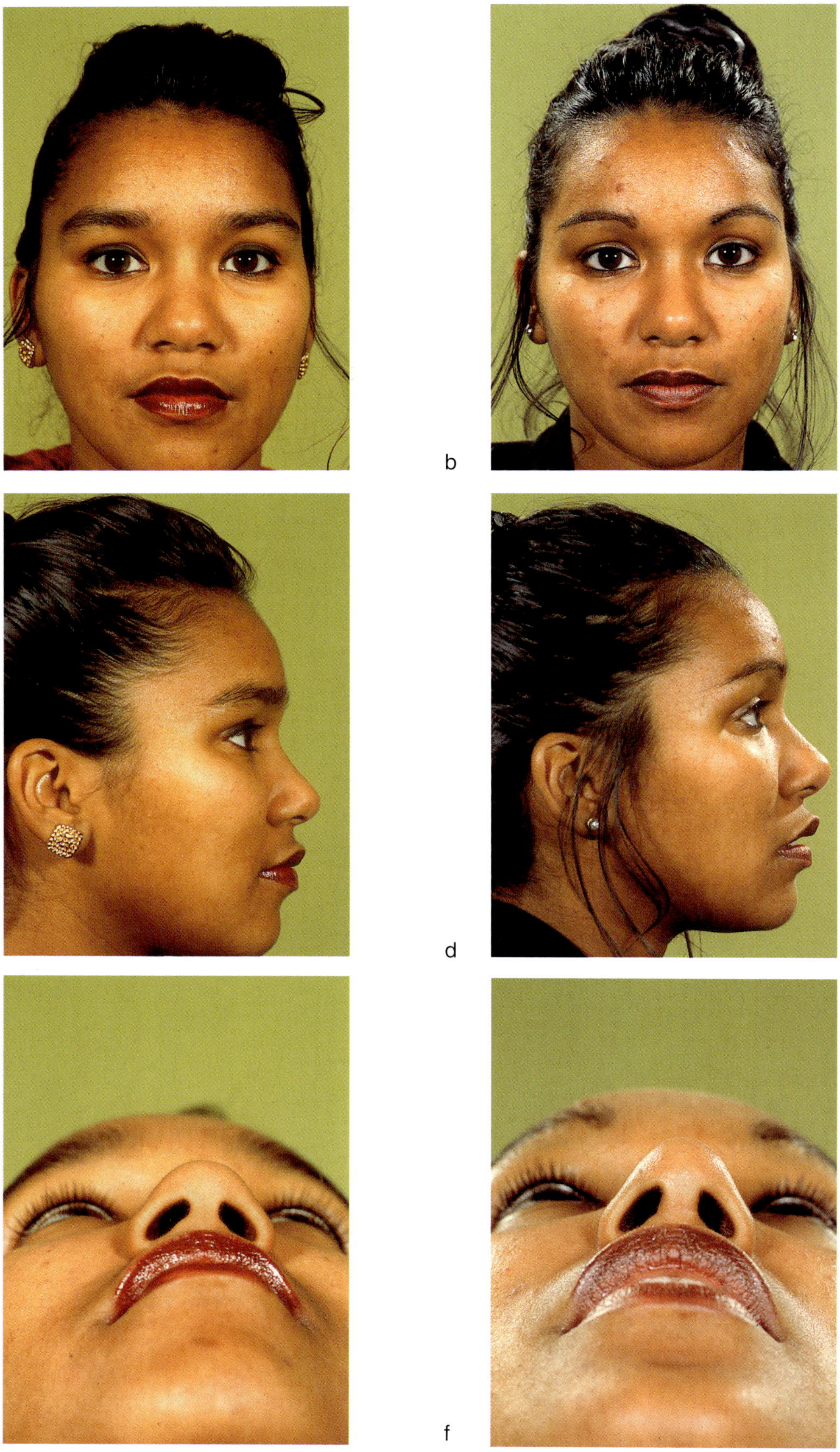

a b c d e f

Fig. 18a-f. Pre- and post-operative views of a patient with a bulbous tip with lack of projection. An external rhinoplasty was performed for more tip projection and refinement with the use of autogenous grafts (columella strut and shield graft) from septal cartilage.

11: SURGERY OF THE OSSEOCARTILAGINOUS VAULT

G.J. Nolst Trenité

Introduction

Looking at the sequence of operative steps, most rhinoplastic surgeons prefer to perform surgery of the osseocartilaginous vault after tip surgery. One of the main reasons for this is that, by applying an external nasal dressing immediately after osteotomy, edema and ecchymosis can be prevented or at least diminished. Another reason is that, in order to obtain an aesthetic balance, in certain cases it is easier to adapt the form of the osseocartilaginous vault to the form of the tip, rather than vice versa. In this chapter, surgery of the osseocartilaginous vault is divided into five sections:

- hump resection
- osteotomies
- management of special bony pyramid problems
- radix nasi surgery
- cartilaginous vault surgery

Hump resection

The nasal hump consists of a cartilaginous and a bony part. In most cases, the bony part of the hump is much smaller than the cartilaginous part. With the endonasal approach, intercartilaginous incisions are connected by a transfixion incision to obtain ample access to the hump. It is important to dissect carefully between the upper and lower lateral cartilage in order to prevent postoperative irregularities of the lateral nasal wall. The intercartilaginous incision from lateral to medial, just caudal of the nasal valve, must be carried around the anterior septal angle. The two intercartilaginous incisions will then be connected by a partial transfixion incision, unless there is a specific indication for a complete transfixion incision. With a complete transfixion incision an important support of the tip in its connection between the medial crura and the anterior edge of the nasal septum will be disturbed (Fig. 1a,b). The next step is to free the cartilaginous part of the hump from the overlying soft tissues. With careful and sharp dissection (No. 15 blade) in the supraperichondrial surgical plane, damage to the musculus transversus nasi, together with unnecessary scarring and bleeding, will be prevented (Fig. 2).

After freeing the cartilaginous vault from the overlying soft tissues, the periosteum is incised at the caudal end of the nasal bone and elevated with a Joseph elevator (Fig. 3a,b). There is no need to elevate the periosteum very far laterally. The procedure should be limited to the area of

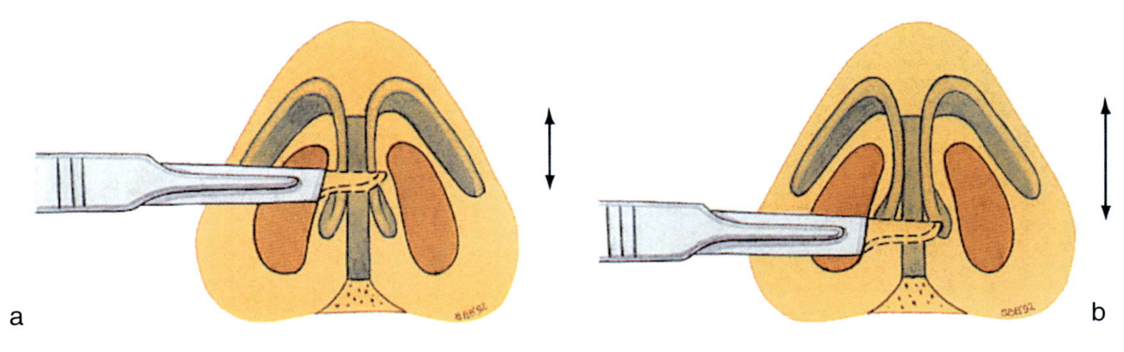

Fig. 1a. partial transfixion incision. *b.* complete transfixion incision.

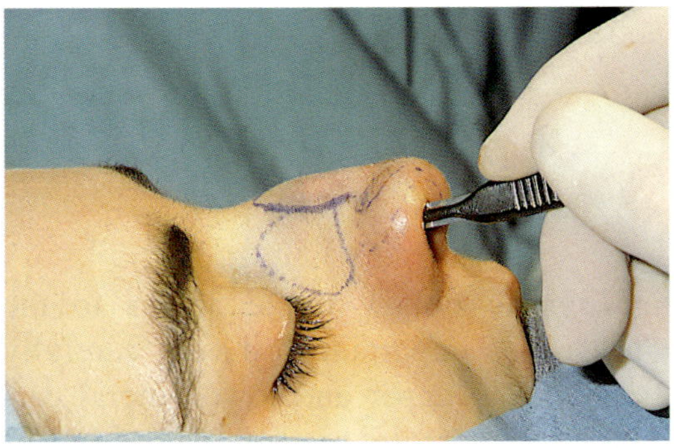

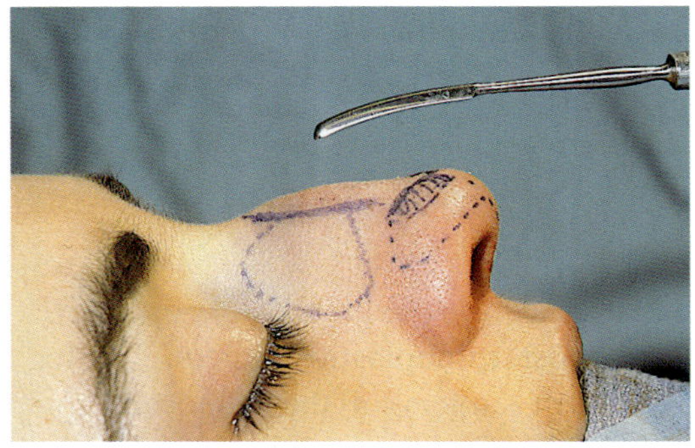

a

Fig. 2. Sharp dissection in the surgical plane (close to the perichondrium) to free the cartilaginous dorsum from the overlying soft tissue.

Fig. 3a,b. Elevation of the periosteum of the nasal bone (only of the hump area) with a Joseph elevator.

b

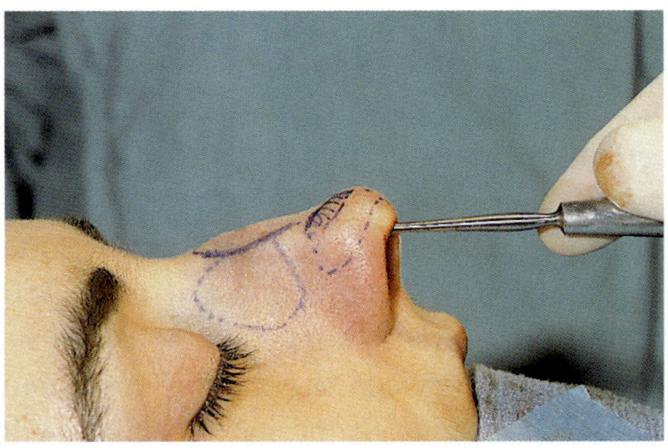

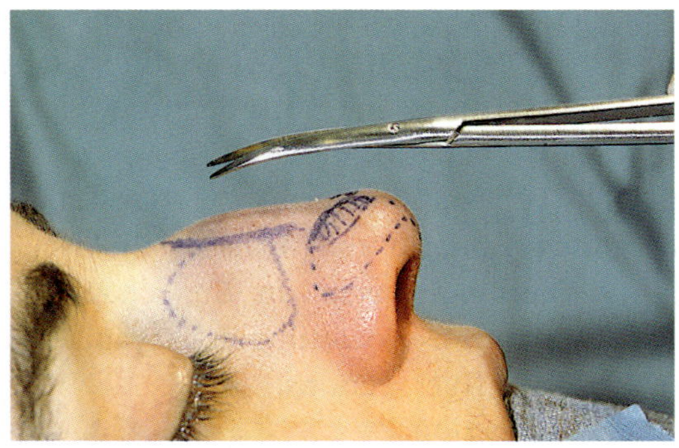

Fig. 3b.

Fig. 4. Dissection of the periosteum attached to the sutura intranasalis.

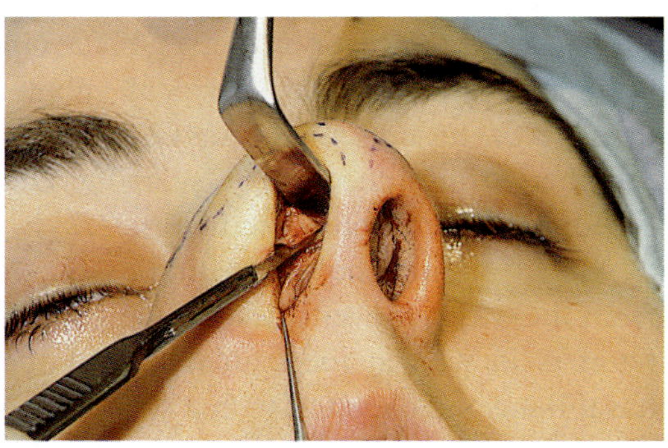

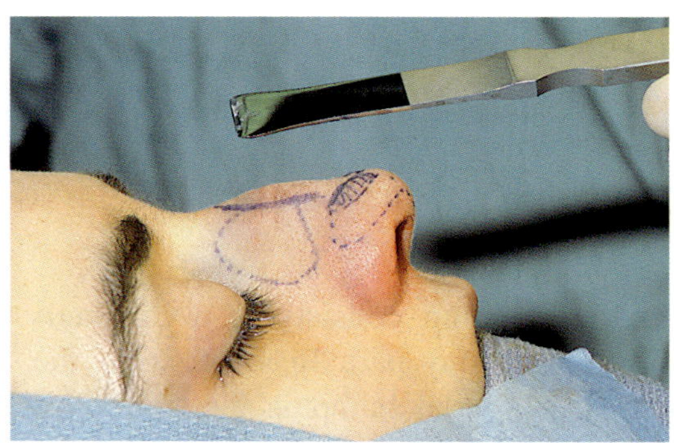

a

Fig. 5. Incising the cartilaginous vault under direct vision at the 'planned' resection line.

Fig. 6a,b,c. Resection of the osseocartilaginous hump with a 14 mm hump osteotome.

b

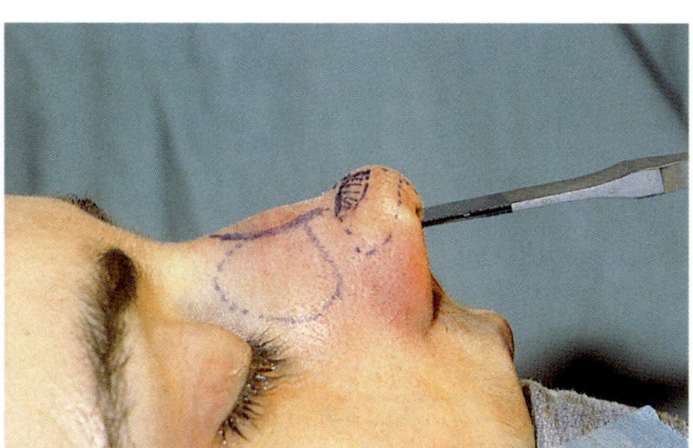

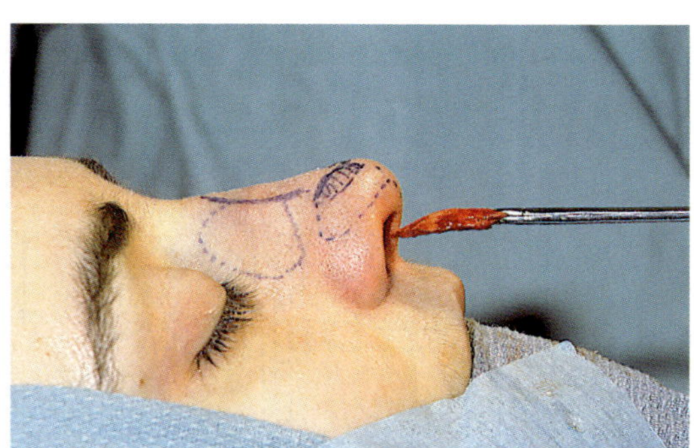

c

Fig. 6b,c.

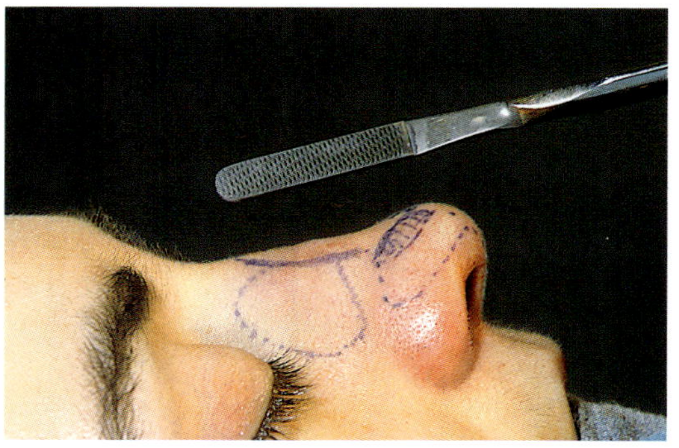

Fig. 7. Smoothening of the bony surface after hump resection with a medium-fine (tungsten-carbide) rasp.

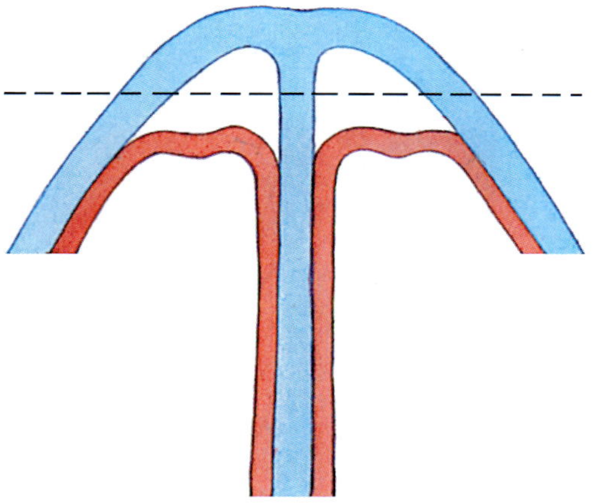

Fig. 8. Stripping of the mucoperichondrium at first on the posterior side of the cartilaginous vault in case of a large hump.

the hump to be resected. Periosteum attached to the sutura intranasalis can simply be cut from the bony vault with a pair of long scissors (Fig. 4). With an 'Aufricht' retractor in place, the cartilaginous vault can now be incised by a through-and-through incision (No. 15 blade) from cephalic to caudal at the 'planned' resection line (Fig. 5).

Using this cartilaginous cutting face as a guideline, the hump osteotome is introduced to loosen the bony part at the hump, followed by the removal of the osseocartilaginous hump 'en bloc' (Fig. 6a,b,c). A (medium-fine) tungsten-carbide or diamond rasp is now used to smoothen the bony surface (Fig. 7) and, if necessary, some extra shaving of the cartilaginous dorsum is carried out to obtain the desired supratip-tip relation. In case of a small hump, it is easier to start shaving off small pieces of the cartilaginous hump to the desired level and then to use a down-cutting rasp to lower the bony dorsum.

When a small bony hump is removed with a rasp, it is certainly less important to elevate the periosteum, the more so as this kind of bony hump resection guarantees a smooth contour of the bony pyramid. When removing the cartilaginous part of a very large hump, stripping off the mucoperichondrium at first on the posterior side of the cartilaginous vault (extramucosal technique), will prevent postoperative irregularities of the dorsum due to damage to the mucoperichondrium (Fig. 8).

There are various additional important points to consider in hump resection:

- Pay attention to the difference in thickness of the overlying soft tissue, which is at its thinnest at the rhinion (the caudal point of the ossa nasalia) (Fig. 9).
- Check whether the nose dorsum shows any small irregularities after hump resection, which should be meticulously smoothed over.
- Check whether enough cartilage has been resected from the anterior edge of the upper lateral.
- Remove all loose bone particles, especially after rasping.
- Correct over-resection by replacing the excised hump after trimming to the appropriate size (Skoog's method), or use an autogenous septal cartilage graft.

A frequently occurring postoperative complication is the 'polly beak', which can be divided into:

- The soft-tissue 'polly beak' (Fig. 10a). This arises when dissection in the surgical plane is not made carefully enough, resulting in scarring of the overlying soft tissues.
- The cartilaginous 'polly beak' (Fig. 10b). This is caused by too little resection of the cartilaginous part, or by a

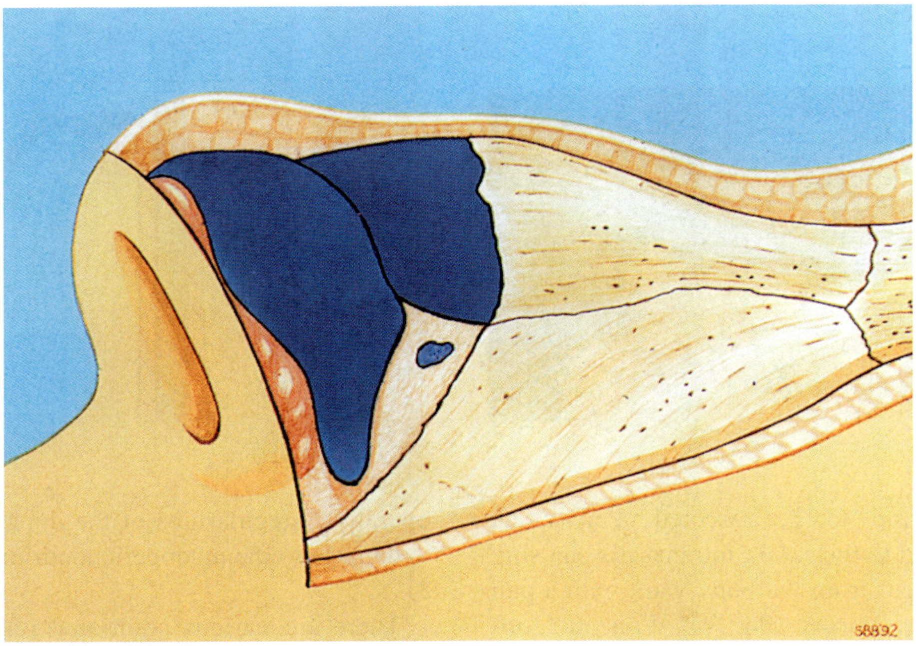

Fig. 9. Illustration of the difference in thickness of the soft tissue lying over the osseocartilaginous vault.

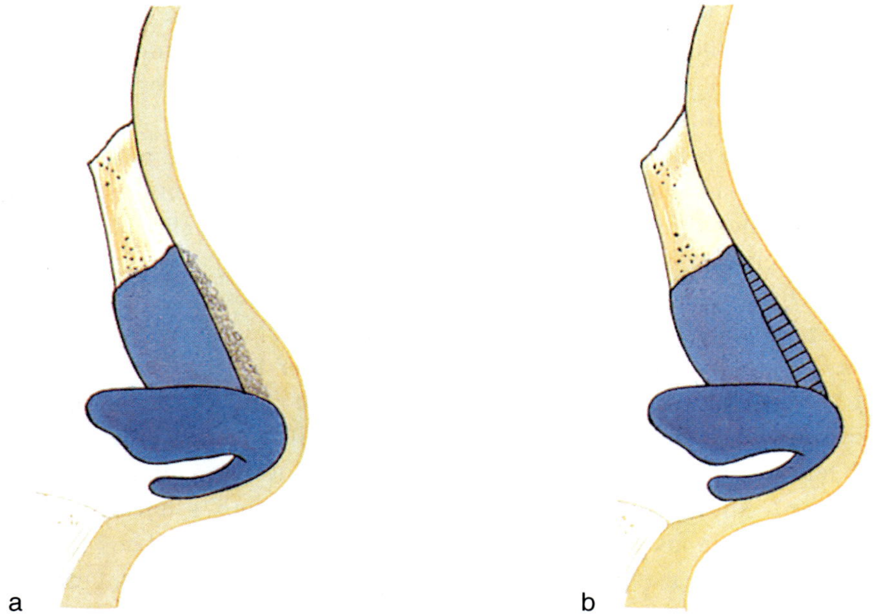

Fig. 10. a. Soft tissue 'polly beak'. *b.* Cartilaginous 'polly beak'.

relatively excessive resection of the bony part of the hump.

– The relative 'polly beak'. This is the result of the tip drooping, due to tip surgery in which the tip support was insufficiently guaranteed (Fig. 10c).

Osteotomies

Osteotomies are required to mobilize the bony pyramid for in-fracture, out-fracture or realignment. With traditional techniques and instruments, mobilization of the bony pyramids results in serious edema and ecchymosis.

The technical refinements of the last

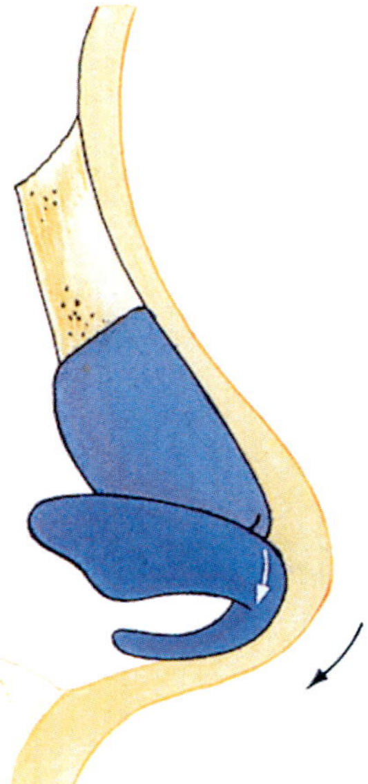

c

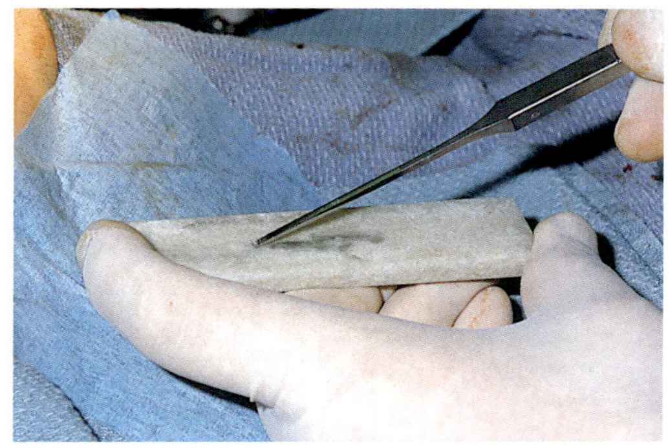

a

Fig. 10c. Relative 'polly beak'.

Fig. 11a. Sharpening of the micro-osteotome 'durante operationem'.

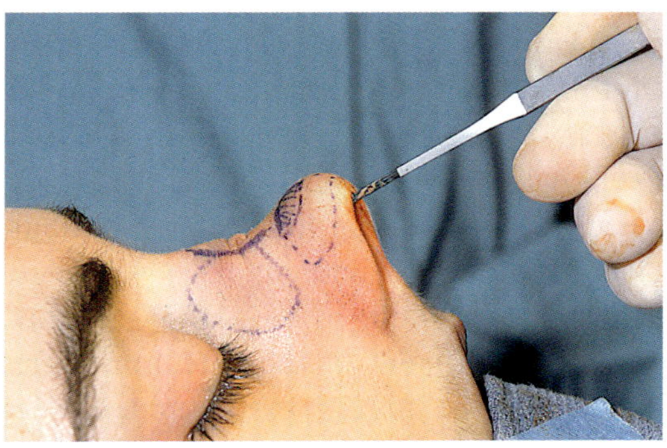

b

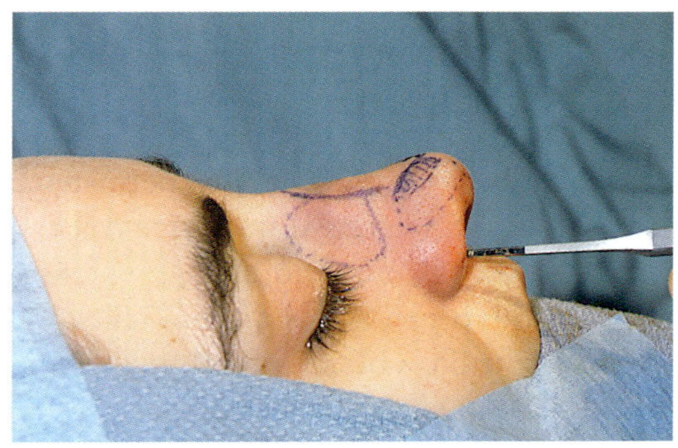

c

Fig. 11b,c. b. Medial-oblique osteotomy. *c.* Low lateral osteotomy.

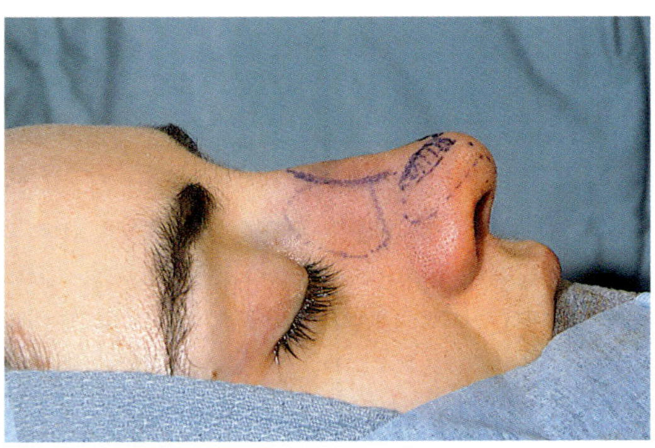

d

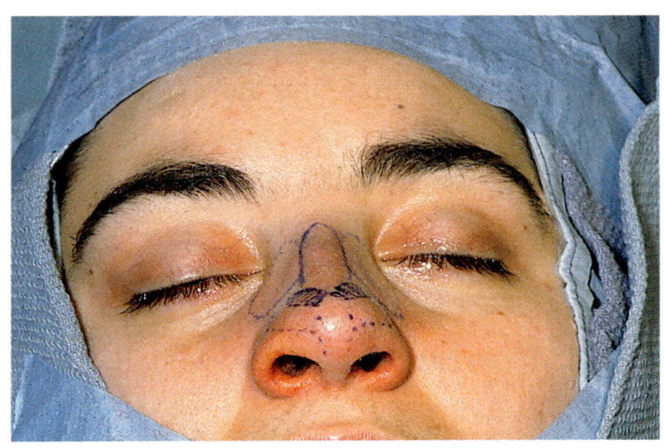

e

Fig. 11d,e. d. Dorsum of the nose after hump resection and micro-osteotomies. *e.* Readjusted bony vault after infracture of the nasal bones.

decade have produced a considerable reduction in ecchymosis and edema, resulting in quicker and better healing. The most important factors are:

- precise placement of the local vasoconstrictive and anesthetic solution
- the use of micro-osteotomes
- preservation of periosteal attachment
- medial-oblique osteotomy to eliminate transverse osteotomy

Well-placed local anesthesia (see Chapter

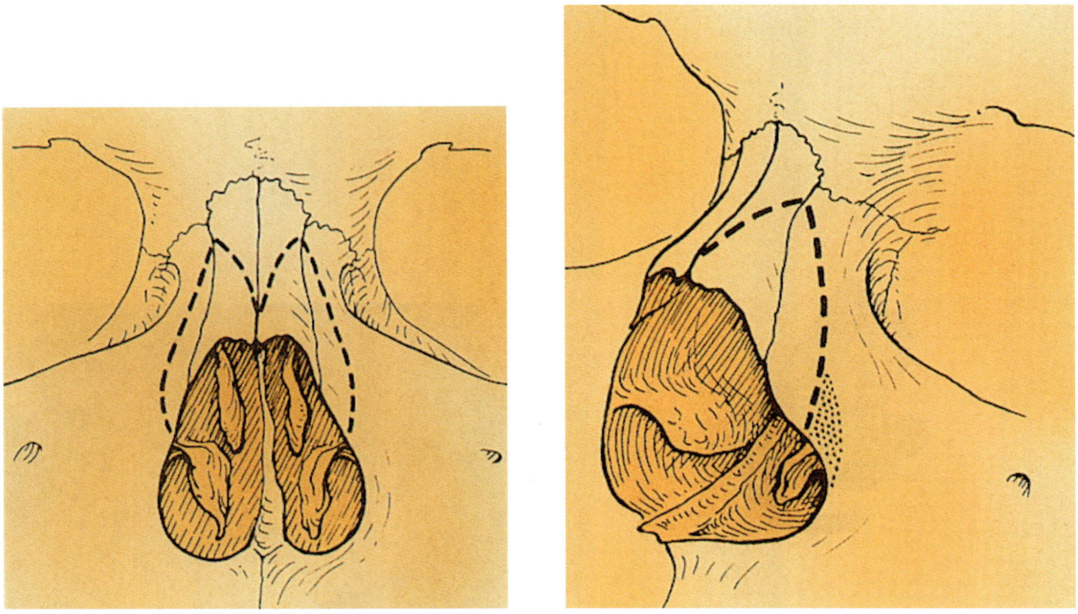

a b

Fig. 12a,b. a. Osteotomy pathway (dotted line) of medial-oblique and lateral osteotomies. *b.* Bony ridge at the base of the lateral wall of the piriform aperture (dotted area) to be preserved in performing a low lateral osteotome followed by infracture of the nasal bone.

4) at least 15 minutes prior to the surgical procedure (on the bony pyramid) is very helpful in reducing bleeding.

With the micro-osteotome if necessary sharpened during surgery (Fig. 11a), it is not necessary to elevate the periosteum. This gives less surgical trauma and leaves the periosteum intact to a large extent in which way it can act as an internal splint. When a medial-oblique osteotomy is combined with a slightly curved lateral osteotomy, there is no need for the traditional transverse osteotomy (Fig. 11b). The crossover point of both osteotomies should not be (and aesthetically there is no need) more cephalic than the intercanthal line, thereby avoiding the thick bone of the radix nasi (Fig. 12a). It is important to leave the (external) periosteal and (internal) mucoperiosteal lining intact as far as possible. Lateral osteotomies can be performed *percutaneously* as well as *intranasally*.

The micro-osteotome will be inserted through the soft tissue of the lateral wall of the piriform aperture, starting at the ascending process of the maxilla at the superior margin of the inferior turbinate. For a low lateral osteotomy, it should then proceed laterally, preserving a bony ridge at the base of the lateral wall of the piriform aperture (Figs. 11c,d,e, and 12b). In this way, any possible narrowing of the airway by in-fracture of the os nasale can be prevented (Fig. 11e). It should then proceed, slowly bending from lateral to medial, as far as the intercanthal line where the medial-oblique osteotomy is carried out. Readjustment of the osteotome after sliding off the bone, prevents unnecessary lesions of the periosteum. A 2-mm osteotome is often sufficient. When the bone is thicker than normal, a 3-mm osteotome is indicated.

In percutaneous lateral osteotomy, a skin incision of 23 mm is made halfway along the planned osteotomy line, after which small point-osteotomies are made cephalically and caudally along the osteotomy line (Fig. 13a,b). Although the percutaneous technique is rather more traumatic than the intranasal one, it gives excellent control. In order to prevent a hematoma, it is wise to put pressure paranasally on both sides at the level of the skin incision after this procedure (three to five minutes).

Additional *intermediate osteotomies* are

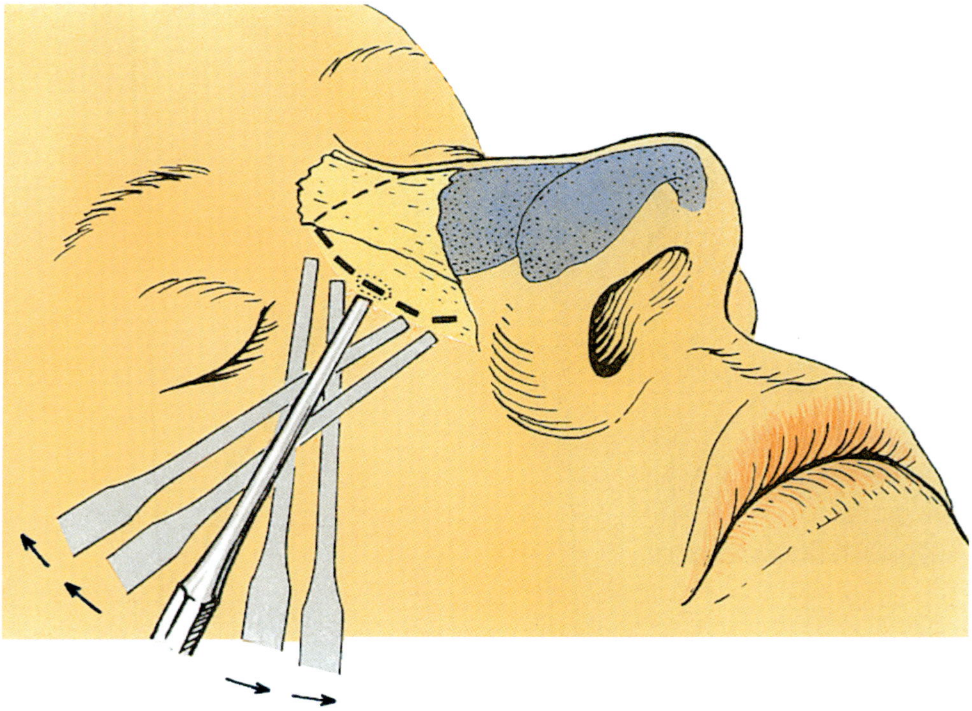

a

Fig. 13a. Percutaneous lateral osteotomy making small point osteotomies along the planned osteotomy line.

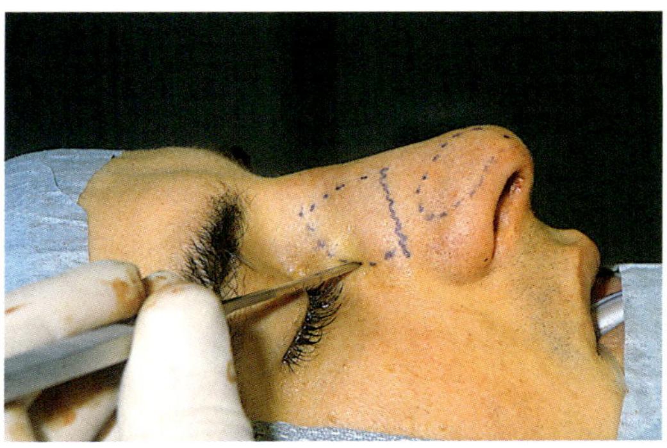

b

Fig. 13b. Percutaneous lateral osteotomy through a skin incision halfway along the planned osteotomy line.

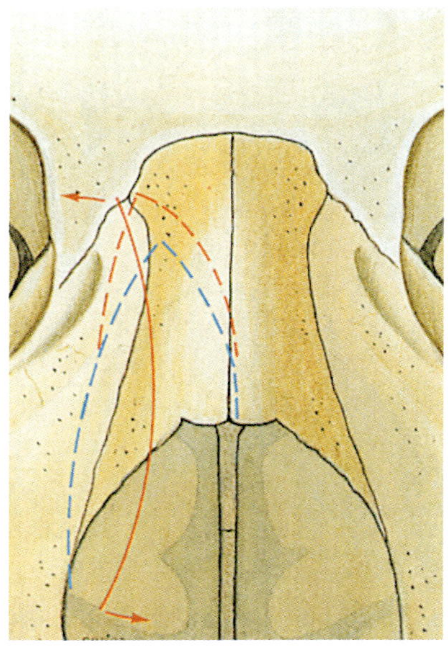

Fig. 14. Rocker phenomenon due to too far cephalically performed osteotomies (red dotted lines).

indicated in an asymmetric bony pyramid. If the traditional transverse osteotomy is indicated, this can either be done percutaneously via a small incision at the level of nasion or an incision in the eyebrow with a micro-osteotome, or intranasally via the lateral osteotomy line, with a special transversely curved osteotome.

Complications which can occur in osteotomies of the bony pyramid are the following:

- An osteotomy carried out insufficiently, after which the bony part springs back into its original position.
- 'Rocker phenomenon' which can occur in osteotomies carried out too far cephalically. When the concave bony part, now curved medially, is repositioned

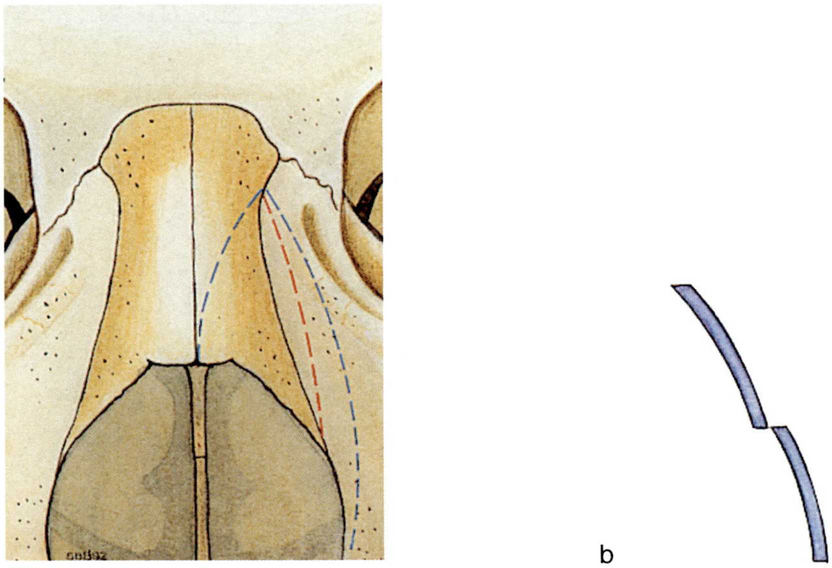

a b

Fig. 15a,b. Staircase phenomenon due to a too far medially performed osteotomy (red dotted line).

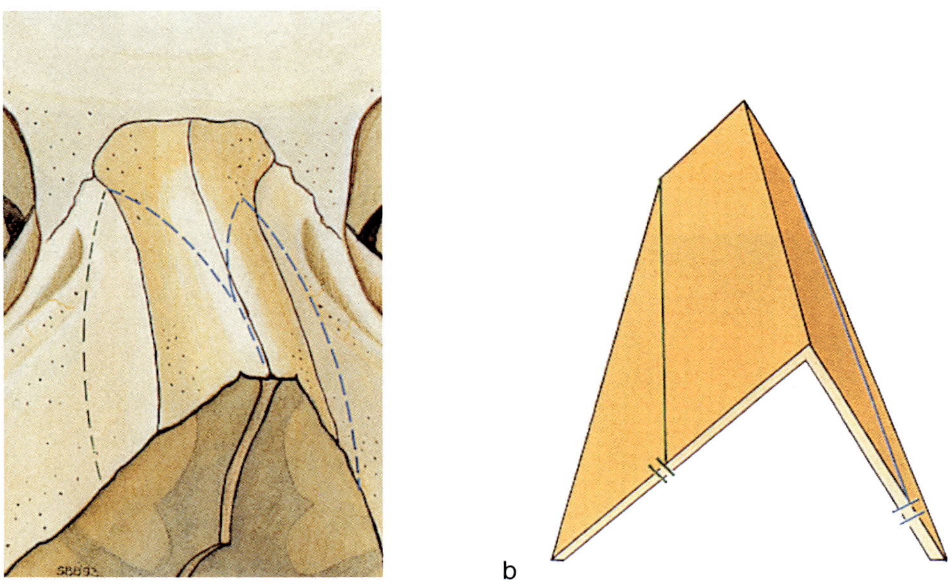

a b

Fig. 16a,b. More medially placed lateral osteotomy (green dotted line) to correct moderate asymmetry of the bony pyramid.

on the caudal or cephalic side, the other part will project (Fig. 14).

- Lateral osteotomies carried out too far medially, in which a staircase phenomenon arises (Fig. 15a,b).
- Callosus (which often disappears spontaneously).

Management of special bony pyramid problems

An asymmetric bony pyramid due to lateral deviation

In a strong deviation of the nose, there may be a large difference between the size of the left and right os nasale, in which case exact repositioning in the midline after standard osteotomies is not possible. If these asymmetries are not too large, a

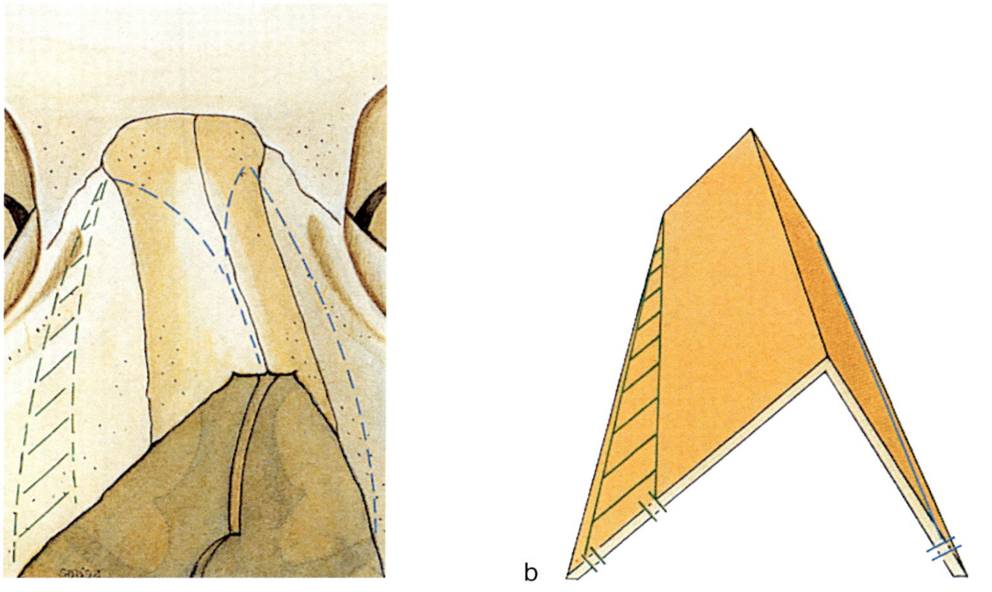

a b

Fig. 17a,b. Resection of a bony wedge (green striped area) in case of severe asymmetry of the bony pyramid.

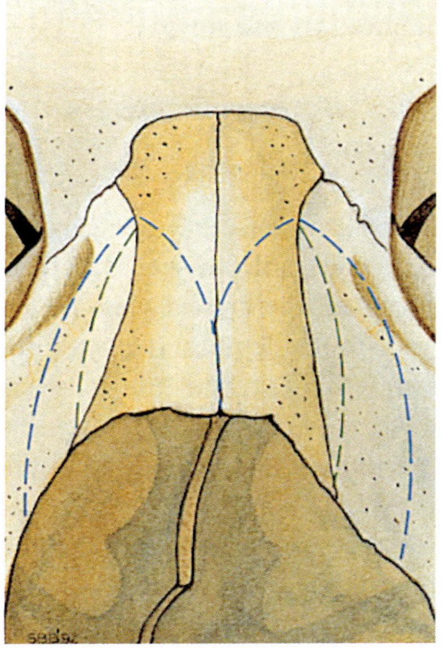

Fig. 18. Supplementary intermediate osteotomies (green dotted lines) to remodel concave and convex bony side walls.

lateral osteotomy, placed more medially on the long side, is often sufficient (Fig. 16a,b). In a very seriously asymmetric bony pyramid, a wedge resection is indicated, whereby a bony wedge is removed on the lateral side of the longest side wall (Fig. 17). When removing a bony wedge, the periosteum will have to be stripped off both sides of the wedge in order to be removed. To obtain adequate repositioning, the septum will also have to be mobilized and corrected, otherwise the chance of the deviation reappearing postoperatively is high.

Abnormally curved nasal bones

In case of a concavity or convexity of a side wall, it is necessary to perform one or more intermediate osteotomies to remodel the bony pyramid (Fig. 18).

Broad trapezoid bony pyramid

With this type of bony pyramid, infracture is not possible by medial-oblique and lateral osteotomies alone. Therefore, a medial wedge resection is mandatory on both medial parts of the nasal bones (Fig. 19).

Radix nasi surgery

The role of the radix nasi is often underestimated in the aesthetic balance of the facial complex. In *frontal* view, the width of the radix nasi should be in good alignment with the natural curve from eyebrow to lateral nasal bone.

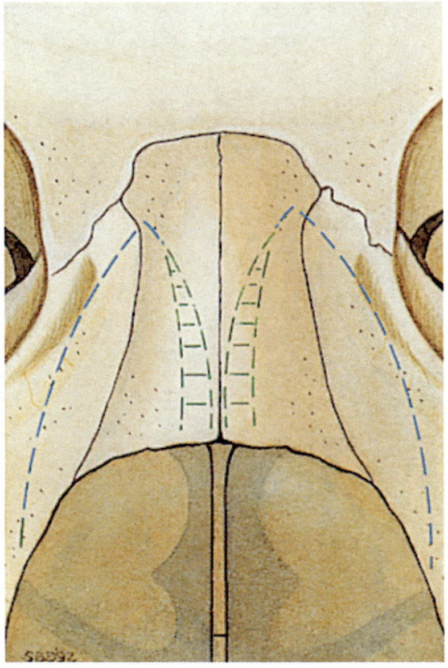

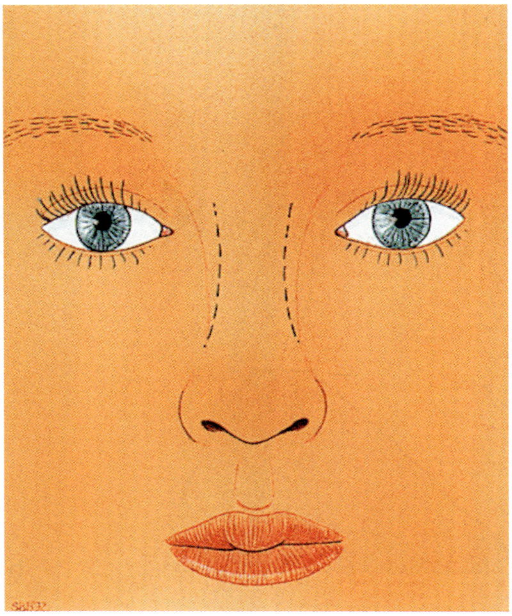

Fig. 19. Resection of medial wedges (green striped areas) to correct a broad trapezoid bony pyramid.

Fig. 20. Proposed correction (dotted lines) of too wide a radix nasi.

Too wide radix nasi is very uncommon and can be corrected by in-fracture, after osteotomies have been placed more cephalically (above the intercanthal line) (Fig. 20). In particular after rhinoplasty, when osteotomies have been placed too cephalically and after too much infracture of the bony pyramid, the radix nasi often becomes too narrow. This can be corrected with out-fracture after re-osteotomies.

In profile, the radix nasi also plays a role in the aesthetic balance of the face, and is characterized by the naso-frontal and naso-facial angles.

A change in the horizontal or vertical position of the deepest depression of the root of the nose (nasion) has a direct effect on the apparent projection and length of the nose. A change in the position of the radix nasi, which is a relatively small surgical procedure, will have a great impact on the appearance of the nose. A dorsal onlay graft gives the nose a longer appearance and the (unchanged) nasal tip a shorter one (see Chapter 7, Fig. 4a,b). Deepening of the naso-facial groove using a chisel or glabella rasp has the opposite effect.

Cartilaginous vault surgery

Resection of the caudal border of the upper laterals

This is indicated as an additional procedure after a considerable shortening of the nose, due to which the caudal parts of the upper laterals protrude into the vestibulum. Care should be taken not to overshorten the upper lateral cartilages, as this may lead to unnatural narrowing of the middle third of the nose. Besides an unaesthetic appearance, over-resection of the upper lateral cartilages may result in functional problems, due to inspiratory collapse of the weakened lateral nasal wall. When shortening the nose, it is a good rule not to resect more from the caudal end of the upper lateral than from the septum (Fig. 21).

Other indications for caudal resection of the upper laterals are internal valve problems caused by pathological returning of the caudal end of the upper lateral, which interfere with normal internal valve functioning.

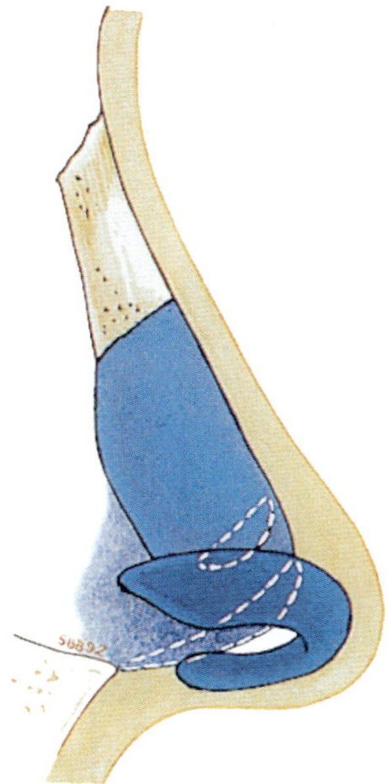

Fig. 21. The resected cartilaginous part of caudal border of the upper laterals and caudal septum in a nose shortening procedure should be approximately of equal length.

Narrowing the cartilaginous vault

In some cases, the cartilaginous vault is trapezoid in shape, due to the flat anterior part of the upper laterals. Resection of a small paraseptal strip of cartilage on both sides will narrow the cartilaginous vault. The technique used for adequate exposure of the cartilaginous dorsum in combination with extramucosal dissection is the same as the one used for resection of a large hump.

Widening the cartilaginous vault

Spreader grafts to widen the cartilaginous vault are indicated for aesthetic reasons when there is a very narrow mid-nose or because of functional problems caused by too sharp an angle (smaller than 10 degrees) of the internal valve. Small strips of autogenic septal cartilage are the first choice as graft material. Using the intranasal approach, they should be placed in an extramucosal pocket between the septum and the lateral cartilages. However, the external approach gives far better control. For technical details see Chapter 9.

In Figures 22-25, pre- and postoperative views of patients are shown who underwent osseocartilaginous vault surgery.

Fig. 22a,b. A patient who underwent a humpresection followed by medial oblique, (endonasal) lateral micro-osteotomies and infraction with moderate edema and ecchymosis two days postoperatively (*a*); and already resolving ecchymosis six days postoperatively (*b*) just before removal of the Denver splint.

a

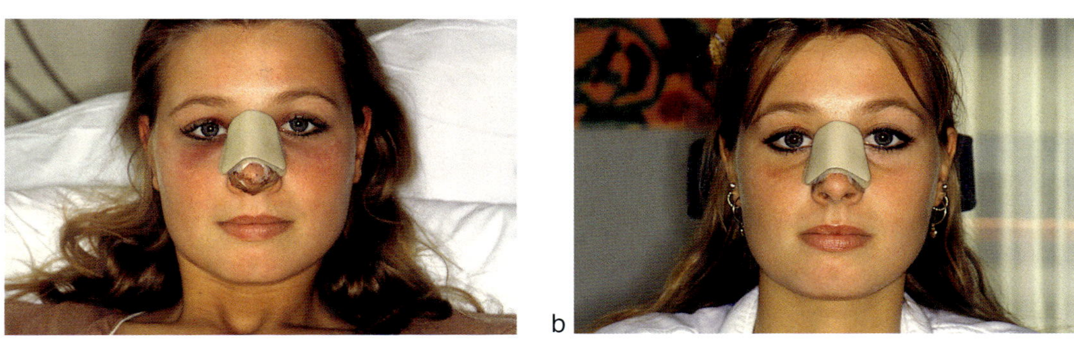

b

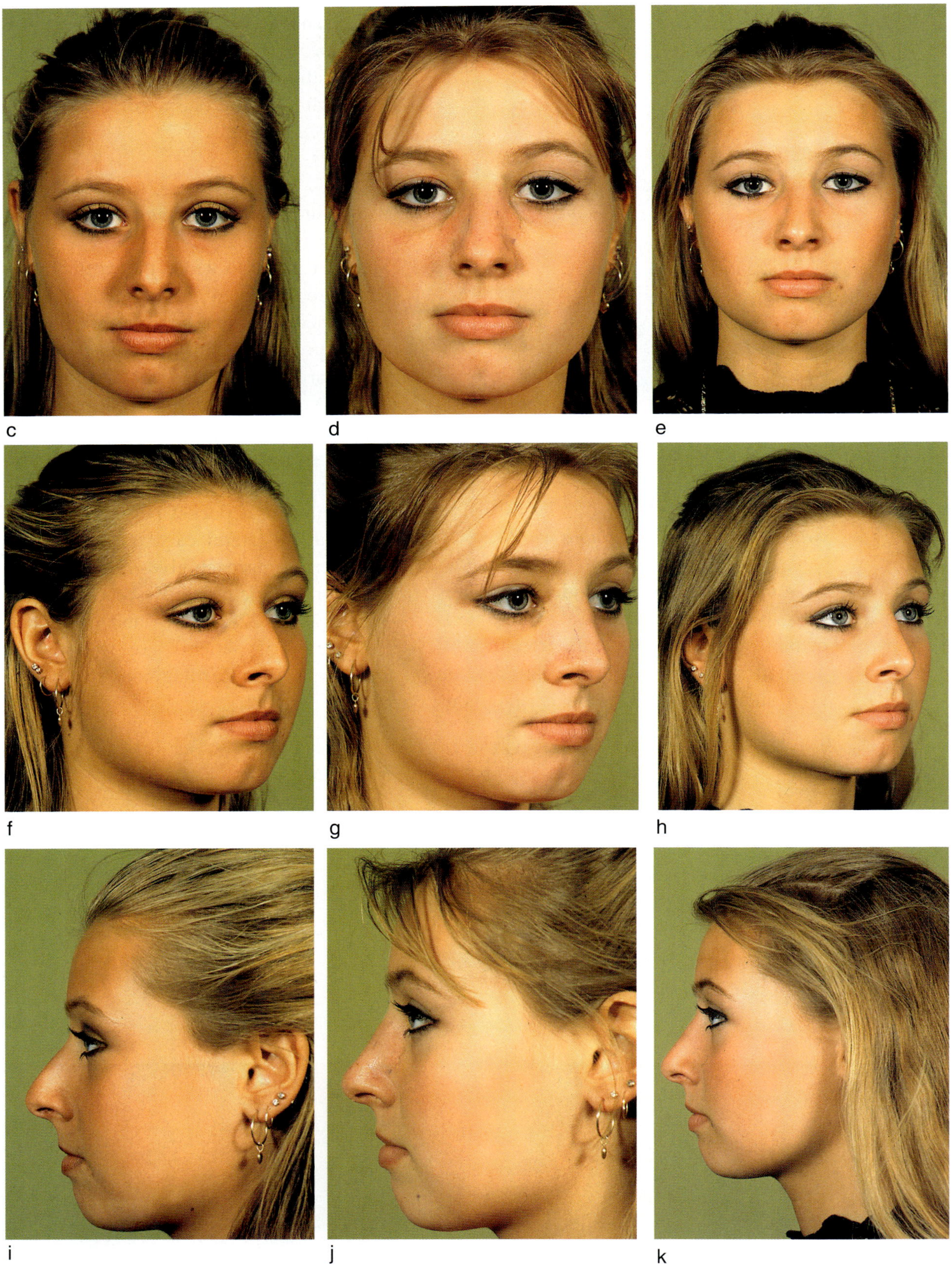

Fig. 22c-m. Pre- (*c,f,l*) and short-term (*d,g,i*) (six days postoperatively after removal of the Denver splint) and long-term (*e,h,k,m*) postoperative views of the same patient (*a,b*) who underwent a hump resection followed by predial-oblique, (endonasal) lateral view-osteotomies and infraction of the nasal bones.

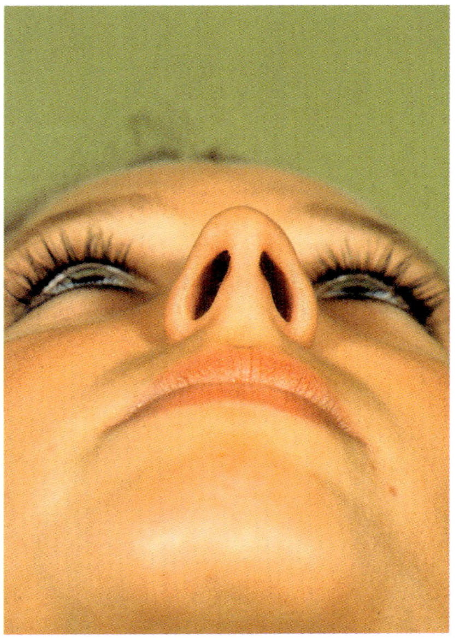
l

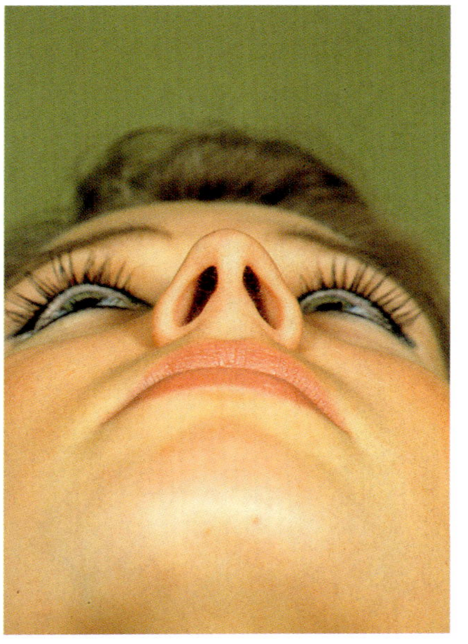
m

Fig. 22l-m

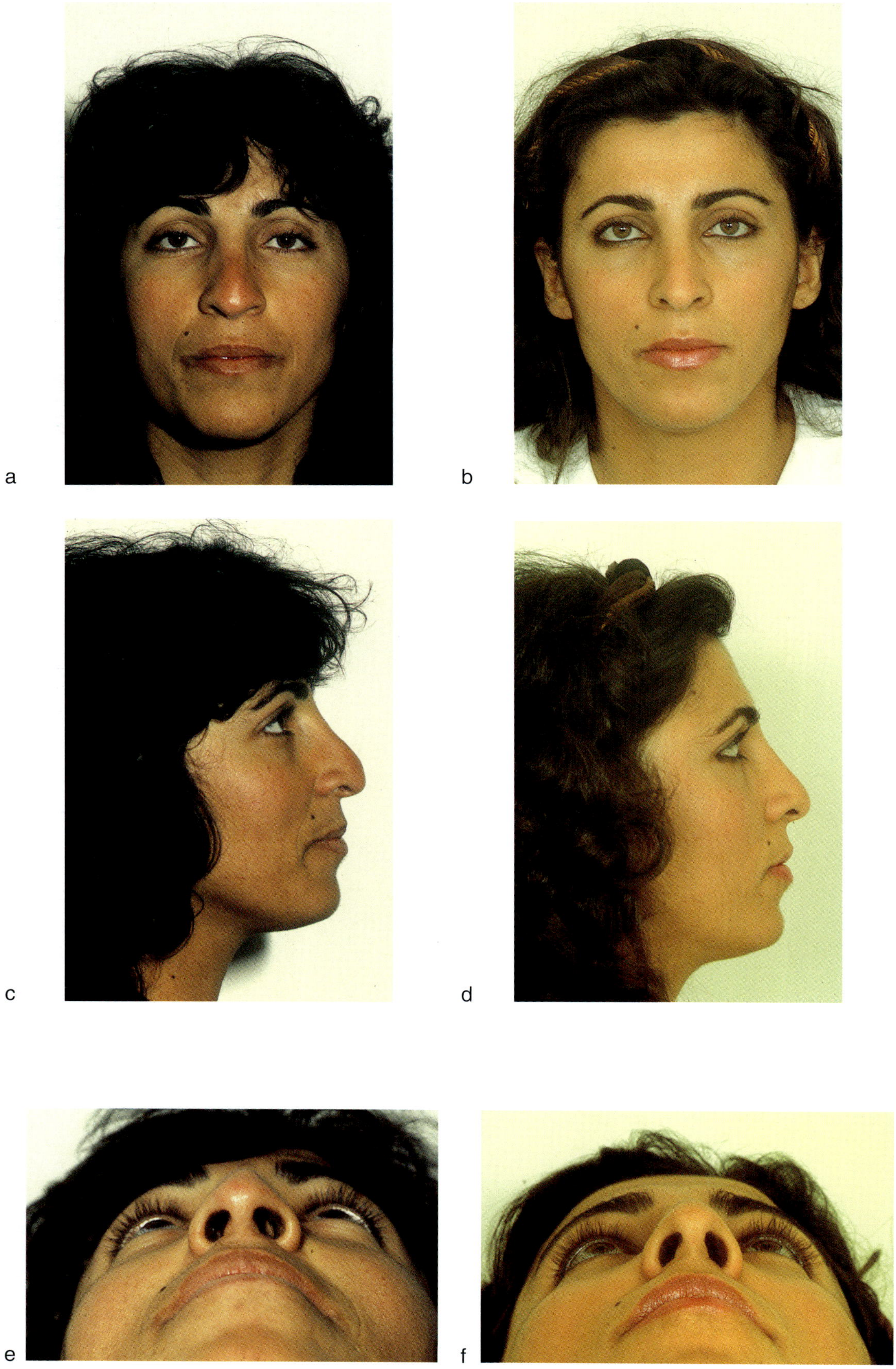

Fig. 23a-f. Pre- and post-operative views of a patient who underwent a revision rhinoplasty to correct her cartilaginous polly beak.

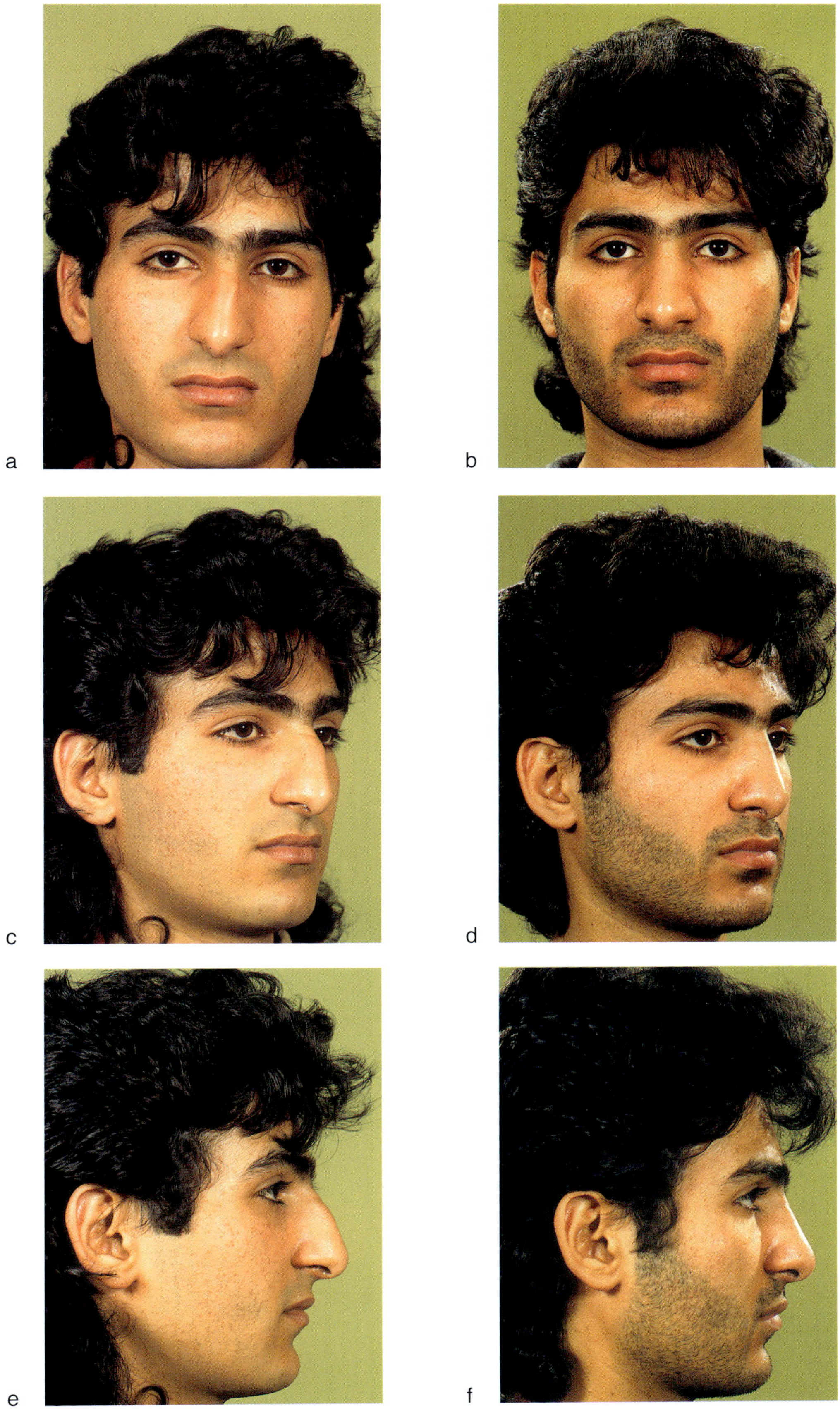

Fig. 24a-f. Pre- and postoperative views of a patient with a tension nose due to overdevelopment of the cartilaginous septum who underwent a rhinoplasty by the endonasal approach to reduce the osseocartilaginous vault and to correct a slight downward rotation of the tip with resection of a caudal strip of septal cartilage.

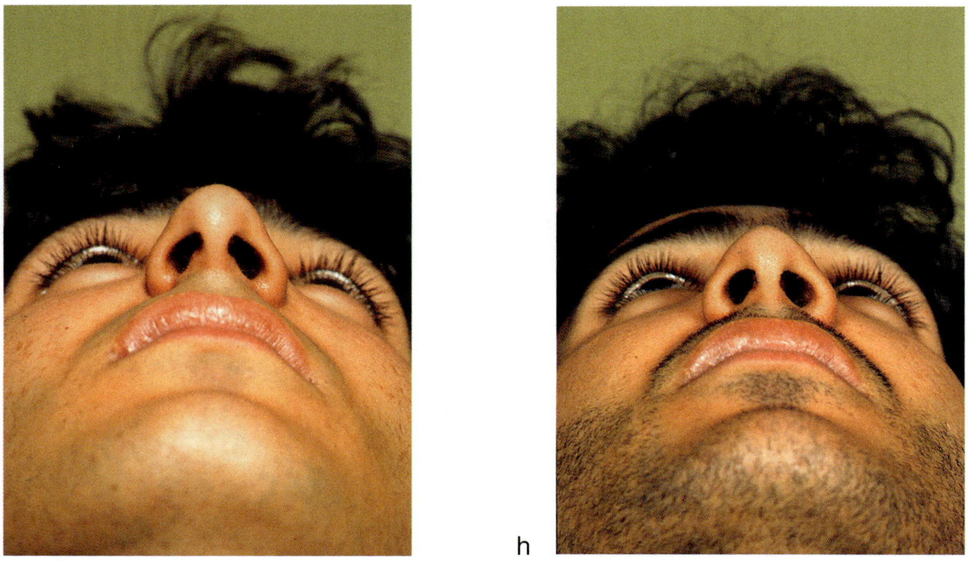

g h

Fig. 24g-h

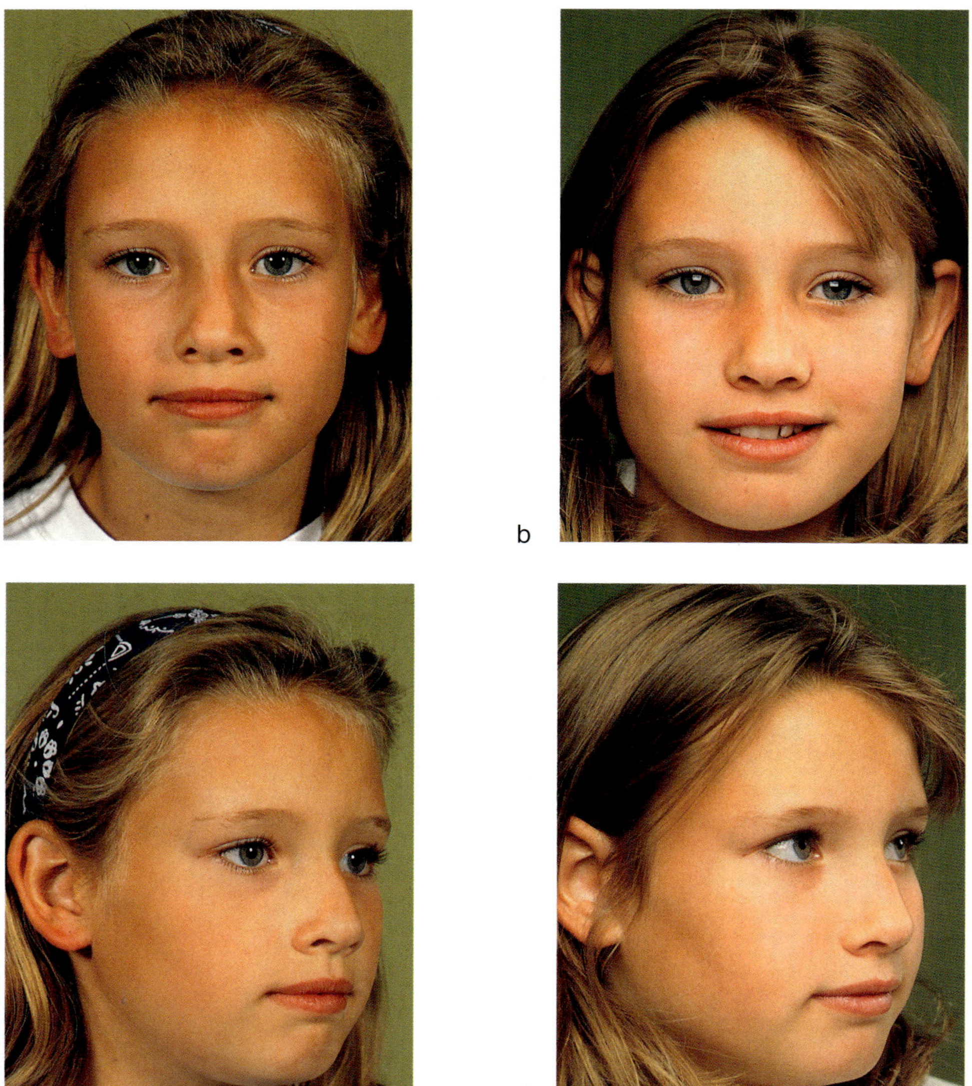

a b c d

Fig. 25a-f. Pre- and postoperative views of a ten-year-old girl who underwent an endonasal septorhinoplasty due to a posttraumatic septal deviation with nasal airway impairment and a gradually increasing deviation of the nasal dorsum. Realignment of the dorsum was performed with medial oblique and (endonasal) lateral osteotomies. When performing rhinoplasties in children, the surgeon should be aware that operating on a growing nose can interfere with midfacial growth. He has to weigh up the possible advantages (psychological and growth directional) against possible disadvantages (growth inhibition). From the experimental work of the Verwoerd group, we know that, in contrast to surgery of the cartilaginous vault, mobilization of the nasal bones does not lead to specific morphological anomalies in further growth (see Chapter 20).

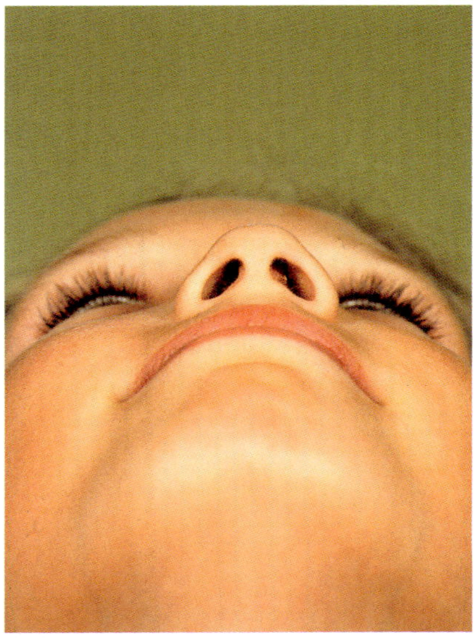

e

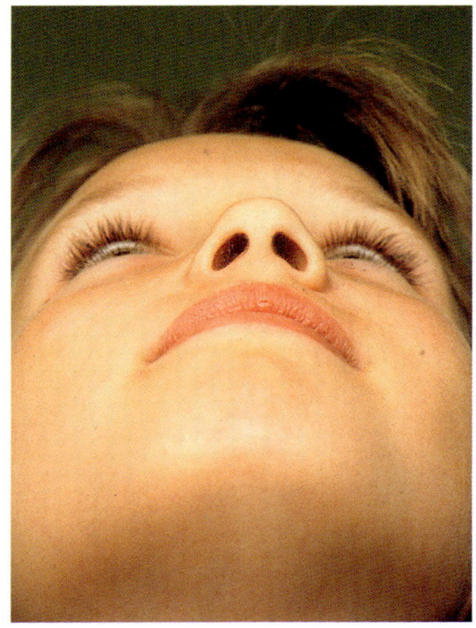

f

Fig. 25e-f

12: OPEN-TIP RHINOPLASTY

H.D. Vuyk and T.D. Zijlker

Introduction

The open approach for rhinoplasty offers excellent exposure of the various components of the nose *in situ*, enabling the surgeon to operate with precision and confidence. With careful attention to columellar skin flap elevation and closure of the incision, skin necrosis and visible scar formation are very unlikely sequelae. The extra time spent on the exposure is important for increased insight into nasal deformities, leading to more detailed reconstructions.

Indications for the open approach depends on the surgeon's preference. The open technique may be used in all rhinoplasty cases, except in those where the surgeon is able to diagnose all nasal deformities preoperatively and can correct them satisfactorily with the closed approach.

This chapter describes the technical aspects of the open approach in a step-by-step fashion. Thereafter, a relatively new grafting technique for nasal tip surgery is introduced.

Exposure

The operation may begin with a hemitransfixion incision. Thus, septoplasty and harvesting of cartilage grafting material can be performed before the rhinoplasty. The hemitransfixion incision is made in the membranous septum and is not connected with incisions used in the open approach. Thereafter, the nasal skeleton is exposed using a mid-columellar incision (Fig. 1a). The ultimate scar in the middle columellar region is supported by the intact medial crurae, which diminishes scar contraction. For the same purpose, the incision (No. 11 blade) is not straight over the columella, but broken using an inverted V (Fig. 2). The mid-columellar incision is extended with marginal incisions (No. 15 blade) (Figs. 1b and 3).

The columellar skin flap is elevated superficially to the medial crura with blunt and sharp scissor dissection, leaving as much soft tissue as possible on the skin flap (Figs. 4 and 5). This enhances the viability of the columellar skin flap, while

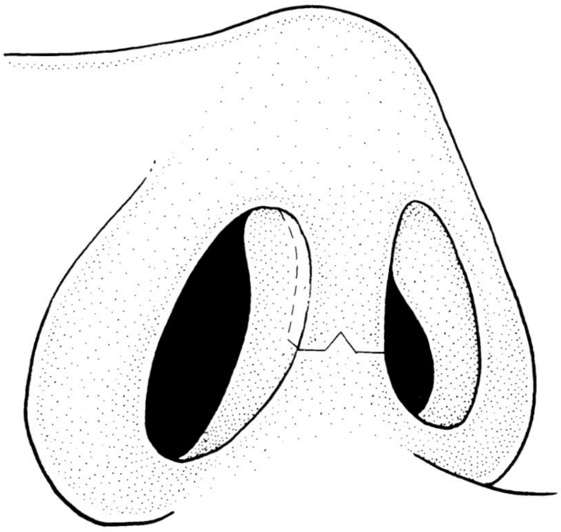

a

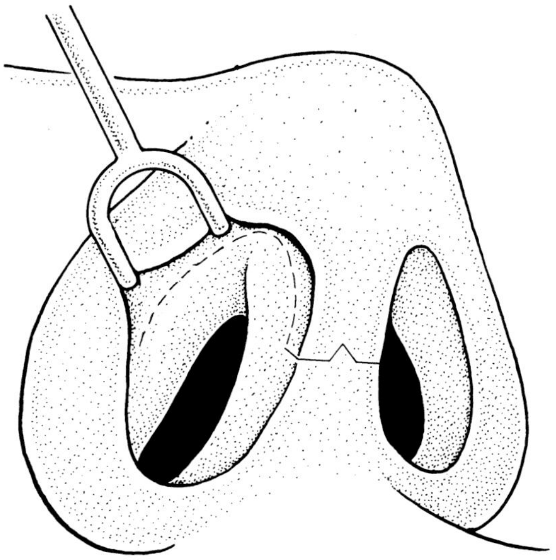

b

Fig. 1a,b. Open rhinoplasty incision schematically depicted, basal view.

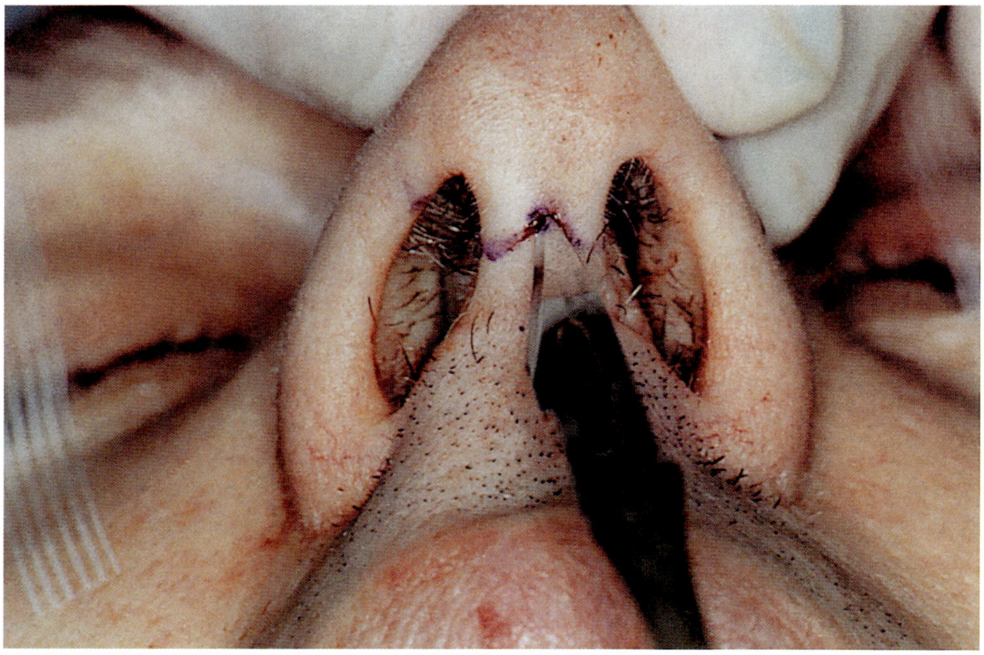

Fig. 2. Mid-columellar broken incision with a No. 11 blade.

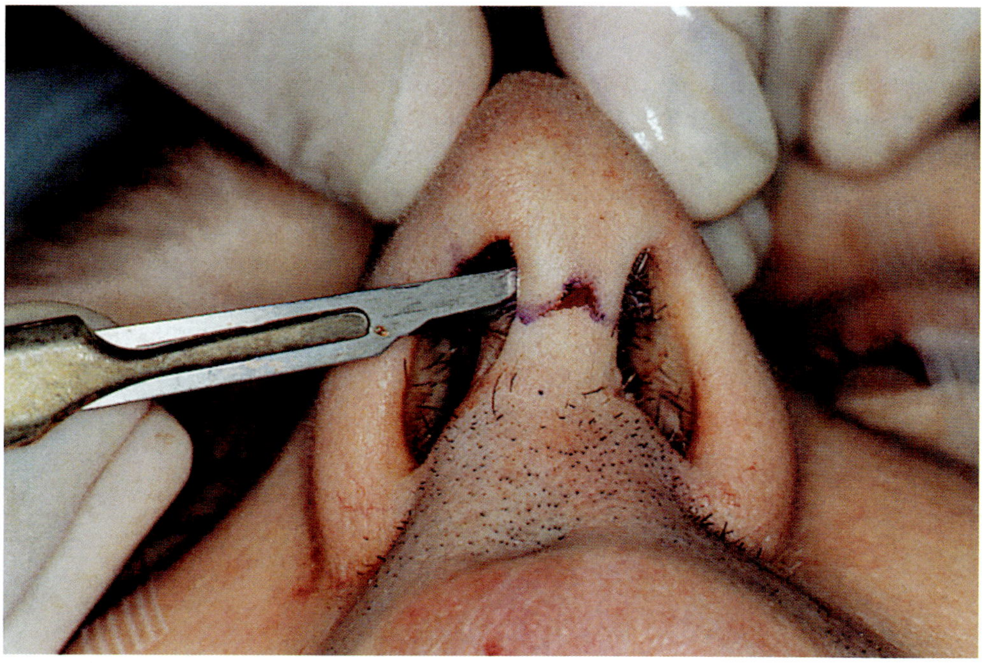

Fig. 3. A No. 15 blade incising the vestibular skin.

the supraperichondrial plane is relatively bloodless. The upper lateral cartilages, lower lateral cartilages and nasal dorsum up to the nasal frontal angle, can be exposed in their undisturbed positions (Fig. 6).

Division of the medial inter-crural ligaments offers extensive exposure down to the premaxillary spine. However, it is preferable to keep the inter-crural ligaments intact and to use the hemitransfixion for work on the septum and nasal spine. After separating the ULC from the septum, the whole septum, including the

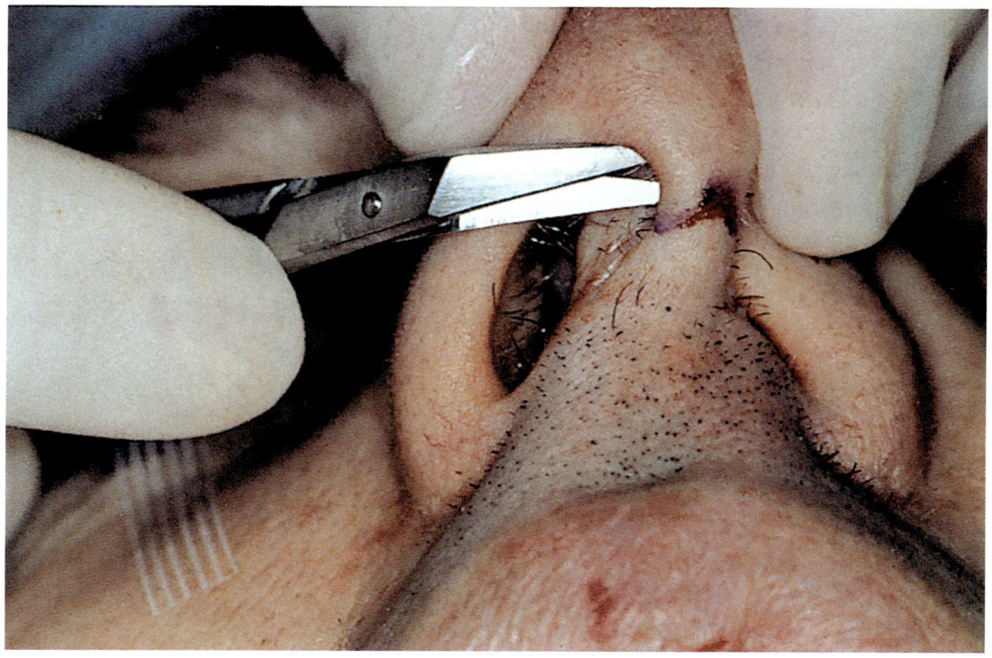

Fig. 4. Elevation of columellar flap with converse scissors.

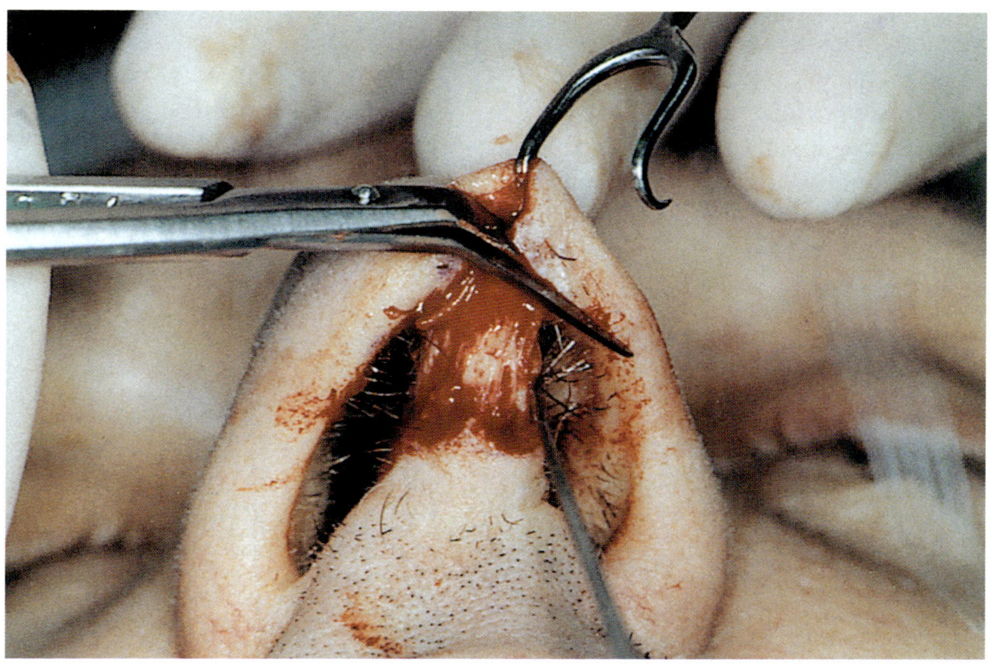

Fig. 5. Skin hook and scissors used to perform marginal incisions and elevate the skin flap under direct vision.

nasal valve, can be viewed from below (comparable to hemitransfixion exposure) and also from above. This may be advantageous in case of dorsal septal deflection, nasal valve problems or septal perforation.

After having achieved wide exposure with the open approach, all rhinoplasty maneuvers deemed necessary can be performed under direct vision with the use of both hands. However, thorough understanding and skill are necessary to achieve good results. The various chapters in this book deal with the technical details of rhinoplasty. All these can be applied using the open approach. The closure of open rhinoplasty incisions will be described in detail here. Thereafter, a new trend in nasal tip surgery which has become popular in combination with the open approach will be described in the second part of this chapter.

Closure

Before closure, the skin at the angle of the lateral marginal incision and horizontal incision is undermined to prevent trapdoor deformities (Fig. 7). Simple 5–0 nylon is used to close the columellar incision precisely (Fig. 8). No subcutaneous sutures are necessary. Meticulous care should be taken in closing wound edges when they are of unequal thickness.

Eversion of skin edges is strived for. Marginal incisions are closed with 5–0 absorbable suture material, as in the routine closed approach. The columellar sutures are removed on day 4, the sutures at the junction of the horizontal columellar and vertical marginal incision on day 7. If significant increase of nasal tip projection occurs, it is advisable to prevent too much tension on the closure line by creating an advancement flap of the inferior columella before closure by extending the vertical marginal incision

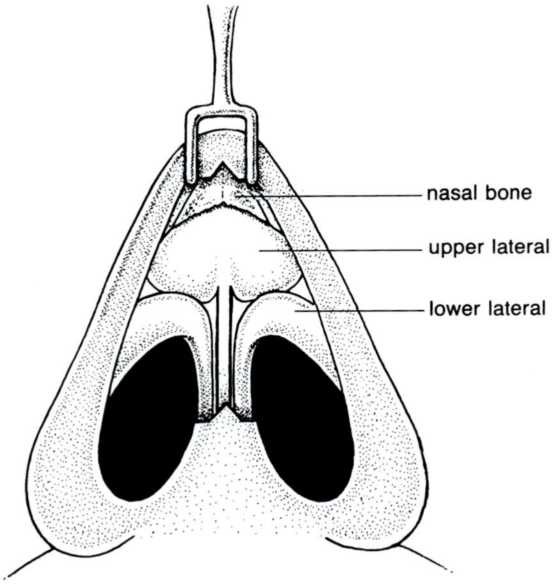

Fig. 6. Undistorted view of lower lateral cartilages, upper lateral cartilages and nasal dorsum.

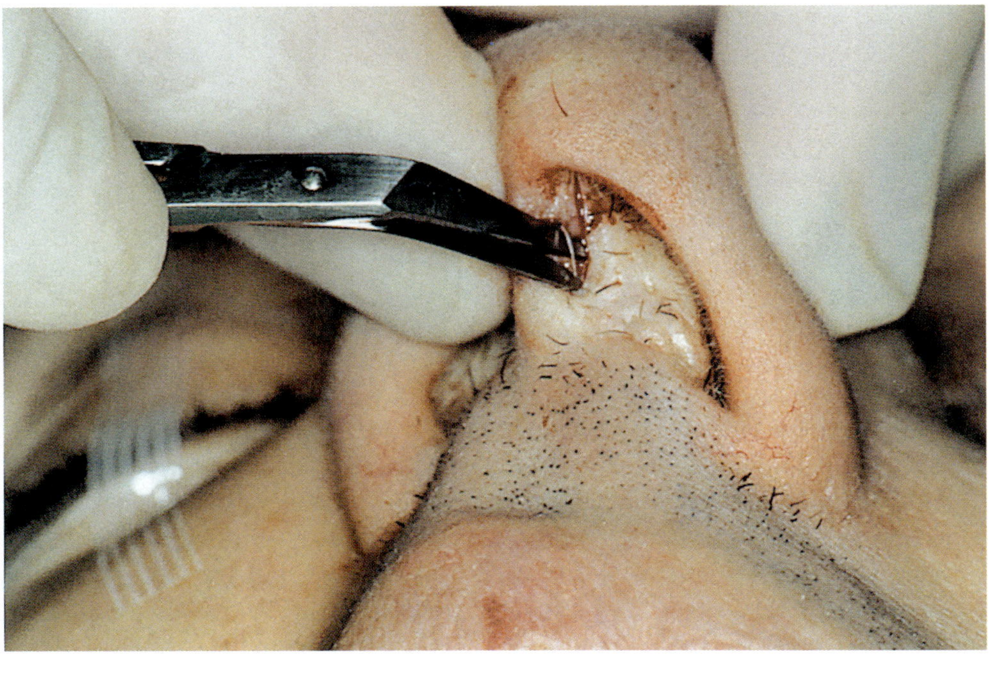

Fig. 7. Undermining of lower columellar wound edge.

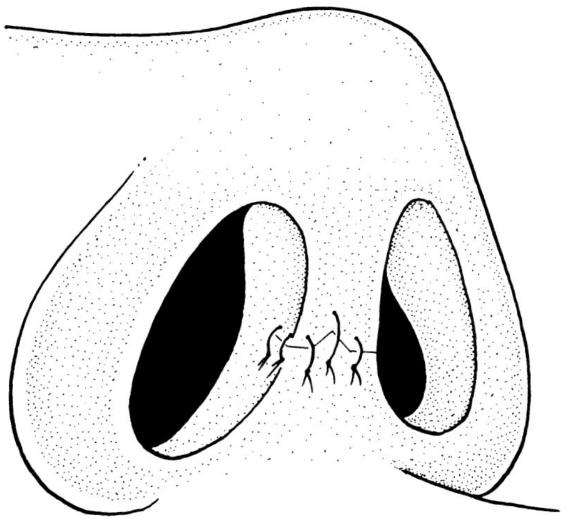

Fig. 8. Closure of open rhinoplasty skin incisions.

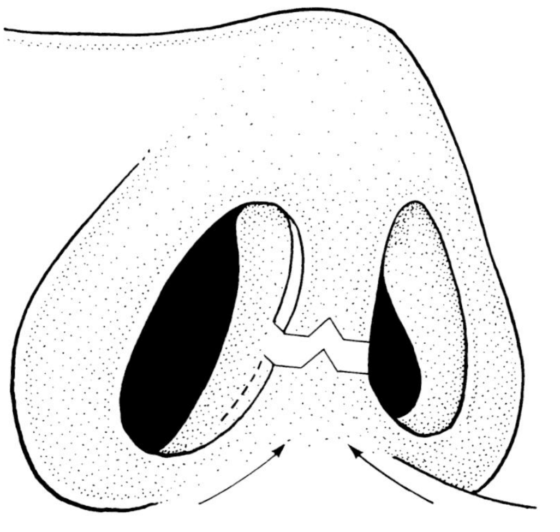

Fig. 9. Advancement flap of columellar base which developed after extending the vertical aspect of the marginal incisions.

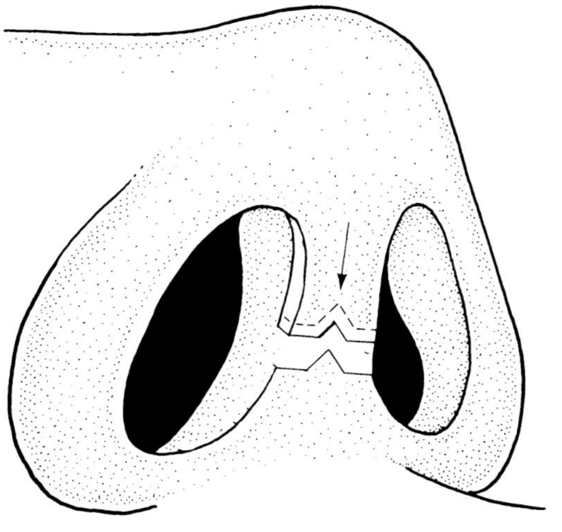

Fig. 10. Shortening of columellar flap.

(Fig. 9). If significant tip deprojection occurs, there may be a tendency for the redundant columellar skin to form a hanging columella. This 1 or 2 mm of excess skin can be excised before closure (Fig. 10).

Cartilage tip grafts

Rhinoplasty has evolved from a predominantly reduction procedure to surgery of a more precise and conservative nature. Emphasis now lies on conservation, reconstruction and even augmentation, and less on reduction. The major unpredictable factor in reduction rhinoplasty is the limited contractibility and pliability of the skin and soft tissues over the nose, especially in patients with thick skin. This uncertain factor can be controlled by creating a stronger projecting underlying nasal skeleton to which the skin and soft tissues can adapt themselves. Moreover, a stronger profile conforms with modern aesthetics. The key to a modern high dorsal profile is adequate and balanced nasal tip projection. Cartilage grafting of the nasal tip and columella may give control over nasal tip projection which is otherwise hard to obtain. Shape and rotation may also be improved with grafting techniques. The open approach has greatly facilitated and improved cartilage tip grafting techniques. As cartilage tip grafting complies with modern rhinoplasty principles, the technique will be described in detail.

Graft harvesting

Autogenous cartilage grafting material has distinct advantages over other grafting material for nasal reconstruction, because of its superior long-term survival rates, easy availability and low risk of infection. Septal cartilage is ideal for tip grafting due to its proper flat shape and stiffness. It can be harvested through a Killian incision leaving the attachment of the medial crura

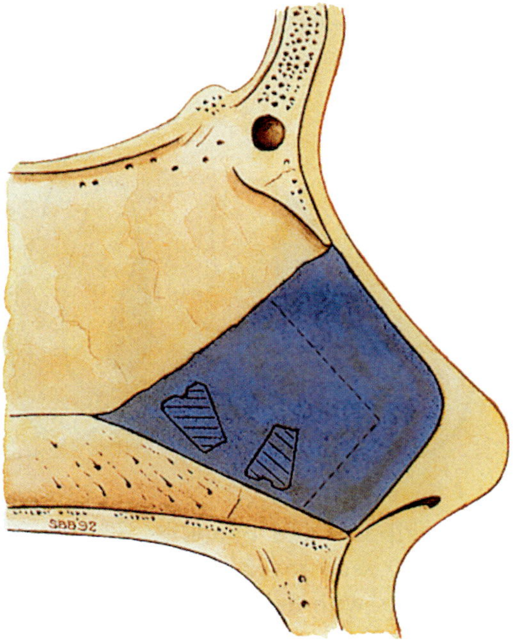

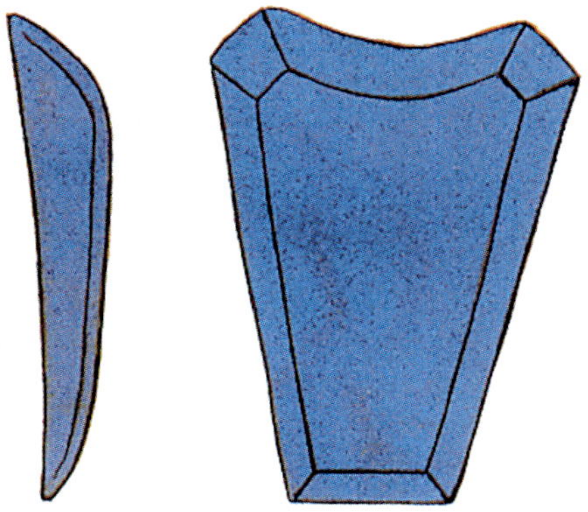

Fig. 11. Cartilage harvesting from the septum.

Fig. 12. The three-dimensional sculptured tip graft.

to the septum intact, or via a hemitransfixion incision when the caudal septum needs modification. The graft is best taken from the thick areas of the septum lying at the junction of the perpendicular plate and the vomer (Fig. 11). Other parts of the septum, leaving a dorsal and caudal strut of at least 1 cm, can be used as a columellar strut. If insufficient septal cartilage is available, cartilage may be obtained from the concha of the ear. For technical details see Chapter 7.

Tip grafts are preferably taken from the area adjacent to the ear canal, including the thickened part of the cavum conchae in the graft. This part shows a helpful curvature which, when judiciously used, can mimic the double break of the nasal tip. However, septal cartilage is preferred to ear cartilage, as the latter is more pliable and generally more strongly curved.

Sculpturing

The shape and size of the graft should be individually adapted, varying with each nose. A flat rectangular piece of cartilage is carved so that one end is notched in the center, leaving the blunted corners approximately 6–8 mm apart to form two tip-defining points (Fig. 12). The graft narrows away from the tip so that the width of the base is 3–4 mm. The length of the graft varies, but is usually about 10–12 mm. In some cases, the graft may extend along the entire length of the columella to increase support and/or augment a retracted columella. The thickness of the graft may vary from 1–3 mm. The most inferior portion of the graft is thinned and the edges are bevelled to blend the tip graft into the underlying structures. A double tip graft may be used to increase dorsal length and to add strength to weak grafts, such as those from the ear. Final precise sculpturing can be performed *in situ* after fixation of the graft to the alar cartilages.

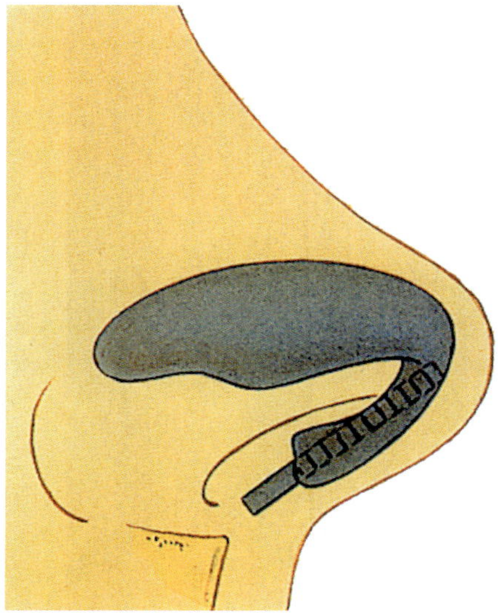

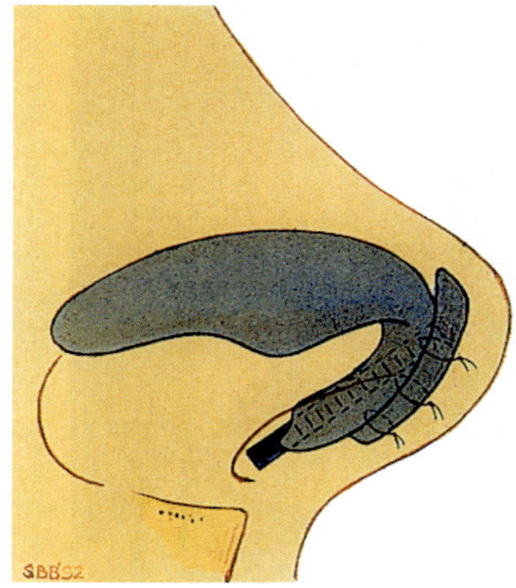

Fig. 13. The columellar strut.

Fig. 14. Sculptured tip graft sutured to the underlying alar cartilages.

Grafting

A stable basis is a prerequisite for tip grafting. A columella strut is used in all cases, lending strength to the medial crura and increasing its potential support. The graft extends from 1–2 mm above the nasal spine to the level of the angle, just below the domes of the alar cartilages (Fig. 13). This sandwich construction is fixed to the septum with an absorbable mattress-type suture.

To create a symmetrical bed for the graft, and especially if there is a hanging columella, the caudal margins of the medial crura may be trimmed. Sculpturing of the lateral crura can be performed, taking care to leave a strip of cartilage of at least 8 mm in width to prevent weakening of the graft base. The tip graft is secured by from four to six prolene sutures (Ethicon 8697) to the underlying domal and crural cartilage (Fig. 14). The exact position depends on the specific indications defined preoperatively. The graft can be sculptured *in situ*. In thin-skinned patients, in particular, the graft should blend imperceptively into the surrounding structures to prevent unnatural points and ridges.

Indications

Cartilaginous grafting of the nasal tip may be indicated in cases which require additional support, projection, contouring or camouflaging. In general, lack of adequate tip projection is the main indication. With tip grafting, the nasal dorsum can be maintained at a higher level, leading to a stronger, more natural appearing projecting structure. Provided the graft is well-shaped and positioned, a defined shape for the domal region of the tip may be produced. Using the tip graft's interdomal width, the degree of tip definition and infratip lobular shape can be controlled. In patients with thick skin and weak lower lateral cartilages, tip grafting is the only precise method to add definition to the domal area.

Asymmetries or irregularities can be camouflaged, making the graft especially suitable for cleft-lip surgery. After transection of the domes of the alar cartilages, tip grafts may be used for camouflaging the sharp edges of the divided alar cartilages. The dorsal length may be increased by 2–3 mm by using a very thick or sometimes double-layered tip graft.

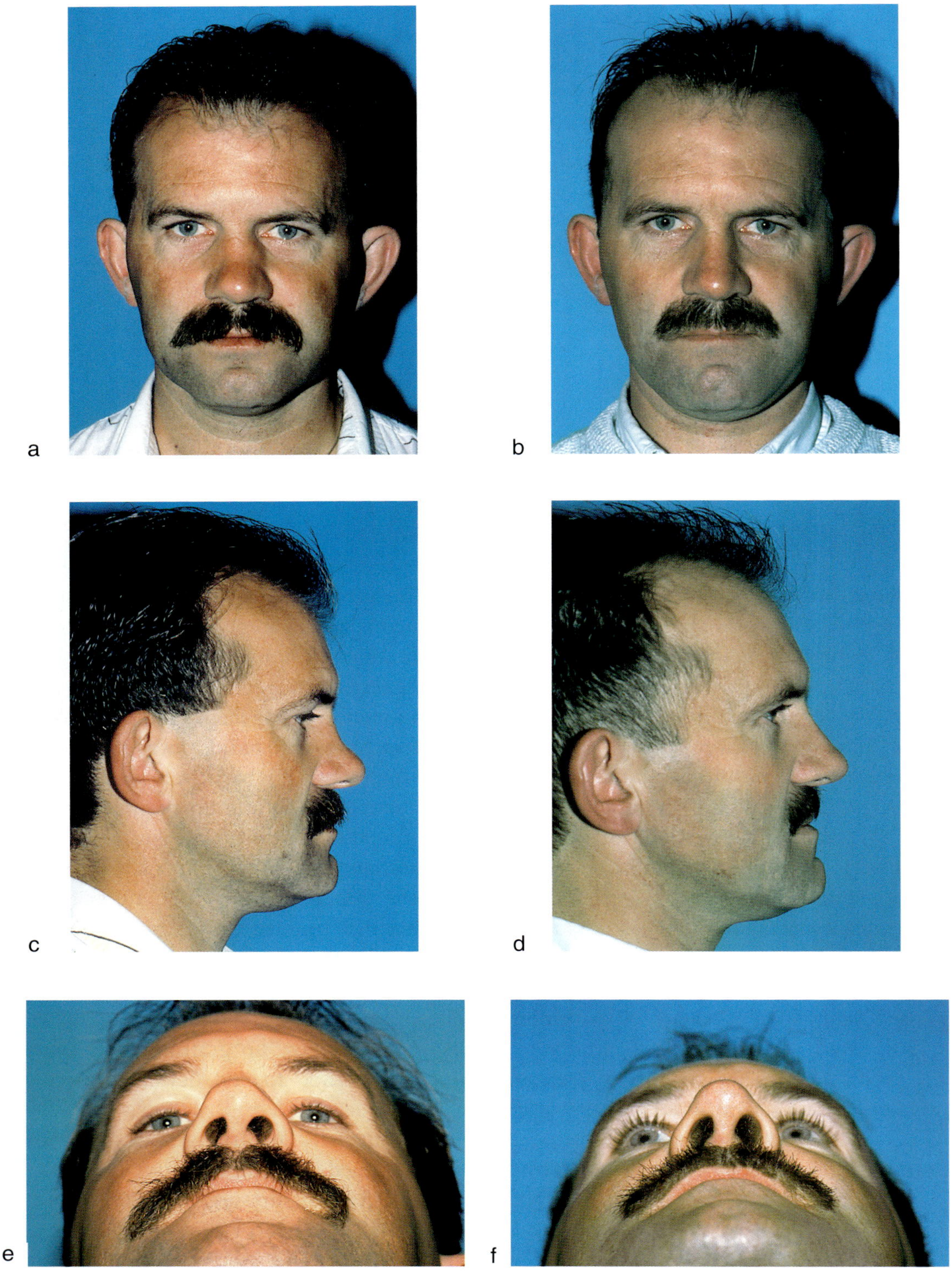

Fig. 15a-f. Pre- and postoperative views of a male patient. Round tip restructured after deprojection with an overlap of medial crura, cephalic trim and reprojection with columellar strut and tip graft. Additionally an infracture was performed on the left side and the whole nasal norsum was augmented with an autogenous conchal cartilage graft.

This small increase in dorsal length or counter rotation of the nasal tip can significantly improve the overall appearance of a short or over-rotated nose.

Conclusions

The open approach offers excellent exposure in rhinoplasty. This advantage more than outweighs the (avoidable) risks

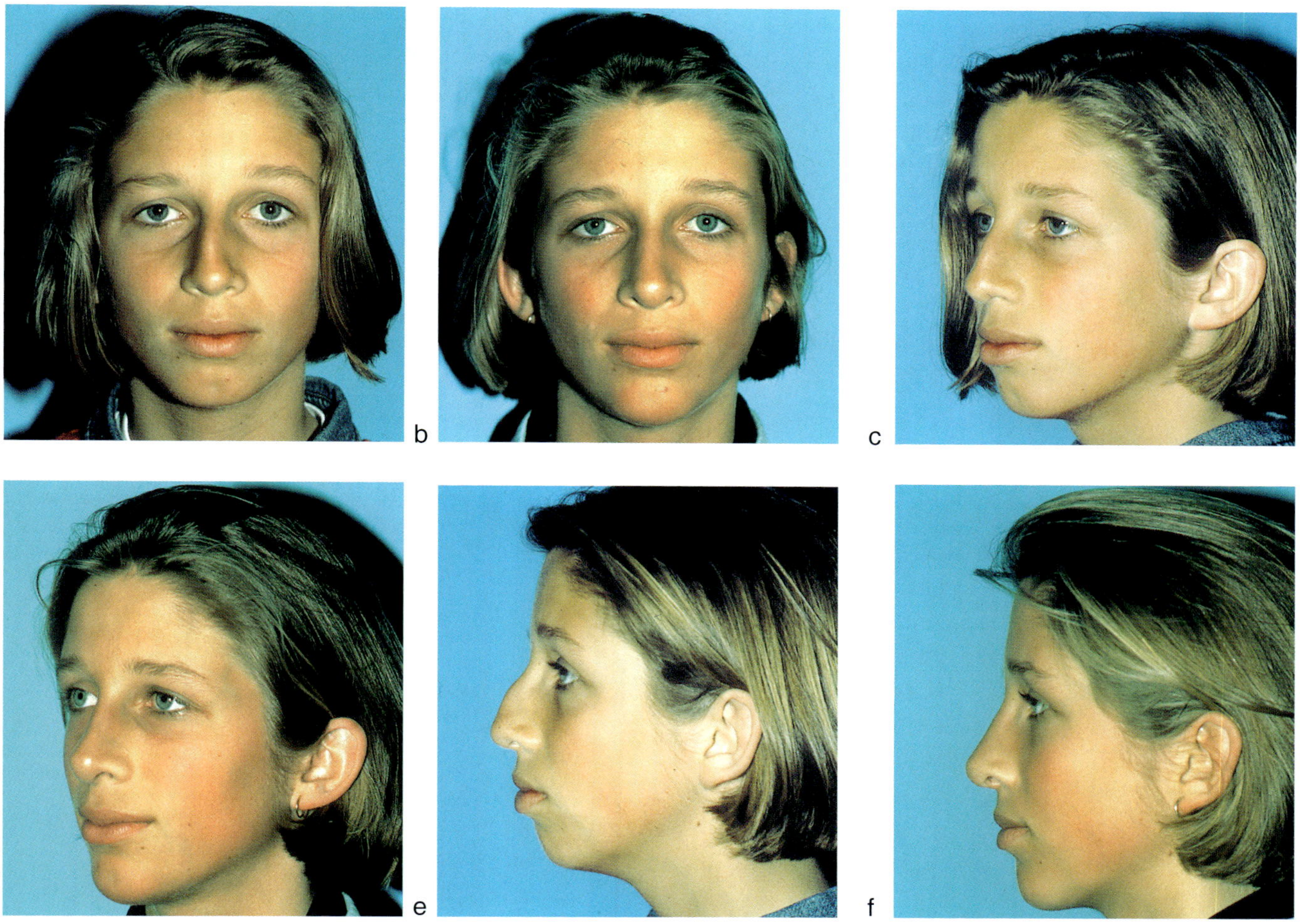

a b c d e f

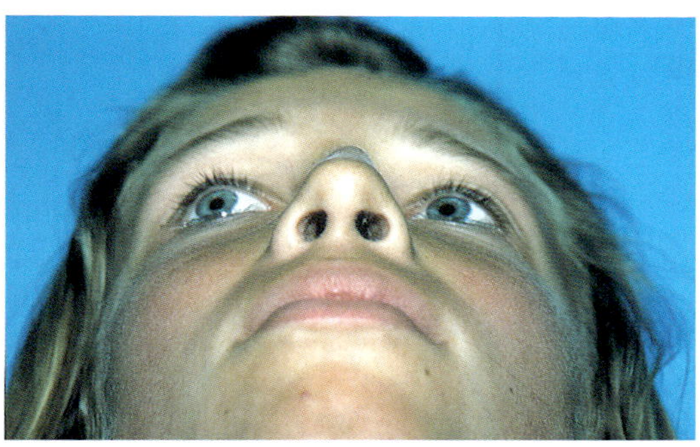

g

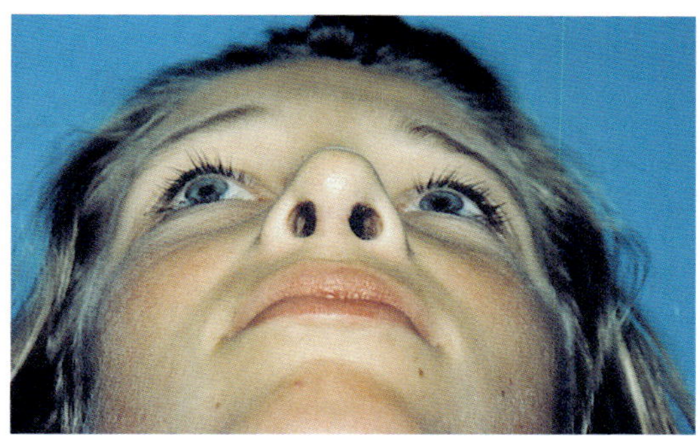

h

Fig. 16a-h. Pre- and postoperative views of a female patient with an underprojected nasal tip, hump and deviation on the left side. The nasal tip projection was increased with premaxillary plumping, columellar strut and double trip graft. The hump was resected and osteotomies were performed to realign the bony pyramid. Additionally augmentation mentoplasty was performed.

of columellar skin flap necrosis and an ugly scar. Cartilaginous tip grafting, using the open approach, may become an important part of the surgeon's armentarium. The potential for increased control over support, projection and contour can lead to satisfactory and predictable results in patients with difficult aesthetic nasal problems. With proper attention to detail, tip grafting can indeed be a gratifying and safe adjunctive procedure in tip rhinoplasty.

In Figures 15 and 16 pre- and postoperative views are shown of two clinical cases in which open-tip rhinoplasty was performed.

13: EXTERNAL RHINOPLASTY
The benefits and pitfalls

G.J. Nolst Trenité and B.C. Vinayak

Introduction

In the last decade, the external approach has gained enormous popularity in rhinoplastic surgery. The possibility to assess anatomical deformities by direct inspection of the nasal cartilaginous and bony framework and the much easier bimanual sculpturing under direct vision have added a further dimension to rhinoplasty, bringing a range of opportunities to the surgeon who masters the technique and exploits its specific advantages. The choice of an external approach depends not only on the specific pathological anatomical findings but also on the ability of the surgeon to achieve an adequate correction. This has especially stimulated less experienced surgeons to choose the external approach even when a less traumatic approach (the non-delivery or delivery) is indicated. In the decision to use the external approach the rhinoplastic surgeon should incorporate the possible sequelae related to this approach. Especially in rhinoplastic procedures the enhancement of a predictable satisfying result demands the most atraumatic surgical procedures. In this chapter, we will present some historical aspects and principles of open-structure rhinoplasty, before considering the advantages with particular reference to grafting in the areas of the bony pyramid, middle nasal vault and the nasal tip, and to specific indications such as revision rhinoplasty, the crooked nose, septal perforations, the tension nose and cleft-lip nasal deformities. Beside benefits there are also pitfalls related to the external approach, which will be also emphasized in this chapter with the goal of shortening the long and arduous path of the learning process in rhinoplasty.

Historical aspects

The terminology referring to this approach enjoys a number of synonyms, *viz.*: the 'elephant trunk' incision (1920) of Harold Gillies[1], the trans-columella incision (1934) of Aurel Rethi[2], the decortication technique (1962) of Sercer[3], the 'external approach' (1974) via the 'butterfly' incision of Goodman[4], and 'open-rhinoplasty' (1969) as synonymous with 'external rhinoplasty', popularized by Anderson[5,6]. The term 'open-structure' (1990) was introduced by Johnson and Toriumi[7]. All these names are largely descriptive, apart from 'open-structure rhinoplasty' which encompasses the philosophy behind the approach.

External incisions in rhinoplasty are not new and have been used in one form or another in all early descriptions of rhinoplasty. The first description of rhinoplasty is believed to have stemmed from India in 600 BC with the works of Sushruta and Samhita[8], in which external incisions and an open approach were practised. The endonasal approach was introduced by John Roe in 1887[9], and Jacque Joseph, a German orthopedic surgeon, in 1904[10], and was to become standard practice in all rhinoplasty procedures, and it remains an important aspect of the majority of cases performed today. The first description of an external rhinoplasty via a transcolumella incision, which has developed into the modern technique, was given by Rethi[2] in 1934 and subsequently by Sercer[3] from Zagreb, using the decortication technique in 1958. In 1970, Padovan, Sercer's disciple, presented his experience of external rhinoplasty in New York. Goodman was impressed and advocated the external approach and described it most elegantly in 1974 with a modified transcolumella incision, as the well-known 'butterfly' incision[4]. Goodman's original description featured all the key points of incision placement, development of flaps and other surgical techniques. Publications over the last 22 years have mainly served to emphasis the salient points in Goodman's original description and the plethora of publications on the topic are a testimony to the recognition of the true value and potential of this approach, and its adoption by some of the most experienced facial plastic surgeons in the world. Recent refinements regarding incision placement and surgical technique have overcome some of the earlier criticisms of a facial scar, delay in resolution of the tip skin edema, loss of tip projection, and extra operating time. The additional nasal tip edema is thought to be due to interruption of the lymphatic and venous drainage due to the transverse columella incision, as well as to the division of the fibrous connections which exist between the skin and the underlying cartilages. The extra operative time is due to the time taken to develop a skin and soft tissue flap, as well as the time taken for meticulous closure of the butterfly incision.

Indications

After assessing the deformities the surgeon has to choose the appropriate approach which enables him to perform a specific sculpturing technique. A decision table such as that advocated by Tardy[11] can be very helpful (Table 1). The choice of the appropriate surgical approach will prevent unnecessary pitfalls.

Special indications for the external approach are:

- congenital deformities such as the cleft lip nose
- extensive revision surgery
- severe nasal trauma
- elaborate reduction and augmentation procedures
- tip deformities such as excess bulbosity and/ or asymmetry
- the need for extra tip rotation
- the correction of extreme overprojection in situations where the surgeon is not able to assess the proper pathology which causes the nasal deformity

The use of the external approach for minor deformities which easily can be corrected by a less traumatic approach (see Table 1) is inappropriate.

Principles of external rhinoplasty

External rhinoplasty by exposing the pathology and allowing open access for corrective surgical maneuvers, lends itself well to a philosophy of conservatism of the structural support of the nose with an emphasis of augmentation and reorientation of the supportive structures as opposed to reduction and resection[12]. However, certain general points need to be considered. The patient who allows the surgeon to make an external incision deserves every effort on the part of that surgeon to respect this privilege by taking great care with proper incision placement and meticulous wound closure[13]. An inverted-V notched mid columella incision is placed such that it is supported by the caudal margin of the medial crura. It is then connected to bilateral marginal incisions. Subsequent dissection should be in the relatively bloodless subperichondrial and subperiosteal plane, leaving as much soft tissue as possible on the skin flap, thus preserving its viability. In this way the lower laterals, upper laterals and bony dorsum can be exposed to the nasofrontal angle in their undisturbed positions[14]. Division of the medial intercrural tissue offers exposure to the caudal septum and premaxillary spine, but it should be left intact (if exposure is not indicated) as this intercrural attachment is one of the support mechanisms for the nasal tip. By

Table 1

Approaches	*Incisions*	*Indications*	*Techniques*
non delivery	– transcartilaginous or intercartilaginous	– slight bulbosity – minimal tip rotation	– cephalic resection lateral crus (complete strip)
delivery	– intercartilaginous and marginal	– moderate bulbosity – extra tip rotation – bifidity – asymmetry	– cartilage resection – scoring and morcelization – alar (domal) suturing (complete or interrupted strip)
external	– broken columellar and marginal	– congenital deformities – extensive revisions – severe nasal trauma – elaborate reduction and augmentation – shield graft – columella strut	– cartilage resections lateral/medial crura – alar cartilage modifications and reorientation (complete or interrupted strip)

dividing the upper laterals from the septum the whole of the septum is accessible from the cephalic as well as the caudal aspect, allowing treatment of nasal valve problems, dorsal septal deviations and septal perforation repair. External rhinoplasty, therefore, provides very extensive exposure for both septal and rhinoplasty surgery (Fig. 1a-h). Other benefits include binocular vision, use of both hands, control of bleeding with diathermy, accurate diagnosis and precise sculpturing of struts, battens and plumping grafts and placement of sutures for graft stabilization as well as being a very useful teaching tool[15]. As intercartilaginous incisions are not used, the valve area is preserved. It is important to appreciate that the disruption of the skin soft tissue envelope from the lower lateral cartilages and the division of the medial inter-crural ligamentous fibrous tissue leads to loss of some of the minor tip support mechanisms, and therefore loss of tip projection should be anticipated in all cases[7]. The tip projection can be maintained by a sutured-in-place columella strut[15] which strengthens the leg of the tripod formed by the conjoined medial crura (Fig. 2). The strut also corrects buckled medial crura, strengthens weak medial crura, corrects tip asymmetries and provides a stable base for the application of tip grafts.

Pitfalls in external rhinoplasty

Incisions

When performing an external approach the broken transcolumellar incision is most commonly used. When performed in the appropriate way and closed meticulous with adequate suture material (6/0 ethilon or prolene), there will be no conspicuous scar (Fig. 3a,b) which makes the columella incision in itself no contra-indication for the external approach[16]. The following points should be considered in external approach incisions to prevent sequellae:

– the broken columella incision should be situated anterior to the medial crural footplates with, as preferred site, the narrowest distance (halfway along the

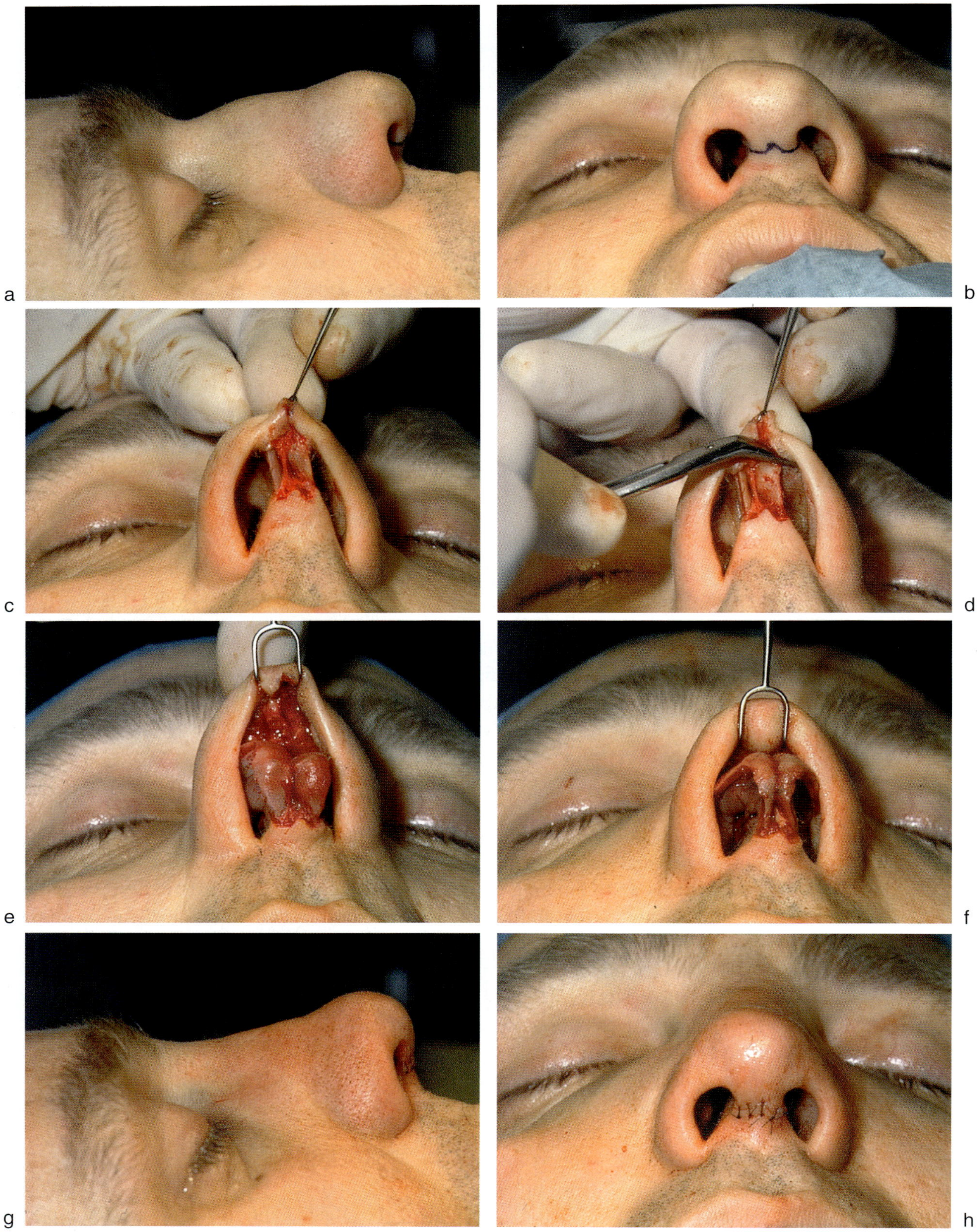

Fig. 1. External rhinoplasty of a post-traumatic nasal deformation with deprojected, asymmetric, bulbous tip and retracted columella *(a,b)*; development of the columellar skin flap *(c)*; and denuding of the cartilaginous bony nasal skeleton *(d,e)*. This approach allows the pathology to be assessed u128nder direct vision and bimanual. After septal reconstruction, repositioning and refining of the lower laterals *(f)*. The direct postoperative result with normal tip projection, restored columellar show and tip symmetry *(g,h)*. Care has been taken meticulously to suture the broken columella incision.

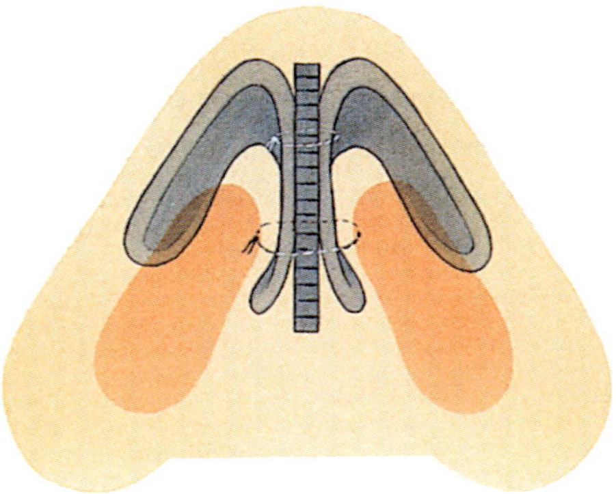

Fig. 2. Columella strut of autogenous septal cartilage for extra tip support fixed by mattress sutures to the medial crura.

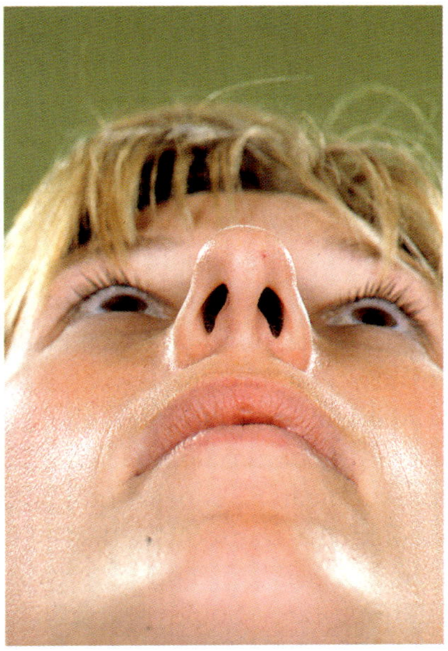

a

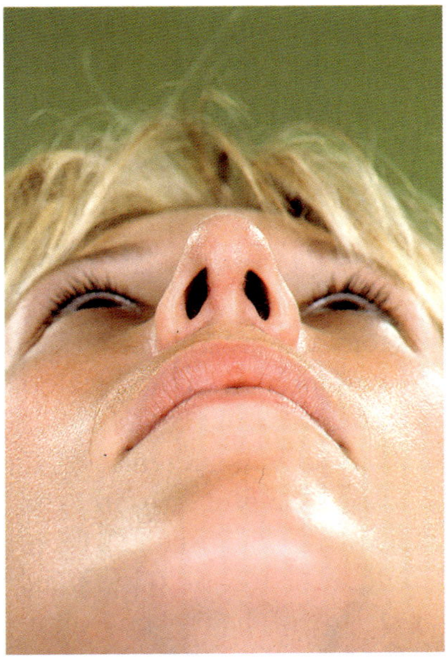

b

Fig. 3a,b. Pre- and postoperative basal views of a reduction rhinoplasty using the external approach. The transcolumellar scar is inconspicuous.

columella) between the nostrils (see Fig. 1a,b)

- the integrity of the caudal end of the medial crura just beneath the incision should be guarded to prevent disruption of the integrity of the medial crura. In general the vertical columella part of the marginal incisions should be placed 1.5-2 mm inside the vestibulum
- the least traumatic way to extend the marginal incisions is to identify the caudal end of the medial crura first, the caudal end can then be used as a guide to extend the marginal incision more laterally using Converse scissors with a spreading movement hugging the caudal end, followed by cutting the overlying soft tissue (see Fig. 1d). To obtain adequate exposure of the nasal skeleton, the marginal incision should be extended at least halfway along the vestibulum. In case of too short a columella in relation to the intended tip projection, a V incision at the base of the columella to perform a V-Y procedure is indicated. When this lengthening procedure is not sufficient a graft procedure should be performed.

Although many other columella incisions have been described, the broken transcolumellar incision is the most appropriate and gives the least visible scar. (see Fig. 3a,b).

Dissection of the soft tissue envelope

To prevent unnecessary peroperative bleeding and to enhance the healing process, dissection in the right surgical plane is obligatory. The dissection starts in the direct supraperichondrial or even subperichondrial plane in the domal area. Dissection should be conducted in a lateral direction up to the hinge area, hugging the lower lateral, with further extension in a cephalic direction to the scroll area. To free the cartilaginous vault, it is easy to make a 'fausse route' into the superficial muscular aponeurotic system (SMAS). To prevent this, the surgeon should start dissection in the midline between or just cephalic to the domes. It can be helpful to incise the perichondrium at the caudal end of the cartilaginous vault vertically in the midline, after which subperichondrial dissection from medial to lateral and in a cephalic direction should be carried out. If necessary at a later stage, too thick a supratip soft tissue envelope can be thinned, which should be done very conservatively so as not to compromise the blood supply to the overlying skin. A common effect of the external approach is prolonged supra tip edema and sometimes a soft tissue polly beak as a sequela of dissection in the wrong plane disturbing the integrity of the transverse nasal muscle.

Dissection of the soft tissue of the bony pyramid in a subperiosteal plane should start 2-3 mm parallel to and above the caudal end of both nasal bones. It is of great importance to palpate the nasal bone with the instrument before making the incision, to prevent separation of the upper laterals from the bony pyramid, a pitfall which can only be corrected with a camouflaging onlay graft.

Fixation of the columella strut

To restore tip support after separation of the medial crura, the use of a columella strut is obligatory in most cases. The graft is placed in a well-defined pocket between the medial crura, and extends from 2 mm above the anterior nasal spine to the angle between the medial and intermediate crura. The sandwich construction is fixed by mattress sutures which must not be placed above this angle in order to prevent loss of the columella-lobular ('double break') angle[18,19]. To prevent asymmetry at the caudal plane of the columella and asymmetry in dome height, it is important to fix the medial crura in the right parallel position temporarily with a needle after which final fixation with mattress sutures is accomplished.

Redraping of the soft tissue envelope and closure of the skin incision

With the open approach it is more difficult to assess a satisfying supra-tip dip and to acquire the desired tip projection, due to a certain traction of the soft tissue after closure of the broken columella incision. Final assessment of the supra tip area and the tip projection should be made after preliminary closure of the transcolumellar incision. If the result is not satisfying, adjustment is still possible either by a slight cartilage vault reduction and, in case of insufficient tip projection, by adding an onlay tip graft through the marginal incision (endonasal approach), or a shield graft which can be sutured into place after reopening the transcolumellar incision.

In case of grafting procedures for augmentation, care should be taken that the overlying soft tissue has sufficient circulation. Whitening of the skin over an augmentation graft is a warning sign, which should not be neglected. A slight reduction of the graft will prevent possible skin necrosis.

Closure of the transcolumellar incision

Meticulous closure should be carried out with appropriate suture material (6/0 ethilon or prolene). Care should be taken that closure is without tension. To prevent tension it is helpful to start with a subcutaneous 6/0 PDS suture. There should be slight eversion of the wound edges. After closure of the broken columella skin incision, the surgeon should make sure of a smooth skin line of the columella from a basal and lateral view. Removal of the skin sutures should be done five to seven days postoperative.

The bony pyramid in open-structure rhinoplasty

The added benefits of visualization and an open approach in correcting upper-third deformities may not be immediately obvious and, indeed, during an open approach, the bony pyramid is often dealt with by palpation with little effort being taken to visualize the bony vault and, therefore, there is little difference with the closed approach. However, if more effort is made to illuminate and dissect in the upper third, then this too is amenable to more accurate diagnosis and precise correction, including the placement of soft tissue implants such as temporalis fascia in thin-skinned individuals, as well as the avoidance of irregularities which can arise from the closed procedure. Optimizing surgery of the upper third by the open approach requires careful dissection in the correct surgical plane, in an attempt to achieve a bloodless surgical field. The dissection should not extend more than halfway along the lateral wall[20]. The key points in the dissection are avoidance of disruption of the keystone ('K') area and a subperiosteal dissection. In order to preserve the K area, the periosteal dissection starts with two incisions 2-3 mm parallel to and above the caudal end of both nasal bones. A systematic examination is then made of the individual components of the bony vault. The size, shape and position of both nasal bones and bony septum, as well as the thickness of the overlying skin-soft tissue envelope in the region of the rhinion and nasion, are assessed individually and in relation to their effect on the nasofrontal angle and the width, height, dorsal profile and contour of the upper third.

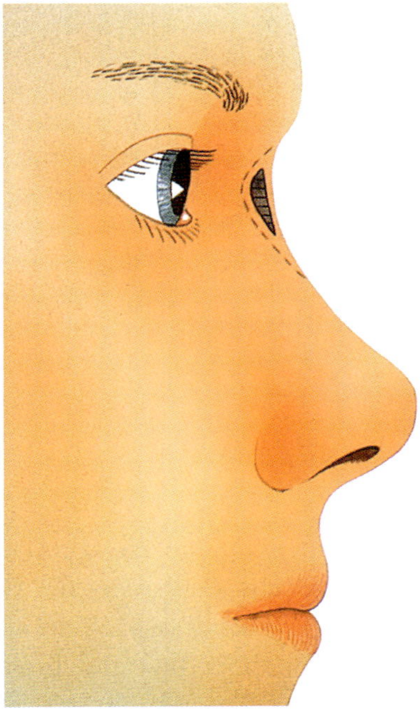

Fig. 4. Autogenous cartilage graft (striped area) to lengthen the nose and to correct the apparent over-projection.

Even minor alterations to the nasofrontal angle can have a profound effect on the overall nasal aesthetics. The open approach allows the use of a burr or reduction of the soft tissue envelope at the nasion to deepen the angle. Conversely, the angle can be deepened or set in a more cephalic position by precise application of soft tissue onlay grafts of temporalis fascia or slivers of autogenous cartilage (Fig. 4).

When altering the height or width of the nose, it should be borne in mind that, in terms of 'apparent' appearance, the width and height of the nasal pyramid have an inverse relationship. The principles and techniques of lateral, medial-oblique and intermediate osteotomies are the same for both the endonasal and open approaches (see Chapter 11). Intermediate osteotomies are often needed in the presence of excessively curved nasal bones (convex, concave, or a combination of both), or a deviating nose with one nasal bone higher than the other, or when narrowing a wide nose which is of normal height (Fig. 5). The position of the medial osteotomy affects the position of the junctional line between the dorsal subunit and the lateral nasal wall. This line should run smoothly from the brow, and depends on the nasal dorsal unit not being too wide or too sharp. When excising a bony hump, it should be remembered that, in the presence of a bony pyramid deviation and unequal height of the nasal bones, the plane of the osteotome must be altered. In addition, excision of a nasal bony hump must take into account the variable thickness of the skin-soft tissue envelope, which means that, to achieve a straight profile, the bony vault must be left relatively high at the rhinion in order to compensate for the thinner overlying skin and soft tissue (Fig. 6).

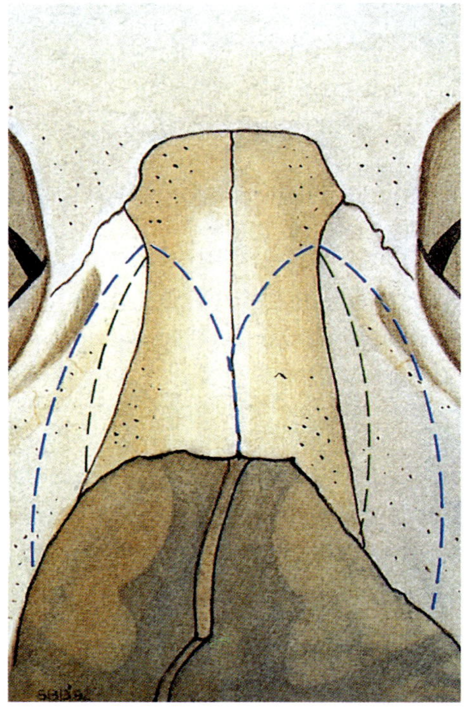

Fig. 5. Supplementary intermediate osteotomies to remodel concave and convex bony side walls.

The middle nasal vault

The 'nasal valve area' is the smallest cross-sectional area in the nasal airway. The boundary is formed by the caudal end of the upper lateral cartilage, the head of the inferior turbinate, the floor of the nose, the nasal septum, and the intervening tissue surrounding the pyriform aperture. The term 'nasal valve' refers specifically to the slit-like opening between the caudal end of the upper lateral and the adjacent cartilaginous septum, normally forming an angle of approximately 10 to 15°. The nasal valve can be altered to some extent by the nasal musculature, and so performs a physiological role in controlling the flow rate of air in the nasal cavity. Rhinoplasty can compromise the nasal valve, particularly in patients with short nasal bones, a high bony-cartilaginous hump and weak upper lateral cartilages[21]. Frequently, there is an additional corresponding aesthetic defect of a 'sunken' or 'pinched-in' middle third. Jack Sheen (1984) recognized these functional and aesthetic problems and their association with the disruption of the 'T' structure of the middle third. He described the endonasal placement of cartilaginous strips, which he called 'spreader grafts', to open up the nasal valve area and angle, thereby improving the flow of air[22] (Fig. 7). The drawback to the endonasal approach is that the graft may shift out of position, or may be difficult

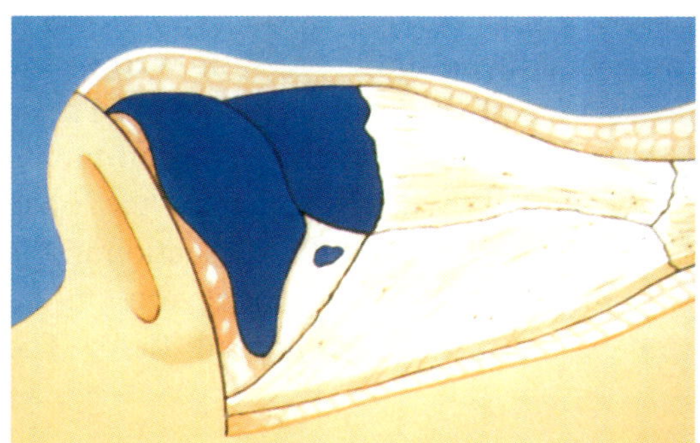

Fig. 6. Illustration of the difference in thickness of the soft tissue lining over the osseocartilaginous vault.

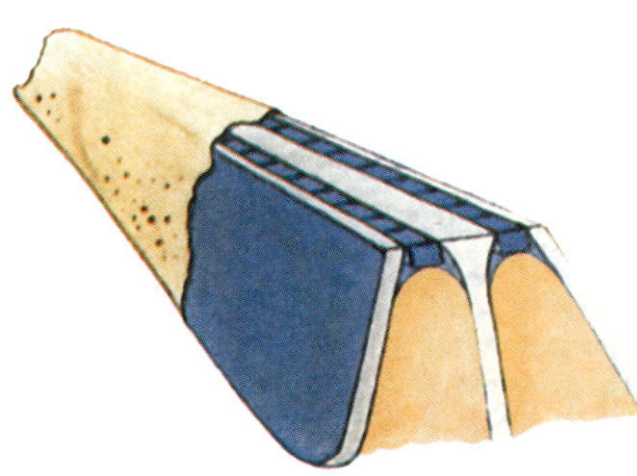

Fig. 7. Spreader grafts of autogenous septal cartilage (striped areas) to restore too narrow a nasal valve and aesthetically too narrow a midnose.

to place in the required position. The open approach allows suture fixation and has certainly made it easier to place these grafts precisely with confidence. In addition, the open approach has allowed the role of spreader grafts to be extended to include: *1.* maintenance or reconstruction of the dorsal nasal roof; *2.* restoration or maintenance of the nasal valve; *3.* straightening and buttressing of a high dorsally deviated septum; and *4.* recreation of the dorsal aesthetic lines (Figs. 8a-h)[23].

The nasal tip by the open approach

The nasal tip has perhaps been the major beneficiary of the open approach since it

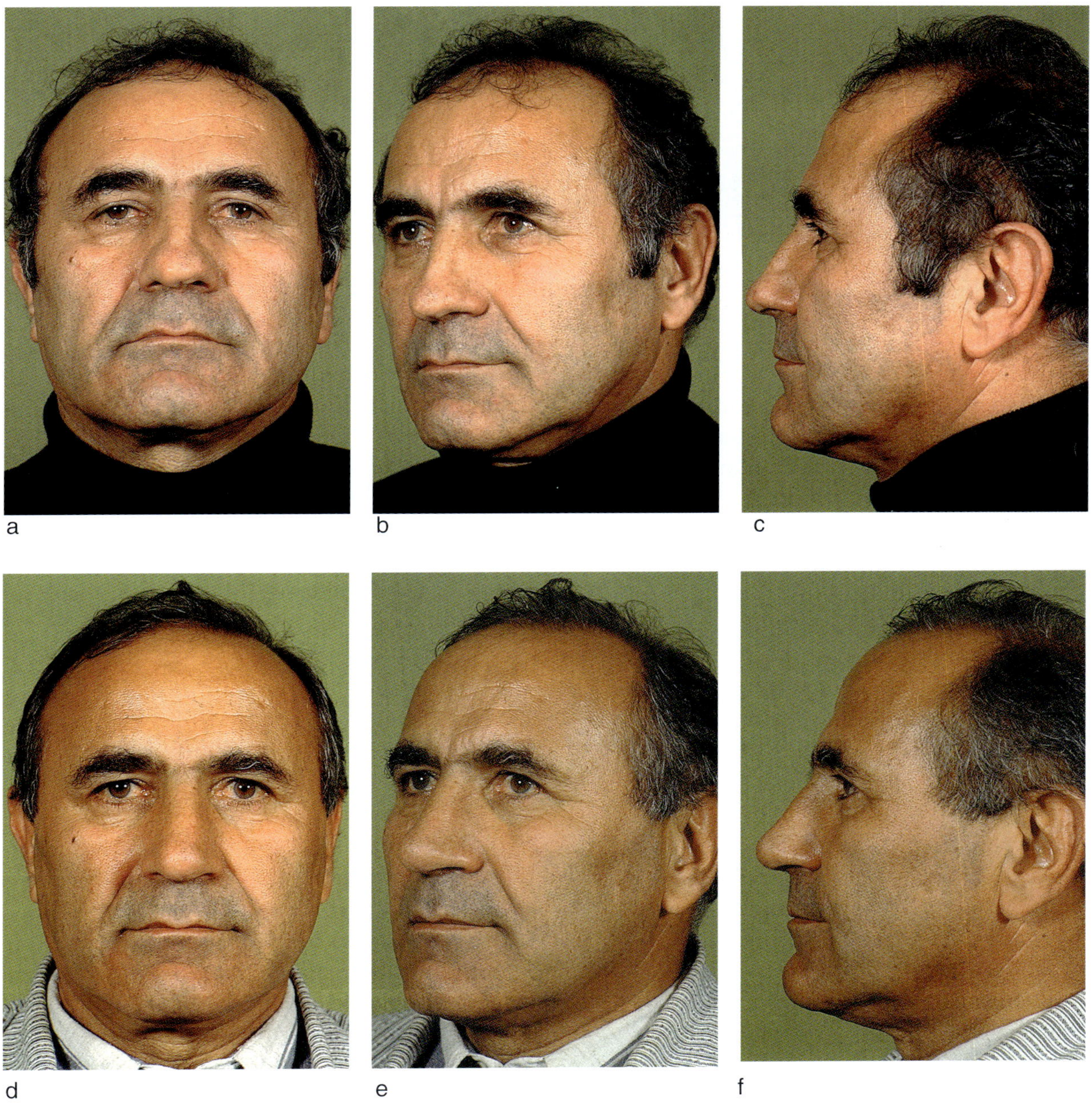

Figs. 8a-h. Pre- and postoperative views of revision rhinoplasty using the external approach in the case of too narrow a midnose and an underprojected asymmetric nasal tip in which spreader grafts, paranasal side grafts, columellar strut and a shield graft were used.

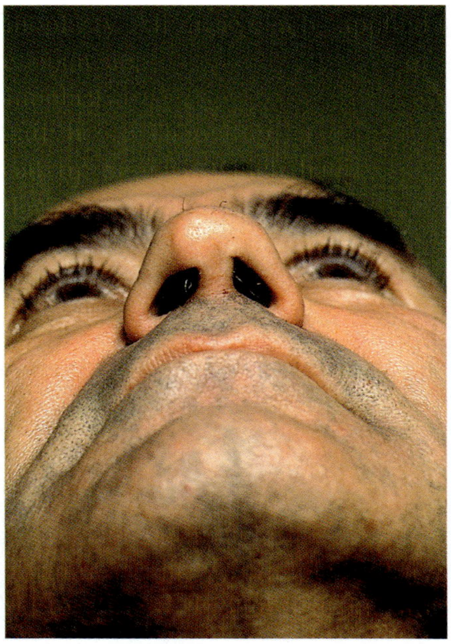

g

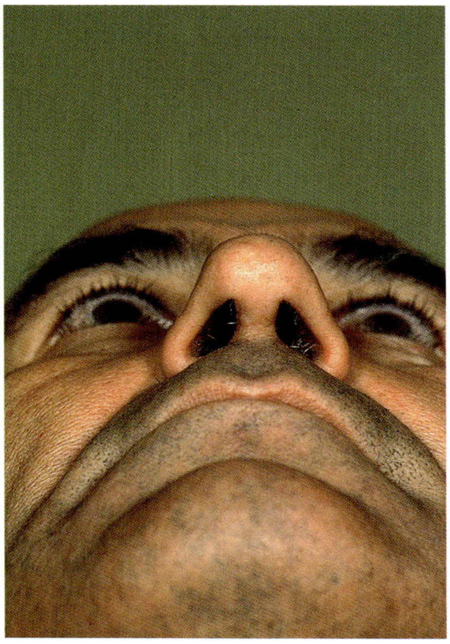

h

Fig. 8g-h.

exposes the structural components of the tip in their natural undisturbed position, allowing an unparalleled opportunity to diagnose the various deformities and asymmetries of the tip, as well as facilitating the surgical manipulation of the tip cartilages and suture fixation of tip grafts. In particular, it allows the correction of even minor asymmetries and so adds an extra finesse to rhinoplasty.

Although many tip procedures may be amenable to a closed approach, open rhinoplasty gives the opportunity to perform all tip procedures with a greater degree of precision, and the confidence of obtaining a good result. To present all tip procedures in this chapter would not be practical and, therefore, we will only feature some of the highlights of tip surgery which benefit most by the open approach, under the heading of tip projection, tip rotation and tip symmetry.

Altering tip projection and rotation by influencing the alar cartilages is based on the 'tripod' theory[5]. This theory states that the structural framework of the nasal tip is based on the two lateral crura and the conjoined medial crura, each forming one leg of the tripod (Fig. 9). This allows an

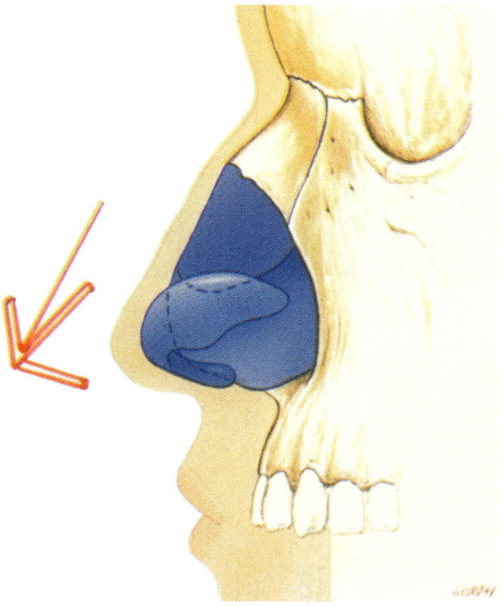

Fig. 9. Tripod complex of the lower third of the nose. The conjoint medial crura comprise one leg of the tripod, while the lateral crura comprise the other two legs.

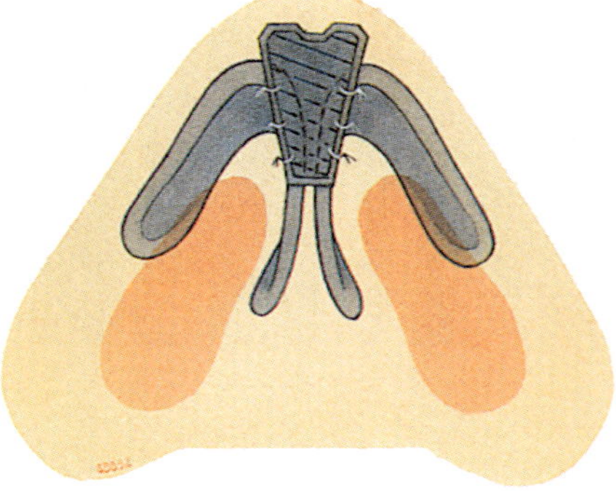

Fig. 10. Shield graft sutured to the medial crura.

understanding of the effect on the tip position by altering the size and position of the medial or lateral crura. For instance, if the medial and lateral crura are reduced in length, the tip is deprojected, whereas if they are augmented, projection is achieved. Superior rotation is achieved by shortening the lateral crura or, alternatively, by lengthening the medial crura causing rotation at the 'hinge' region.

Lateral crural procedures, such as lateral crural retrodisplacement for superior rotation of the tip[24] and the lateral crural steel[26] for more tip projection, can be performed in a more controlled fashion by using the open approach[11,25,26]. It is difficult to perform this procedure with a high degree of symmetry when using the closed approach.

The importance of the medial crura in nasal tip surgery has been described by Goldman[25]. Although the original descriptions are based on a closed approach, which was practised at that time, the open approach makes the procedure easier with more precise transection at the dome or another point in order to achieve the desired projection and remove bifidity whilst obtaining symmetry. The open approach also allows the additional symmetrical positioning and suture fixation of a shield graft, as described by Sheen[27] (Fig. 10).

Revision rhinoplasty

Revision rhinoplasty is undoubtedly one of the most challenging operations undertaken by the facial plastic surgeon. Various authors have reported an increase in the number of revision cases, which may be a reflection of the greater popularity of rhinoplasty and the enhanced expectations and discrimination of both the surgeon and patient[28,29].

Failure of rhinoplasty may be the result of inadequate or overzealous surgery or, in some cases, be related to patient factors, such as unfavorable healing. Patient dissatisfaction can also arise from a lack of rapport between patient and surgeon, or from a conceptual discrepancy between the patient's desired and the realistic outcome. These same factors also account for failure of revision rhinoplasty, but the problem is compounded by the greater difficulty of achieving the desired result with each subsequent revision. The need for revision may arise from either inadequate or overzealous primary surgery. This can produce either localized loss of contour or loss of the support mechanism (which may be associated with functional problems). Minor contour defects are very amenable to using precise pocket grafting via an endonasal approach, as described by Tardy[31]. This is sometimes required for refinement after an otherwise successful result. However, in the majority of patients referred to us (as a tertiary referral center for rhinoplasty), the problem usually involves the major supporting structures. In such cases, corrective surgery either requires reduction or addition of tissues. In the few cases that require simple reduction, we would advocate an endonasal approach if possible. However, those requiring reconstruction are usually best treated by the open approach in view of the better exposure for precise diagnosis, structural grafting and relocation of tissue, including augmentation (using autogenous material whenever possible) with the aim of producing predictably favorable long-term results (Fig. 11a-f).

Crooked nose

When excising a bony hump in the presence of a bony pyramid deviation and unequal height of the nasal bones, the plane of the osteotome must be altered. The excised hump can be resculptured and replaced as an onlay graft in order to camouflage any dorsal irregularities and

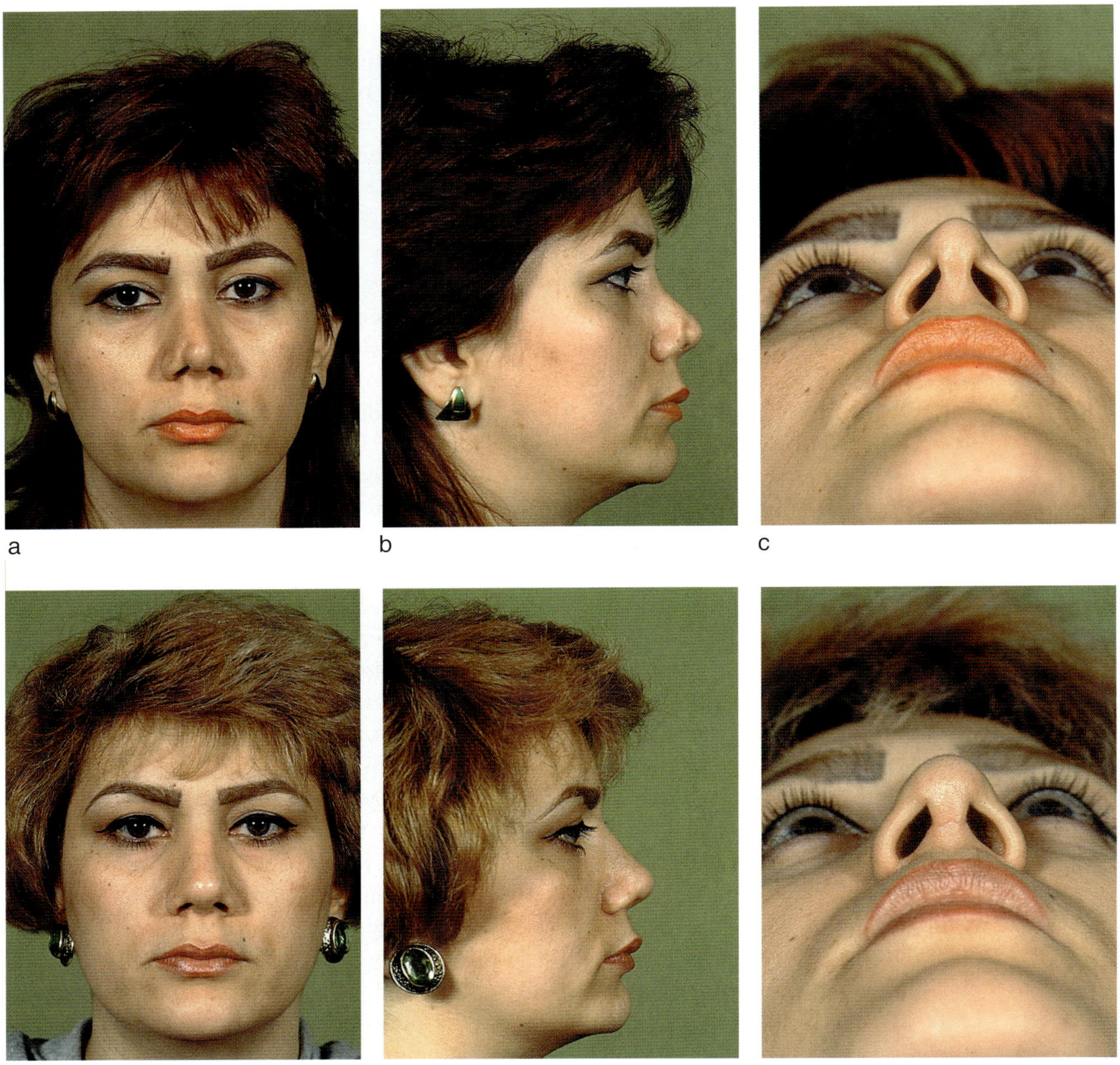

a b c

d e f

Fig. 11a-f. Pre- and postoperative views of a revision rhinoplasty with the external approach to correct for overzealous resection of the lateral crus and surrounding soft tissue.

provide a smooth dorsal profile[30]. The osteotomies are performed in a sequential manner. For example, if the nose deviates to the right, the first step is to mobilize the left nasal bone and reposition it in its normal position; the next step is to position the bony septum in the midline; and, finally, the right nasal bone is repositioned in its normal position[20]. The sequence is reversed for a nose which deviates to the left.

When the lower two-thirds of the nose are crooked after a septoplasty to correct any caudal septal deviation, this is usually due to a C-shaped dorsal deviation of the nasal septum, possibly complicated by previous surgery which disrupts the union of the upper laterals to the septum. In mild cases, the dorsal aspect of the septum is shaved on the convex side and sutured to the upper lateral cartilage, if necessary together with cross hatching on the concave side. If this is not sufficient to correct the deviation, a unilateral spreader graft is placed between the dorsal septum and the upper lateral cartilage[19]. The spreader

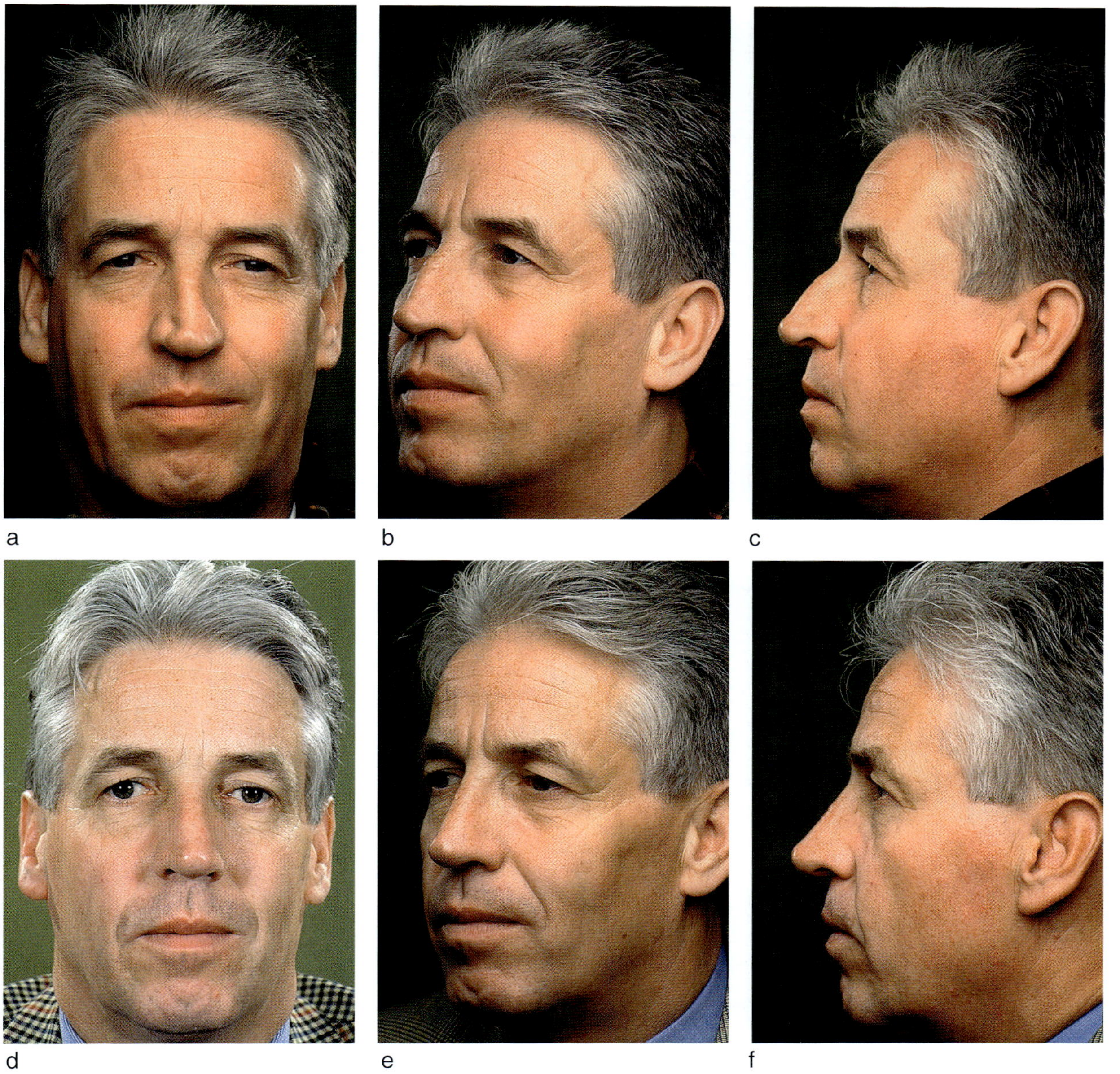

Fig. 12a-f. Pre- and postoperative views of a rhinoplasty in the case of a crooked lower third of the nose, using the external approach in which a spreader graft was used to straighten the cartilaginous dorsum.

graft acts as a stent as well as opening the nasal valve area. Any residual deformity is corrected by an onlay graft (Fig. 12a-f).

Septal perforation

As mentioned above, the open approach allows unique exposure of the septum, both from the cephalic and the caudal aspect, thus facilitating the repair of large septal perforations[32-37]. A full discussion of septal perforation repair is outside the scope of this chapter (see Chapter 18).

Tension nose

The term 'tension nose' was first coined by Cottle[38] and denotes a high nasal dorsum with stretching of the overlying skin and soft tissue, together with a highly arched and narrow nasal vault. Another constant finding is an overgrowth of the quadrilateral nasal septum[39] along both the

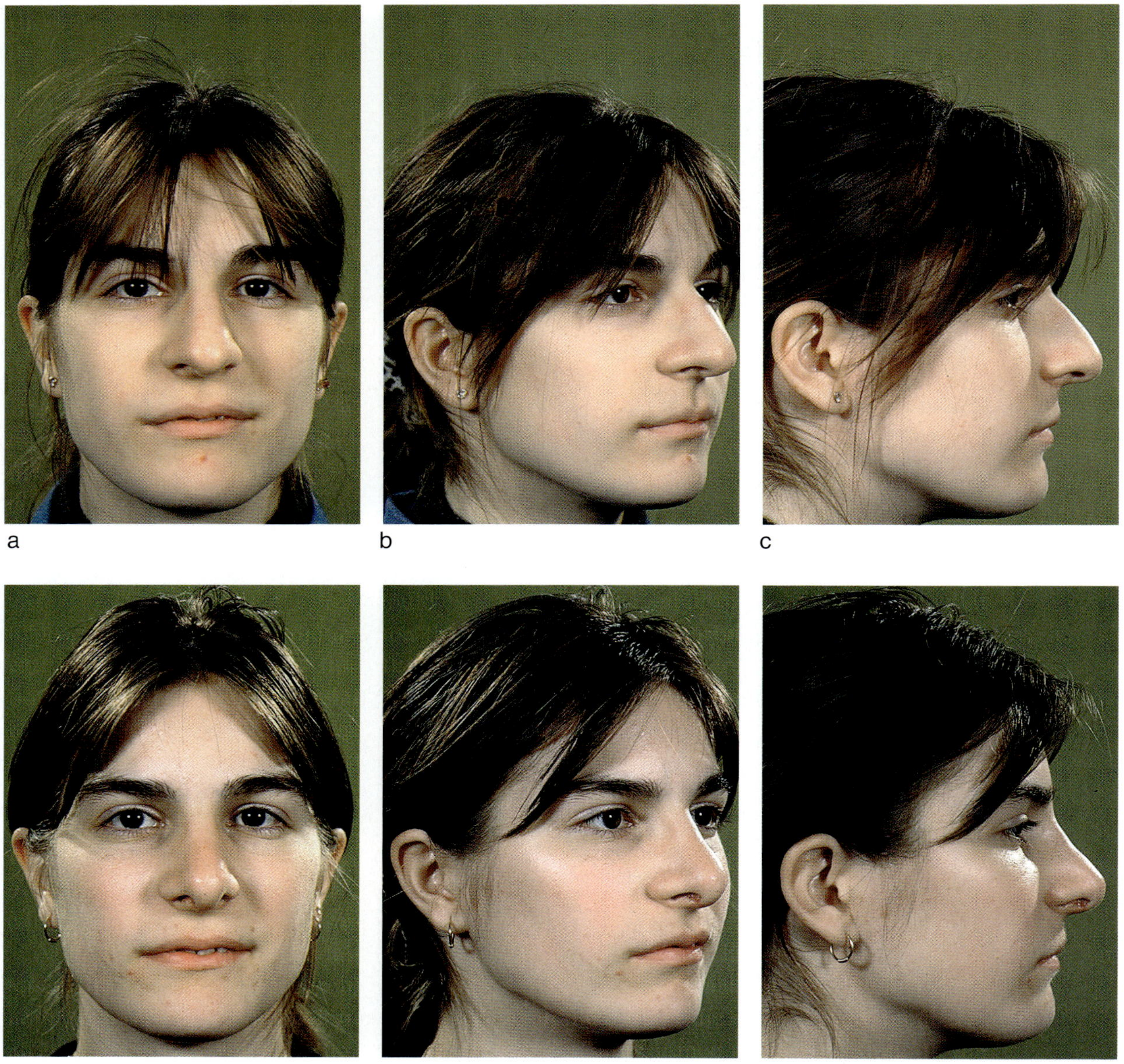

a b c

d e f

Fig. 13a-f. Pre- and postoperative views of a tension nose with overgrowth of cartilaginous nasal septum and lower laterals.

dorsum and caudal aspects, which exerts a 'pedestal effect' by pushing the lower lateral cartilages in a forward and downward direction, causing a blunting and anterior displacement of the nasolabial angle and shortening of the upper lip, since the anterior nasal spine is commonly also long. In a study by Johnson[39], the incidence of tension nose in primary rhinoplasty was 46%. Johnson describes a method of tip deprojection by excision of excessive elements of the nasal septum and anterior spine, followed by reprojection of the domes using tip grafts and suture techniques. Such measured modifications can be performed with precision using the open approach (Fig. 13a-f).

Cleft lip nasal deformities

The severity of primary nasal deformities is directly related to the severity of the cleft lip. Nasal deformities affect the nasal

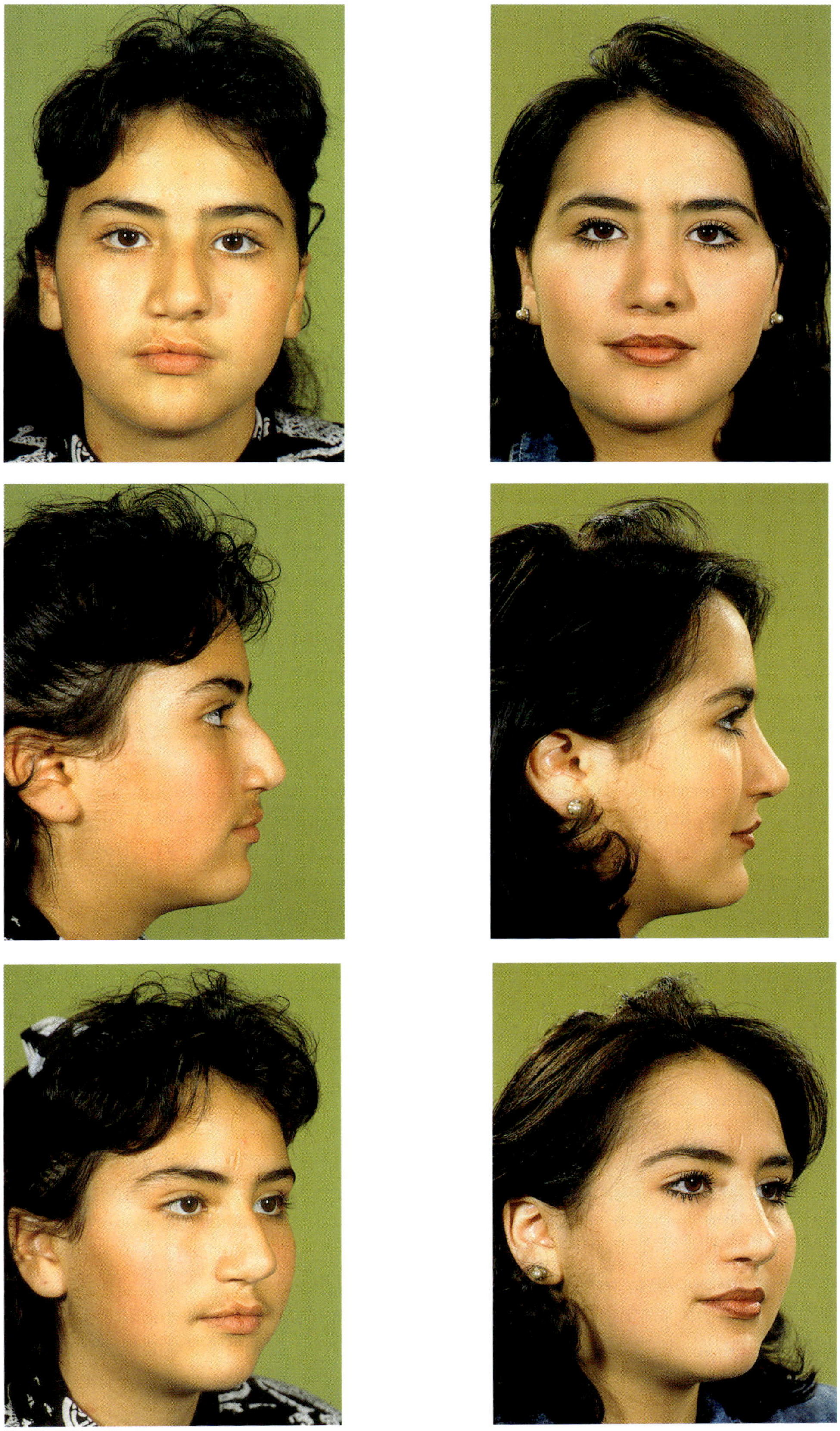

a b c d e f

Fig. 14a-h. Pre- and postoperative views of a patient with a unilateral cleft who underwent an external rhinoplasty to improve tip symmetry by repositioning the right lower lateral, fixed to a columella strut with mattress sutures. Improved projection was achieved through a shield graft. The right alar base was endorotated and medialized with a modified Z-plasty. To improve aesthetic harmony, a pseudo hump was resected, followed by micro osteotomies to realign the bony pyramid.

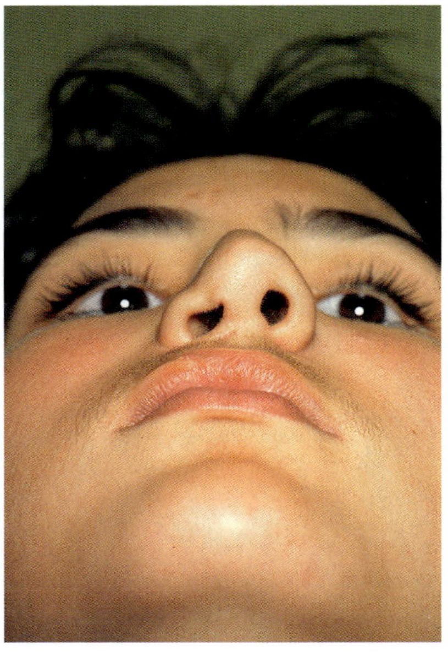

g

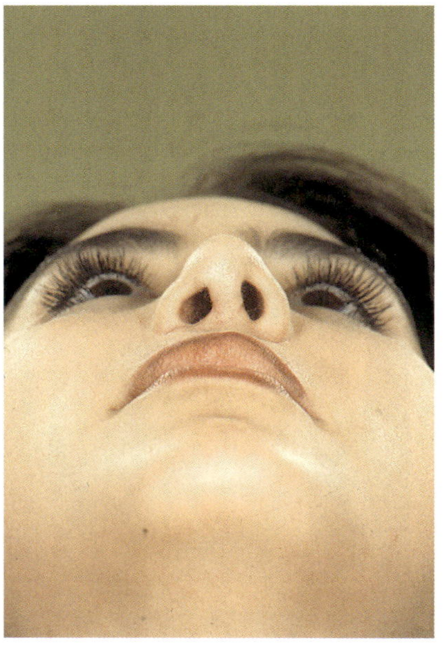

h

Fig. 14g-h.

and vestibular skin as well as the cartilaginous and bony skeleton. Cleft-lip-nasal deformities can be classified into unilateral and bilateral[40], and form a characteristic pattern (see Chapter 15). Rhinoplasty in a cleft lip patient, particularly in the presence of an alveolar cleft, is challenging and frustrating, due to the limitation of the final postoperative result[41]. The secondary, and hopefully definitive, nasal construction should be performed using the open-structure technique in the presence of severe tip asymmetry. The use of conservative techniques allows the procedure to be performed before puberty. However, the surgeon has to weigh up the psychological and future nasal directional growth benefits against possible inhibition of mid facial growth[40,43]. A V-Y procedure to lengthen the columella is usually needed in bilateral cleft deformities, and this should be borne in mind when pacing the incision[42]. A complete cleft will be associated with hypoplasia and retroposition of the maxilla on the cleft side. If mild, a cartilaginous graft can be used for support in order to relocate the alar base, while in severe cases, a maxillary advancement will be needed. The key to correcting tip asymmetry is a stable and symmetrical base formed by the columella strut. The alar cartilage on the cleft side must first be dissected free, after which it can be repositioned and sutured to the columella strut (more antero-cephalic)[40,45]. This does not alter the lateral alar base displacement. A Z-plasty to reposition and to endorotate the ala at the cleft side is often obligatory[40]. Finally, a shield graft is positioned, which further increases tip projection, enhances tip definition and camouflages minor tip asymmetries (Fig. 14a-h).

Conclusions

External rhinoplasty has proven to be a valuable part of the armentarium of the rhinoplastic surgeon. Especially in more difficult nasal tip deformities, the external approach allows the surgeon to analyze the skeletal abnormalities with direct binocular vision. It enables him to correct deformities with bimanual manipulation and direct suturing of graft material. Dissection in the right surgical planes and meticulous suturing with the appropriate suture material will prevent unnecessary sequelae of this surgical approach, such as prolonged supratip edema and aesthetically unacceptable transcolumellar scars. Nevertheless the rhinoplastic surgeon should bear in mind that he should choose the least traumatic approach to enable him to apply the appropriate techniques to correct the specific deformities to enhance predictable satisfying long-term results.

14: WEDGE RESECTION IN ALAR BASE SURGERY

G.J. Nolst Trenité

Introduction

Alar base reduction performed at the end of the type of rhinoplasty in which the tip height is lowered, resulting in some alar flare, is often underestimated in connection with the impact on the overall aesthetic result. It should be handled as if it were an initial procedure with good analysis of the problem and an adequate operative plan. The goal in alar base surgery should be to create an aesthetic balance and prevent an unnatural appearance and functional impairment.

Preoperative considerations

In the basal view, the nasal tip should approximately have the form of an equilateral triangle formed by tip lobule, alar lobules, nostril sills and columella base (Fig. 1).

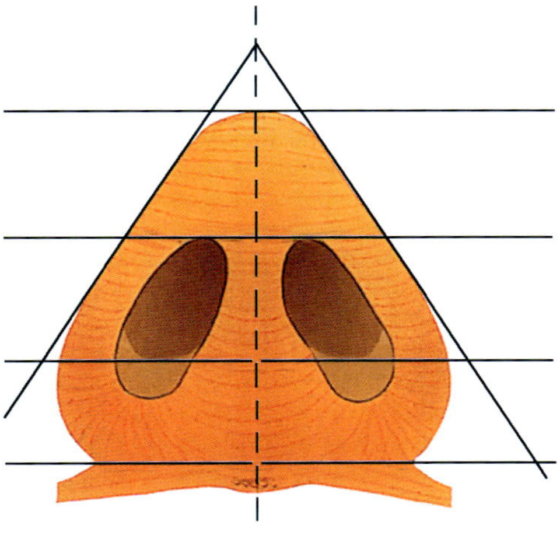

Fig. 1. Basal view of the nose which should have the form approximately of an equilateral triangle with the lobular, intermediate and basal parts of the columella as three equal segments.

The nostrils are oval-shaped in an oblique position in the Caucasian adult nose, while they are rounder and in a more horizontal position in Negroid and Asian noses. The large variety of alar base configurations demands differentiation in the shape, type and position of the wedge being resected. The wedge can be *V-shaped*, *inverted V-shaped* or *rectangular-shaped* (Fig. 2a,b,c). Depending on the shape of the wedge, it will consist of only alar skin or of alar with vestibular skin and underlying soft tissue. The position of the wedge resection can be more medial or lateral on the nasal base. The choice of a particular kind of wedge depends on the proposed type of reduction. There are three basic types of reduction:

- alar flare reduction
- nostril size reduction
- a combination of both

In cases of alar flare with a more or less normal nostril size, an inverted V-shaped wedge with the apex in the nostril groove, consisting of alar skin only, has to be excised (Fig. 3a,b). To reduce an oversized nostril with minimal alar flare, V-shaped wedge excision with the apex

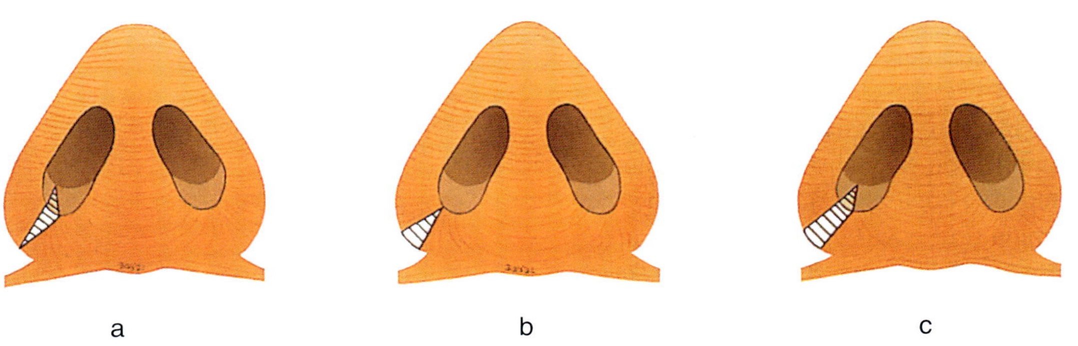

Fig. 2a,b,c. The three basic types of wedge in alar base reduction. *a.* V-shaped. *b.* Inverted V-shaped. *c.* Rectangular shaped.

a
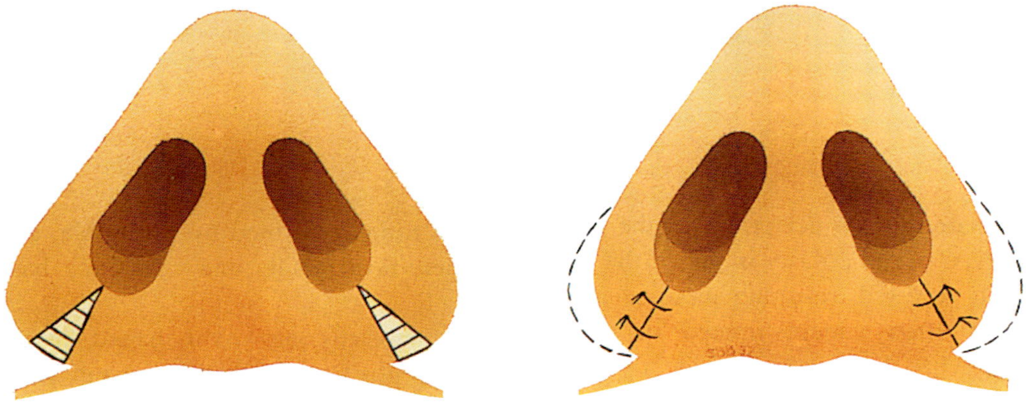
b

Fig. 3a,b. Alar base reduction in case of alar flare only.

a
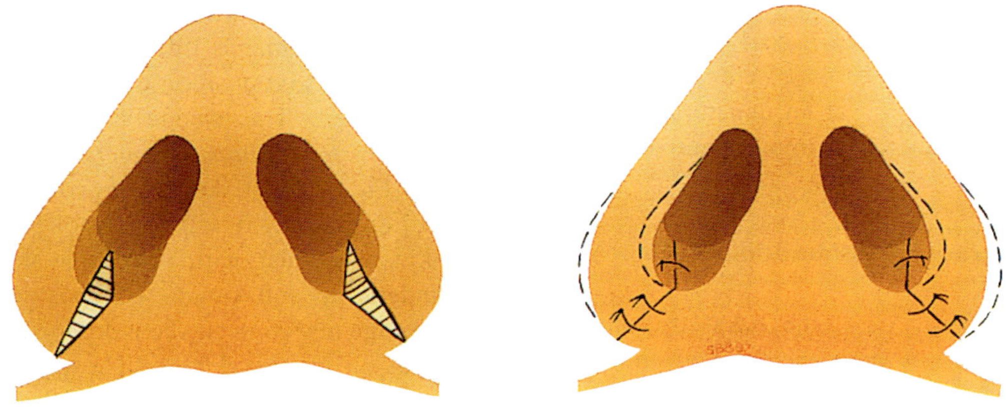
b

Fig. 4a,b. Reduction of oversized nostrils only.

a
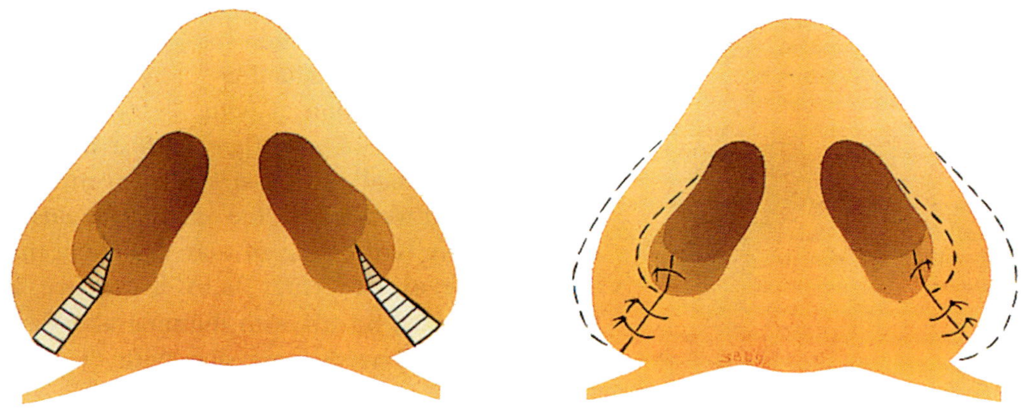
b

Fig. 5a,b. Correction of alar flare in combination with oversized nostrils.

in the alar groove, consisting of both alar and vestibular skin, is indicated (Fig. 4a,b).

When an oversized nostril exists in combination with alar flare, a rectangular-shaped wedge excision should be performed (Fig. 5a,b). In planning a resection of the alar base, the surgeon should prevent:

- imbalance between nostril size and alar lobule
- asymmetry and visible scarring
- notching of the nostril sill

Technique

After exact outlining of the wedge to be resected on the skin (Fig. 6a,b), local anesthesia (lidocaine 2% and epinephrine 1:100,000) is deposited in the alar base and alar rim without disturbing the contour. The skin incisions are made, holding the alar lobule with the thumb and forefinger (Fig. 7a,b). In the case of resection of the vestibular skin, the skin margin in the nostril should be slightly bevelled to prevent inversion of the skin after suturing. To prevent notching, it is helpful to break the straight line of the incision at the nostril sill with a 'hockey stick'-type incision, to conserve the natural rounding of the nostril sill (Fig. 8). Although it seems logical to place the posterior incision in the alar groove of the alar facial junction, to hide the scar, there is then more chance of unwanted scarring than when the incision is placed approximately 1 mm more on the lobular side. The wound should be meticulously closed with 6/0 nylon in the nostril sill and alar area (Fig. 9). It is not necessary to close the vestibular skin completely, as this can facilitate the drainage of residual blood and wound exudation.

a
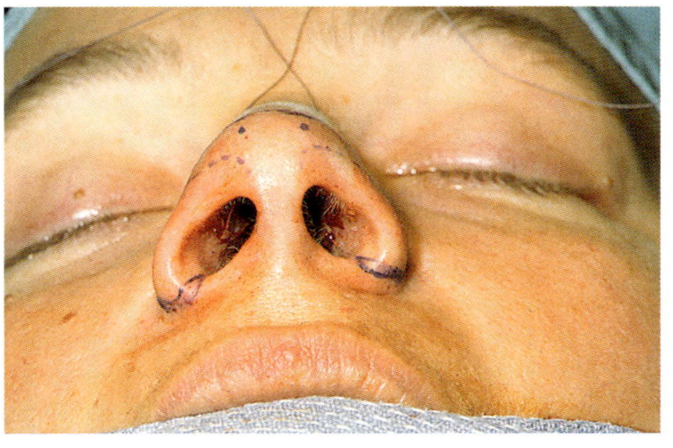
b
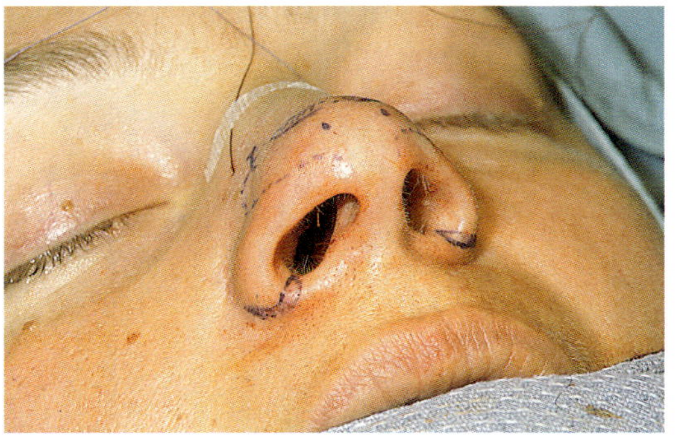

Fig. 6a,b. Outlining of the wedges to be resected on the skin.

a
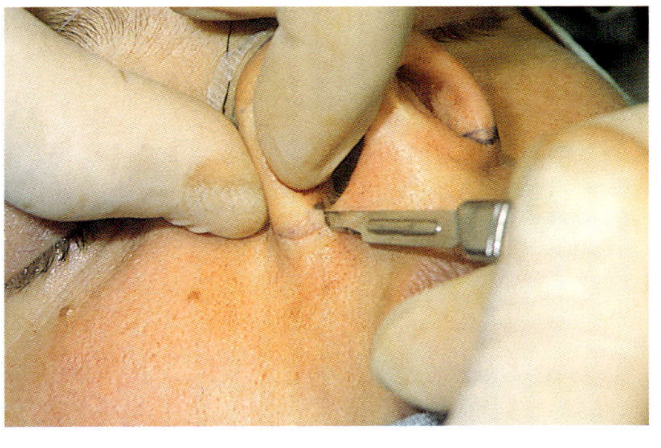
b
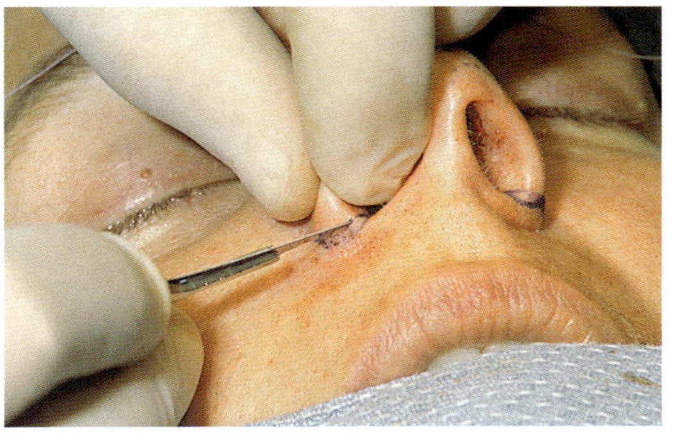

Fig. 7a,b. Initial skin incisions.

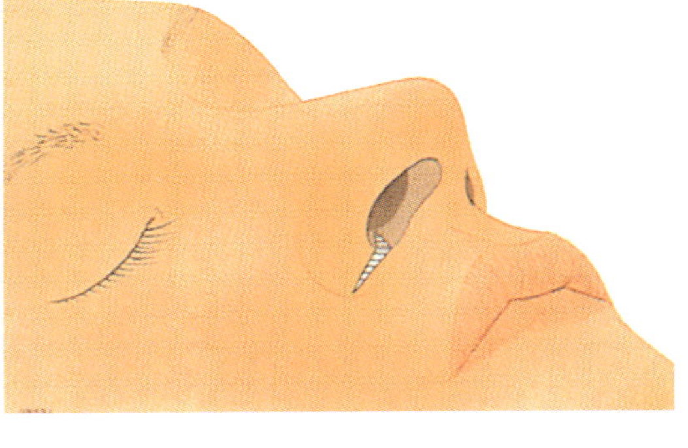

Fig. 8. 'Hockey stick'-type incision to break the straight line of the incision.

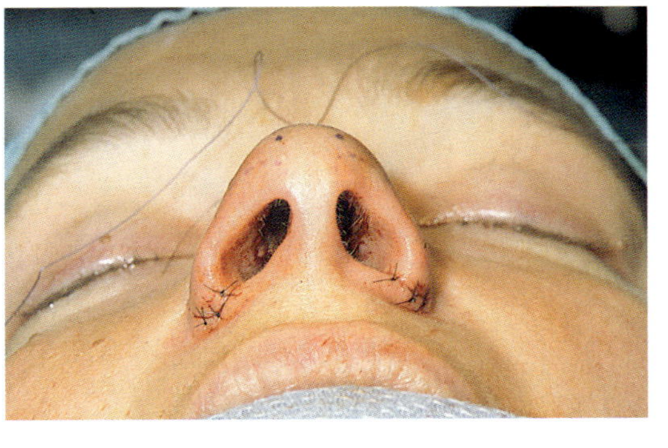

Fig. 9. Skin closure with 6/0 nylon sutures.

PART III: CAPITA SELECTA

15: SECONDARY SURGERY OF THE CLEFT- LIP NOSE

G.J. Nolst Trenité

Introduction

Rhinoplasty in the cleft-lip patient (and especially in combination with an alveolar cleft) is very challenging due to its complex pathology, and is also frustrating due to its limitations in the final postoperative result.

The characteristic anatomical changes already present in fetal life are secondary to the cleft-lip syndrome itself. Depending on the lip repair technique used, the deformity of the nose will become more or less pronounced in the postoperative period, during facial growth. Therefore, reallocation of the alar base to create as symmetrical and normal a position as possible and for the bilateral cleft combined with a lengthening procedure for the short columella, may help in preventing some of the surgical and psychological problems in the future.

Although there is a traditional reluctance to perform a rhinoplasty on a growing nose, as this can interfere with midfacial growth, the use of new atraumatic (conservative) operative techniques has created the tendency to correct nasal deformities before puberty. The surgeon has to weigh up the possible advantages (psychological and growth directional) against the possible disadvantages (growth inhibition). Positive short-term results can be 'overshadowed' by growth disturbances during the puberty growth spurt.

a

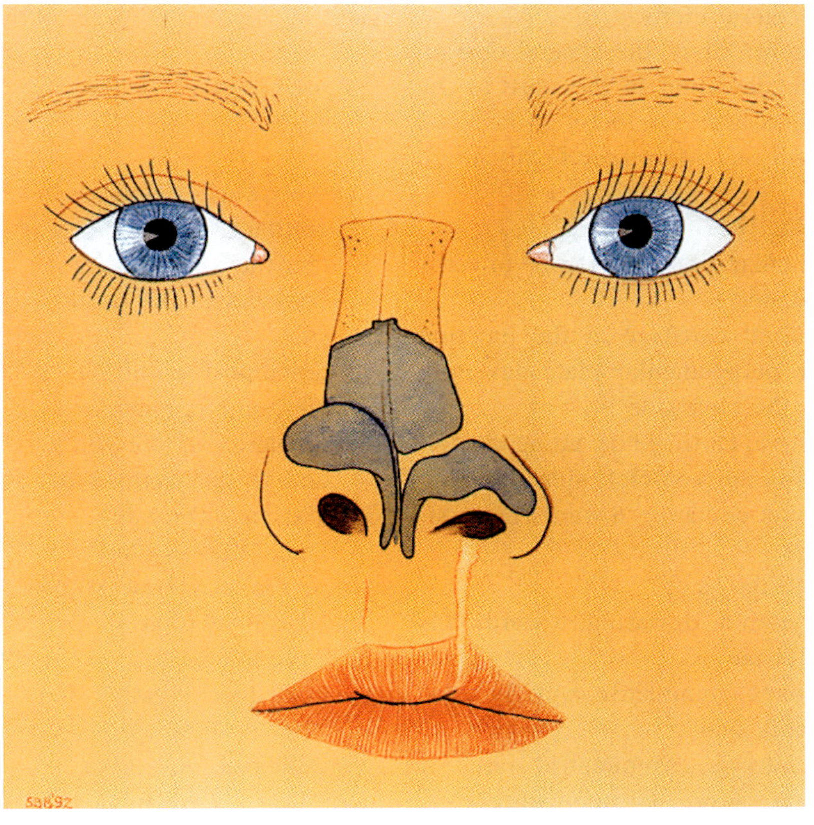

Fig. 1a. Unilateral cleft: deviation of the nose to the non-cleft side and asymmetry of the nasal tip.

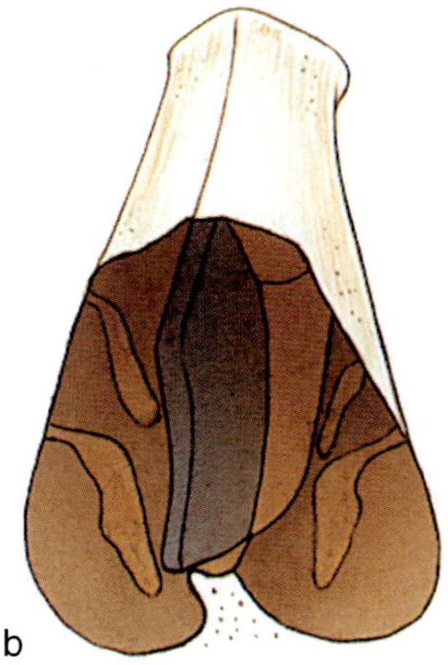

b

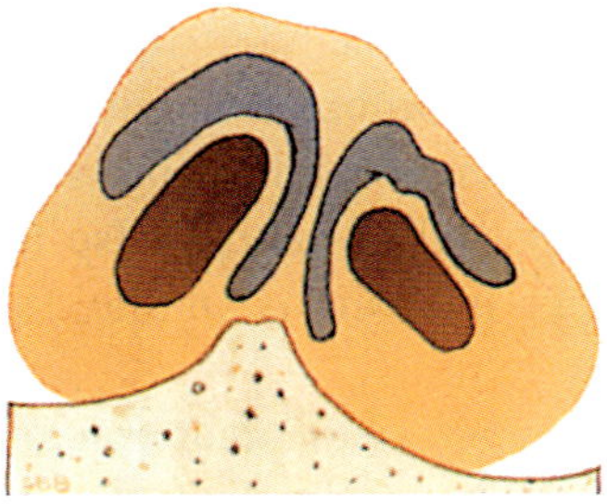

c

Fig. 1b,c. b. Characteristic septal deviation in unilateral clefts. *c.* Downward displacement of alar cartilage, down position of the medial crus, lateral displacement of ala base at the cleft side and tendency to bifidity.

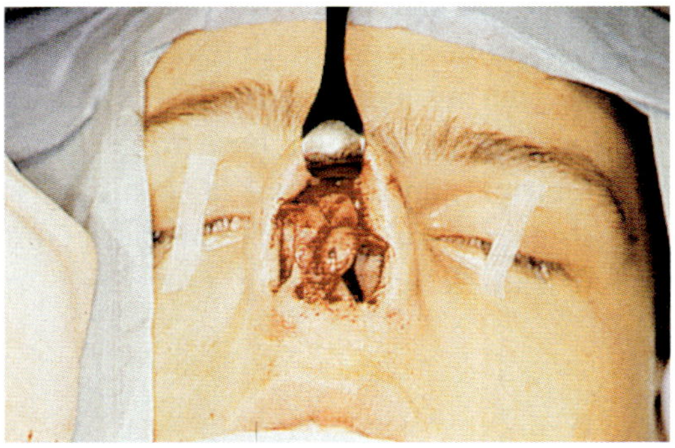

d

Fig. 1d. External approach in unilateral cleft showing typical asymmetry of the lower lateral and disjunction of upper and lower lateral at the cleft side.

Pathological anatomy

Preoperative assessment of the nasal deformity is of the utmost importance when dealing with a secondary correction of a cleft-lip nose. There are certain anatomical characteristics of the nose (in varying degrees) in patients with unilateral and bilateral clefts:

In *unilateral clefts*, the general characteristics are deviation of the nose to the non-cleft side, and asymmetry of the nasal tip (Fig. 1a,b,c,d). More specifically, these are:

septum (Fig. 1b)
- perpendicular plate deviating towards the cleft side
- quadrilateral cartilage at the junction with the perpendicular plate deviating towards the cleft side
- quadrilateral cartilage deviating caudally towards the non-cleft side
- nasal spina deviating towards the non-cleft side

dorsum (Fig. 1a,d)
- bony pyramid deviating towards the non-cleft side
- nasal bones asymmetric and flattened at the cleft side
- upper laterals asymmetric and a disturbed junction between upper and lower laterals at the cleft side tip (Fig. 1c,d)

- downward displacement of the alar cartilage at the cleft side
- tendency for bifidity
- buckling of the lateral crus at the cleft side
- down position of the medial crus at the cleft side columella (Fig. 1c)
- deviation at the top to the cleft side and at the base to the non-cleft side alar base (Fig. 1c)
- lateral (up- or downward) displacement of the alar base resulting in a more horizontal rotation of the nostril at the cleft side
- inadequate rotation

In *bilateral clefts*, the general characteristics are a very short columella with

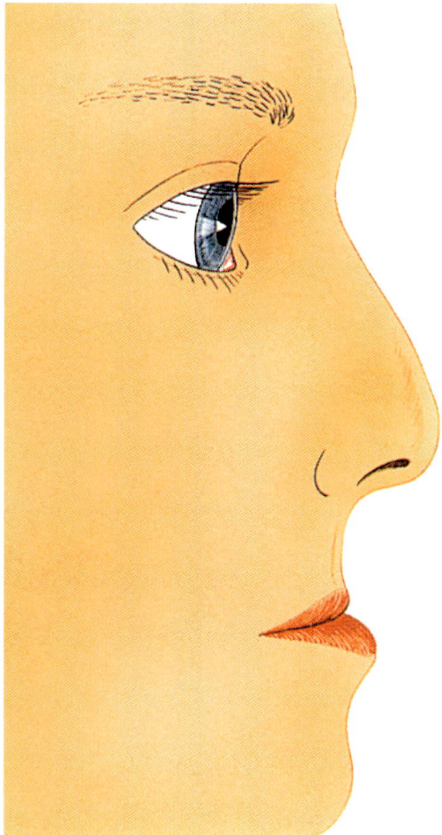

a

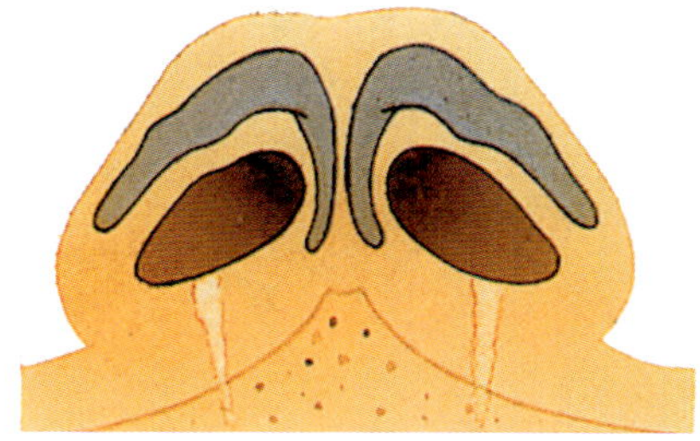

b

Fig. 2a,b. a. Bilateral cleft: lack of nose projection due to a short columella with downward tip rotation. *b.* Bifidity, short columella, buckling of the lateral crura and lateral displacement of the alar bases resulting in a horizontal rotation of the nostrils.

downward tip-rotation and lack of nose projection (Fig. 2a,b). More specifically, these are:

septum – no specific deviation
– disturbed caudo-ventral outgrowth

dorsum – lack of projection with flattening of the osseo-cartilaginous vault
– disturbed junction between upper and lower laterals

tip – bifidity
– downward rotation of the alar cartilage
– buckling of the lateral crura

columella – very short

alar base – lateral displacement of the alar bases resulting in a horizontal rotation of the nostrils
– inadequate rotation

These anatomical characteristics are most obvious when there is a large complete cleft. In these cases, there is hypoplasia and retroposition of the maxilla at the cleft side, resulting in a lack of maxillary support. In mild cases, a cartilaginous graft can be used to give a foundation for the reallocated alar base. In severe cases, a maxillary advancement technique is indicated.

Early surgical procedures, such as mucoperiosteoplasty in uni- and bilateral clefts and forceful retraction of the protruding premaxilla in bilateral clefts to facilitate surgical closure of the cleft lip, result in extra midfacial growth inhibition. The use of an orthopedic device (the growth stimulator), as developed and advocated by Weil, and postponing of the surgical procedure for as long as possible stimulates normal midfacial growth.

Operative techniques

After the preoperative analysis of the pathological anatomy causing the nasal deformity, the operative procedure is outlined. In view of the complexity of the pathology, it is helpful to divide the procedure into the following parts:

- septal surgery
- tip surgery
- osseo-cartilaginous vault surgery
- maxillary augmentation
- alar base reallocation

Although the sequence of the operative steps may change according to individual

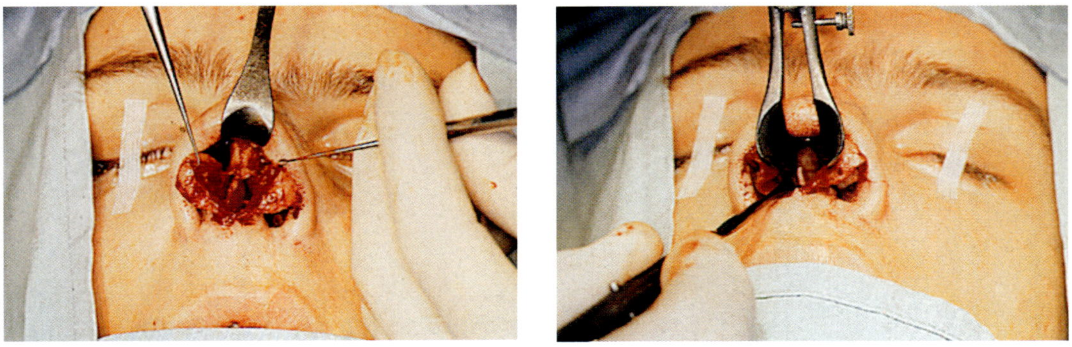

a b

Fig. 3a,b. a. External approach in unilateral cleft patient showing the characteristic deviation of the caudal septum towards the non-cleft side. *b.* Harvesting of an autogenous cartilage graft to be used as a columella strut.

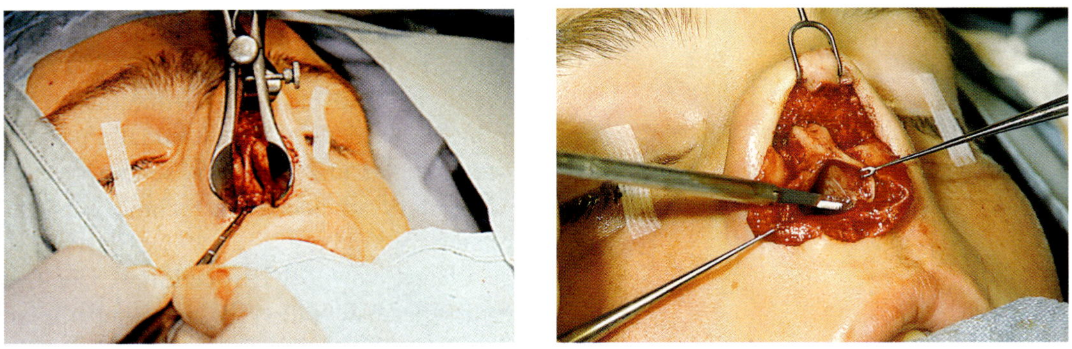

c d

Fig. 3c,d. c. Anterior nasal spine deviated towards the non-cleft side. *d.* Scoring of the caudal part of the cartilaginous septum at the concave (non-cleft) side.

cases and personal preference, it should be as logical as possible.

Another basic starting point in the procedure is which approach to use: closed or open. In general, the open (external) approach is indicated in cases with severe deformity of the nasal tip, which needs extensive reconstruction. The closed (intranasal) approach is useful in patients with mild nasal tip deformities.

The use of the following grafts and implants is often indicated in rebuilding the nose:

- columella strut for tip projection
- shield graft or onlay tip graft for tip definition
- dorsal graft for dorsal height
- premaxillary implant to restore maxillary support for the nose (ala)

Autogenous septal or ear cartilage grafts are the first choice over allogenic and nonbiological (xenogeneic) material. For maxillary augmentation, xenogeneic material such as proplast or goretex can also be used.

Surgical procedures in unilateral cleft lip patients

Septal surgery

The standard Cottle procedure: hemitransfixion incision, followed by subperichondrial and subperiosteal tunnelling at both sides is appropriate in both open and closed approaches. In the open (external) approach, the direct approach to the septum after separating the intercrural ligaments is a good alternative (Fig. 3a).

After the tunnelling procedure, separation of the quadrilateral cartilage from the premaxilla and vomer is carried out (in most cases the quadrilateral cartilage is displaced from the premaxilla towards the non-cleft side). The next step is a vertical chondrotomy to separate the perpendicular plate from the quadrilateral cartilage, followed by limited resection of cartilage to make repositioning possible in the midline. Then osteotomies of the vomer and perpendicular plate are carried out to facilitate luxation towards the mid-

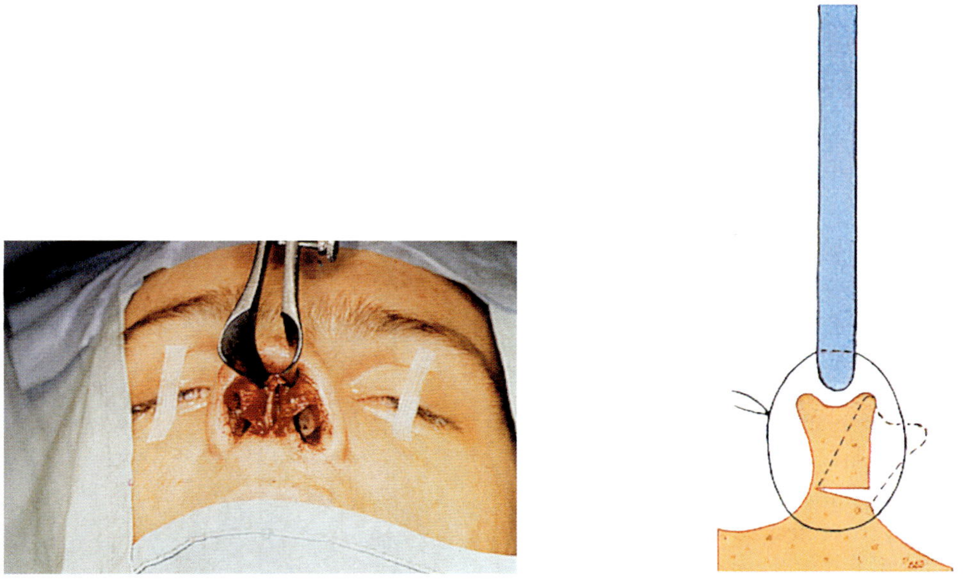

Fig. 3e,f. e. Realigned caudal septum and anterior nasal spine. *f.* Fixation suture after realignment of the nasal spine.

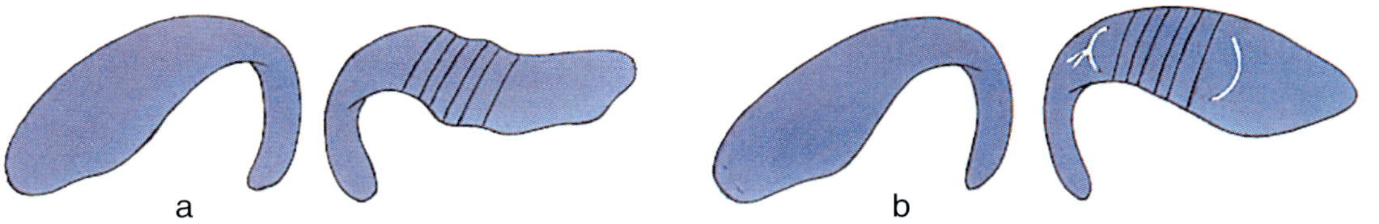

Fig. 4a,b. a. Scoring of the buckled lateral crus. *b.* Adjustment mattress suture after scoring procedure.

line (in most cases the quadrilateral cartilage deviates into the nasal passage at the cleft side at the junction with the perpendicular plate) (Fig. 1b).

Realignment of the caudal part of the quadrilateral cartilage (deviating to the non-cleft side) is performed by superficial vertical parallel chondrotomies at the non-cleft side, breaking the spring and, in this way, creating bending of the cartilage to the opposite side (for standard septoplasty procedures see Chapter 6). This is followed by repositioning of the anterior nasal spine from the non-cleft side to the midline, after a horizontal osteotomy and fixation by sutures to prevent redeviation of the caudal septum and the anterior nasal spina (Fig. 3a–f).

If necessary, autogenous cartilage grafts can be harvested from the quadrilateral cartilage (Fig. 3b), taking care not to disturb the septal support of the nasal dorsum and tip. Left-over cartilage (crushed or not) should be replaced between the mucoperichondrium blades to prevent a possible septal perforation.

Tip surgery

Closed (delivery) approach for mild asymmetry of the nasal tip: Intercartilaginous incisions are made 2 mm caudal to the internal valve extending around the caudo-cephalic border of the septal cartilage (No. 15 blade), and marginal incisions are made along the caudal border of the lateral crus, the dome and the upper part of the medial crus. The lateral crura are freed with curved pointed scissors at the non-vestibular side, from the overlaying soft tissue. The next step is delivery of the lower lateral cartilages for inspection and comparison (for standard surgical procedures see Chapter 10).

The lateral crus is sometimes buckled

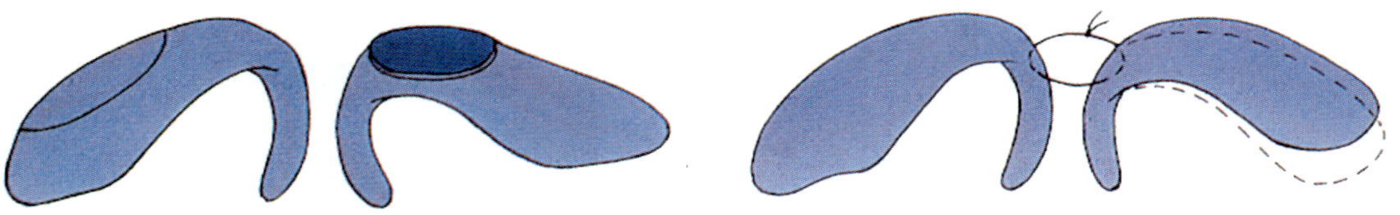

Fig. 5. Resection of the cephalic part of the lower lateral at the non-cleft side to augment the dome at the cleft side.

Fig. 6. Mattress suture to reposition the lateral crus (cleft side) in a more medial and prominent position.

at the cleft side. This should be corrected by scoring the cartilage and, if necessary, a supplementary adjustment mattress suture (Fig. 4a,b). In most cases, the lateral crus at the non-cleft side is larger in the cephalo-caudal direction. To create better symmetry, a small piece of cartilage from the cephalic side of the lateral crus should be resected. This piece of autogenous cartilage is very useful as an onlay graft to augment the dome at the cleft side, when repositioning of the lower lateral cartilage does not give an optimal result (Fig. 5). To reposition the lower lateral cartilage at the cleft side, the vestibular skin is separated from the lateral crus (with curved pointed scissors). The whole lateral crus is now repositioned more medially and upward (cephalic) to give a more prominent symmetric dome. It is fixed with mattress sutures (PDS 5/0) to the lower lateral cartilage on the normal side (Fig. 6).

Sometimes it is necessary to dissect the lateral crus free of its lateral attachment to create satisfactory repositioning. A columella strut of autologous septal cartilage in a pocket between the medial crura is often useful to obtain extra tip support. The junction of the lower lateral and the upper lateral cartilage is disturbed to a greater or lesser extent at the cleft side. By suturing the cephalic border of the lower lateral to the caudal border of the upper lateral cartilage, the lower lateral is brought into a normal upward rotating position. After reallocation of the alar base (at the cleft side) more medially, a final Z-plasty at the lateral side of the intercartilaginous incision is sometimes necessary to correct an oblique band (Fig. 7).

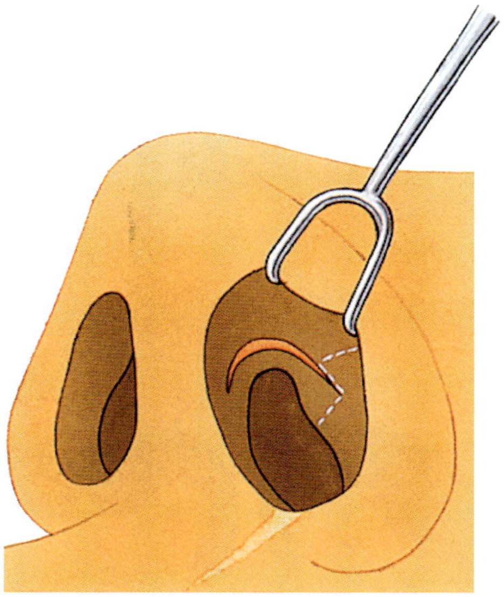

Fig. 7. Z-plasty of the vestibular skin after repositioning the lateral crus.

Open (external) approach for severe asymmetry of the nasal tip: A broken columellar incision is made, taking care not to damage the underlying cartilage (Fig. 8a,b). This incision is connected to marginal incisions following the caudal border of the lower lateral. Careful dissection of the columellar skin flap is performed with Converse (hooked) scissors. With light upward traction of the skin flap, it is quite easy to free the anterior side of the lower laterals by blunt dissection up (avascular) to the dome and in a lateral direction, extending the marginal incisions (with the scissors) along the caudal border of the lateral crus, then in a cephalic direction in a surgical plane adjacent to the cartilaginous vault (Fig. 9a,b,c).

The next step is to free the lateral crus from the vestibular skin at the cleft side (with curved pointed scissors) (Fig. 10a,b). A columellar pocket is made by dissection between the medial crura, in which

Fig. 8a,b. a. Broken (asymmetric) columellar incision. *b.* Completing the columellar skin incision while medial crura are protected by a pair of curved pointed scissors in a subcutaneous pocket.

a 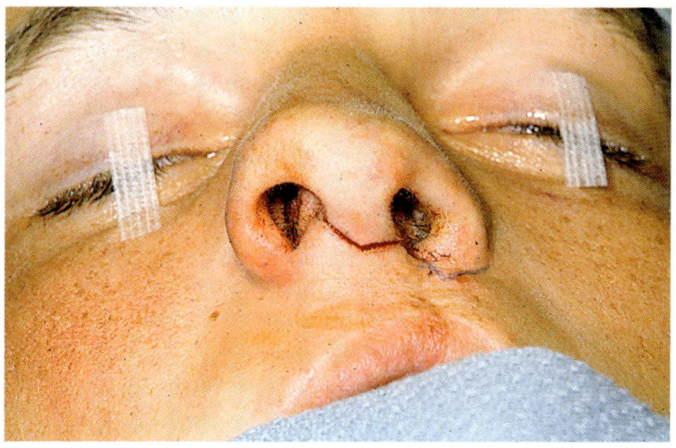

b 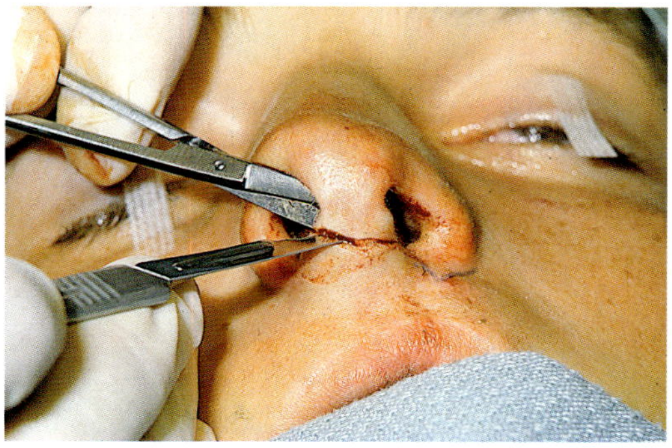

Fig. 9a,b. a. Dissection of the columellar skin flap. *b.* Freeing the lateral crus (subperichondrial) in a lateral direction.

a 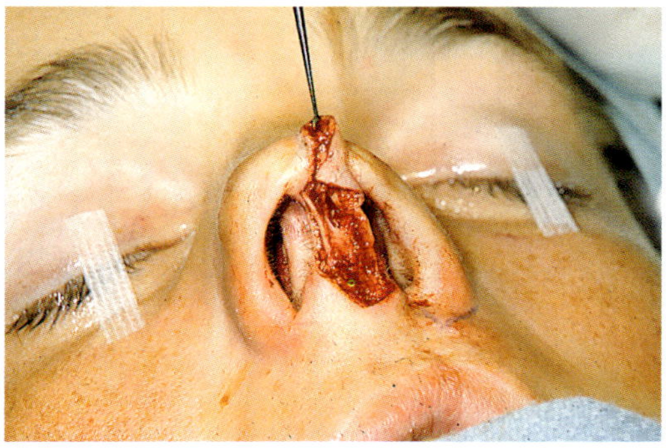

b 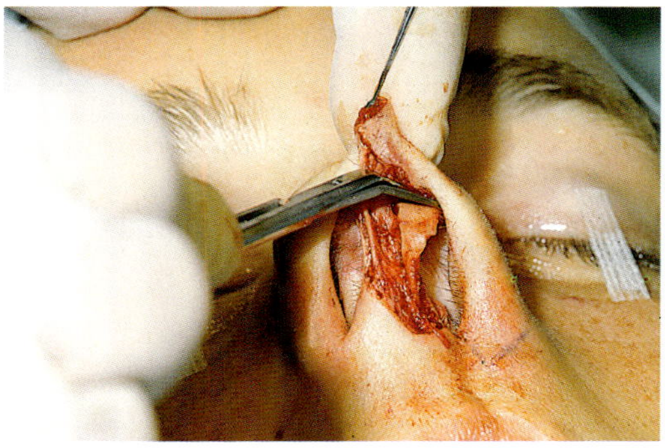

Fig. 9c. Cartilaginous vault dissected free and separated from medial crura to approach the caudal end of the septum.

Fig. 10a. Dissecting the lateral crus free from the vestibular skin.

c 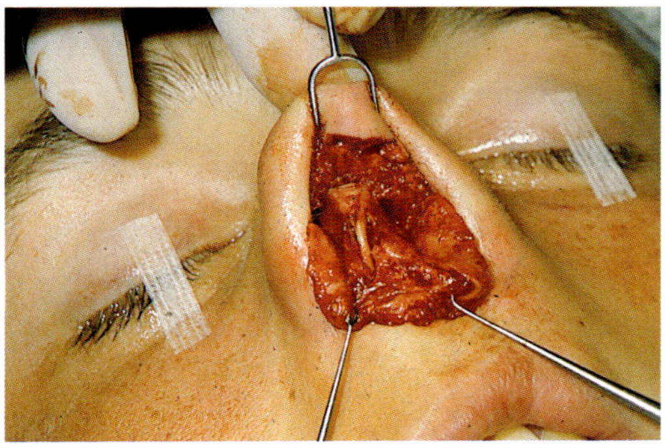

a 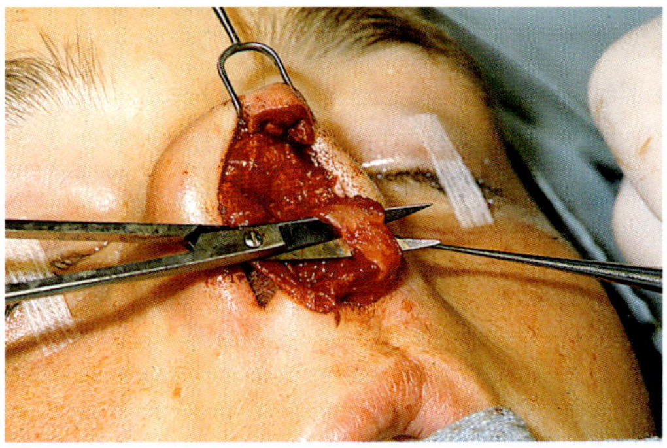

Fig. 10b. Lateral crus freed completely for repositioning.

b 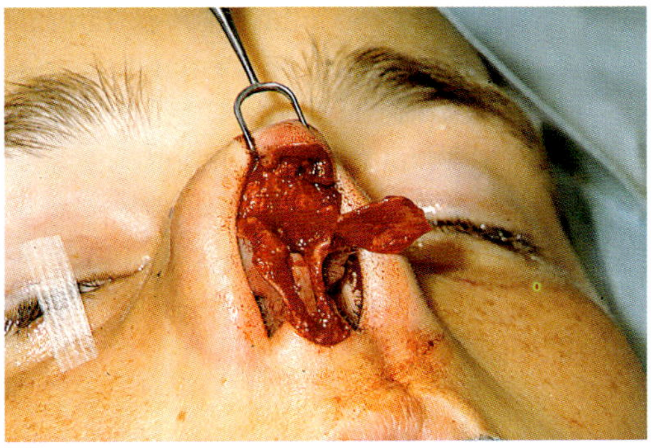

an autologous cartilage graft is placed (columella strut). The lower lateral cartilage on the cleft side is moved into a new more medial and prominent position, and sutured with the lower lateral of the normal side to the columellar strut (Fig. 11). If necessary, the lateral crus (at the cleft side) which compared to the broad lateral crus (at the nasal side) is often buckled, is remodelled and repositioned as described in the section on the closed

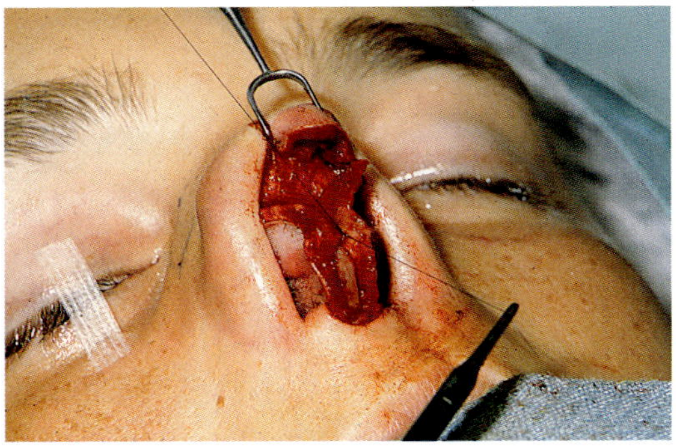

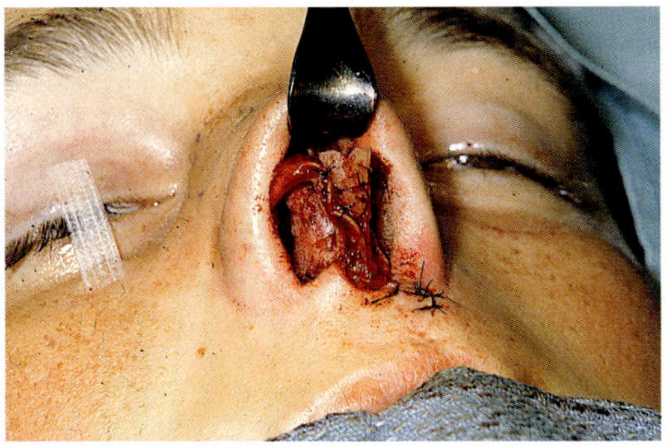

Fig. 11. Lower lateral at cleft side is sutured in a more medial and prominent position (6/0 nylon).

Fig. 12. Shield tip graft sutured in place.

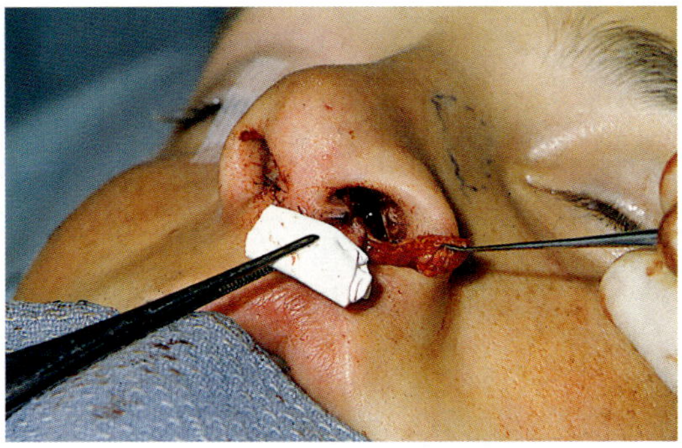

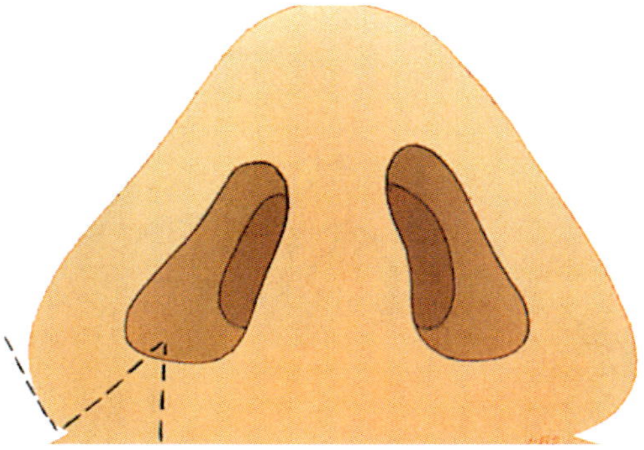

Fig. 13. Maxillary augmentation with goretex at cleft side.

Fig. 14. Z-plasty to relocate the alar base in a more medial position.

approach to the tip (Fig. 4a,b). When this stage tip definition is not satisfactory, a shield graft such as that described in Chapter 12 can be used. Depending on the thickness of the skin, a sharper or less sharp double pointed shield should be used (Fig. 12).

Osseo-cartilaginous vault surgery

In both open and closed approaches, the cartilaginous and bony dorsum can be corrected with the standard rhinoplasty technique described in Chapter 11.

Maxillary augmentation

Hypoplasia and retroposition of the maxilla (at the cleft side), as a result of a complete cleft, should be corrected to form a firm base for the nose and to contribute to the aesthetic result of the rhinoplasty. Different biological and non-biological materials can be used as autologous cartilage: processed irradiated bovine (xenogeneic) cartilage, hydroxyl apatite, mersilene or goretex. A simple technique is to use the alar-base incision, already necessary for reallocation of the alar base, followed by preoperation of a premaxillary supraperiosteal pocket, in which the graft or implant can be placed (Fig. 13).

Alar base reallocation

Most frequently, the alar base is lateralized, which results in abnormal horizontal rotation of the nostril. Although there are many different techniques to reallocate the alar base, a simple Z-plasty is useful for medializing the lateralized alar base (Fig. 14) and, in certain cases, for lateralizing the alar base when the nostril is too narrow.

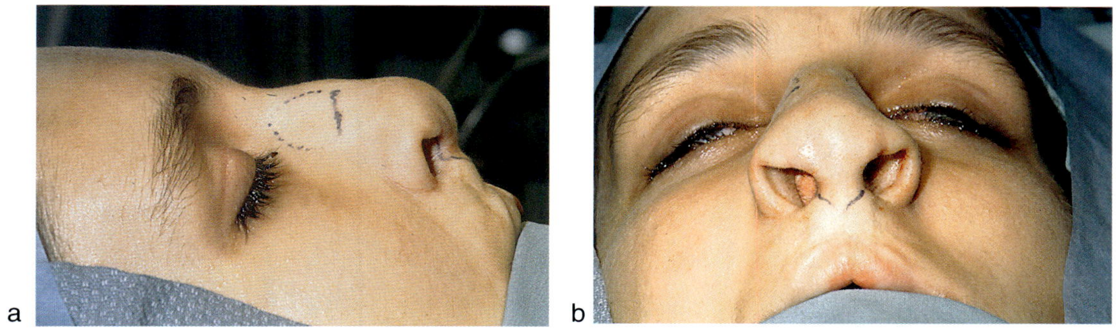

Fig. 15a,b. Preoperative lateral and basal views of a bilateral cleft patient.

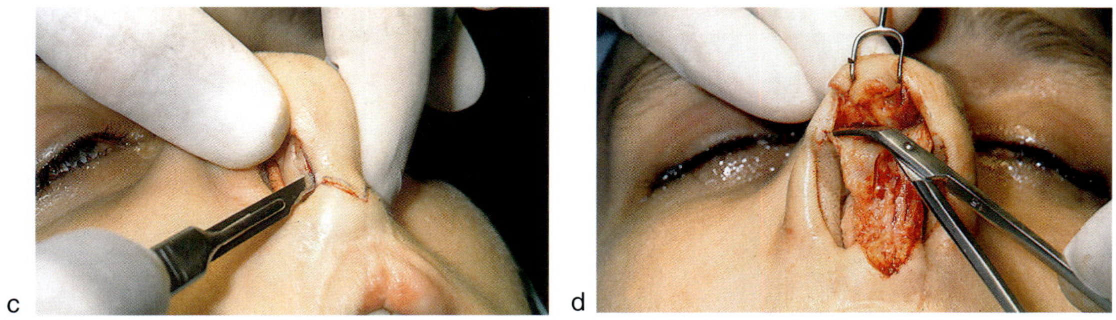

Fig. 15c,d. Columella V incision followed by dissection in a supraperichondrial plane with Converse scissors.

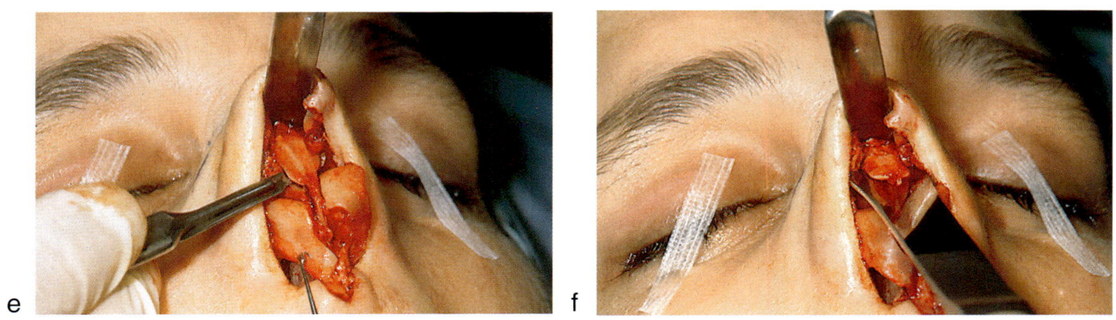

Fig. 15e, f. Hump resection.

Surgical procedures in bilateral cleft lip patients

Septal surgery

As there is, in most instances, no septal deviation due to the cleft syndrome, septal surgery is only necessary for harvesting an autologous cartilage graft or in case of post-traumatic septal deviation. For the technique to be used, see Chapter 6.

Tip surgery

The very short columella and downwardly rotated tip, which result in a lack of tip projection (Fig. 15a,b), make an open (external) approach the most appropriate. The most important goals are:

1. to lengthen the columella in order to make adequate tip projection possible;
2. to eliminate bifidity and, if necessary, remodelling of the lower lateral cartilage.

Instead of making a broken mid-columellar (butterfly) incision, V-Y advancement technique incisions are used to lengthen the columella (Figs. 15c,j,k and 16a,b,c,d). With the modified columella skin flap, the procedure to expose the nasal cartilaginous and bony skeleton for remodelling and repositioning of the lower lateral cartilage, is the same as that described for

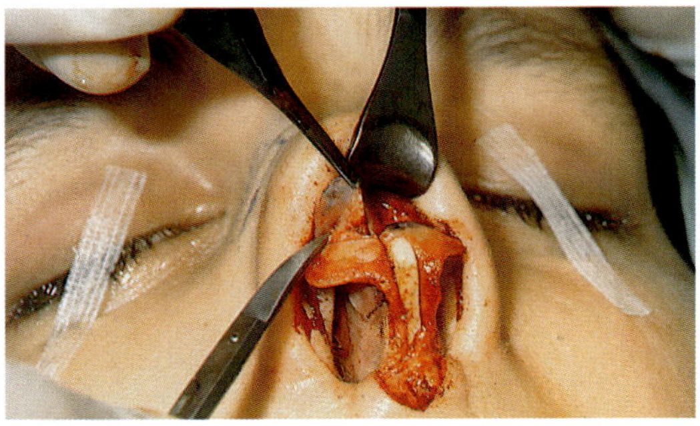
g

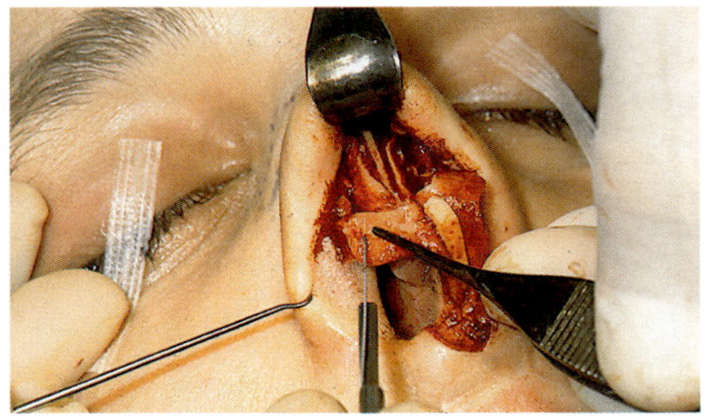
h

Fig. 15g,h. Resection of the cephalic part of the lateral crus and superficial scoring of the cartilage.

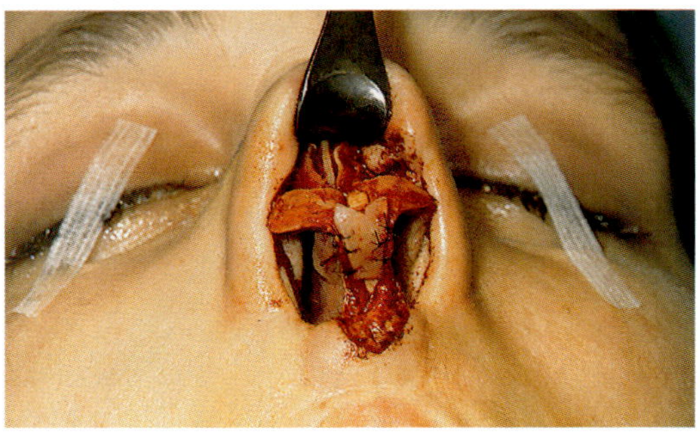
i

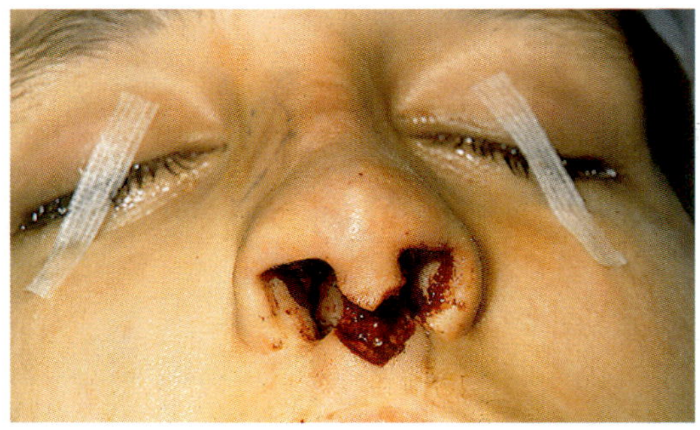
j

Fig. 15i,j. i. Shield graft sutured in place. *j.* V-Y advancement procedure to lengthen the columella.

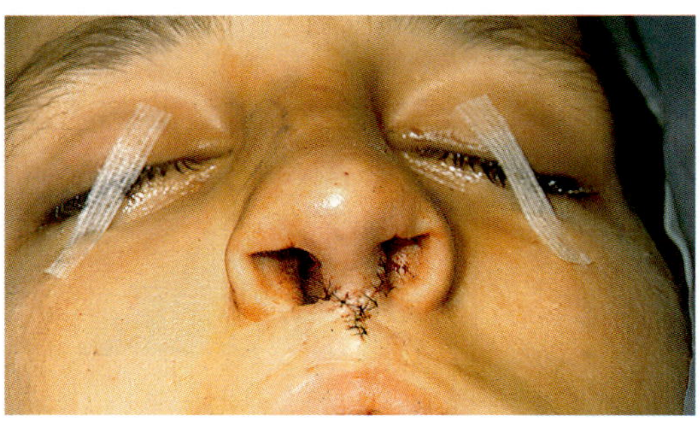
k

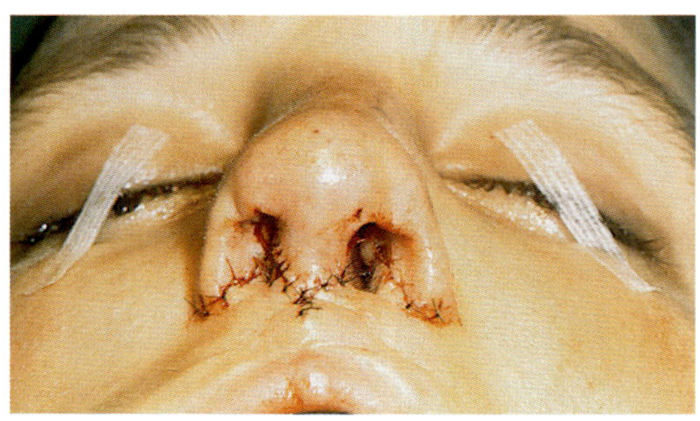
l

Fig. 15k.

Fig. 15l,m. Direct postoperative situation after vestibular and alar base wedge resections.

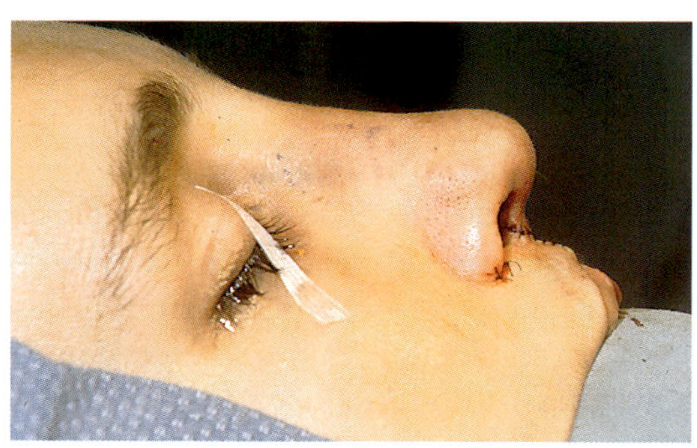
m

Fig. 15m.

unilateral clefts. Buckling of the lateral crura is often present and can be corrected by scoring and adjustment mattress sutures. A columella strut is even more important for restoring tip projection in bilateral than in unilateral clefts, as is the use of a shield graft for tip definition (Fig. 15d–o).

Osseo-cartilaginous vault surgery

In most cases of bilateral cleft, the bony and cartilaginous dorsum is straight, broad and low. Standard rhinoplasty procedures

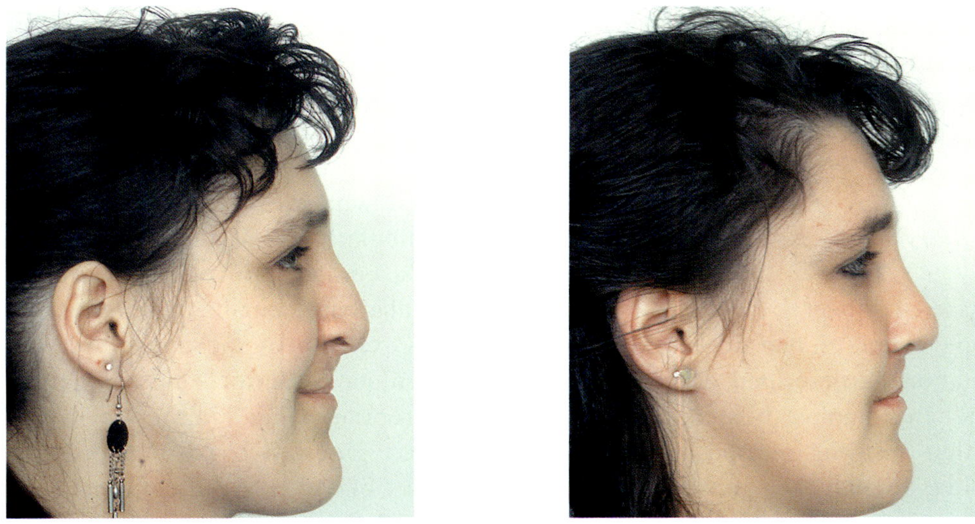

n o

Fig. 15n,o. Pre- and (long-term) postoperative profile view. Compared with the direct postoperative lateral view, there is a slightly diminished tip projection and columellar show.

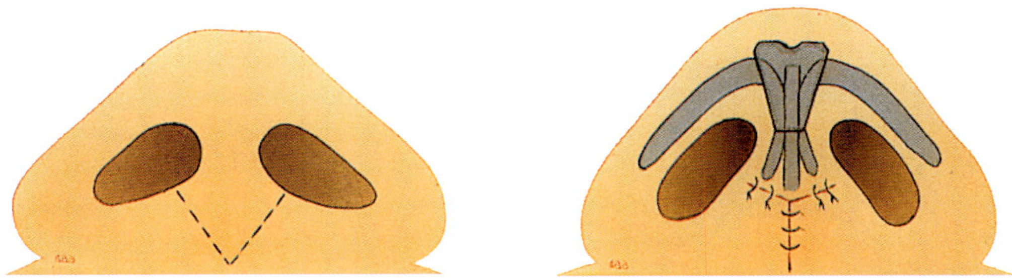

a b

Fig. 16a-b,c-d. V-Y advancement procedures to lengthen the columella.

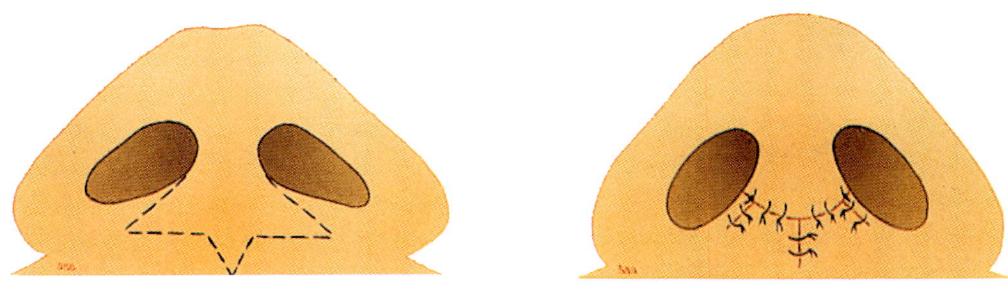

c d

Fig. 16c-d.

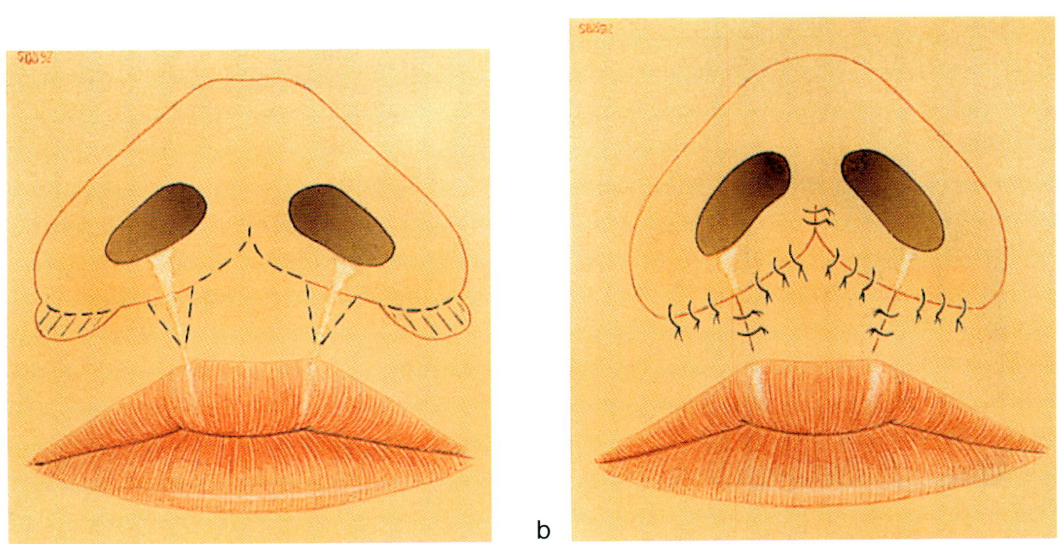

a b

Fig. 17a-b. Crone's technique for lengthening the columella, medial rotation of the alar base and excision of scar tissue on the upper lip.

are used to narrow and augment the dorsum. Autogenous septal and concha cartilage grafts are the first choice for dorsum grafts.

Maxillary augmentation

In case of bilateral cleft patients with a complete cleft on one side, maxillary augmentation as described earlier is appropriate. In complete bilateral clefts, there is often a strong retropositioning of the maxilla, for which a maxillary advancement technique is indicated.

Alar base reallocation

The lateralized alar base on both sides can be medialized with Z-plasties as described earlier and, if necessary, combined with wedge resection of alar and vestibular skin. If there is an indication for a combination of medial rotation of the alar base, lengthening of the columella and excision of the upper lip scars, the technique described by Crone is very appropriate (Fig. 17a,b).

In Figures 18-21 pre- and postoperative views of secondary rhinoplasty in unilateral cleft lip patients are shown.

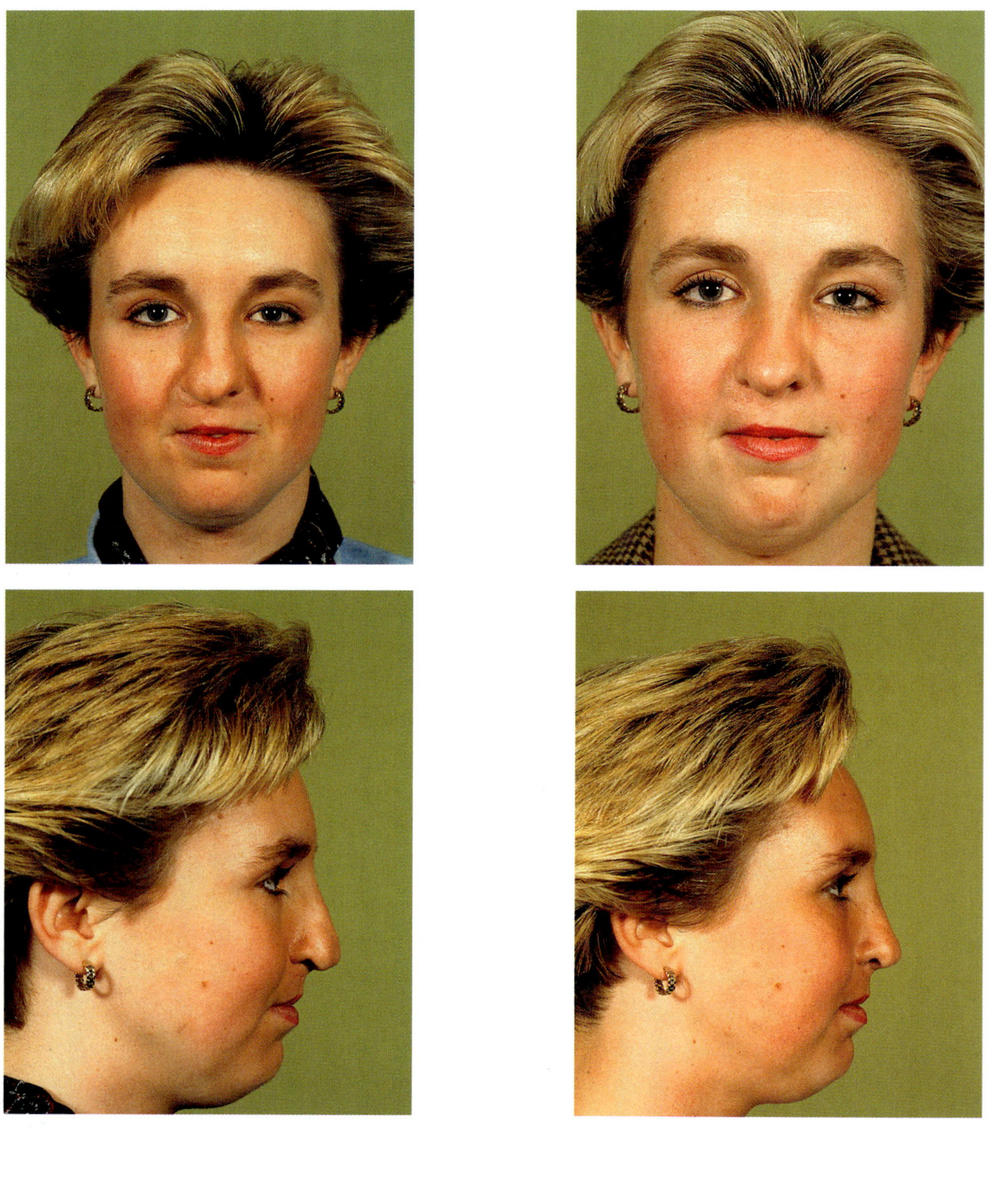

a b c d

Fig. 18a-h. Pre- and postoperative views of a patient with a unilateral cleft who underwent an external rhinoplasty to correct the asymmetric and underprojected tip and an osseo-cartilaginous deviation of the dorsum to the non-cleft side. Postoperatively, a custom-made vestibulum device (*g,h*), was worn day and night for six weeks, and thereafter for six weeks only at night.

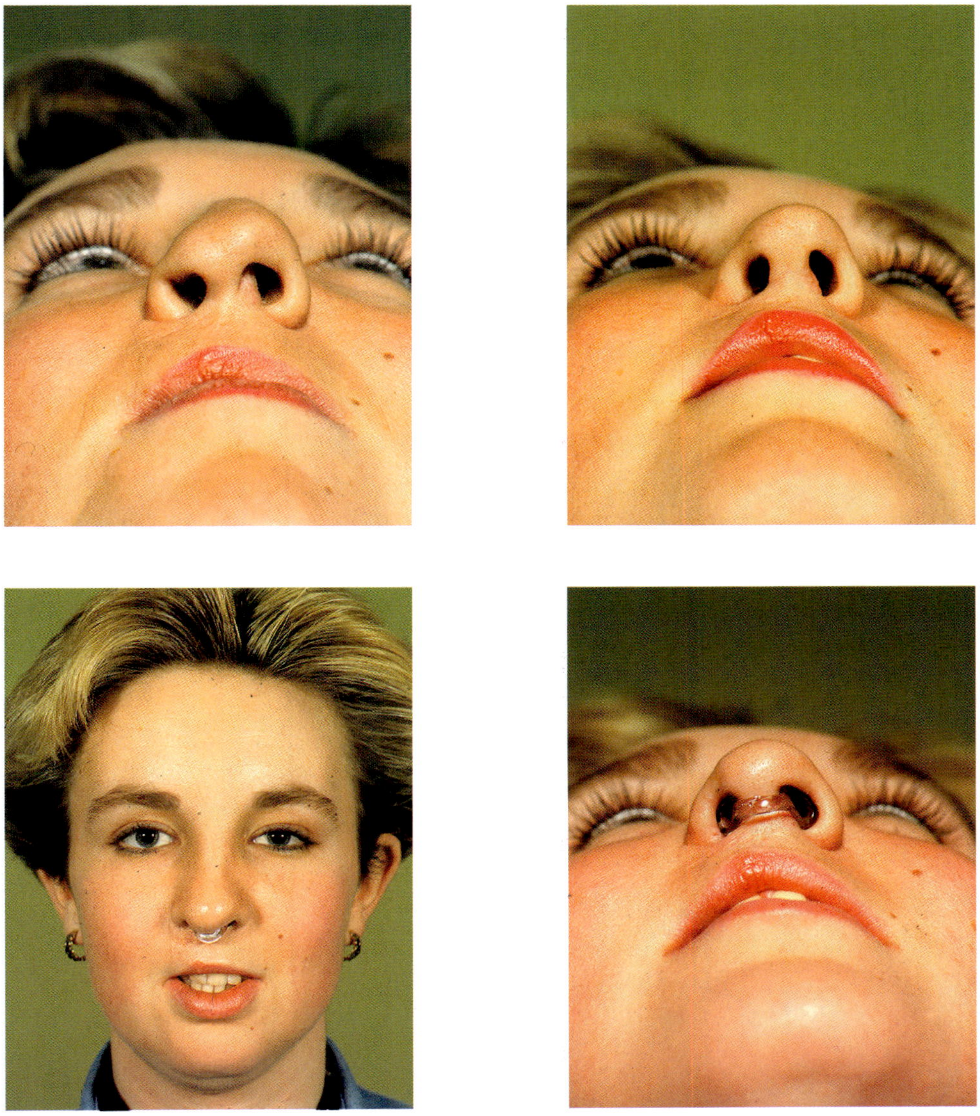

e f g h

Fig. 18e-h.

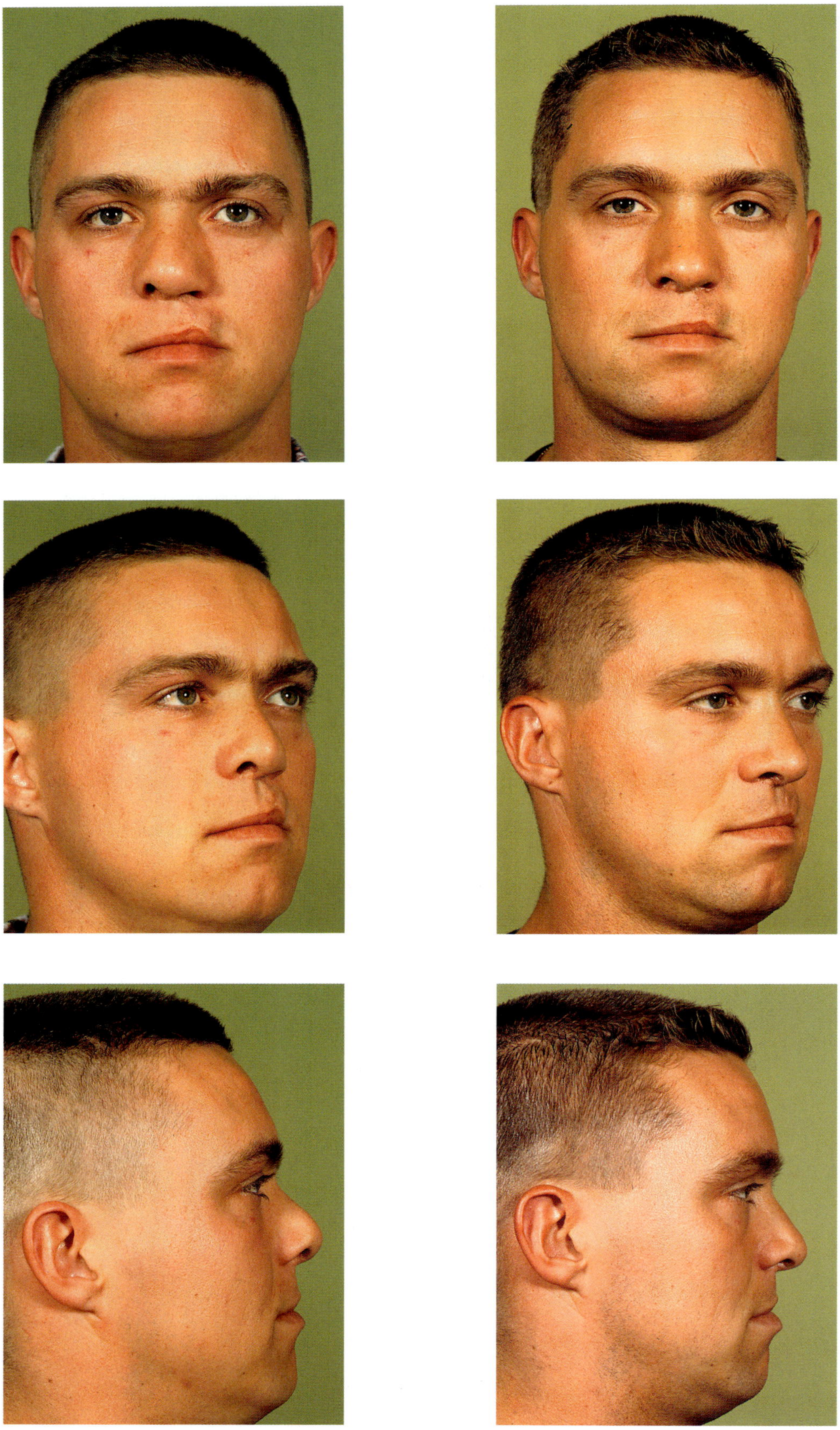

a b c d e f

Fig. 19a-h. Pre- and postoperative views of a case of secondary rhinoplasty in a unilateral cleft lip nose. The external approach was chosen to correct the asymmetry of the tip to lengthen and rotate the nose upward with a columellar strut, a columellar onlay graft and a shield graft. Realignment of the nasal dorsum was performed with micro-osteotomies.

Fig. 19g,h.

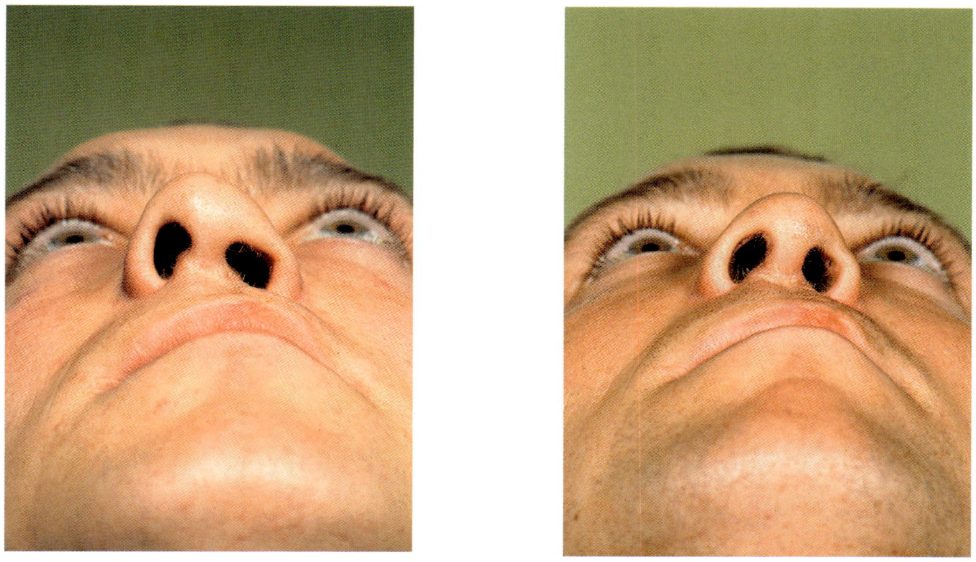

g h

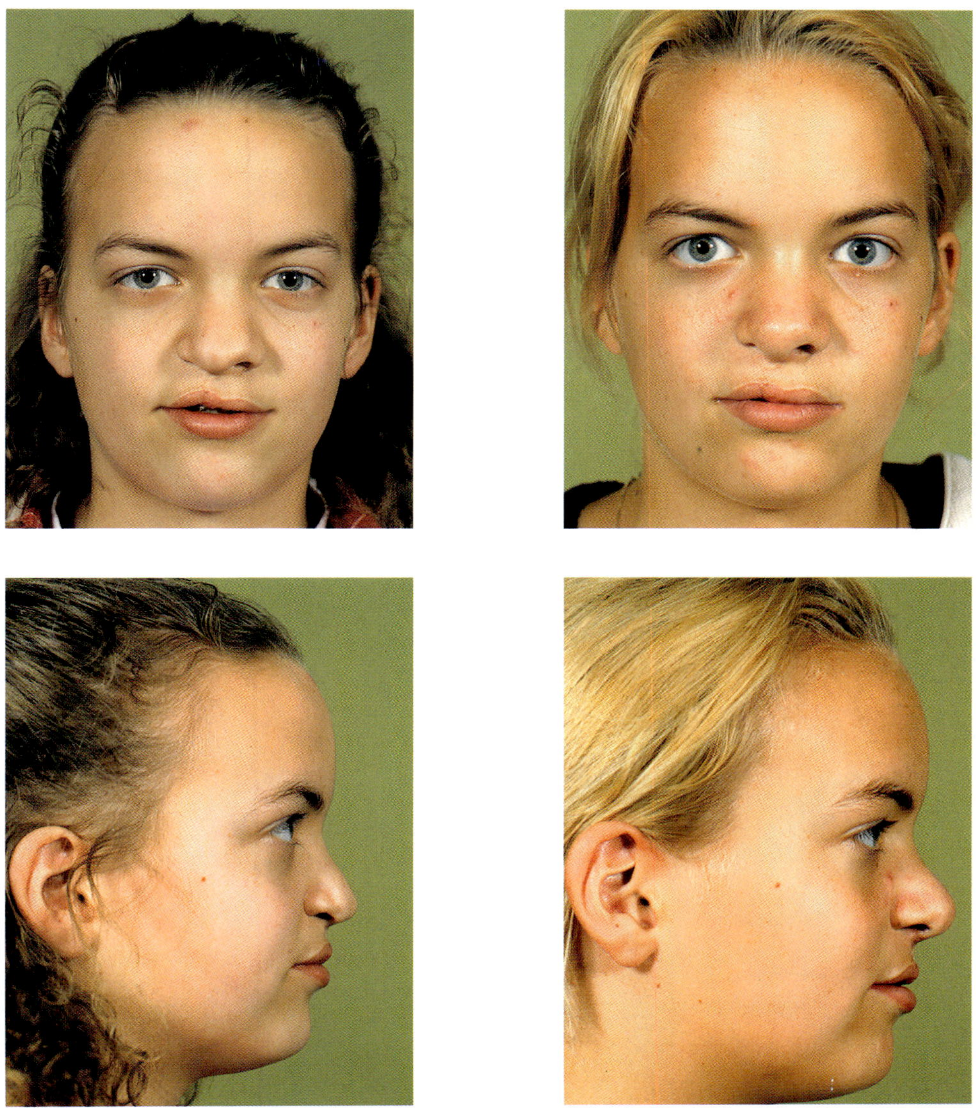

a b c d

Fig. 20a-h. Pre- ad post-operative views of a 14-year-old girl with psychological and functional problems due to the typical unilateral cleft lip nose deformity. Through an external approach, the septal deviation was corrected, followed by repositioning of the distorted lower lateral at the cleft side and endorotation of the alar base. Tip projection was restored with a columella strut and a shield graft.

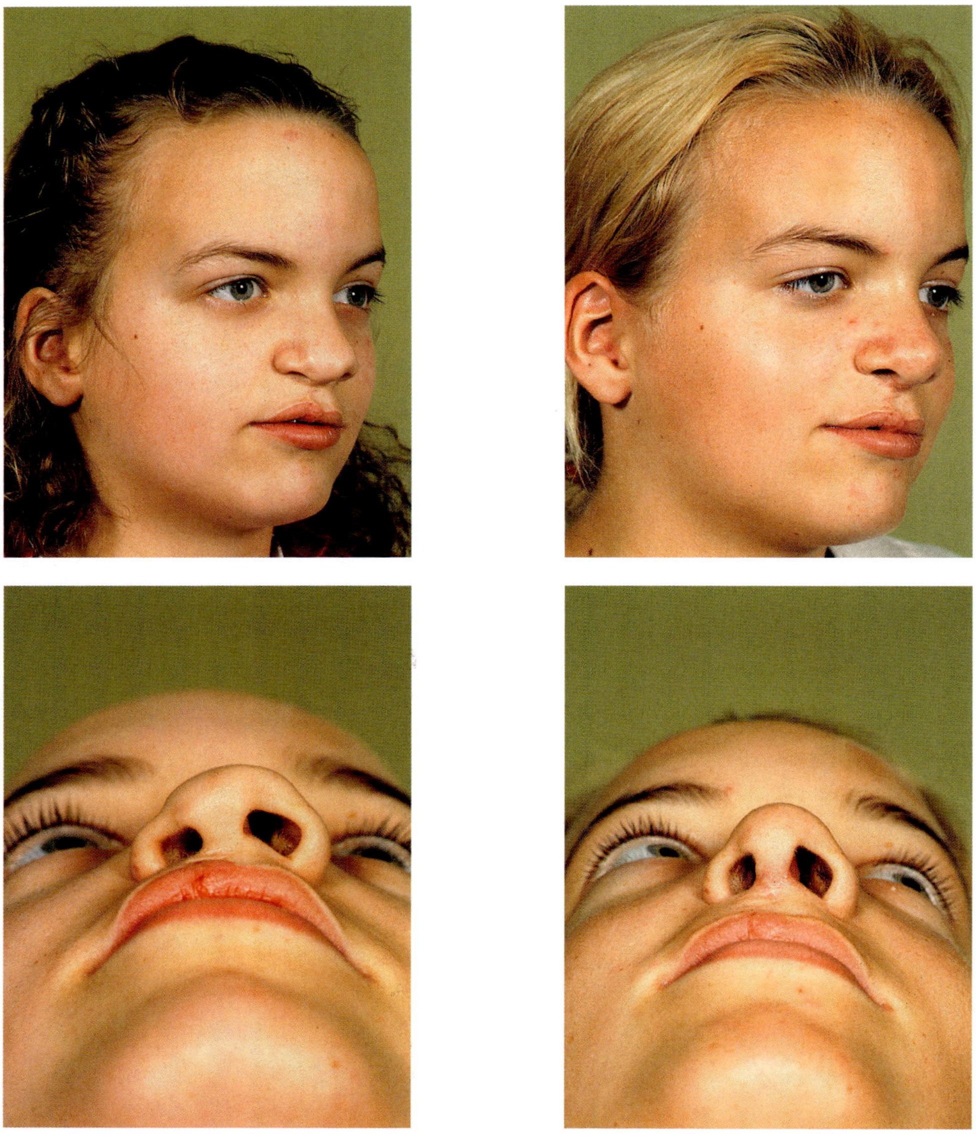

e f g h

Fig. 20e-h.

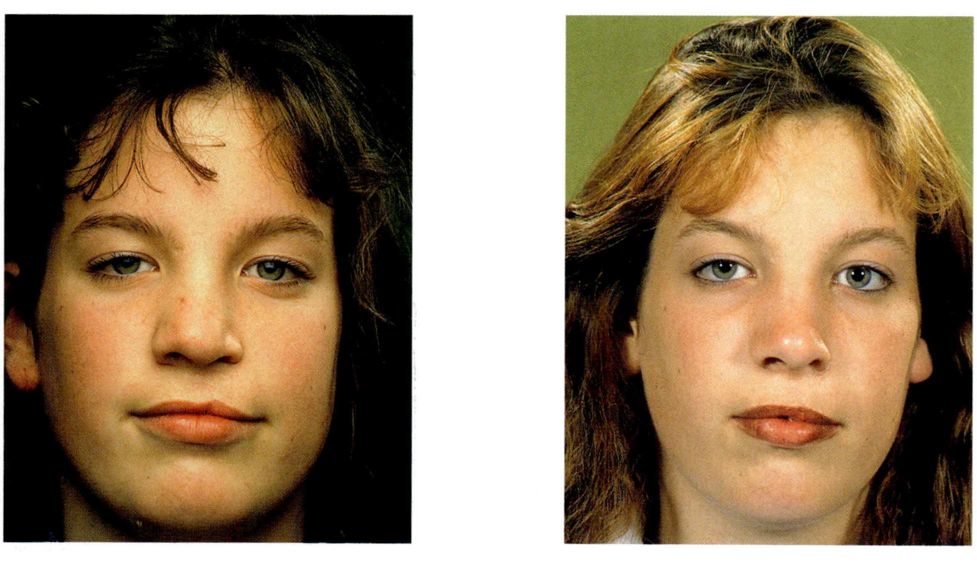

a b

Fig. 21a-h. Pre- and postoperative views of a 15-year-old girl who underwent an external rhinoplasty to correct a moderate characteristic unilateral nasal deformity. Although no complete symmetry of the nostrils was achieved, she lost her disturbing cleft lip stigma.

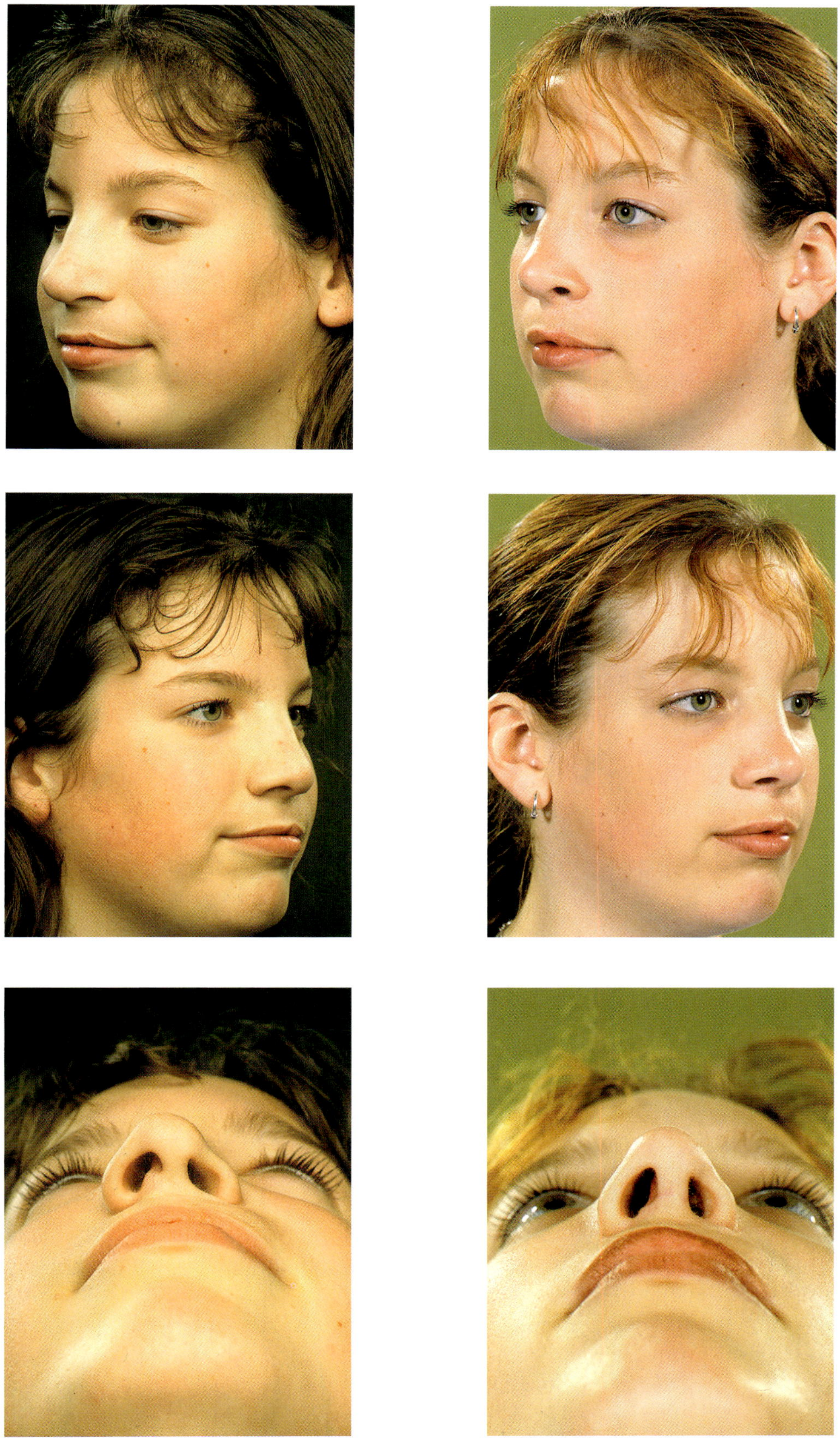

c d

e f

g h

Fig. 21c-h.

16: THE OVER-PROJECTED NASAL TIP

T.R. Bull

It is well known to rhinoplasty surgeons that reducing a projecting nasal tip is not easy. In certain circumstances it may present a very difficult surgical problem. If the skin overlying the cartilages is thick, and the anatomy of the nasal tip is unaesthetic in that it is bifid or square as well as being over-projected, fairly radical tip surgery can be carried out without problem. Not infrequently, however, with a projected tip the skin is thin and the cartilage is strong with a nasal tip that is narrow and pointed. The overall anatomy of the nasal tip is over-projecting, with the anatomy of the dome and projecting aspects of the lateral and medial crura in themselves being aesthetic. Reduction of the projecting tip in these instances presents a problem. In most cases, the dome requires to be retroplaced either by a Lipsett technique or by removing equal portions of the lateral and medial crura, leaving the cartilage at the dome intact. With these techniques, the anatomy of the dome will not be altered. It is extremely uncommon for removal of the upper or cephalic aspect of the alar cartilage to suffice in reducing a markedly projecting tip sufficiently and surgery to this aspect of the cartilage alone is not adequate. The purpose of this analysis of the projecting nasal tip, however, is to draw attention to the role of the anterior nasal spine.

When assessing management of a case of a projecting nasal tip, palpation of the anterior nasal spine is helpful. If there is a prominent spine, the entire tip of the nose may be 'lifted' forward by the spine and reduction may recede the tip by as much as 3–4 mm. An X-ray of the anterior nasal spine is also helpful (Fig. 1).

The anterior nasal spine

The position of the feet of the medial crura is frequently influenced by the anterior nasal spine. If the spine is unduly prominent, the feet are thrust forward and their position is altered in the tip view of the nasal vestibule. The septum too is lifted forward. If the nasal spine has been fractured, there is deviation into one nasal vestibule carrying both the feet of the medial crus and the nasal septum to one side. In these instances, it is well known in septoplasty that fracture of the nasal

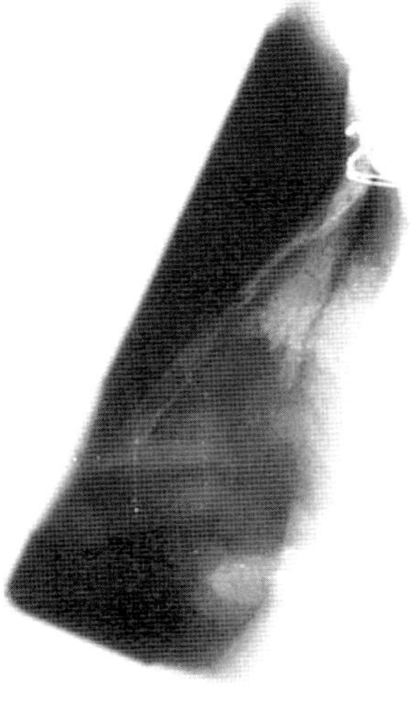

Fig. 1.

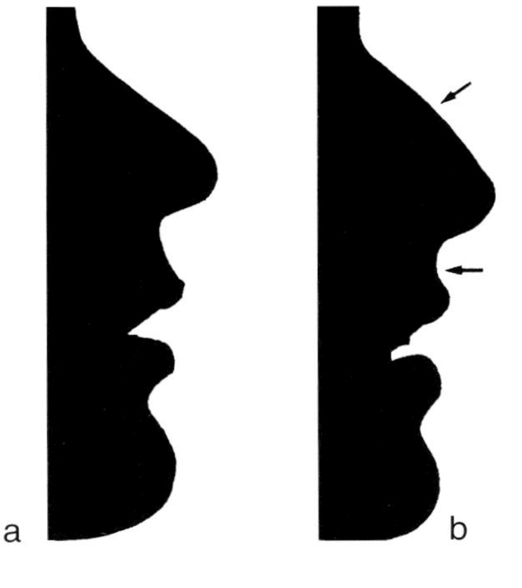

Fig. 2a,b.

spine is required to achieve a mid- line position of the nasal septum. It is, however, the prominence of the anterior nasal spine and the position of the feet of the medial crus which are relevant to the projected nasal tip.

There are other anatomical factors associated with the projected nasal tip, when the contributory factor to this – and it may be the sole cause – is a projecting anterior nasal spine. There is webbing of the naso-labial angle and a shortening of the upper lip (Fig. 3a). Finally, there is not infrequently a very active pull of the musculus depressor septi. On smiling, the tip of the nose is pulled down, making a septal prominence in the supra-tip area and also a curling and shortening of the upper lip is apparent (Fig. 2a,b). A marked gum show is also commonly present. Also, it is necessary to examine under the upper lip to see whether there is a very marked and possibly 'tight' median frenulum.

Surgery for the projecting nasal tip in those cases in which there is no prominence of the anterior nasal spine, requires a Lipsett technique or a variation of this to recess the nasal tip. If, however, the nasal spine is prominent, this alone may require correction to reduce tip projection without surgery to the alar cartilage – the anatomy of which is frequently aesthetic. On other occasions with a grossly projecting nasal tip, surgery to both the anterior nasal spine and the alar cartilages is necessary.

Excision of the anterior nasal spine

Infiltration in the region of the nasal spine with a vasoconstrictor is necessary as this is a particularly vascular area. The transfixion incision is carried down to the anterior nasal spine with dissection to expose the anterior nasal spine. A coarse rongeur is needed to remove the anterior nasal spine and it is frequently helpful if

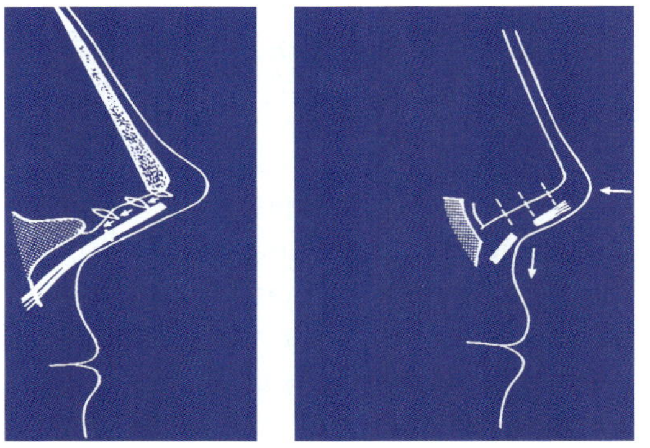

a b *Fig. 3a,b.*

the adjacent prominence of the cartilaginous nasal septum is dissected and removed. A freeing of the upper lip via this incision to break the attachments of the base of the muscular depressor septi is carried out. A retrograde dissection into the columellar is needed further to divide the fibers of this muscle (Fig. 3b).

These steps achieve a marked alteration in the anatomy of the projecting nasal tip. Not only is the projection recessed but also the feet of the medial crus come to lie in a more aesthetic position (Fig. 4a,b). The anatomy of the upper lip is also changed. A lengthening of the upper lip results as does a diminution of the webbing of the naso-labial angle. In most cases the upper lip is short and this is a benefit, but it must also be noted that in those slightly more unusual cases where the upper lip is already long, the decrease in nasal tip projection is counter-balanced by some lengthening of the upper lip with excision of the anterior nasal spine.

Division of the muscle finally makes a difference to the nasal tip on talking and smiling. Mobility of the nasal tip is reduced when this muscle is divided, and on smiling the prominence in the supra-tip region of the nasal septum is absent. Also conspicuous is the change in the upper lip which is released to be longer and does not curl on smiling. There may also be less gum show. The musculus depressor septi, however, is only one of the factors relevant in gum show and the

Fig. 4a,b.

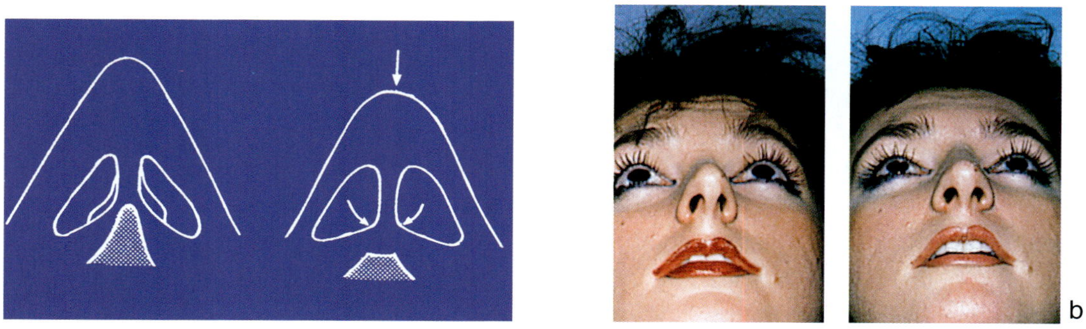

a b

anatomy of the incisor teeth, maxilla and levator labii superioris may also be relevant. There are occasions, however, when division of this muscle alone suffices to bring about a change in a short upper lip and a gummy smile. A large tight upper lip frenulum is released either by a Z-plasty or by a V-Y plasty. This is a further factor in releasing the upper lip.

Suturing

The placing of the sutures between the caudal septum and columella has been said to influence nasal tip projection. If the sutures are placed low on the caudal septum, and high on the columella, the tip position is recessed: if the sutures are placed high on the septum and low on the columella, the tip will be projected. Most rhinoplasty surgeons, however, will maintain that this placing of sutures may influence the tip position on the operating table, and the ultimate position of the tip will revert. In other words, the tip suturing technique is, in itself, ineffective in controlling tip projection: this too is my view.

The suture position may, however, be very relevant if the anterior nasal spine is excised. If there is a space into which the tip can be lowered, sutures placed low in the septum and high on the columella may effectively recess the tip (Fig. 3a,b). With excision of an enlarged anterior nasal spine, if the sutures between the septum and columella are placed obliquely, the projecting tip will be receded or retrodisplaced. Either permanent or absorbent sutures will result in the tip being retrodisplaced into the area previously occupied by the anterior nasal spine.

Summary

Attention is drawn to the role of the enlarged or prominent anterior nasal spine and its relevance to tip projection. In some cases, excision of a large anterior nasal spine alone will suffice for retrodisplacement of the nasal tip.

17: AUGMENTATION RHINOPLASTY

I.S. Mackay

Augmentation of the nose frequently presents a greater surgical challenge than reduction rhinoplasty. Generally, with the latter, providing the surgeon takes the necessary steps to correctly assess the degree of reduction that is required, performs this carefully and uses the now well-established and safe techniques, few problems should be encountered. The same is not true for augmentation, where grafts may become infected, extrude, absorb, twist, buckle, move or present unsightly irregularities at their edges. With an autogenous graft, there is the added possibility of problems at the donor site with infection, pain or other disfigurement.

Synthetic grafts overcome the latter difficulty, but are more likely to extrude and can feel 'unnatural'. There are, however, certain circumstances in which a synthetic graft may provide the best option.

The first human bone graft to the nose was described in 1861 by Ollier, who carried frontal bone as part of a forehead flap reconstructive rhinoplasty. Konig described the first cartilage graft using costal cartilage as a nasal implant in 1896 (Wallace). In 1900, Professor van Mangoldt of Dresden used costal cartilage in a 16-year-old boy with congenital luetic saddling (de Jong).

Numerous synthetic materials have been used for nasal implants:

1828	gold and silver	Rousset
1904	paraffin	Eckstein
1925	ivory	Maliniac
1931	cork	Dahmann
1939	marble	Zeno
1948	acrylic	Wolf and Lloyd

More recent synthetic grafts are Silastic (varying from hard to spongy in form), polyamide mesh (Supramid), Proplast and calcium triphosphate (Ossoplast).

From a surgical point of view, those cases where augmentation may be considered can be grouped as follows:

Saddle accentuated by a hump

A minor supratip depression which is accentuated by sometimes even a small hump and where removal of the hump is

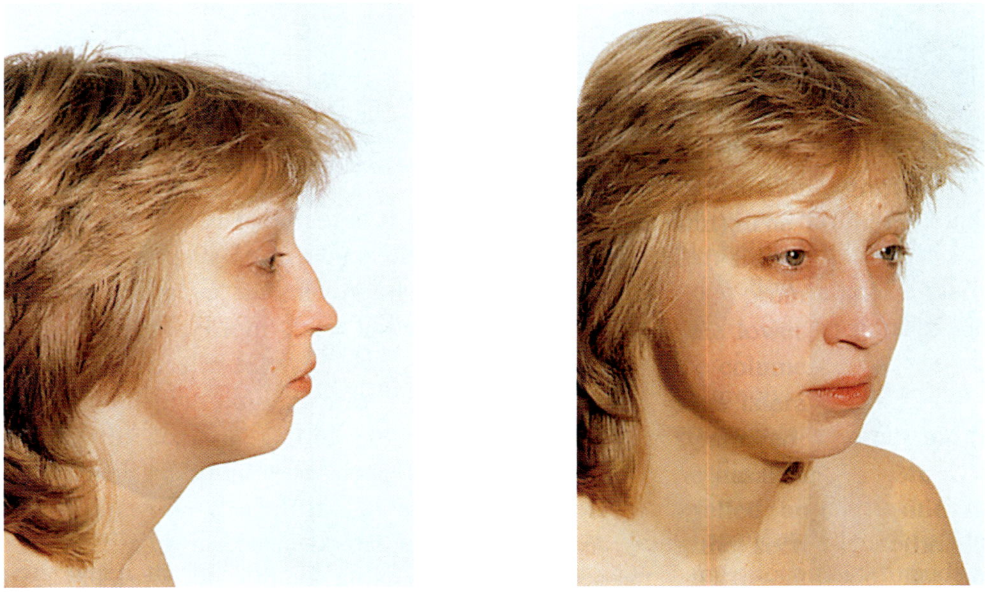

Fig. 1. Pre- (*a,b*) and post- (*c,d*) operative views showing a small saddle accentuated by a hump where reduction of the hump reduced the need for augmentation to a slither of cartilage in the supratip region (combined with chin augmentation using a Silastic implant).

a

b

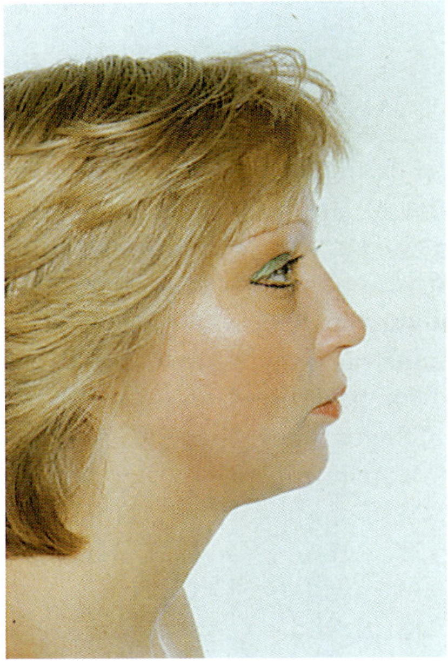

c

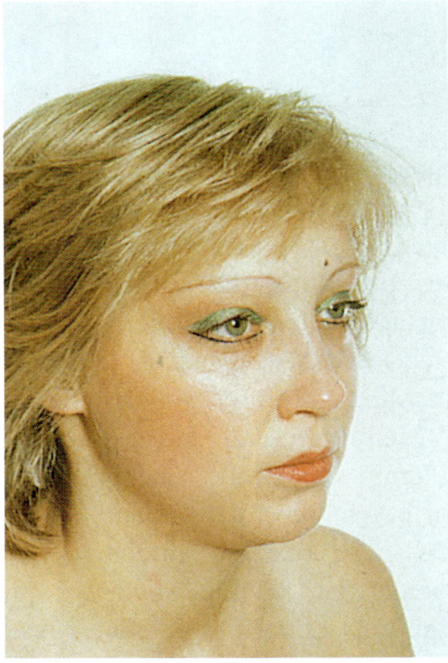

d

Fig. 1c,d.

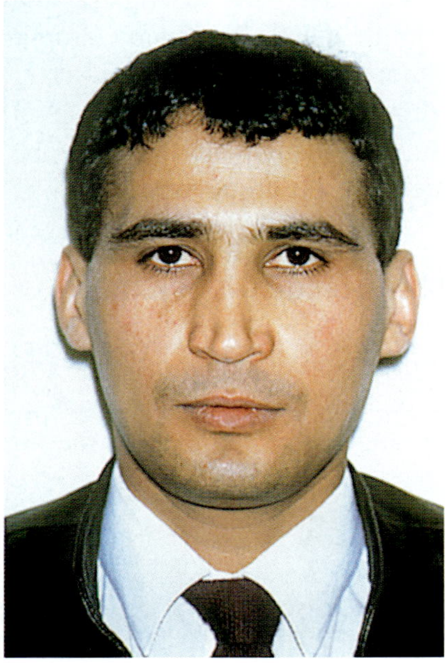

a

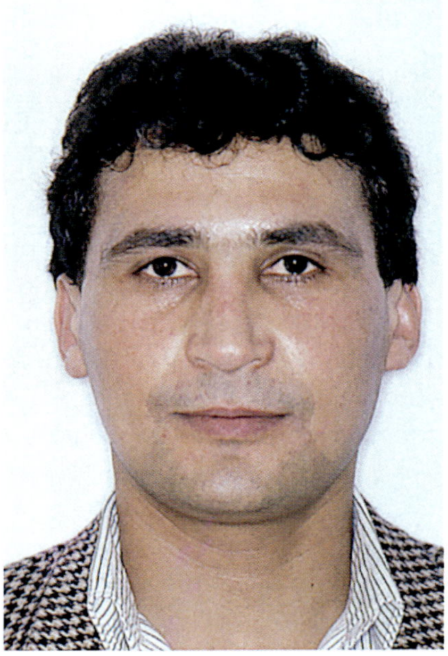

b

Fig. 2. Pre- (*a*) and post- (*b*) operative views demonstrating the use of auricular cartilage as a filler to augment minor depressions in a revision rhinoplasty.

all that is required to restore the profile. This is particularly applicable to females in whom a smaller nose may even be seen as an advantage (Fig. 1).

Minimal depression requiring 'filling'

A small depression in the supratip region or elsewhere in the nose may simply require a little padding to fill in the depression. It is tempting in this situation to use an injectable filler such as collagen, but the improvement is often short-lived. Injection with more permanent 'fillers' may have a useful role in the future, but long-term follow-up with these is not yet available. In this situation, an autogenous graft such as temporalis fascia or thin strips of cartilage is advantageous. The lower lateral nasal cartilage is particularly suitable for this purpose (Fig. 2).

Fig. 3. Pre- (*a,c,e*) and post- (*b,d,f*) operative views demonstrating a moderate saddle deformity corrected with a 'sandwich' of layers of auricular cartilage to the dorsum and septal cartilage harvested posteriorly and implanted anteriorly to augment the columella.

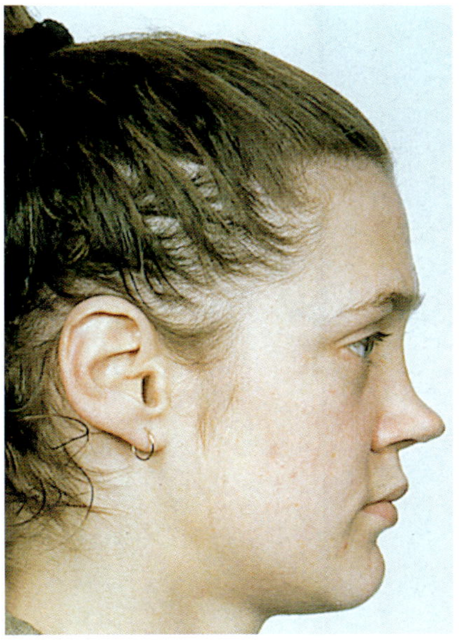
a

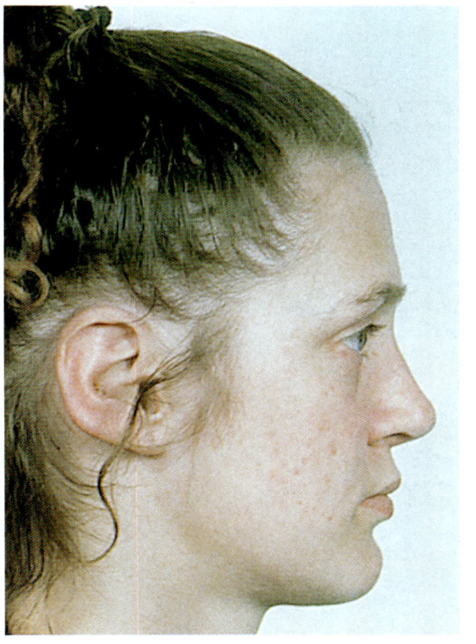
b

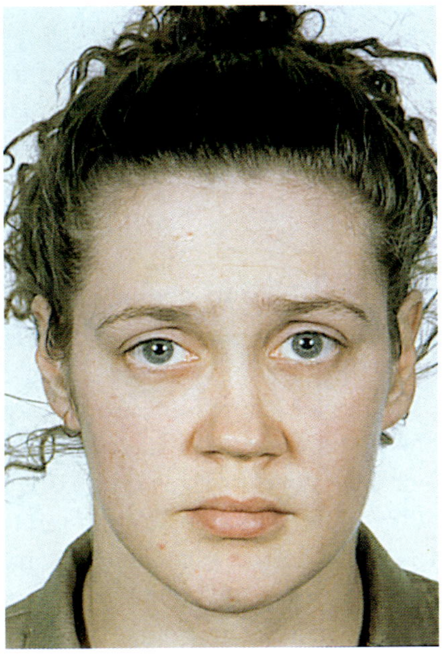
c

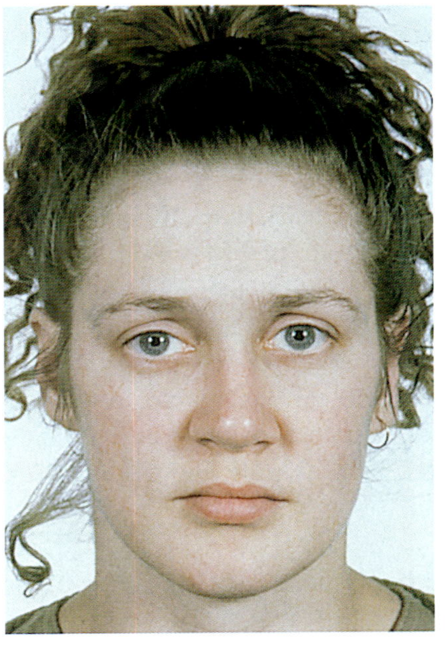
d

Fig. 3c,d.

Moderate sized saddle

The small to moderate sized saddle can be corrected using conchal cartilage from the ear or nasal septal cartilage, if this is still available.

Septal cartilage is particularly suitable for augmenting the columella when support is required; even quite large saddles can be corrected using layers of cartilage sutured together as a 'sandwich' and if necessary covered with a layer of temporalis fascia to soften the edges which may otherwise be visible, especially in a patient with thin skin (Fig. 3).

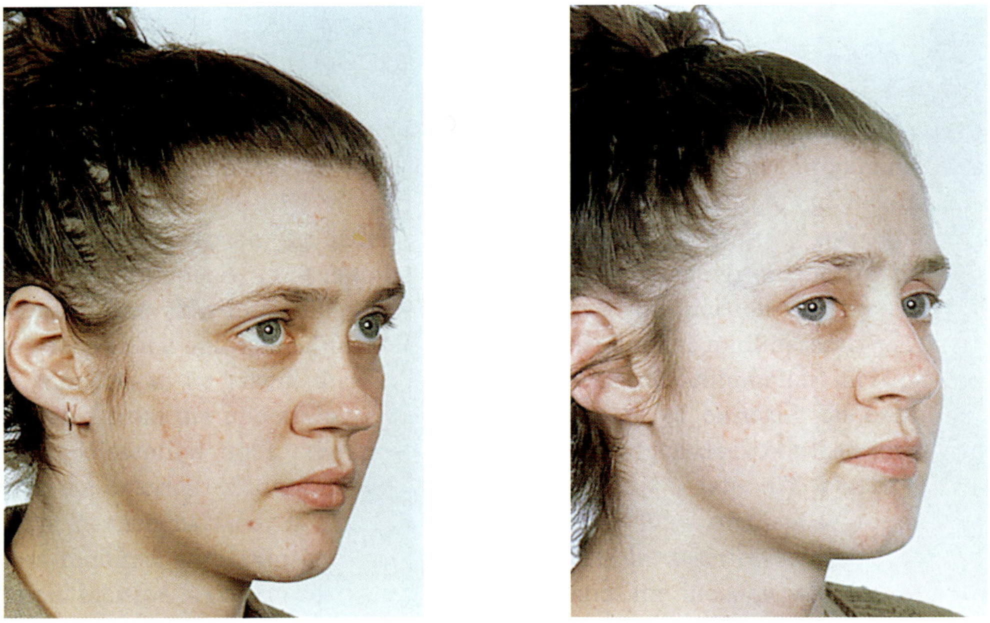

e f

Fig. 3e,f.

Large saddle

It is the gross saddle, where there would be insufficient material available from the ear or septum, which presents the major problem and where most controversy lies. In this group, there is often loss of nasal bone in addition to loss of cartilaginous support of the nose. Here the choice lies between iliac bone graft, which may absorb, rib cartilage, which may twist and change shape, or a synthetic material, which may extrude and be lost.

Saddle associated with lack of septal support

Where there is lack of septal support, particularly at the tip of the nose, this should be corrected by replacing missing septal cartilage, either with septal cartilage harvested more posteriorly or conchal cartilage from the ear. If this is not corrected, it may lead to protrusion or extrusion of the graft at the root of the nose, due to the cantilever effect. An added advantage of correcting lack of septal support by replacing missing cartilage is that this usually results in a very much smaller defect which can then be corrected by a small conchal cartilage graft.

Saddle secondary to granulomatous or other disease

The saddle which results from granulomatous disease, such as sarcoid or Wegeners, or such conditions as relaps-ing perichondritis, presents a particular problem. Clearly, in the first instance it is important to undertake all steps to make the diagnosis and treat the underlying cause.

Having completed this, however, one must then set about correcting the defect and it is in this group that synthetic materials may play a major role. They can be inserted with minimal operative intervention under local anesthesia and should not change shape or themselves be susceptible to the disease process (Fig. 4).

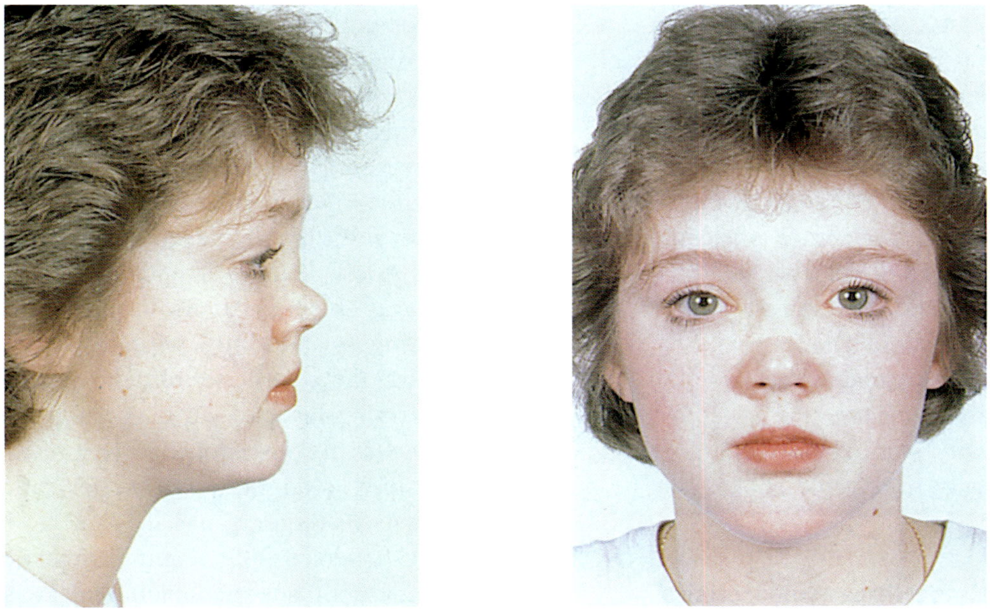

a b

Fig. 4. Pre- (*a,b*) and post- (*c,d*) operative photographs demonstrating the use of Silastic to correct a saddle secondary to granulomatous disease.

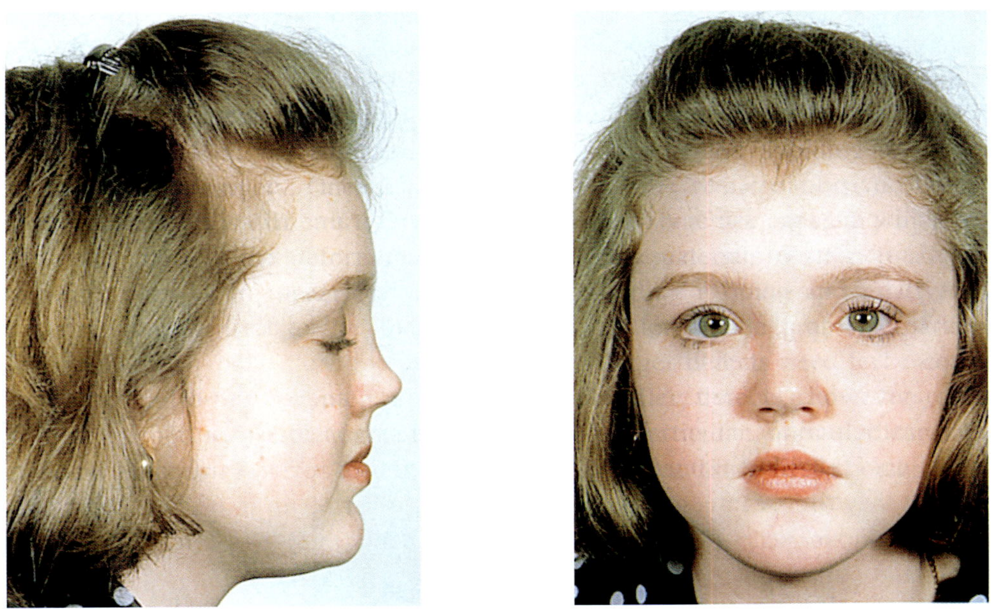

c d

Fig. 4c,d.

Deviation of the nose

Deviation of the nose may require correction of the septum, the nasal bones and possibly the tip of the nose. At times, however, despite all this, the nose will still not look straight and some form of camouflage technique will be required. Frequently this will be combined with septal surgery or some other rhinoplasty technique, and septal cartilage or lower lateral nasal cartilage may be readily available to use to good effect to augment one side of the nose, leading to an 'impression of straightness'.

Implants and graft options

So far, the perfect graft material has not been found. It should be:

1. non-toxic, non-carcinogenic and non-allergenic
2. non-destructive to adjacent tissue and should not impede healing
3. look and feel 'natural'
4. non-resorbable
5. easily available
6. easy to shape
7. easily sterilizable
8. easily removable should this be necessary

Autografts

Bone

Bone has probably been the most commonly used material for nasal augmentation for over 100 years. It is not, however, free from possible complications: a painful donor site, the use of a hard material in a soft part of the nose, and the necessity for a recipient bony bed to be made available so that revascularization is possible and even then the graft may, and frequently does, resorb. Infection, as with all grafts, may occur involving total or partial loss of bone. Superficial skin breakdown may follow infection of a graft with conspicuous scarring, particularly with thin and tethered skin from previous trauma or surgery.

Cartilage

Autologous (autogeneic) cartilage appears to be a satisfactory material and is particularly suitable for correcting small to medium sized defects when cartilage can be harvested from the concha of the ear or septal cartilage. Neither of these donor sites is usually associated with significant postoperative pain or other problems. The use of diced or morselized cartilage has been advocated, but it is apparent that absorption is more frequent with fragmentation. When more material is required, the rib may be chosen as the donor site; this, however, can be painful, may rarely lead to a pneumothorax and the graft may twist. Mowlem confirmed twisting in about 50% of cases. Removal of both the perichondrium and superficial underlying layer of cartilage from the rib graft was recommended to ensure that it remained straight. In a series of 300 patients undergoing nasal costal cartilage graft, however, 20% required revision for a variety of reasons, including twisting (Gibson).

Banked bone and cartilage has also been used and bovine cartilage, originally introduced by Stout in 1933, has enjoyed a revival of interest. The techniques for preserving and sterilizing these tissues either by boiling, Merthiolate, 70% alcohol, freeze-drying, irradiation or other manoeuvres, are necessary, but it has been demonstrated that foreign body reaction is more vigorous with these grafts which tend to be replaced in time with fibrous tissue or become heavily calcified. Bovine cartilage tended to resorb in ten of a series of 12 implants. Cadaver rib cartilage stored in Cialit (similar to Merthiolate) was followed up in 63 patients after nasal augmentation. In 12 of these implants, there was a recurrence of the deformity either due to infection, extrusion or absorption. The material was firm and brittle and, radiologically, 50% became calcified (Gibson).

Dermofat and dermis grafts

Dermofat and dermis grafts were first described in 1920 and used in 1932 for nasal augmentation. The major problem with these grafts is judging the degree of absorption that may occur. Thompson estimated approximately 20% absorption, while Reicht allowed for a 10% reduction in volume. A further disadvantage, as with all soft implants, is that it is not possible to fashion and shape the graft.

Synthetic grafts

Muhlbauer, while advocating the use of homologous (allogeneic) rib cartilage to augment the nose, believes that synthetics should be used only as a 'last resort', as there is a tendency for infection and extrusion. A Silastic graft, however, does have certain advantages. It is not associated with a painful donor site, if it does become infected it can be easily removed, it is a simple matter to insert, and this can easily be undertaken under local anesthesia.

Milward, reviewing 76 cases, found it unsatisfactory in 27 cases, but it is interesting to note that none were lost in the nine patients in whom Silastic was used to correct a saddle deformity in which the graft was inserted via an external midline columellar incision. Rozner described 22 cases in which Silastic was used and where only two were lost, while Marvin reported 24 cases in which an L-shaped strut of Silastic was used via a midline columellar incision and no cases were lost.

A review of the fate of Silastic nasal implants in 87 cases over a ten-year period with a minimum period of follow-up of one year (average follow-up 3.5 years) was reported in 1983 (Mackay). The type of Silastic prosthesis, whether firm or soft, did not appear to affect the result, but introduction of the graft via an intranasal vestibular incision was shown to be less satisfactory than a midline vertical columellar incision.

Polyamide mesh has been used to augment the cartilaginous portion of the nose. One hundred and eighty-six cases with a minimum follow-up of one year were reported for saddling, only three of which were lost to follow-up; of the 186 implants performed, there was no incidence of superficial skin loss and the nose remained soft and mobile, resisting trauma and the 'marking' from the minor trauma of wearing glasses (Stucker). Polyamide mesh, however, simply acts as a filler and the shape cannot be accurately fashioned, which is a considerable limiting factor in its use for more major augmentation. Reliable long-term studies demonstrate its eventual near-complete absorption.

Surgical technique

Harvesting of autografts

The donor site

Nasal septal cartilage is an excellent graft material particularly suited to providing support. Relatively large areas of septal cartilage can be excised without fear of further saddling, providing this is removed posterior to an imaginary line joining the anterior nasal spine to the osseocartilaginous junction. Several layers may be sutured together to form a sandwich which can then be carved into shape to fill the defect. The edges of such a graft need to be meticulously thinned and bevelled, using a sharp blade to prevent these edges producing sharp ridges which can be felt and seen, particularly under thin skin. The nasal septal mucoperichondrial flaps can be sutured with through-and-through mattress sutures which usually negate the need for any nasal packing, although care should be taken not to over-suture or to tie these too tight as this can result in necrosis and a septal perforation.

The pinna provides an excellent site from which to harvest autogenous cartilage for nasal augmentation. Areas of cartilage of up to 3.5 cm long can be excised from the conchal cartilage without any change in the shape of the ear, providing the anti-helical fold is kept intact. This can be achieved via a posterior or anterior approach, the latter being preferred if a composite graft is to be taken, incising the skin immediately anterior and deep to the anti-helical fold. If cartilage alone is to be taken, the skin can be elevated from the underlying cartilage by blunt dissection up to the posterior edge of the external auditory meatus. The cartilage is then excised. If a composite graft is required with skin and cartilage, the initial incision is continued through the cartilage, which is then elevated from the underlying skin of the posterior surface of the pinna. The skin and cartilage composite graft is then excised and the defect made good by fashioning an island graft of postauricular skin which is pulled through from posteriorly to anteriorly and meticulously sutured in place.

Once hemostasis has been achieved, the skin incision can be carefully secured with fine sutures. Tardy has described a simple and effective dressing of two layers of Telfa sandwiched on either side of the donor site bed and overtied with a single through and through nylon bolus suture, which provided firm compression for 48 to 72 hours. With this, no head bandage or other dressing is required.

The techniques for harvesting bone are well established. With iliac crest bone grafts, the postoperative pain, possibility of hematoma or infection and the ultimate scar, are obvious disadvantages. Meticulous suturing can make the scar minimal and removal of the medial table of the iliac crest or central portion minimize the deformity. Costal cartilage grafts also have similar problems of harvesting, with the added possibility of a pneumothorax.

The recipient site

The technique for introducing the nasal graft varies. Converse favors the cartilage-splitting incision for introducing the graft. This was thought to be the incision of choice for all grafts, except those which need to extend from the tip of the nose when a rim incision was preferred. Apart from minimal midline scarring, however, the external columellar incision has the advantage of ensuring an exact midline pocket which does not lead into the nasal vestibule. A laterally placed intranasal incision may predispose to an oblique pocket. In a series reporting the fate of Silastic, the incision was the main factor contributing to success or failure. Of 23 cases in which Silastic was inserted via an intranasal incision, ten were unsatisfactory either because of infection, extrusion or poor alignment. In 62 cases inserted via an external midline columellar incision, all remained satisfactory (Mackay).

Whenever possible, the recipient pocket should be fashioned in such an exact way that the graft can be placed into this pocket as a perfect fit. The pocket is then closed and no more stabilizing sutures are required. In other instances, however, it may not be possible to achieve this, particularly when augmentation is combined with other procedures undertaken at the same time, or if an external approach has been used.

In this situation, the graft can be placed on the outside of the nose, but in the position it will be required. Using 4/0 plain catgut with a 1-cm straight cutting needle, the latter is passed through the graft and into the skin, marking both graft and skin. The suture is then passed through the graft at this point, a knot is tied to prevent this from pulling through and, using a retractor, the needle is passed intranasally then out through the point previously marked in such a way that the graft can now be

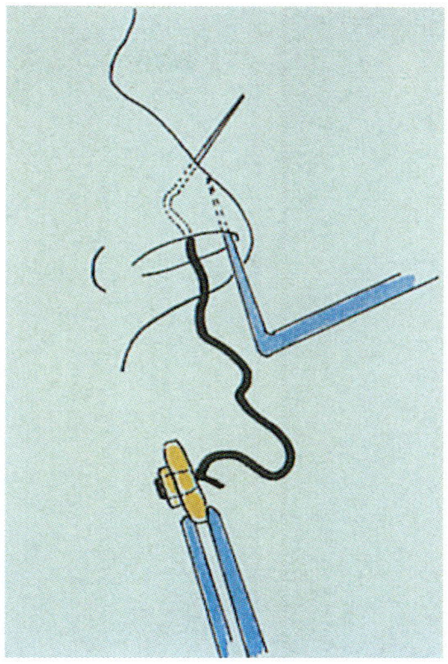

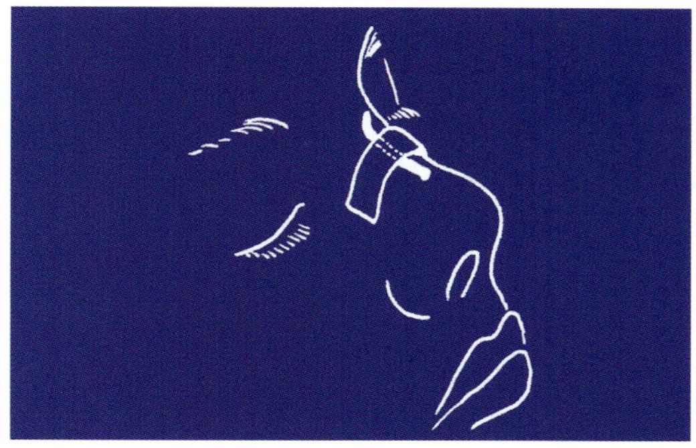

Fig. 5. Cartilage 'sandwich' sutured and secured with a 4/0 plain catgut suture.

Fig. 6. The suture can be secured with an adhesive dressing.

inserted into the nose, and then secured by careful traction on the suture. It is unnecessary to tie any further knots as the suture can simply be strapped to the skin with a half- inch Steri-strip (Figs. 5 and 6).

An important point to remember is to mark the site at which any augmentation is required prior to surgery. Once the skin has been elevated, it is difficult to be sure of the exact site and the deformity may 'disappear', only to 'reappear' once the skin has reattached itself to the underlying structures.

There is no uniformly accepted view as to the best method to use to augment the nose. Some authorities prefer to use synthetic materials, some cartilage, while others will continue to use bone. Few would deny that if the perfect synthetic material were available, then this would be the obvious choice, being easily available and in large quantities to fill any defect, without the problems of infection or extrusion, and avoiding a donor site. So far, this remains elusive. There are, however, some occasions in which today's synthetic materials offer real advantages in providing a quick and relatively simple solution to the problem, particularly when larger defects need to be corrected. For smaller defects, however, cartilage and, in particular, auricular cartilage remains the author's first choice.

18: SURGICAL MANAGEMENT OF LARGE SEPTAL PERFORATIONS

Rodolphe Meyer

Introduction

Today, practically all septal perforations should be closed surgically. Only a hole in the posterior bony part of the septum, which is extremely rare, may remain untreated because it does not cause any problems.

I have completely abandoned the button, which I introduced in 1972, and small flap methods in favor of surgery that should allow the closure of all kinds and sizes of perforations. Total closure of the perforation is always the goal. The choice of surgical procedure is determined by the size and position of the defect. In the last 15 years, I have developed two methods: one for closure of perforations of up to 5 cm in diameter, as a one-step operation, and the other for larger defects (of more than 4 cm in diameter) as a three-step procedure.

The extramucosal technique is especially valuable in treating perforations of up to 5 cm in diameter, because it enables their closure in one step even if, occasionally, an additional small bilateral buccal flap is needed.

One-step procedure for septal perforations of up to 5 cm in diameter

To close perforations of up to 5 cm with a one-step method, it is necessary to mobilize a large area of the mucoperichondrium and to use adaption sutures free of tension from the perforation edges. In order to make this possible, the transfixion incision is first extended downwards and laterally, parallel to the edge of the piriform aperture, along the floor of the nose to the inferior concha on the lateral nasal wall.

Proceeding from the transfixion incision, the mucoperichondrium is dissected from the septal cartilage over a large area. The mucoperiosteum of the nasal floor is detached laterally as far as the inferior nasal meatus. Finally, the external skin over the upper lateral cartilage is mobilized. This cartilage can now be severed at its fusion point with the cartilaginous septum, along its entire length. The result of the procedure up to this point, is a hose-like structure consisting of mucoperiosteum and mucoperichondrium with the upper lateral cartilage attached. The perforation located there collapses due to the elimination of tension. The hole which is round or oval becomes a slit (Figs. 1, 2a and b).

To reduce the size of the actual cartilage defect in the lamina quadrangularis, I use one of two methods, depending on the location and nature of the perforation. If the hole is not too deep posteriorly and its greatest diameter is perpendicular to an imaginary line of the floor of the nose, I make resections of cartilage strips above and below the edges of the perforation, parallel to its greatest diameter. As a result of this reduction, the lamina quadrangularis is divided into two parts: the caudal part can be fully mobilized and pushed back and up against the cranial part. This decreases the size of the perforation, which can be further closed by inserting a dried layer of parietal fascia. If the patient's nose has a hump and he agrees to a reduction of the dorsum, and if the greatest diameter of the perforation is parallel to the imaginary sagittal line at the floor of the nose, I resect horizontal cartilage strips in front of and behind the perforation. In this way, an anterosuperior septal plate is separated from a posteroinferior septal plate. The upper plate can be pushed down onto the lower plate following mobilization at the dorsum, in the same manner as was taught by Cottle and Loring[1] (Fig. 1).

One-step procedure for antero-caudal septal perforations

In cases of septal perforation of up to 5 cm in which there is little space between the defect and the columella, it is difficult to join the columella or the remnant of the membraneous septum with the dissected mucoperichondral flap on both sides.

With the perforation closed and sutured, the bilateral flaps sometimes cannot be advanced more than the caudal-most edge of the perforation in the cartilage. The bare anterior pillar must then be covered with skin or buccal mucosa, either as a graft or transferred as a flap. When there is only a narrow strip of membraneous septum to be covered just behind the columella, I use a skin graft from the postauricular region. In more difficult cases, I prefer the bilateral use of buccal mucosal grafts, and, in special cases, I apply two simple gingivolabial flaps without delay. In such cases, I close the perforation with extensive extramucosal dissection, and finish covering the septum anteriorly with two small gingivobuccal flaps (Figs. 2B, 3c and d). The small gingivobuccal flap has to cover the bare submucous area of the remnant of the membraneous septum close to the columella, in order to close the gap between the columella and the dissected mucoperichondrial flap which contains the closed perforation. This is done on both sides, thus avoiding a columellar retraction (Fig. 3e).

Three-step procedure for septal perforations larger than 5 cm

For closure of perforations larger than 5 cm in diameter, I advocated a composite buccal flap 29 years ago. This method was first presented at the Swiss ENT Congress in May 1968 by my assistant, Dirlewanger[2]. Later, we were pleased to read that a similar technique had been demonstrated by Akyildiz[3] at the Rhinology Congress in Zagreb in September 1968. In 1969, Hertig and Meyer[4] published the procedure as Meyer's method. It was described again in 1972[5]. Smaller flaps without cartilage reinforcement were adopted for small perforations only by other authors.

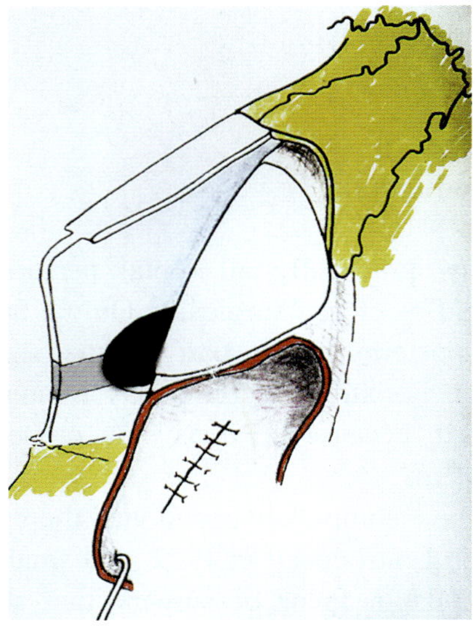

Fig. 1. One-stage procedure with extensive mucoperichondrial and mucoperiosteal dissection for closing the oval perforation which has become a slit due to traction.

Meyer's method[4] is indicated for the repair of severe septal defects of more than 5 cm in diameter. It is a three-step procedure in which a spoon-shaped flap from the oral vestibule, and including a piece of cartilage, is inserted into the perforation, and then severed from its pedicle once its three-layered plate has taken to the septum. The surgical procedure includes the following three steps:

1. During the first step, I prepare the flap in the mucous membrane of the oral vestibule. The flap, which will later consist of a pedicle and an oval piece of cartilage covered on both sides by mucous membrane, starts in the gingivobuccal fold of the oral vestibule, next to the frenulum above the upper row of teeth. A piece of cartilage is taken from the entire concha of the ear, without substantially deforming the pinna. The cartilage piece is then flattened by radial incision and placed into a submucous pocket in the oral vestibule in front of and below Stenson's duct (Fig. 5c). Next to this, another flap is cut inferiorly in the mucous membrane. This tiny flap retains a proximal base and is folded under the existing submucous pouch, but in a deeper layer, not completely touching the cartilage graft pocket. The cartilaginous reinforcement is now between two walls of mucous membrane, one on the superficial oral side and

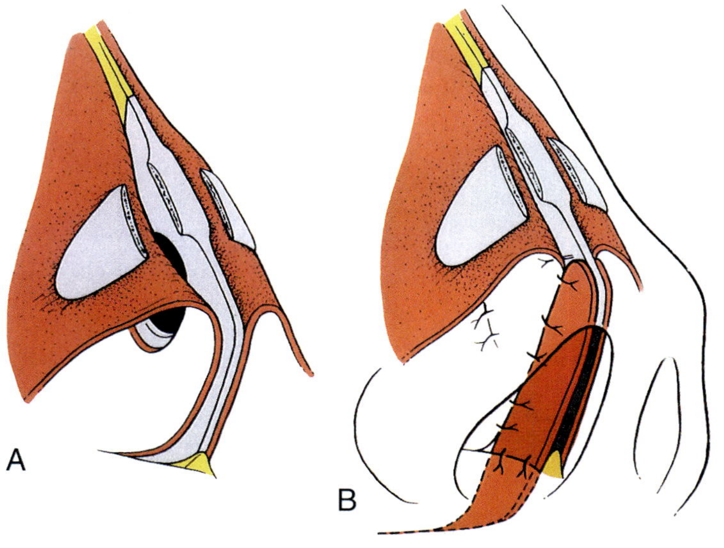

Fig. 2. A. One-stage procedure, with in addition, *B.* Bilateral buccal mucosal flaps to be interposed between the columella and the two dissected mucosal flaps.

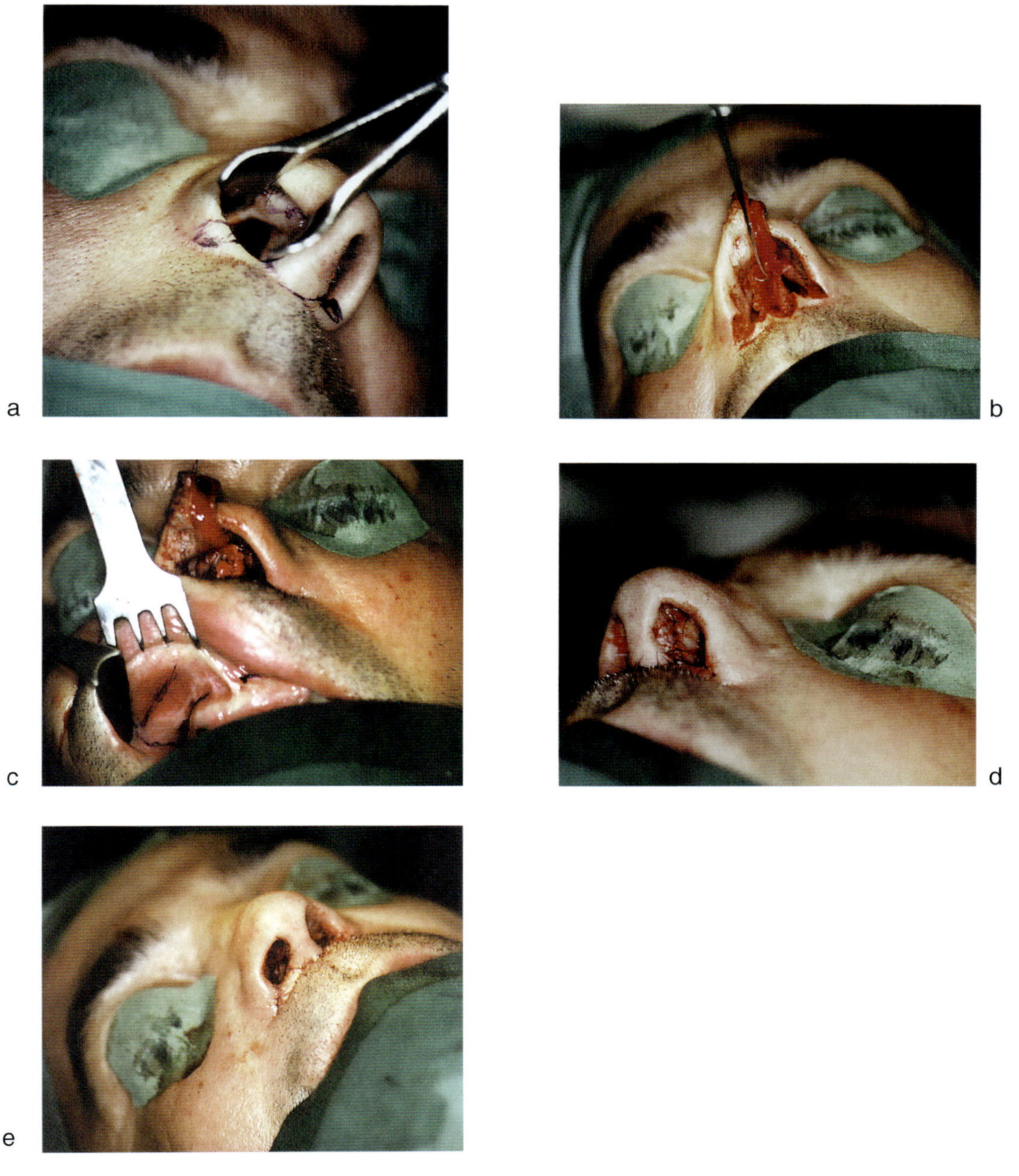

Fig. 3a. A 50-year-old man with a septal perforation of 5 cm in diameter. *b.* After elevation of the columella and bilateral alotomy, the two mucoperichondrial and periosteal flaps are dissected for closure of the perforation in the mucoperichondrium, and will receive a fascia graft between them. *c.* Right buccal flap outlined. *d.* Left buccal flap sutured between the columella and the left mucoperichondrial flap after closure of the perforation. *e.* End of the operation with the buccal flap interposed behind the columella.

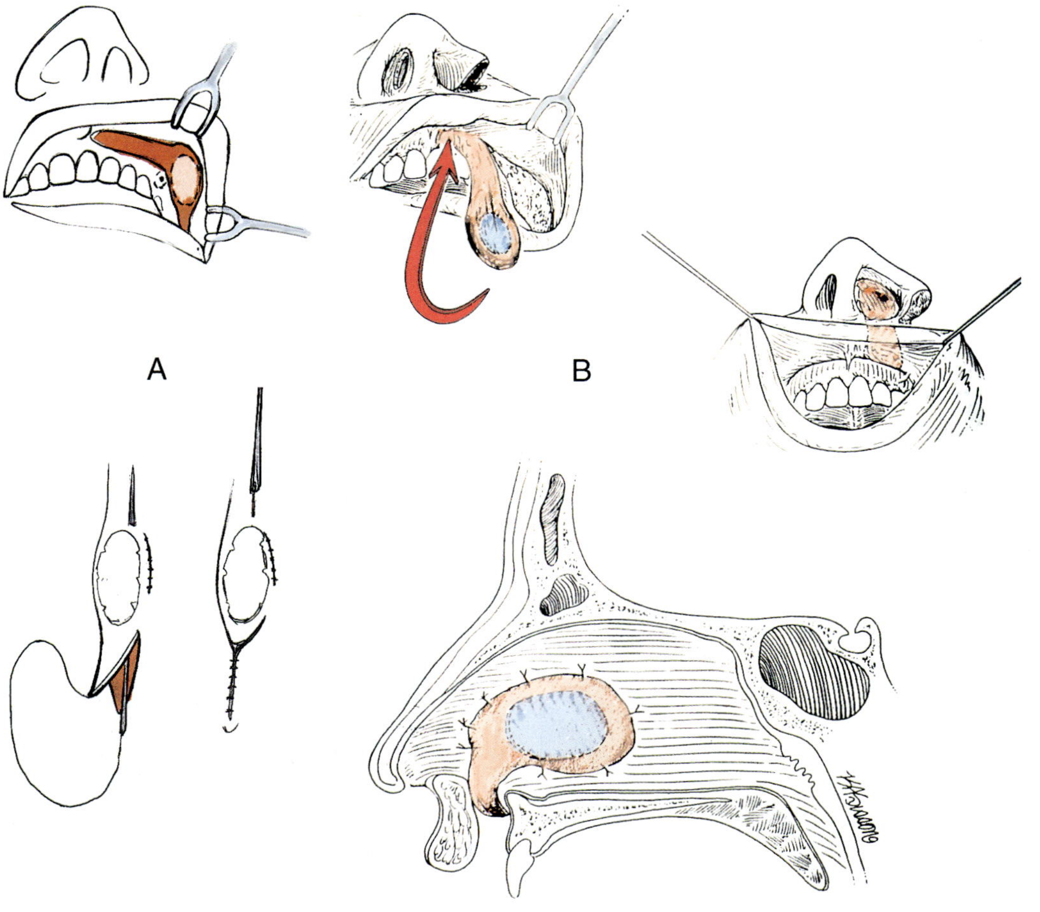

Fig. 4. A. Closure of a large septal perforation in a three-stage procedure with a gingivo-buccal flap. First stage: the three-layered compound flap, reinforced with ear cartilage, is outlined and elevated at the buccal extremity. The incision for insertion of the cartilage graft is sutured. The distal extent of the compound flap is cut in a V-shape and is turned behind the cartilage graft in another deeper submucosal pocket. The conchal graft is spread and flattened and lies in a very superficial submucosal pocket. The reverse flap is placed in the deep pocket and lines the cartilage graft. A transmucosal suture holds the flap extremity. Closure of the donor area of the distal aspect of the flap. *B.* Second stage of the procedure: the compound flap is mobilized and ready to be introduced into the nasal cavity. Transfer of the flap to the septal defect through a tunnel in front of the nasal spine. The flap is sutured into the septal defect. The pedicle can be discarded during the third stage.

the other on the non-oral side. The defect at the donor site of the small distal mucosal flap is closed by approximation. The pedicle of the whole buccal flap, beginning at the frenulum, is tubed by moulding a longish horizontal roll of mucosa and submucous tissue, using interrupted small incisions and mattress sutures (Fig. 4A).

2. After about five weeks, during the second step, the spoon-shaped flap can be cut and fed into the nasal cavity to fill the septal defect through a tunnel running along the anterior nasal spine. The donor site is then closed by approximation. In order to facilitate suturing the mucous membranes of the buccal flap to the edges of the perforation, it helps to incise the base of the columella and, if necessary, also the alar base (one or both). The columellar base incision extends back to the anterior lower edge of the perforation, so that the portion of the septum located in front of the defect can be raised together with the columella, thereby creating a wide opening to access the perforation. If the mucous membrane on both sides of the flap is now sutured to the cleaned-up edges of the perforation, the columella and the ventral portion of the septum are automatically brought back to their original positions. The columellar base is again sutured to the philtrum and to the medial edge of the vestibule on both sides. Occasional alotomies are also sutured (Fig. 4B).

3. The patient is left to heal for a further five weeks, after which the third step can be carried out on an outpatient basis. The division of the pedicle is usually performed under local anesthesia. At the same time, the three-layered flap in the septum can be thinned if necessary, and correction of an alar collapse (Figs. 5g and 6f) or of a concomitant saddle nose (Fig. 6) can be added. In some cases, the third step is not necessary because of postoperative shrinking of the pedicle in and above the premaxillary tunnel. For large and extremely large

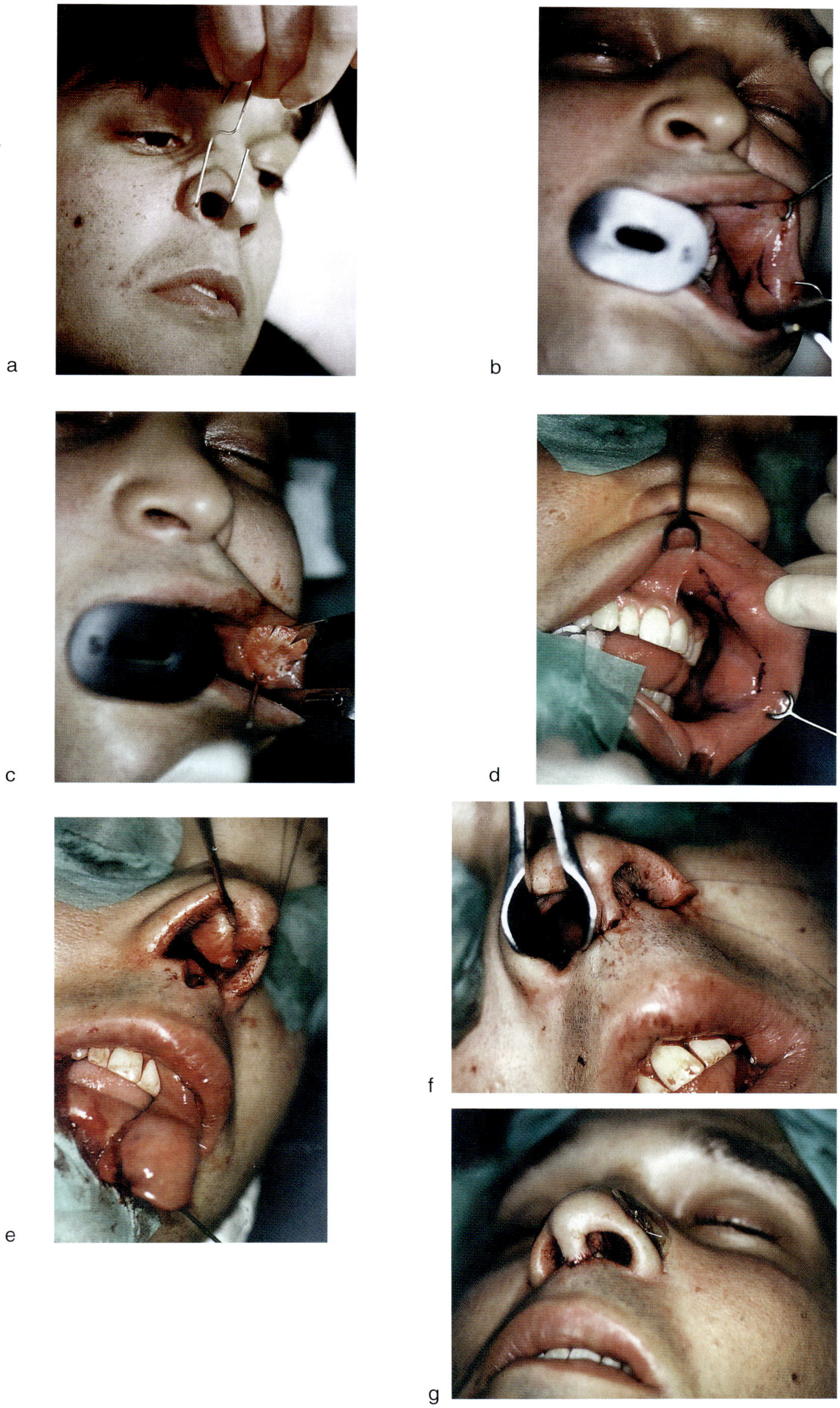

Fig. 5a. A 25-year-old man with a large septal perforation requiring a three-stage procedure for closure. *b.* Outline of the composite buccal flap. The operation is performed under analgetic sedation (Propofol). *c.* Insertion of the flattened conchal cartilage into the submucous pocket for reinforcing the flap. *d.* The buccal flap is about to be elevated and transferred. *e.* The flap is elevated and ready for passing through a gingivo-nasal tunnel to the septal defect. *f.* Insertion and suture of the flap into the large perforation. *g.* Thinning of the neoseptum and contemporaneous correction of the bilateral collapse by cartilage grafting and transalar sutures. At the time the septum was lost, the collapse was not manifest but was caused by that loss.

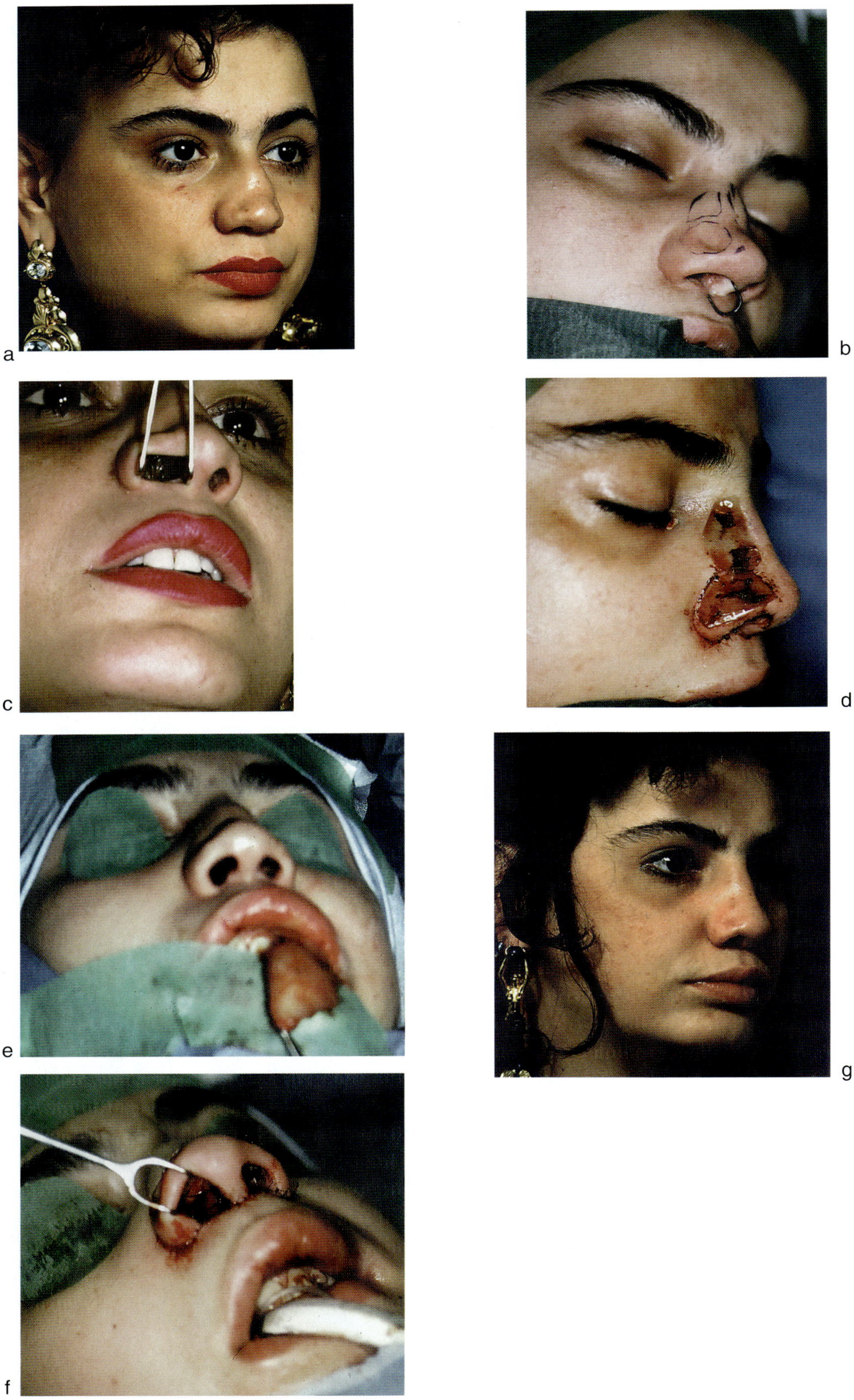

Fig. 6a. A 21-year-old girl with a saddle nose and complete destruction of the septum, due to drug abuse. *b.* Nasal cavity without septum, full of black crusts. *c.* Well-vascularized extensive composite buccal flap about to be transferred. *d.* Suture of the flap for reconstruction of two-thirds of the septum, suture of the columellar base and of bilateral alotomy. *e.* Third stage with elimination of the pedicle in the gingivonasal tunnel and correction of the saddle nose with an ear-conchal graft, and of the bilateral collapse with cartilage grafts slices and transalar sutures. *f.* The end of the third stage. *g.* The external result.

perforations, the staged composite buccal flap is the only procedure described in the literature which can achieve a reliable closure. Even when, in rare cases, a posterior asymptomatic slit remains, the procedure is worth doing. In all difficult cases, I inform the patient that such a slit might occasionally have to be left as an incomplete result. However, all patients agreed to undergo the complex three-step surgical procedure.

Septocolumellar reconstruction

For septocolumellar reconstruction, I refrain from using a labial or nasolabial flap and prefer the frontotemporal flap, which leaves inconspicuous scars in the donor area (Figs. 7c-g). The frontotemporal flap has its best indication in septocolumellar repair. The columella and septum are the most difficult parts of the nose to reconstruct. Cartilage-supported tongue flaps[6], arm flaps[7], and cheek flaps[8], are not versatile and sophisticated enough to be modelled to conform to the fine shape of the apicocolumellar structures. For this purpose, in 1968 I advocated the use of a frontotemporal flap which I had already been using for other kinds of reconstructions since 1963[5,10-13].

In cases of septocolumellar loss of tissue, I do not know of any other technique which is as appropriate as the frontotemporal flap. I have refined the original technique for alar repair, described by Schmid and Widmajer[6] in 1961, for special use in apicocolumellar and septocolumellar reconstructions[14].

The septocolumellar repair flap is cut in the frontotemporal region and is composed of a bipedicle carrier flap at the upper border of the eyebrow, and a rectangular flap at the temple. This temporal component, which joins the lateral pedicle of the bridge flap, is lined by a cutaneous or mucosal graft, and carries a cartilage graft from the ear concha. During the first stage, the superciliary carrier flap is cut as a skin strip 4 mm in width, with the incision bevelled outwards to include a greater width of subcutaneous tissue. This subcutaneous layer is backed by a strip of split skin which is carefully sutured to both the skin edges of the flap. The donor defect of the bipedicled limb is closed by pulling down the mobilized skin of the forehead. At the same time, I form a superficial subcutaneous pocket in the temporal region through an incision at the lateral orbital rim, and I place the auricular graft into this pocket. Through a second incision, near the temporal hair-bearing skin, I dissect a second pocket in a deeper subdermal layer of the skin. This pocket, which does not communicate with the first one, is partially lined with a cutaneous or mucosal graft from the cheek, leaving the deeper raw surface covered with gauze only. The edges of the graft are sutured to the incision. During a second stage, five to seven weeks later, the rectangular temporal flap composed of three layers, skin cartilage and mucosa, is transferred to the septocolumellar defect by means of the superciliary carrier flap. To facilitate the suturing of the rectangular flap, and the modelling of the tip, columella and septum in the proper position, I usually have to open the vestibule by using a wide basal alotomy or a paramedian dorsal incision. Both external layers of the flap are meticulously sutured to the freshened edges of the internal septonasal defect. After a further three or four weeks, during the third stage, the nourishing bridge flap is divided at its proximal and distal ends, and the septal part of the inserted flap can be thinned.

In one exceptional case with a loss of two-thirds of the columella and the whole septum, I had to resort to an extended frontotemporal flap, which required four stages for reconstruction and, on one side, an incision continuing from the alotomy up along the lateral osteotomy line. In this case, an additional triangular flap was outlined and elevated at the lateral end of the rectangular temporal flap in order that it

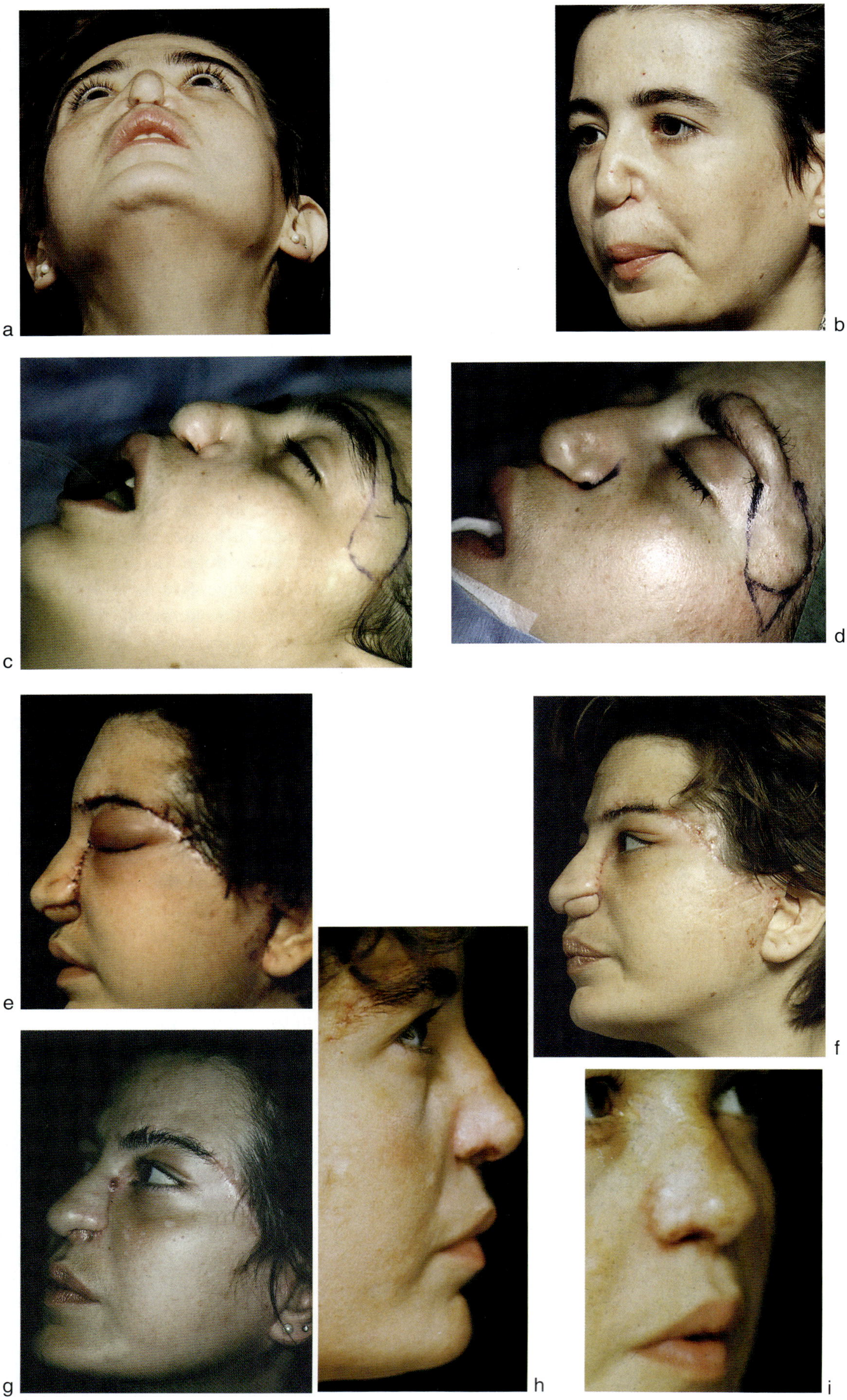

Fig. 7. a and *b.* External nose constriction, total loss of the septum and partial loss of the columella, due to drug abuse in a 29-year-old female. *c.* First stage with preparation of a frontotemporal flap for columellar and septal reconstruction. Outline of the flap before insertion of an ear-cartilage graft into a subcutaneous pocket for reinforcement. *d.* Second stage with the flap ready for gradual transfer. The distal triangular part of the flap will be folded and turned behind the cartilage graft. *e.* The patient after the third stage with the flap completely transferred for combined septocolumellar reconstruction and closure of the donor area. The final flap transfer necessitated a partial left rhinotomy. *f.* The patient after the third stage. *g.* The result after the fourth stage. *h* and *i.* Late result after 5 stages.

could be folded over the lateral distal end, thus building a three-layered columella and anterior septum. The proximal part of the rectangular flap was lined with buccal mucosa. During the third stage, the flap had to be inserted through an enlarged bony fissure in the left lateral osteotomy line. A fourth stage was necessary for fixing the septum in the midline of the cavity.

Nowadays, it is important that large perforations in iatrogenic, and particularly in cocainoman patients can be closed, in order to stop crust formation, repeated bleeding and dry pharyngitis. In many cases, concomitant external deformities also have to be corrected.

19: THREE-STEP RECONSTRUCTION OF SADDLE NOSE DEFORMITIES

G. Rettinger

The term 'saddle nose' simply describes a depression of the nasal dorsum without analyzing the degree and the structures involved. Frequently the deformity is limited to the dorsum and can be dealt with using cartilage grafts[3,6,14] or regional cartilage flaps from the lobular cartilages[5]. These methods are reserved for minor deformities. Congenital or acquired saddle noses are in fact complex deformities which need detailed analysis before reconstruction[13]. A therapeutic concept is presented, based on the notion that dividing one major problem into three minor ones enables the surgeon to reverse the pathological process and restore proper anatomical relationships, thereby restoring nasal breathing function.

Analysis of the saddle nose deformity complex

There are many different types of saddle nose which require specific surgical treatment[13]. The following characteristics describe the most frequent findings and omit certain entities, such as maxillonasal dysplasia, 'pig snout nose', and other rare disorders[11].

To evaluate saddle noses, it is necessary to understand certain fix points and lines[4]. For example, tip projection is expressed by the nasofacial (NF) angle (the angle between the facial plane and the line from nasion to the tip defining point; normal ranges between 30° and 40°, Fig. 1b, insert). A specific and definite nasofrontal angle is required to make meaningful measurements of tip projection. When the nasofacial angle is less than 30° and the dorsum projects above the line between the nasion and the tip of the nose, this situation is called a pseudohump (Fig. 1b, insert).

The frontal view (Fig. 1a and Table 1a) mainly demonstrates a broad dorsum, tip and nasal base (ala lateral to a vertical line through the medial canthus). With a depressed nasofacial angle, the epicanthal folds hide a normal medial canthus. This is due to redundant skin which may be present.

The lateral view demonstrates a decreased projection of both the dorsum and tip (Fig. 1b and Table 1b). The columella is retracted and the nasolabial (NL)

Fig. 1a.

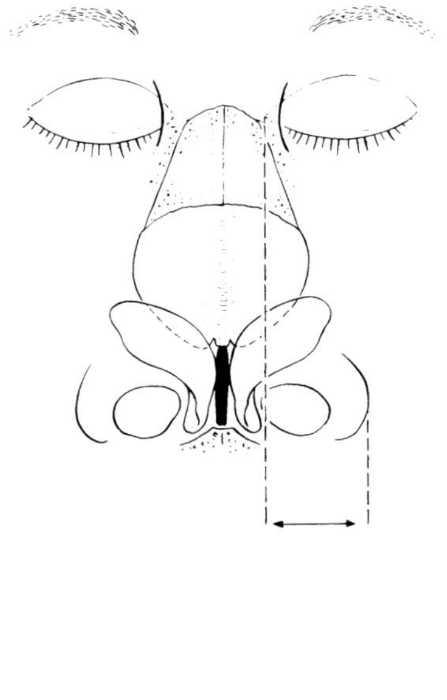

Table 1a.

Front view

- wide dorsum
- wide alar base
  (alar lateral to vertical line through medial canthus (↔))
- epicanthal folds

Fig. 1b.

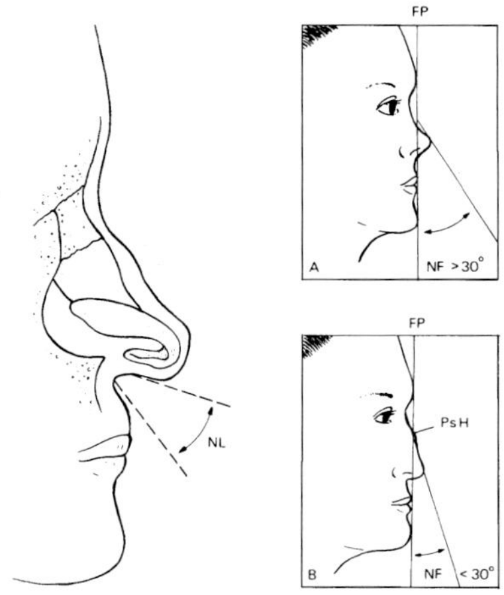

Table 1b.

Side view
- low dorsum
- decreased tip projection
  naso-facial angle NF (between facial plane FP and line through nasion – tip, normal {~ 35°) [insert A]
- retracted columella
  naso-labial angle NL < 90°
- short columella
- hidden columella
  (not visible on side view)
- rounded and long upper lip
- pseudo hump PsH when bony pyramid is normal [insert B]

Fig. 1c.

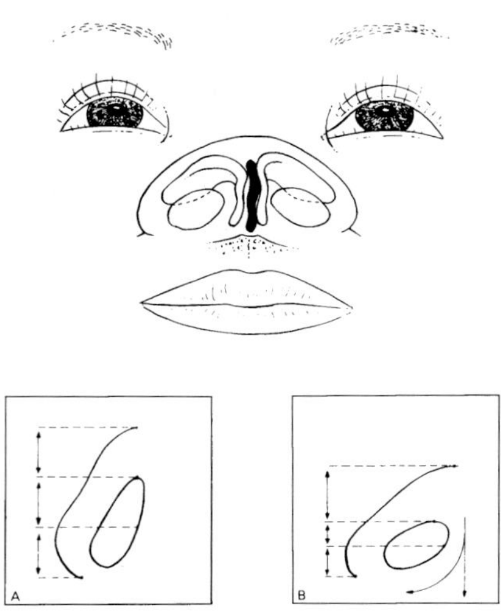

Table 1c.

Base view
- rounded nostrils
- alar insertion perpendicular to cheek
- short and broad columella
  (medial crura curled)
- wide interdomal distance
- disproportion of normally equal distances between tip, anterior border of nares, midcolumella and alar base
  Insert A = normal
  Insert B = pathological
- decreased tip projection causes elongation of nostril sill and upper lip (arrows in insert B)

Fig. 1d.

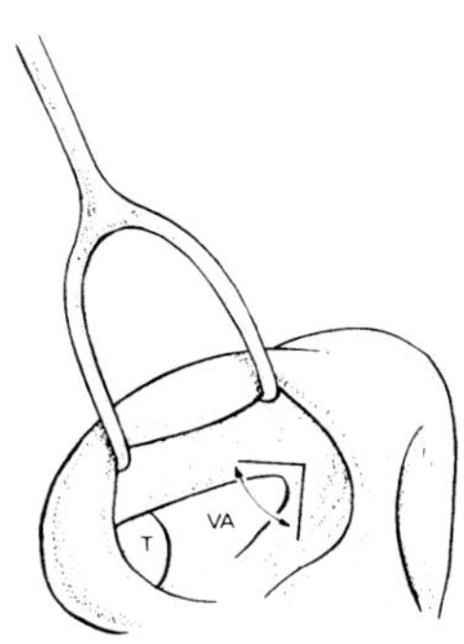

Table 1d.

Vestibule
- Valve angle (VA) 90°
  (ballooning)
- Hypertrophy of inferior turbinate (T)
- Deflections of septal remnant

angle is acute (Fig. 1b and Table 1b). The basal view is also changed in a uniform way (Fig. 1c and Table 1c). The tip projection is decreased and a short columella results. In addition, the base widens with an associated lengthening of the nostril sill (Fig. 1c, insert). A disproportion between the vertical diameter of the components of the nasal base can be measured (Fig. 1c, insert).

The tip defining points are wider than normal, resulting in a rounded lobule

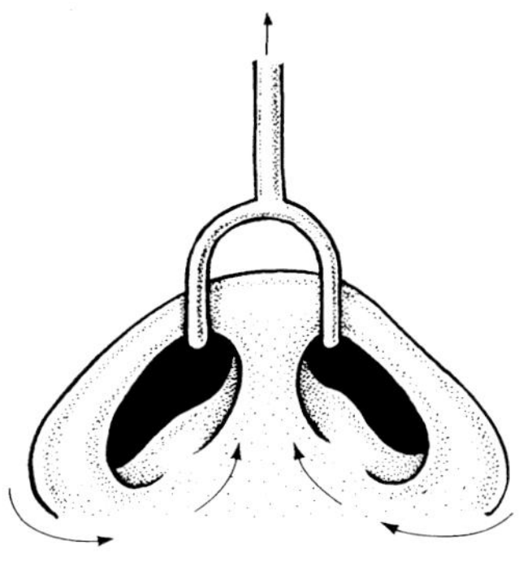

Fig. 2a.

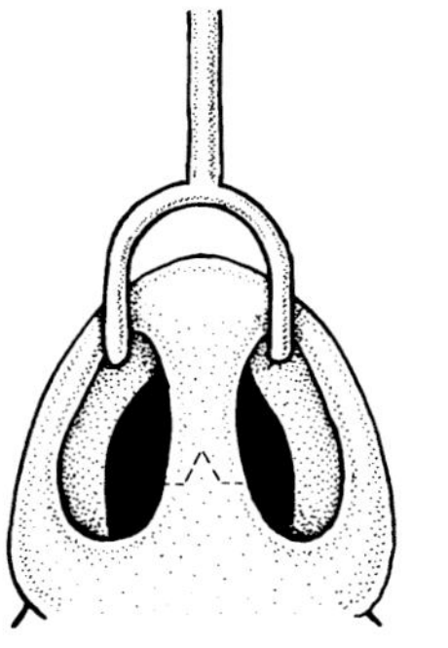

Fig. 2b.

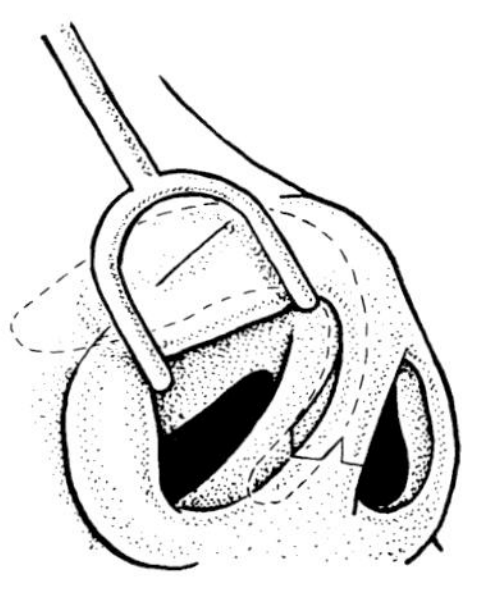

Fig. 2c.

which includes the nostrils. The nasal valve angle is also abnormal and may be 90° or greater (Fig. 1d). The anatomical disturbance of the valve angle (normally 10° to 15°) can account for a portion of the nasal breathing dysfunction. Frequently the inferior turbinates show a pronounced compensatory hypertrophy; in all likelihood, this is an attempt to maintain a normal valve area.

The visible deformities result from abnormalities in the bony and cartilaginous infrastructure. Practically all the abnormal findings of the lower nose are produced by destruction and displacement of the cartilaginous septum alone. The abnormalities of the upper part of the nose are the result of bony pyramid deformities. In conclusion, reconstruction of the caudal nasal septum is both the philosophical and structural pillar 'underpinning' the surgical repair of the saddle nose, together with remodelling of the bony pyramid. Due to severe destruction and loss of tissue, some additional procedures are often necessary.

Surgical procedure

Incisions and approach

With manual elevation of the tip and columella, care must be taken that the skin of the columella is mobile and tension is minimal (Fig. 2a). If this is checked, an inverted-V incision in the lower third of the columella is chosen (Fig. 2b). The intranasal incision should be placed cranial to the lower border of the medial crura, to enlarge the columellar flap for later coverage of the columellar implants (Fig. 2c). At the dome, the incision should meet the caudal margin of the lower lateral cartilage and then follow this margin laterally, like a normal marginal incision. Using hooks for skin elevation (no forceps), the strong fibers near the dome are severed and the skin is easily dissected in an epiperichondrial and an epiperiosteal plane. The vessels between the medial crura and near the lateral parts of the lateral crura are cauterized. The fibrous fatty tissue between the domes and filling the deep groove between domes and upper lateral cartilages is removed and the perichondrium preserved (if the perichondrium is stripped off from the outer surface of the lateral crura, the resulting unilateral scar will contract and create a medial convexity, a so-called 'pinched nose').

After division of the interdomal ligament and the attachments between the medial crura, the remnants of the caudal

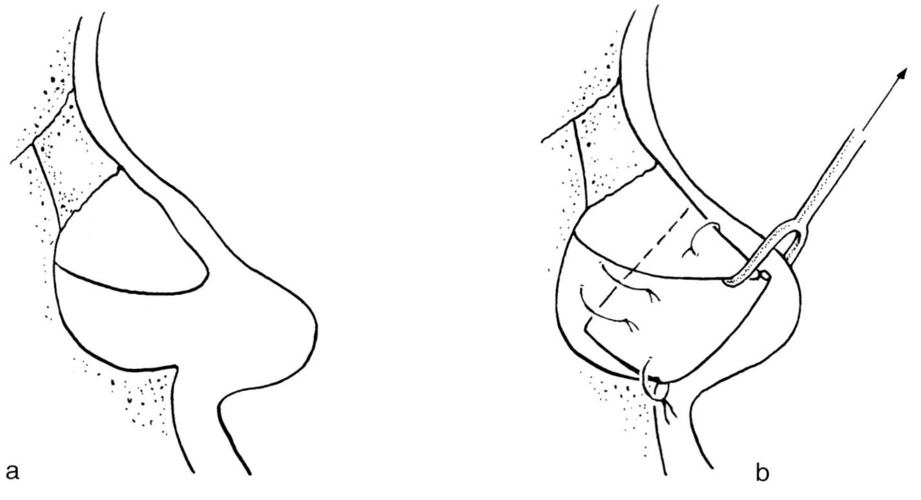

Fig. 3a,b.

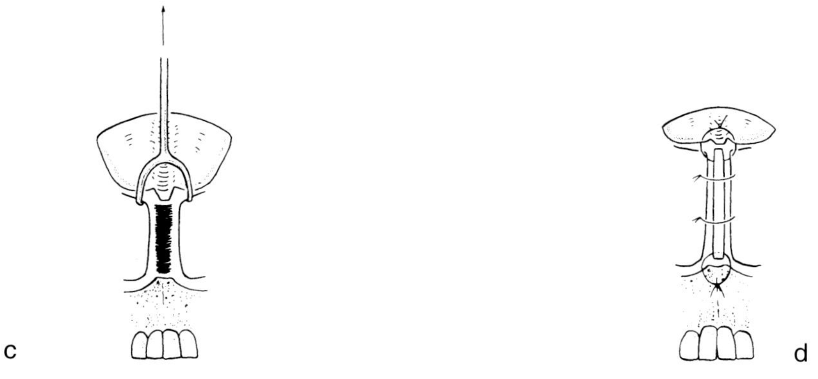

Fig. 3c,d.

septum are exposed by elevation of the mucoperichondrium. The approach to the infrastructure is now completed, after elevation of skin and mucosa from the intranasal surface of the upper lateral cartilages.

Resection and mobilization

The remnants of the cartilaginous septum are removed after transsecting the insertion of the upper lateral cartilages, leaving the cartilaginous dorsum intact. Parts of the bony septum should also be removed for later reconstruction.

The bony pyramid is mobilized by intraseptal, paramedial, lateral and transverse osteotomies[4,8]. In the case of asymmetries, intermedial osteotomies using the incisions already present can be undertaken.

Reconstruction of caudal septum and nasal valve

The caudal septum between premaxilla and cartilaginous dorsum must be straight and stable, since it supports all the surrounding structures such as the nasal dorsum, columella and tip. Autogenous septal cartilage is the material of choice for reconstruction[9]. If it is not sufficient in size or stability, septal bone or autogenous rib cartilage can be used. In the latter case, a central, balanced graft should be carved from the entire rib. The graft should fit exactly into the gap between the premaxilla and the caudal end of the

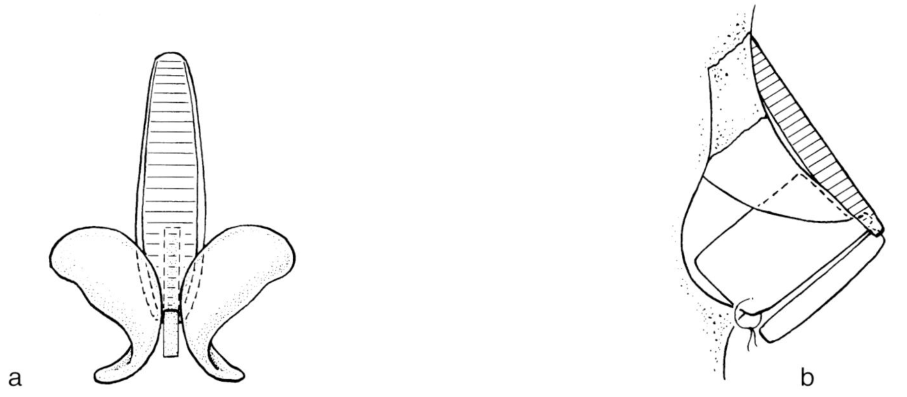

Fig. 4a,b.

upper lateral roof cartilage (Fig. 3a) and should reach at least 5 mm beyond this level. It is best fixed by sutures (Fig. 3b): *(a)* sutures through the graft and soft tissues around the spine prevent the implant from backward rotation; *(b)* sutures through the graft and upper lateral cartilages maintain the graft in the medial sagittal plane. Mattress sutures are placed both through the graft and the mucosa to provide stability, and additionally close the intraseptal space (Fig. 3b-d). Before placement of mattress sutures, the membranous septum should be pulled downward to preserve some lining for columellar grafting (see below).

Reconstruction of nasal dorsum

The narrowing of the bony pyramid and reconstruction of the caudal septum should adequately elevate the dorsum by reversing the initial pathological process. If additional augmentation is necessary, a dorsal cartilage graft can be introduced. Some details are of special importance:

1. The undersurface of the graft should exactly fit the outline of the nasal dorsum. Spaces between the graft and the graft bed can cause distortion secondary to scar contracture.
2. The cephalic part of the graft needs special attention as it tends to shift laterally or lift away from the nasion. Therefore, the implant should be placed in a pocket which is prepared exactly in the midline. The skin over the nasal dorsum is undermined. The nasal bone is exposed and rasped to create a bed for graft fixation. Adequate thinning of the graft is required to avoid any visible or palpable 'steps' or irregularities (Fig. 4a,b).
3. The caudal end of the graft must be thickest in the sagittal plane, as it has to replace the fibrous fatty tissue which was removed during the approach (Fig. 4b). The caudal end of the dorsal graft is shaped like a fork to fit the septal graft in that portion not covered by the cartilaginous dorsum (Fig. 4a,b).
4. The cross-section of the implant is flat where it forms the new dorsum with a gentle curve to the lateral plane (Fig. 4a). The greatest diameter in the frontal plane is at the junction of the cartilaginous and the bony pyramid.

The exactly carved dorsal graft is fixed to the already reconstructed central pillar by a suture through the dorsal graft, upper lateral cartilage, septal graft and all the way back on the contralateral side.

Reconstruction of the tip, columella and nasal base

A medial strut of cartilage is placed in a pocket caudal to the spine with wide undermining of the alar base and fixed in the fork of the dorsal graft, which provides a caudal projection and support for

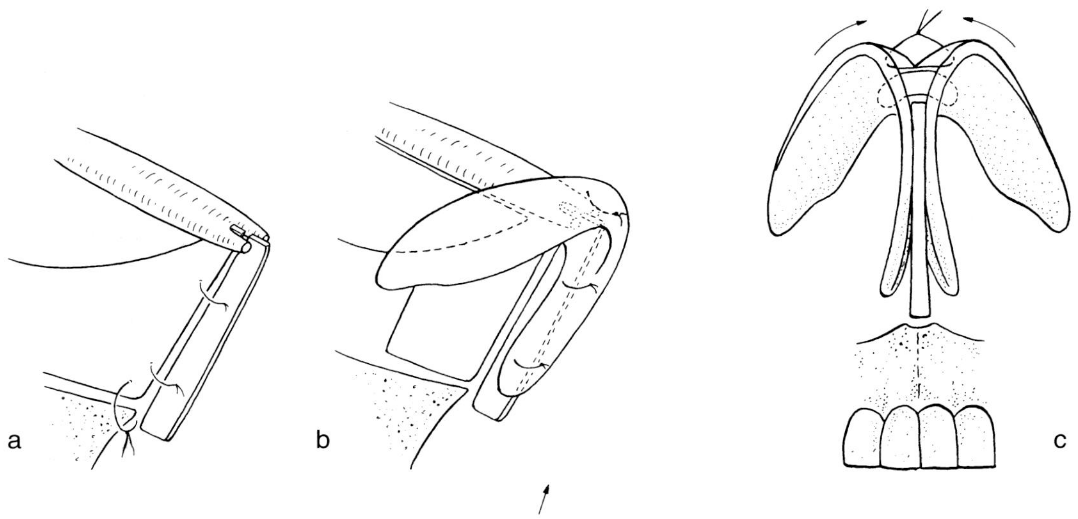

Fig. 5a,b,c.

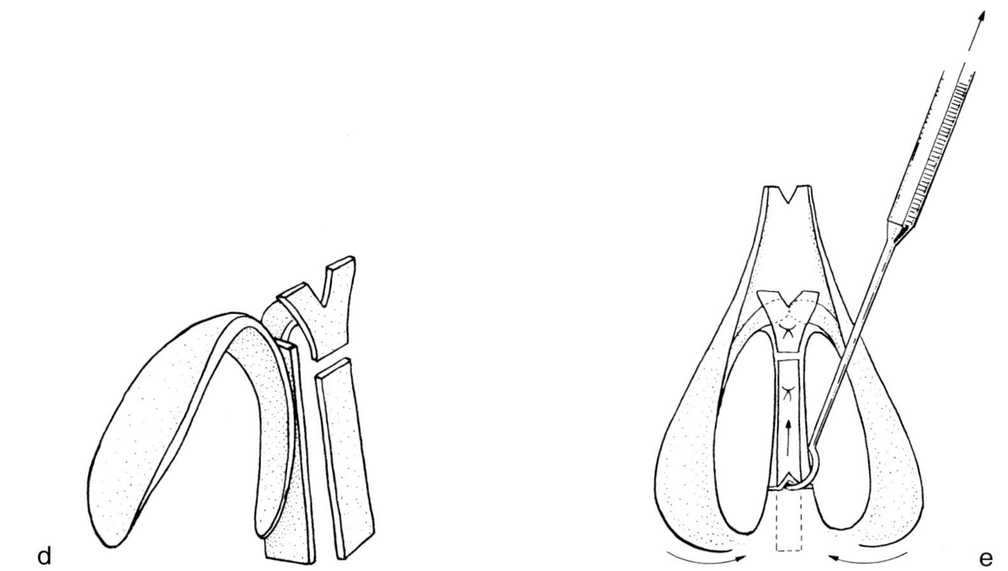

Fig. 5d,e.

the medial crura (Figs. 4b, 5a). These are sutured and fixed with through-and-through mattress sutures, producing two effects: the lower lateral cartilages have a new support and the columella is now in a more caudal position which corrects retraction of the columella. Additional tip support is achieved by a suture through the medial crura, just medial to the domes in a plane anterior to the dorsal graft, thereby reconstructing the previously severed interdomal ligament (Fig. 5b,c).

Two additional cartilage grafts are used as onlay grafts for the tip and columella (Fig. 5d,e). They build up a new refined tip and produce a double break of the columella. The cartilaginous structure prevents retraction and makes the incisional scar rather inconspicuous.

Finally, before skin closure with 6/0 non-resorbable sutures, a suspension suture of the columella base to the premaxillary implant releases tension and moves the nostril sill medially (Fig. 5e).

Comments

With these details, the procedure to correct all the components of a severe saddle nose deformity can be dealt with. They result in a stable and somewhat stiff cartilaginous nose which is nonetheless very acceptable to the patient. The advantage of the open approach is the possibility of dividing the reconstruction into independent steps (septum, dorsum, tip and base). The open approach also allows suturing of the grafts under direct vision. Careful preoperative evaluation and meticulous technique can keep significant complications to a minimum[1,2,7].

Columella

If the columella is very short (*e.g.*, Binder's syndrome), it may be difficult to close the columellar incision after increasing tip projection.

The interposition of a composite graft, as well as an initial columellar lengthening procedure through a VY-advancement flap from the upper lip, may imperil the graft or result in an unpleasant scar. Scars from previous surgery or accidents may endanger the blood supply and cause columellar necrosis. In these cases, a closed technique is preferable. The blood supply to the columella may also be disturbed if an additional Weir resection of the alar base is performed. The Weir procedure should be performed at a second stage, although it is rarely necessary because narrowing of the nasal base is usually achieved by elevation of the tip.

Dorsum

In significant depressions and thin atrophic skin, the mere adequate elevation of the dorsal skin may cause necrosis[10,12]. Wide lateral undermining and the intraoperative 'skin test' of placing a sponge under the dorsum can avoid an unexpected extrusion of the graft through a skin defect. If the possibility of necrosis exists, then controlled tissue expansion (even intraoperative) can create a proper recipient site for the dorsal graft. If the dorsum is short preoperatively, a condition frequently found in growth disturbances due to trauma or septal abscess in childhood, then elevation of the dorsum may result in further cephalic tip rotation ('height of the dorsum is taken from the length of the nose'). In these cases, the nasal infrastructure has to be lengthened. The length of the dorsal implant must be adequate to push the medial crural strut caudally.

A double-layered tip and columellar onlay graft may also be helpful. In most instances, the nasal skin will adapt to these structures, but special care has to be taken with the endonasal skin and mucosal lining. If necessary, the membranous septum may be supplemented by buccal mucosa transposition flaps and the lateral vestibular skin by composite grafts from the concha of the ear.

Finally, it should be mentioned that the open approach causes a long- standing thickening of the supratip area which can only partially be avoided by pronounced tip grafts and the creation of an adequate distance in the levels of the dome and the dorsal graft.

Further details

Concomitant midface and mandibular disorders with malocclusion should be corrected prior to nasal reconstruction. Mild forms of retrognathia seen in nasomaxillary dysplasia can be treated by premaxillary implants or grafts during nasal surgery. Narrowing of the alar base, if still necessary after tip elevation, is better accomplished by a non-resorbable alar

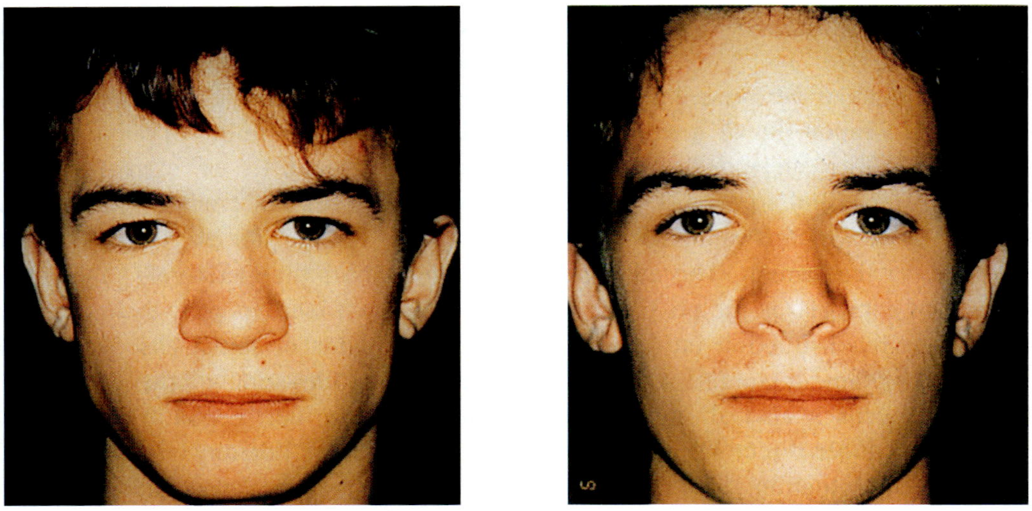

a b

Fig. 6a-f. Saddle nose deformity after trauma (18-year-old patient).
a,c,e. Preoperative views.
b,d,f. Postoperative views.

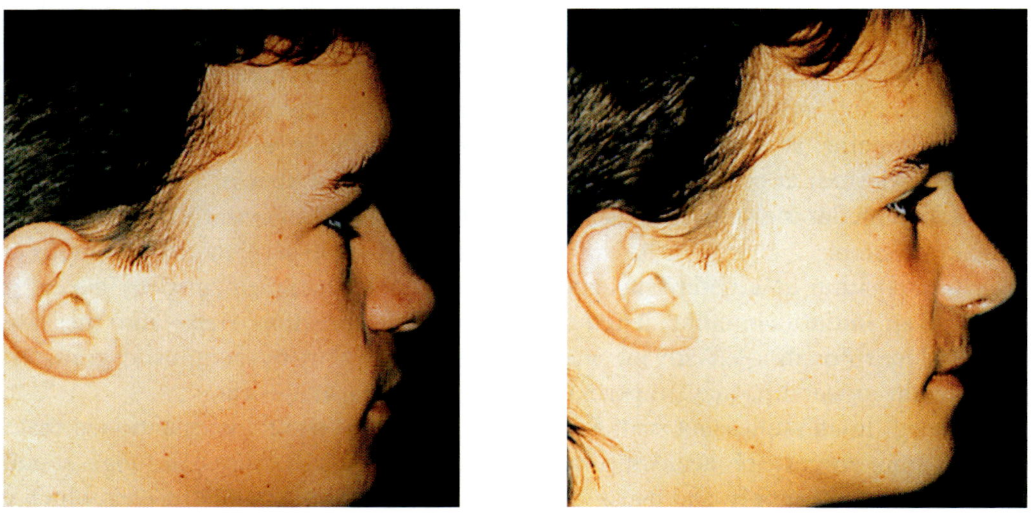

c d

Fig. 6c,d.

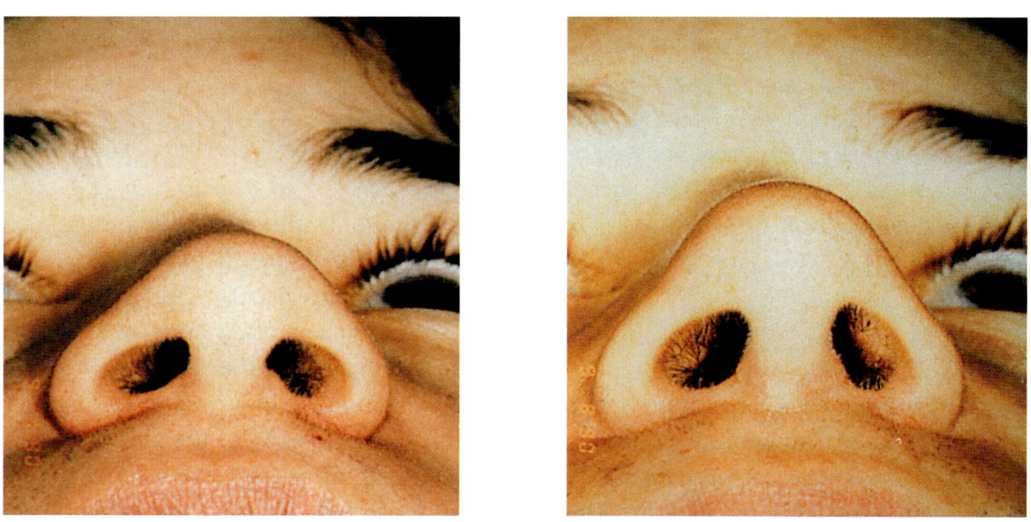

e f

Fig. 6e,f.

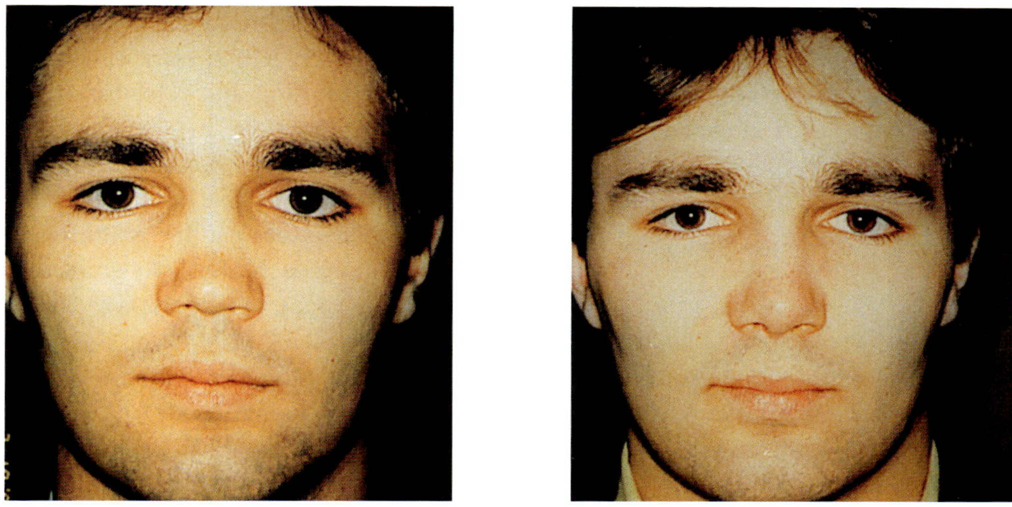

a b

Fig. 7a-f. Saddle nose deformity after trauma and submucous septal resection.
a,c,e. Preoperative views.
b,d,f. After reconstruction with autogenous rib cartilage.

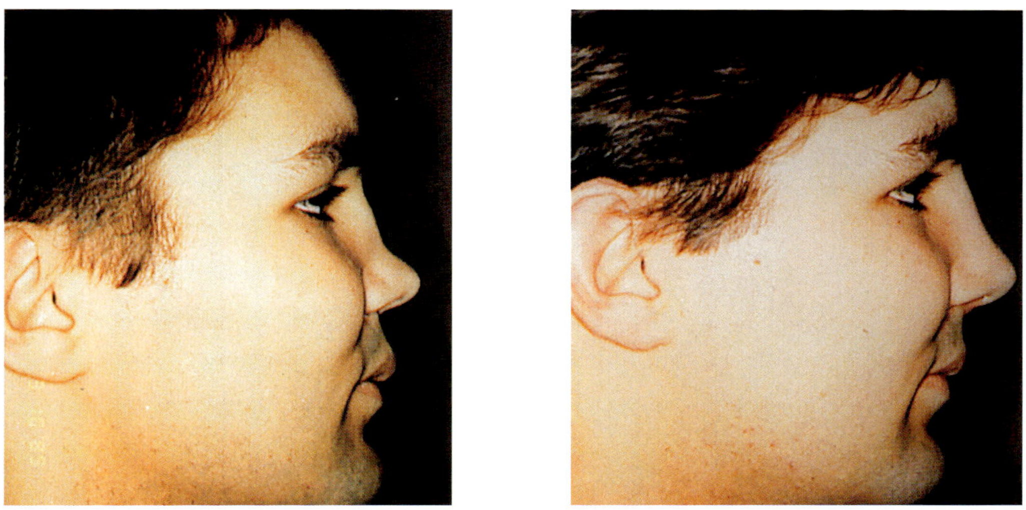

c d

Fig. 7c,d.

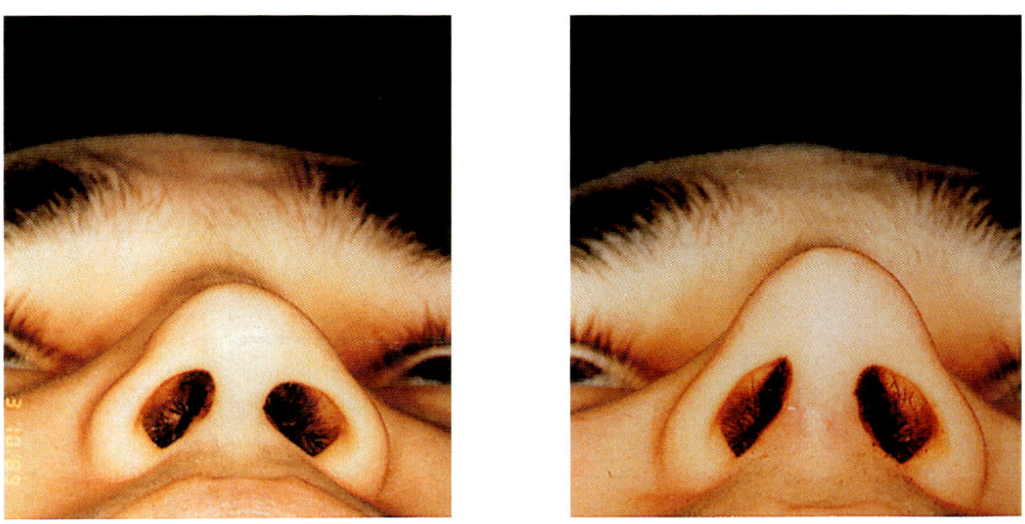

e f

Fig. 7e,f.

base suture than by alar base resection. This technique not only avoids an additional scar near the columellar incision but also releases tension and elevates the columellar base.

Conclusions

Severe saddle noses show a host of detail deformities. Many of these should be dealt with in a rather aggressive way in order to achieve a satisfying result (Figs. 6, 7). The open approach helps to solve the problem by *(a)* dividing the 'big problem' into three minor problems, *(b)* providing direct visualization which helps to maintain symmetry, and *(c)* creating stability by direct suturing and 'closure of empty spaces'.

The prerequisites for good results are thorough preoperative analysis, delicate handling of tissues and the realization that the open approach alone does not replace a surgeon's lack of experience.

Acknowledgement

The author wishes to thank E.B. Kern, MD, Mayo Clinic, Rochester, USA, for reviewing this Chapter.

20: RHINOSURGERY IN CHILDREN
Developmental and surgical aspects

C.D.A. Verwoerd and H.L. Verwoerd-Verhoef

Introduction

For a long time it has generally been accepted that in children surgery of the bony and cartilaginous nasal pyramid, and in particular the nasal septum, should be postponed until the age of 16 years. Yet, it neither seems possible nor advisable to adhere strictly to this rule in all cases.

Rhinosurgery in children can be required for various reasons[3,10,16]. Indications are acute trauma, recent traumatic deformities and a distortion of the nose, which appears highly progressive during growth.

Nasal growth and septum surgery

Numerous observations deal with severe growth anomalies of the nose after submucous resection at a young age. In the latest decennia, however, several authors stated that septal correction does not interfere with nasal growth[1,7]. Subsequently, the trend towards performing rhinosurgery in children has increased substantially. This change in attitude incurs certain risks and is not yet based on long-term follow-up of nasal growth after surgery. Moreover, it became evident that surgery of the growing nose should be based on knowledge of the specific anatomy, developmental mechanics and wound-healing of the supporting cartilaginous and bony structures in children.

Nasal growth and length of follow-up after surgery

Nasal growth continues well after puberty. Growth was found to be completed later in male adolescents (18-20 years) than in female (16-18 years). However, some longitudinal studies demonstrate that growth of the male nose may continue up to the age of 20-25 years[24]. For a correct evaluation of the effects of trauma and surgery a follow-up should be continued for at least some years after puberty. In many case reports the post-surgery observation period is too short. Unfortunately, most clinical studies focus on the development of the nose and neglect adjacent parts of the facial skeleton. In particular growth of the upper jaw can be affected by nasal injury. Therefore, orthodontic and cephalometric data should be included in the follow-up.

In many cases it is difficult or even impossible to decide to what extent the observed nasal development reflects the genetically programmed growth or the effects of trauma and surgery.

Anatomy of the nose in infants

A child's nose differs substantially from the adult nose in size and form (Fig. 1). Also the anatomy of the supporting cartilaginous and bony framework shows significant differences between young and adults. The infant nose is characterized by less frontal projection, a shorter dorsum, flat tip, shorter columella, round nares and a larger nasolabial angle. In proportion to the brain skull, the facial skull in neonates is much smaller than in the adult[4,8,12].

Specific features of the infant nose are:

1. The septum cartilage reaches from the nasal tip to the anterior skull base and sphenoid (Fig. 3). A perpendicular plate has not yet been formed. The upper lateral cartilages extend under the nasal bones over their total length and merge with the cartilaginous anlage of the anterior cranial base (Fig. 2).

2. Septum and upper lateral cartilages form a T-bar-shaped structure, the dorsoseptal cartilage, which is directly based on the sphenoid; it supports the nasal bones and determines the contour of the cartilaginous nasal dorsum. Anteriorly, it is attached to the upper jaw by a fibrous connection with the anterior nasal spine (septospinal ligament).
3. In infants, the vomer is only rudimentary developed; it is represented by a thin bony plate on both sides of the basal rim of the cartilaginous nasal septum and an incomplete lamella of bone between the basal rim and the palatal bone (Fig. 5).

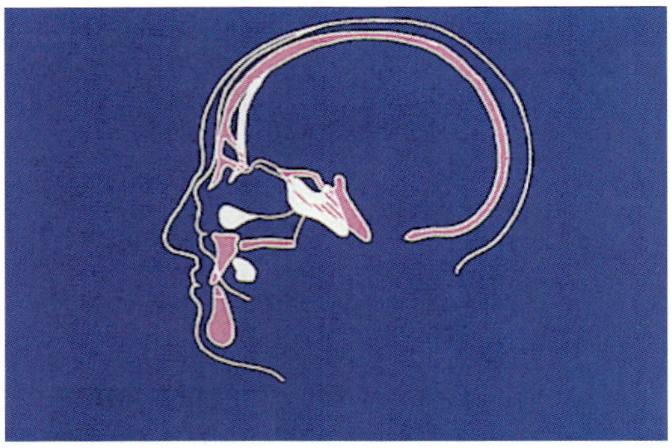

Fig. 1. Schematic drawings in the sagittal plane of the heads of a newborn and an adult. The skeleton parts of the newborn are in white and of the adult in red. The neurocranium of the newborn is magnified to the size of the adult. The neurocranium of both stages are superimposed. The 'extra' growth of the facial skeleton during childhood, in comparison to the brain skull, is reflected in the more prominent nose, and upper and lower jaw of the adult.

Nasal development during childhood

During childhood and early adolescence the facial skull, including the nasal skeleton, grows faster than the brain skull. Consequently, the baby face will change into an adult profile with a more prominent nose, upper jaw and mandible (Fig. 1).

Next to dimensional growth of the nose some structural developments have to be mentioned here.
1 . Ossification of the cartilaginous septum, starting near the anterior skull base will result in the formation of the perpendicular plate (Fig. 4). The vomer is developing by fusion of the bilateral and median anlages (Fig. 5). Finally, the perpendicular plate and the vomer merge at the age of 6 to 8 years.
2. The intracephalic parts of the dorsolateral cartilages show a process of regressive changes during the early years of childhood, leaving only an extension of 3-15 mm under the nasal bones in the adult stage.
3. The junction of cartilaginous septum, vomer and perpendicular plate demonstrates a variety of morphological presentations (Fig. 5)[15, 18]. It is important to recognize that most of the resulting septal cristae and vomeral spines are directly not related to deviations of the nasal dorsum since the growing dorsoseptal cartilage is based on the sphenoid and 'stabilized' in the midline by the upper laterals (T-bar).

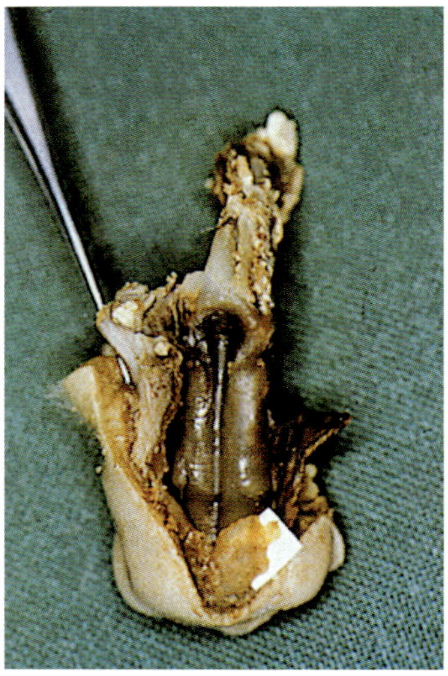

Fig. 2. Nasal dorsum of a human neonatal specimen after removal of the frontal and nasal bones, demonstrating the dorsolateral (= upper lateral) cartilages merging with the cartilage of the anterior skull base. At the end of the supraseptal groove, the cartilaginous crista Galli can be distinguished as a prominence in the sagittal plane. The left lower lateral cartilage is presented on a piece of paper.

Specific 'architecture' of the cartilaginous nasal septum from neonate to adult

In the neonate various parts of the nasal septum demonstrate obvious differences in thickness (Fig. 3)[4, 17]. A zone of thicker cartilage (± 3 mm) spreads from the sphenoid into anterodorsal direction to support the nasal dorsum (sphenodorsal zone). A second zone of thicker cartilage forms the basal rim of the septum, extending from the

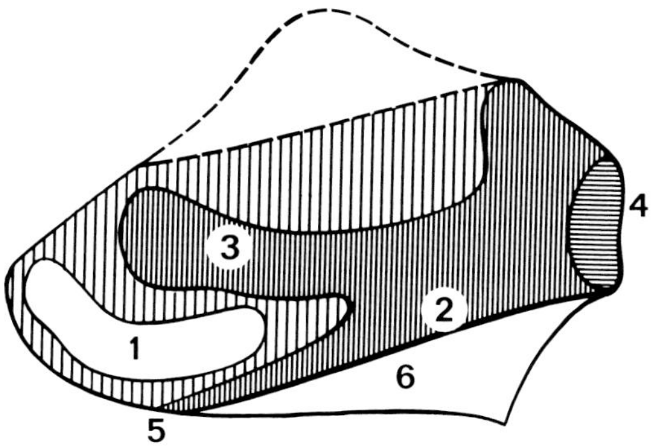

Fig. 3. Thicker and thinner areas of the cartilaginous septum in a neonate (schematic presentation). *a.* Anterocentral area of thin cartilage; *b.* Zones of thicker cartilage: the sphenospinal (basal) zone extends from the sphenoid (4) to the anterior nasal spine (5) and the sphenodorsal zone extends from the sphenoid to the nasal dorsum; the thickness of the cartilage varies from less than 0.75 mm (1), between 0.75 and 1.5 mm (3), between 1.5 mm and 3 mm (2), to more than 3 mm (anterior to the sphenoid) (6). Vomer anlage between the basal rim of the cartilaginous septum and the palate; the most dorsal part of the septal cartilage, including the crista Galli, is delineated by an interrupted line.

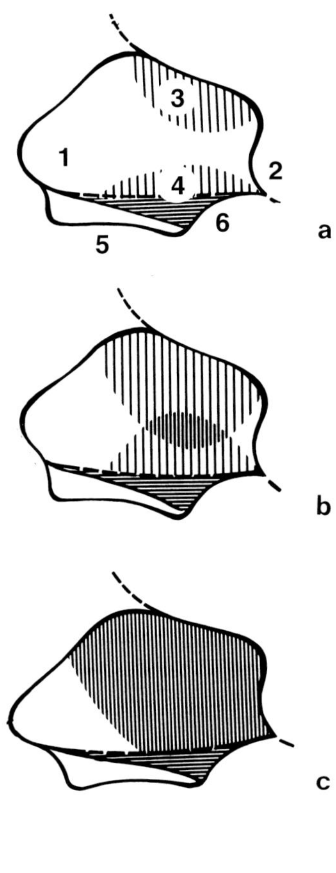

Fig. 4. Median line tracings of the development of the perpendicular plate and vomer. *a.* One to three years of age, the septal cartilage (1) extends as far as the sphenoid (2); first anlage of the perpendicular plate (3) and alae vomeris (4); between the basal rim of the cartilage and palate (5) is the inferior part of the vomer (6). *b.* Ten to 17 years of age, expansion of the perpendicular plate and the bilateral vomeral alae results in the overlapping and merging of these bony structures. *c.* Adult, bony integration of both structures.

sphenoid to the anterior nasal spine (sphenospinal zone). The caudal rim of the septum is only slightly thickened and will contribute to the support of the nasal tip.

An area of extremely thin cartilage (0.4 mm), ventrocaudal in the septum and surrounded by the thicker cartilage of the sphenospinal and sphenodorsal zones, may not be considered to play a role in supporting the nasal dorsum.

Essentially the same pattern of thinner and thicker areas in the cartilaginous nasal septum is found in older children and adolescents. However due to the formation of the perpendicular plate, the support of the sphenodorsal zone of thick septal cartilage shifts from the sphenoid to the thickened caudal edge of compact bone of the perpendicular plate (Fig. 4). The junction between the septum cartilage and the perpendicular plate is extremely tight.

The role of different parts of the septodorsal cartilage in nasal growth

Animal studies and clinical observations pointed to developmental mechanisms, regulating postnatal growth of the nose and other parts of the midface.[19]

The increase of length and height of the nasal dorsum appeared to depend on expansion of the sphenodorsal zone of thick cartilage, which is later based on the caudal edge of the perpendicular plate. Consequently partial or total loss of this zone will cause an underdevelopment of the nasal dorsum, which remains too low and too short).

The thickened basal rim of the septal cartilage (sphenospinal zone) acts as another growth center. A substantial defect in this zone results in retroposition of the anterior nasal spine and maxilla. However, loss of the area of thin cartilage, anteriorly and caudally in the nasal septum, does not appear to interfere with nasal growth!

As the nasal septum and both upper lat-

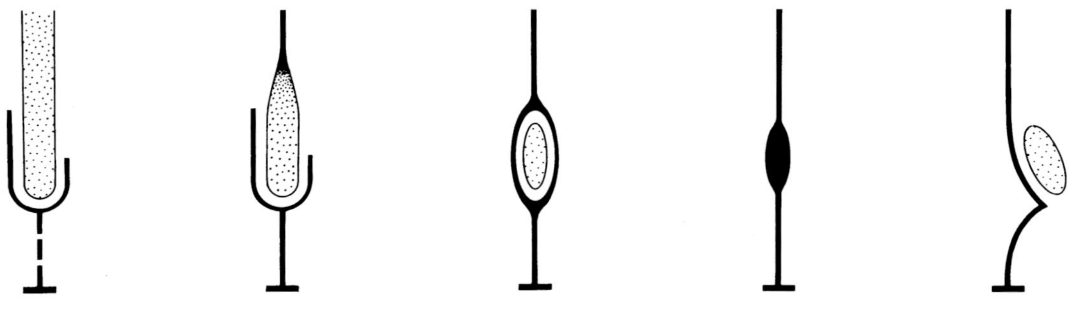

Fig. 5a-e. Schematic transversal section of the septovomeral junction. *a,b:* Development between birth and ten years. *c,d,e:* Variations in the adult stage. *a.* Basal rim of septal cartilage fitting in the vomeral groove, formed by the vomeral alae in the neonatal stage: the inferior part of the vomer, based on the palate, is a thin bony lamella with lacunae; asymmetrical development of the vomeral alae. *b.* Progressive enchrondal ossification of the cartilaginous septum and subsequent remodelling of the bone result in the formation of a thin perpendicular plate. *c.* Both vomeral alae and the perpendicular plate have fused, enclosing a posterior extension of persisting cartilage: sphenoid tail. *d.* Complete ossification of the septal cartilage and bony integration of the vomer and perpendicular plate. *e.* Asymmetrical development of the vomer with formation of a vomeral spine and sphenoid tail, bordered on only one side by a vomeral ala.

eral cartilages form one T-bar-shaped structure, defects or scarring of each of the three components will affect further growth of the whole structure. For the septum this may be evident but also injury to one upper lateral cartilage can result in malformation of the nasal dorsum (narrowing or deviation).

Different types of nasal maldevelopment in patients after (partial) loss of septum cartilage during early childhood are illustrated in Fig. 8,9,10.

Preferred fracture lines and septum deviations

The nasal septum is a composition of septum cartilage, perpendicular plate and vomer. Each of these components has a specific anatomy, featuring thicker and thinner, stronger and weaker parts. In case of trauma the septum tends to fracture at the weakest, most vulnerable sites. This explains the preference in the location of fracturing, as observed in adult patients and children[17].

A common fracture of the nasal septum is the socalled C-fracture. The inferior, 'horizontal' part of the fracture follows the thinner area of the septum, immediately dorsal to the sphenospinal zone. The 'vertical' part is found in the center – the thinnest part – of the perpendicular plate. The superior part, varying in length, is located under the nasal dorsum.

Another presentation of a fracture line involves the most caudal area of the septum, and extends from the insertion of the septospinal ligament through the cartilage to the dorsal rim, just caudal of the attachment of both upper lateral cartilages. A dissociation of the septal cartilage from the perpendicular plate is exceptional.

A fracture of the cartilaginous septum is usually followed by an immediate overlap of the separated parts. During further (sagittal) growth an overlap might lead to a progressive deviation without re-integration of the separated parts (Fig. 6,7)[19].

The preference in localisation of fracture lines is reflected in specific types of septum deviation in children as well as in adults[6,13].

Rhinosurgery, wound healing and growth: experimental evidence

The effects of surgical interventions have been analyzed in animal experiments. The following analasions are in agreement with clinical observations[8, 9, 20, 21, 22, 23].

1. Elevation of the mucoperichondrium on one or both sides does not present any disadvantage in terms of disturbed growth.
The elevated perichondrium may be stimulated by intraseptal blood to produce fibrocartilage which could lead to distortion of the septum. Thus, intraseptal blood collection should be presented.

2. The cutting faces of separated parts of septum cartilage are quickly covered by fibrous tissue, impeding a structural re-inte-

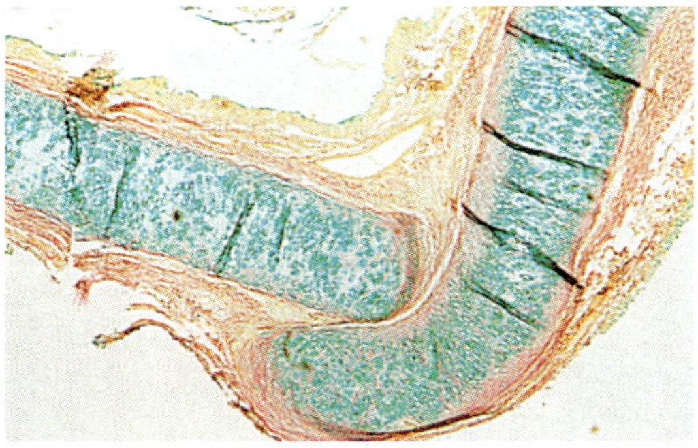

Fig. 6. Horizontal section through the septum of an adult rabbit (24 weeks). Overlapping and angulation of the segments are the result of a septal transection at the age of four weeks. Fusion of the perichondrium, covering the cut ends.

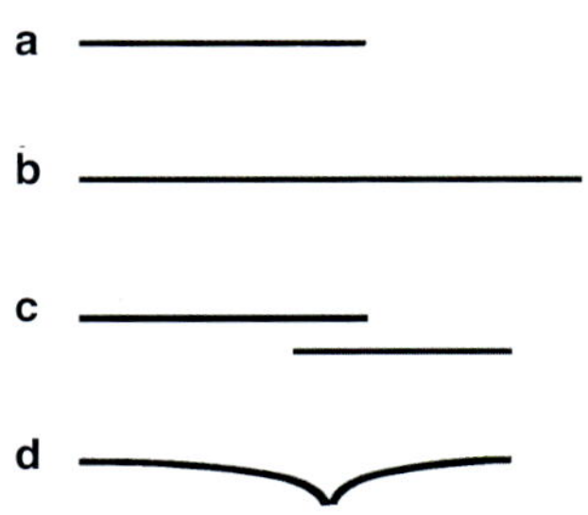

Fig. 7. Schematic impression of the increase in length of the septum under normal *(a,b),* and abnormal *(c,d),* conditions. The growth of the interrupted cartilage with overlapping *(c),* or angulation *(d),* prevents normal lengthening of the total septum and results in an underdevelopment of the nose.

gration of the cartilage. It bears the risk of deviations or angulations.

3. Overlapping edges, occurring after transection of cartilage, should be trimmed for a good end-to-end adaptation.

4. Re-implanted cartilage fragments tend to dislocate and crushed cartilage usually shows progressive deformation during growth.

5. Mobilisation or partial resection of the nasal bones or vomer do not disturb further development!

Rhinosurgery in children

Follow-up studies, and current knowledge of wound healing and growth mechanics have contributed to surgical concepts but still leave many questions unanswered. Therefore, parents and patients should be informed that late results can not be predicted. Even after several years recurrent septum pathology may occur as well as an abnormal development of the nose. Different treatment strategies may be advocated pending the outcome of adequate prospective studies[14,15].

Treatment of recent traumatic deformities in children

Diagnosis

Correct diagnosis of fractures and dislocations of the bony and cartilaginous nasal pyramid is difficult in children, even more than in adults because of the smaller dimensions, the often abundant swelling due to edema and/or hematoma, and less patient cooperation. When in doubt, the examination - inspection and palpation - should be repeated after 2 or 3 days when the soft tissue swelling has diminished, if necessary under general anaesthesia. After decongestion of the nasal mucosa anterior rhinoscopy or nasal endoscopy are mandatory for assessment of the cartilaginous pyramid. Vertical or horizontal fractures are often found. Fractures of the bony nasal pyramid do not occur as frequently in children as in adults because the nasal bones are less prominent and the greater part of the nasal skeleton is cartilaginous. Moreover, the sutures bordering the nasal bones have not yet been ossified and could stretch in case of trauma.

Treatment: Closed reduction

The prevailing method of managing nasal fractures in (young) children is closed reduction under general anaesthesia [14]. A combination of elevation of the nasal dorsum – thereby straigthening the nasal septum – and prolonged digital compression of the nasal bones is usually successful in restoring the nasal morphology. The elasticity of the septodorsal cartilage and its capacity of regaining its original form are essential for the success of this manipulation. Nasal packing is only tolerated by older children and contradicted in young children because they are obligatory nose breathers. Repositioning of splayed or dislocated nasal bones is nearly always possible without an open reduction. In exceptional cases a 2-mm-osteotome may be used to mobilize dislocated parts and produce a satisfactory alignment of the nasal bones.

Treatment: conservative septoplasty

Obvious deformities of the nasal septum after recent trauma, usually in older children, are treated by a conservative septoplasty, within one week after the accident. At surgical exploration, preferably by hemitransfixion incision and unilateral tunnelling, 'clinical' fractures of the septum sometimes appear to be angulations with a rupture of the perichondrium on one side only. Overlapping of fractured edges is a frequent finding.

A fracture reaching from the anterior nasal spine to the dorsal side of the septum just caudal to the upper lateral cartilages, is rather common. Another preferred site is horizontal just superior to the septospinal zone, associated with the vertical fracture of the perpendicular plate.

At anterior rhinoscopy the differential diagnosis with a pre-existing developmental variation, such as disjunction of the septovomeral region, can be difficult. This pre-existing disjunction, not related to a trauma, does not need correction.

After re-alignment of the fractured septum, intraseptal blood accumulation should be removed and the mucosa approximated by through and through suturing. Intranasal Silastic splints can be used to support the septum for one or two weeks.

Surgical treatment of deformities of the septum and nose not related to recent trauma

Severe breathing problems due to septal pathology and external distortion of the nose are generally accepted to be indications for surgery, in particular, when the malformations appear to be progressive during growth.

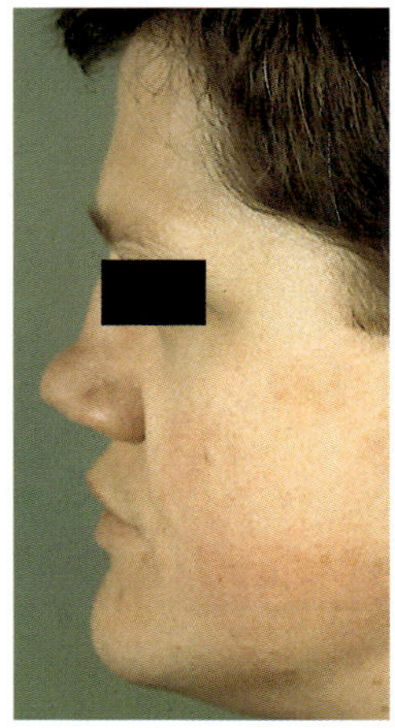

Fig. 8. Facial profile illustrating the development of the nose and maxilla after loss of major parts of the cartilaginous septum (sphenodorsal and sphenospinal zone) during childhood: low and broad nasal dorsum, retroposition of the anterior nasal spine, underdevelopment of the maxilla.

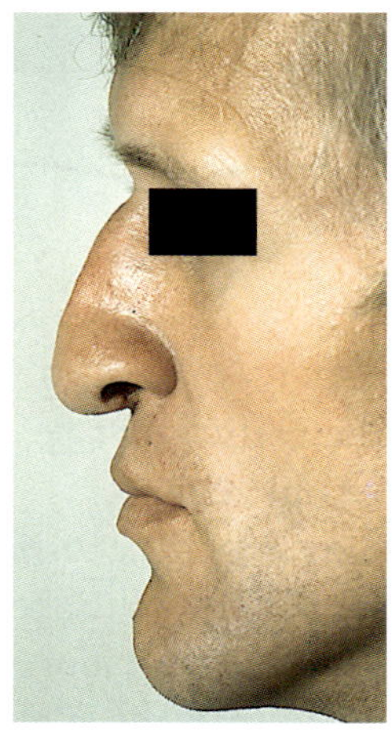

Fig. 9. Facial profile illustrating the development of the nose and maxilla after the loss of the basal part of the septal cartilage (sphenospinal zone) during early childhood: normal prominence of the bony nasal dorsum. Underdevelopment of the maxilla is indirectly responsible for lowering the cartilaginous nasal dorsum; the cartilaginous nasal skeleton of normal dimension is based on a retropositioned maxilla.

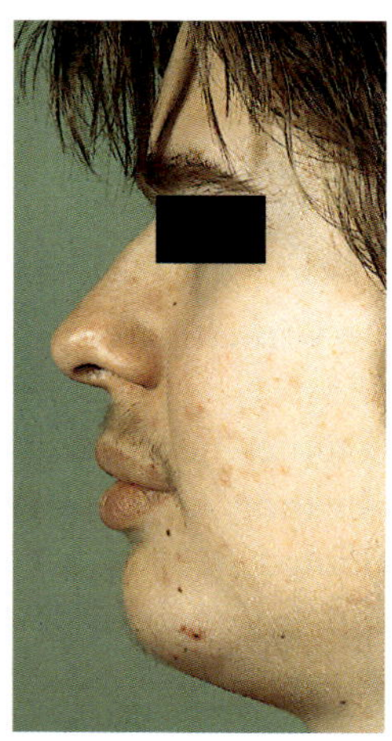

Fig. 10. Facial profile: normal nose development in a young man with a known septal perforation (anterocentral part) from the age of nine years.

External correction is usually postponed until after the adolescent growth spurt although experimental evidence suggest that mobilization of the nasal bones will not seriously disturb growth. Surgery is nearly always restricted to correction of the malformed septum.

The use of magnifying glasses is advised for these procedures in children.

As far as the technique is concerned, a few points should be raised:

1. Hemitransfixion, followed by elevation of the mucoperichondrium (anterior and superior tunnel) on one or both sides is a technique suitable for children. If necessary, an inferior tunnel is made parallel to the maxillary crest. The mucoperichondrium of the nasal floor should never be elevated in order to prevent damage to the incisival nerves.

For correction of only a crista or a vomeral spine the mucoperichondrium is elevated over a smaller area. The mucoperichondrial incision should run just caudal to the crista or spine. To diminish the chance of a complicating septum perforation the cartilage is incised a few millimeters in posterior direction in order to make a tunnel on the other side. Cartilage should be respected as much as possible. The septospinal ligament should preferably left untouched.

2. The vomer may be partially resected without disturbing nasal growth.
3. Resection of a deviating basal rim is not expected to have consequences for the outgrowth of the nasal dorsum. However, in young children (less than 5 years of age) it may lead to a later retroposition of the anterior nasal spine.
4. Posterior chondrotomy or dissociation of the septal cartilage from the perpendicular plate should be avoided as this area is of paramount importance for the support of the growing nasal dorsum.
5. Defects in the cartilaginous septum should be reconstructed as completely as possible, preferably with non-crushed autologous septum cartilage in order to minimize the risk of septal perforation or scar formation between the bilateral mucosal membranes. Suturing will help to prevent dislocation of the implant.
6. A luxated caudal rim of the septum should be brought into a columella pocket where it must be anchored by sutures between the medial crura of the alar cartilages.
7. Separation of the septum from the upper lateral cartilage on one or both sides should be avoided in order to prevent later irregularities of the nasal dorsum due to reactive, new formation of cartilage at the wound surface.

Special post-traumatic conditions

Dorsum haematoma

Rupture of an upper lateral cartilage from the piriform aperture is a difficult diagnosis. In many cases it leads to a dorsum haematoma, caused by rupture of the external branch of the anterior ethmoidal artery, which penetrates the connecting area between the upper lateral cartilages and nasal bones. Observed by anterior rhinoscopy the haematoma is most evident between the caudal edge of the upper lateral cartilage and the cephalic margin of the alar cartilage. Externally the haematoma is often concealed by facial oedema. It is recommended to puncture or drain the haematoma, and approximate a dislocated upper lateral cartilage to the nasal bone by nasal packing.

Septum haematoma and abscess

Septum haematoma and abscess should be treated in the same way as in adult patients. When a larger part of the septum has become necrotic immediate implantation of bank cartilage appears to be an efficient method to prevent a collapse of the nasal cartilaginous pyramid due to loss of cartilage and scar formation. It can not be expected, however, to promote normal growth of the nose. The actual further development will depend on the growth capacity of remaining vital cartilage.

Bank cartilage is thought to bear the risk of contamination; therefore, the use of concha cartilage is preferred nowadays.

Septum perforation

Septum perforation is a rare phenomenon in children. Follow-up of a few patients has suggested that a perforation limited to the thin antero-central area of the septum does not lead to abnormal development of the nose, probably because it does not interfere with the growing framework of thicker zones in the septum (Fig. 3 and 10). Closure of such a perforation incurs the risk of scar formation with negative effects on nasal growth. It is therefore only indicated in exceptional cases with abundant formation of crustae and chronic rhinitis.

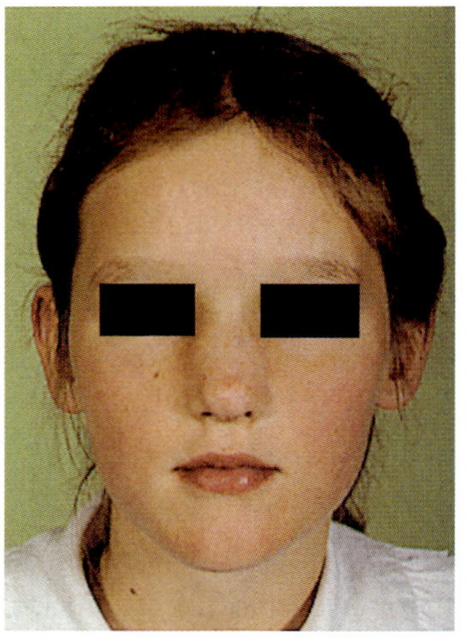

Fig. 11. An 11-year-old girl with nasal deformation after a previous trauma, characterized by: *a.* low and broad bony and cartilaginous pyramid; *b.* flattening and partial median dissociation of the nasal bones; *c.* almost sagittal position of the frontonasal process of the maxilla.

Late maldevelopment of the nose

After nasal trauma a correct diagnosis is most important, because neglected injuries can be the cause of later abnormal development (Fig. 11). Sometimes it takes one or more years before a low and broad cartilaginous and bony pyramid, flattening and partial midline dissociation of the nasal bones, a nearly sagittal position of the frontonasal processes of the maxilla and septal pathology become evident.

The results of surgical correction of such progressive nasal deformities in growing children is often disappointing. A better option is a rhinoplasty after the adolescent growth spurt.

21: REVISION SURGERY

C. Walter

Introduction

It has to be realized that these so-called postoperative failures can result in minor deformities or can end in major disasters, depending on the surgeon's capability and the patient's individual reaction.

In the past, it was said that 3% to 5% of patients operated on needed some revisional surgery. During recent discussions at international meetings, senior surgeons have admitted that nowadays, due to the ever-increasing number of surgeons performing this operation and perhaps also due to the higher expectancy of patients with regard to results, the number of revisions being performed has risen to 20% to 25%.

According to the visible deformity, we can differentiate between:
1. minor deformities
2. medium grade deformities impairing the nasal airway
3. severe deformities with partial destruction of the bony or cartilaginous elements and endonasal strictures in varying degrees of severity

Generally speaking, it is not advisable to reoperate on patients who have undergone nasal surgery until one year has elapsed since the last intervention. As we are now dealing with two, three, four and five-year postoperative results, it can be clearly observed that additional changes and skin shrinkage take place even after three to four years. In cases in which several rhinoplasties have been carried out prior to the consultation, we advise that a year and a half should be allowed to elapse so that suitable tissues can be found. Preoperatively, a clear and detailed analysis of the deformities should be made.

Surgical procedures

After proper evaluation, the operation can be carried out under local or general anesthesia. In all cases of revisional surgery, we add cortisone (Kenacort 40 mg per 100 ml) to the local anesthetic. We feel that this has an advantageous effect on postoperative swelling and healing. The operations are divided into:
1. decreasing surgery
2. augmentation surgery

Approach

The first step in the operation is hemi- or complete transfixion, according to the findings. Complete transfixion is used if we want to reduce the length and width of the septum or the nasal spine, and to rotate the columella along the septal cartilage portion in relation to the upper lip. Hemitransfixion is used when no alteration of the nasal-labial angle should occur.

The anterior nasal spine plays a key role here. Residual septal deviations should be corrected during this approach and it is very important to pay close attention to the size of the inferior and middle turbinates. The latter sometimes contributes more to nasal breathing impairment than the inferior turbinate, and is one of the key factors in insufficient realignment of the septum if not corrected. In such cases, we recommend endonasal partial ethmoidectomy and lateral fracture with partial resection of the middle turbinate in conjunction with corrective measures on the inferior turbinate.

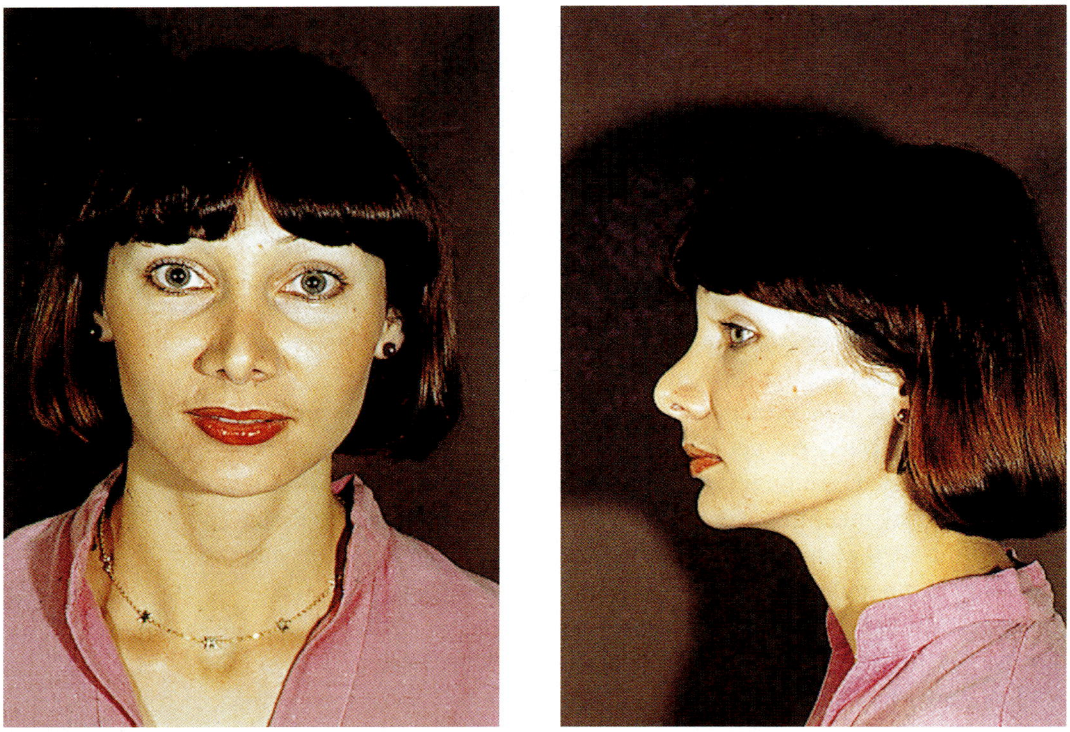

a b

Fig. 1a,b. Typical pollybeak nose after 2 rhinoplasties. Over-resection of the dorsum and lower lateral cartilages (frontal and lateral view).

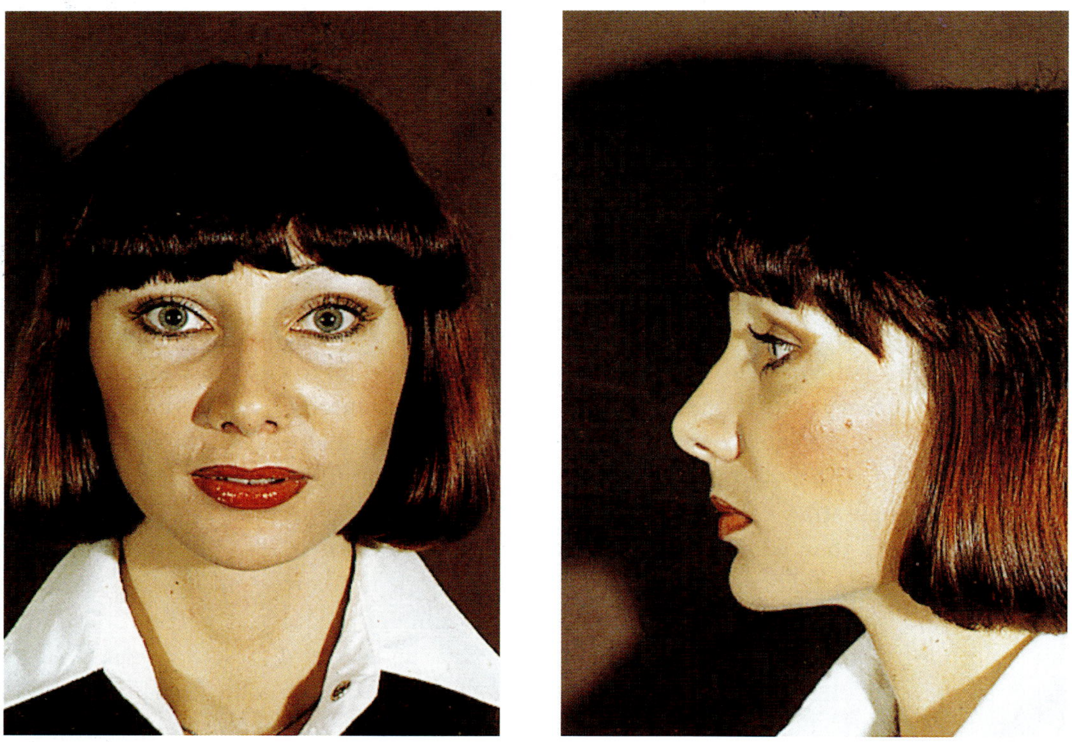

c d

Fig. 1c,d. Postoperative situation after augmentation of the dorsum and tip with autogenous cartilage onlay grafts.

Nasal dorsum

The next step is evaluation of the height of the nasal dorsum. In the typical pollybeak deformity, we often have to deal with an insufficient cartilage reduction in the lower half of the nasal dorsum at the junction of the septum and the attachments of the triangular cartilages. Usually, over-resection of the lower lateral car-

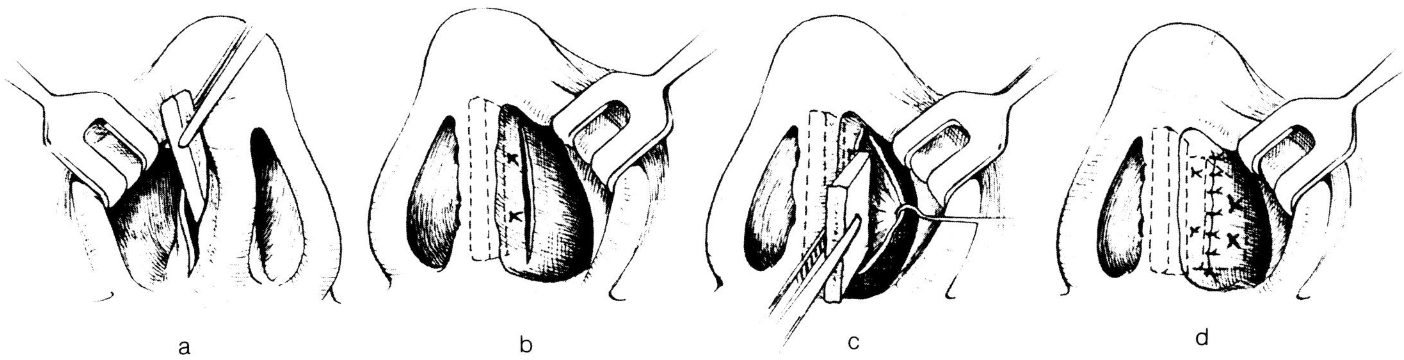

Fig. 2. Insertion of grafts into the columella (*a,b*) and if necessary into the anterior septum (*c,d*) to raise the tip and correct a retracted columella.

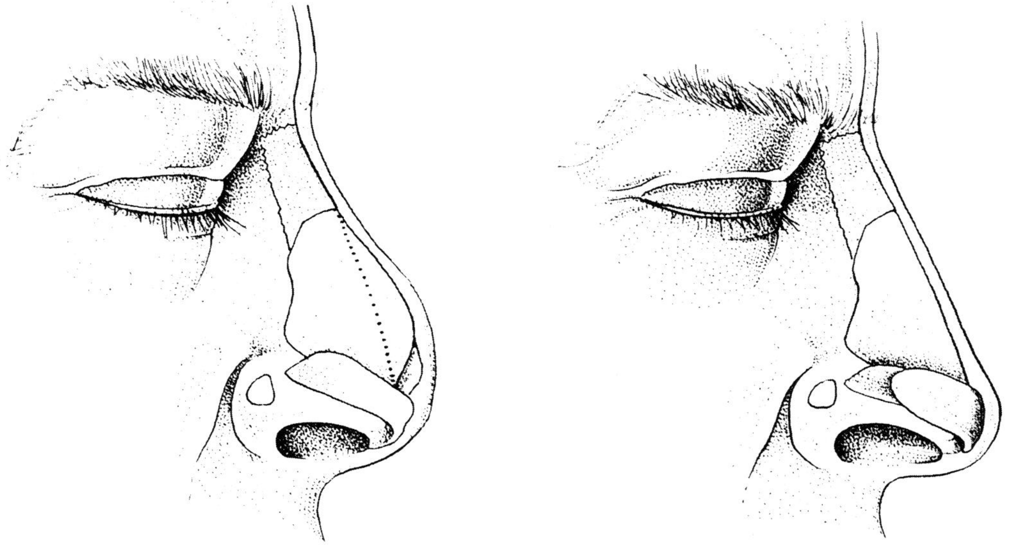

Fig. 3. Cartilage onlay graft to replace resected lower lateral cartilage for tip elevation.

tilages has occurred. The tip is suspended at the septal angle. Any reduction in the height of this structure will cause the tip to drop more. After an initial improvement in appearance, a new pollybeak becomes noticeable after a few months in a nose which is now smaller than before and more disastrously deformed (Figs. 1a-d).

We feel that the intercartilaginous approach gives us a sufficient opening to evaluate the situation properly. Prior to any resection of cartilaginous parts and in that vital internal valve triangle, the surgeon must ensure that sufficient cartilage is present in the lower lateral cartilage area to elevate and project the nasal tip.

If too much of the supporting lower lateral cartilages has been removed by mistake, the surgeon should not lower the dorsum unless he has obtained sufficient tip projection with onlay grafts, buttons or struts into the columella and into the tip region (Figs. 2 and 3). The dorsal pyramid is then uncovered by careful sharp dissection, carefully elevating the periosteum but avoiding injury of the cartilaginous bony junction. This could bring about additional problems by inward displacement of bone or cartilage at this junction after dislocation.

After determining the position of the nasal tip, the next step is realignment of the nasal dorsum. It is always advantageous to cut through the junction of the septal cartilage in the upper laterals in order to free them. In most cases, it is not

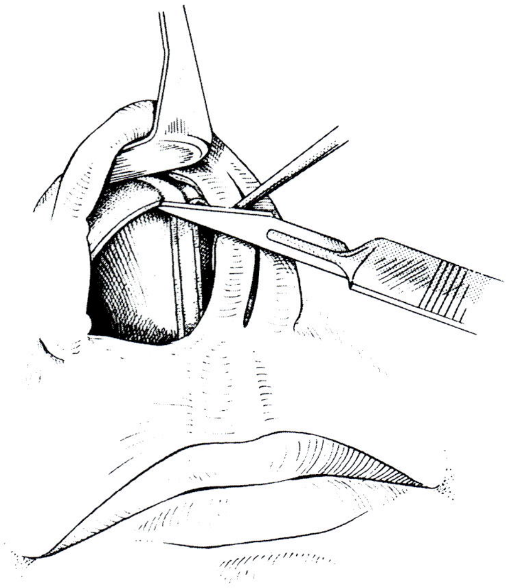

Fig. 4. Separation of the upper lateral cartilages from the septum but not the mucosa.

a

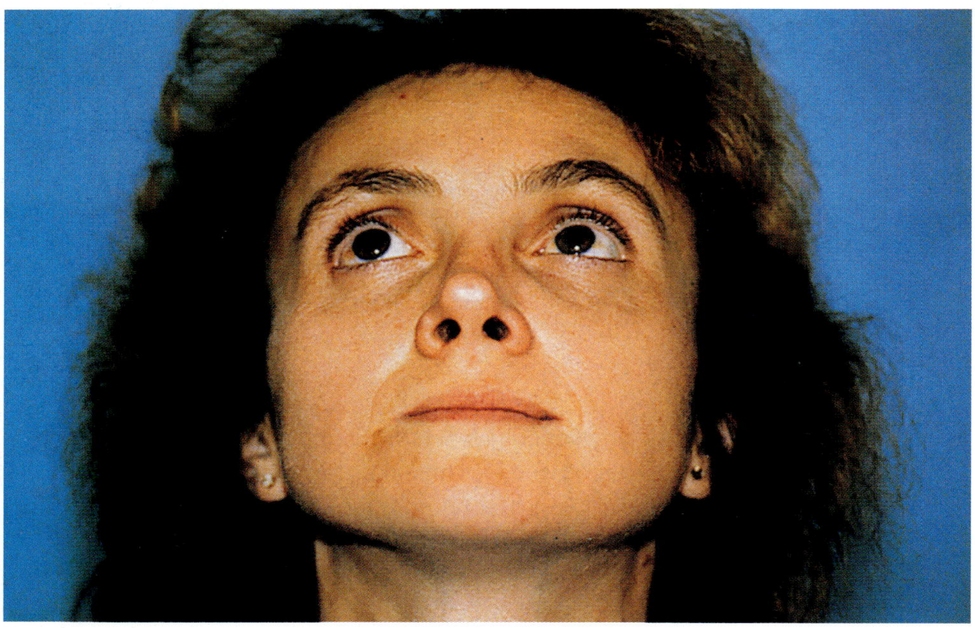

Fig. 5a. Over-resected nose producing alar collapse, shortening and saddling (basal view).

absolutely necessary to go through the mucosa.

Simple severing of the cartilages is often sufficient to narrow the cartilaginous dorsum by freeing these cartilages (Fig. 4). Smoothing of the nasal dorsum (there are often residual irregularities), for which rasps are the usual instruments, should be followed by careful suctioning of the leftover bony particles. Excision of cartilaginous protuberances under direct vision with a scalpel at the junction of the bony and cartilaginous hump is sometimes better than the traumatizing rasp.

If it has been determined preoperatively that the previous surgeon has lowered the dorsum too much, the surgeon should not undermine a wide area of skin, but should only create a small pocket on the dorsal line of the nose, in order to have just enough room for placement of a cartilaginous or bony graft. This can be obtained either from the bony parts of

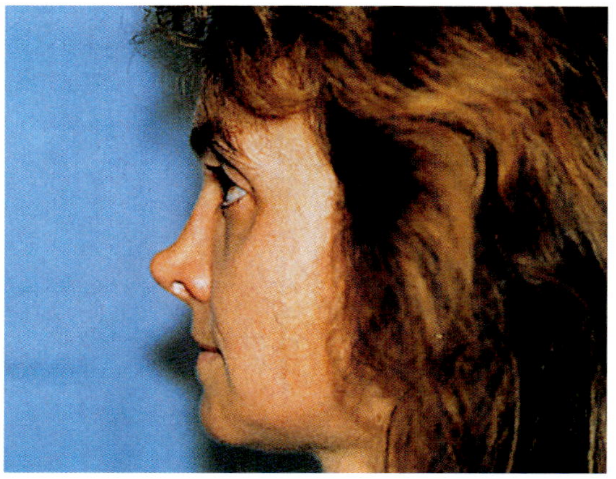

Fig. 5b. Over-resected nose producing alar collapse, shortening and saddling (lateral view).

b

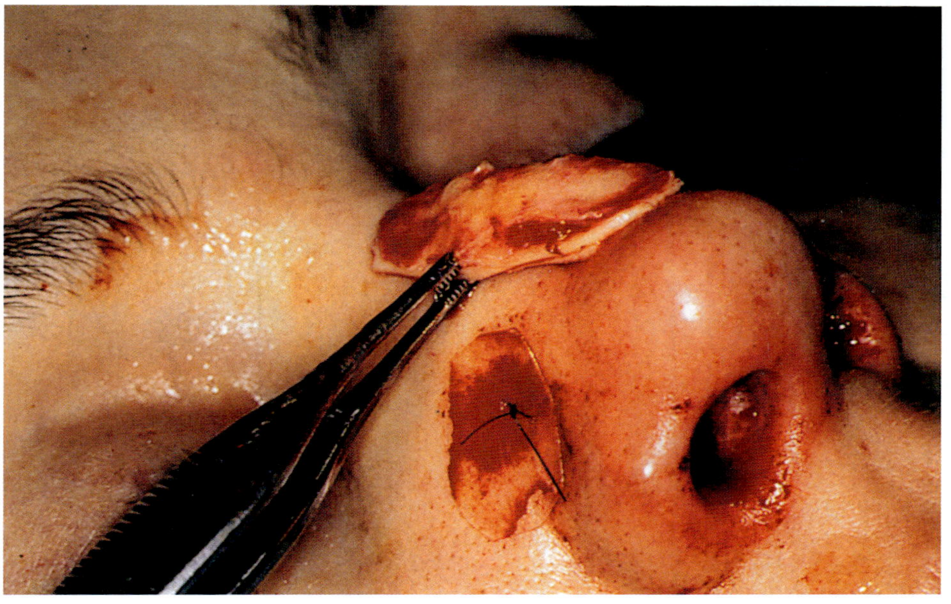

Fig. 5c,d. Operative procedure prior to inserting ear cartilage into the dorsum. The lateral wall has already been reinforced by a cartilage graft. Skin protection from sutures cutting through by silicon plates.

c

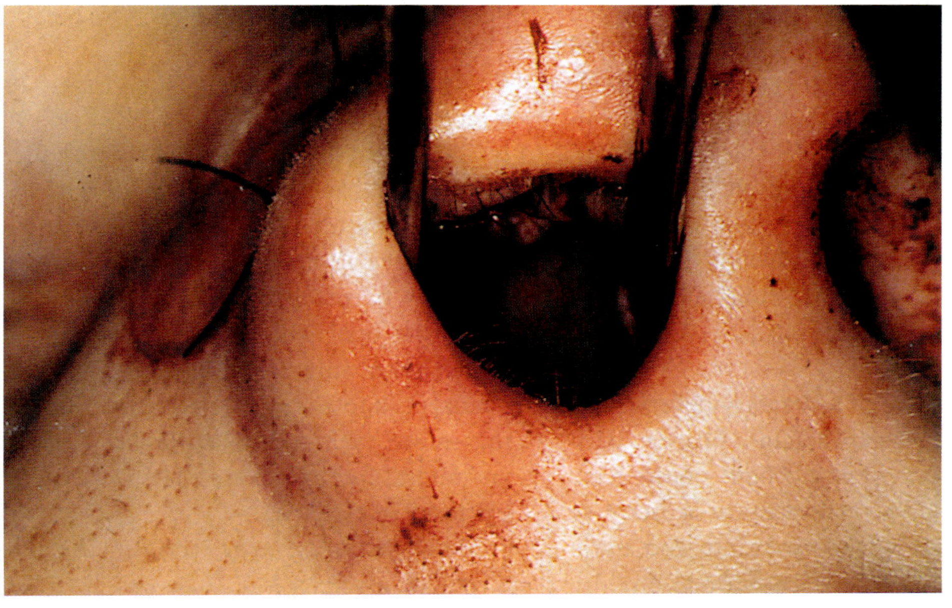

Fig. 5d.

d

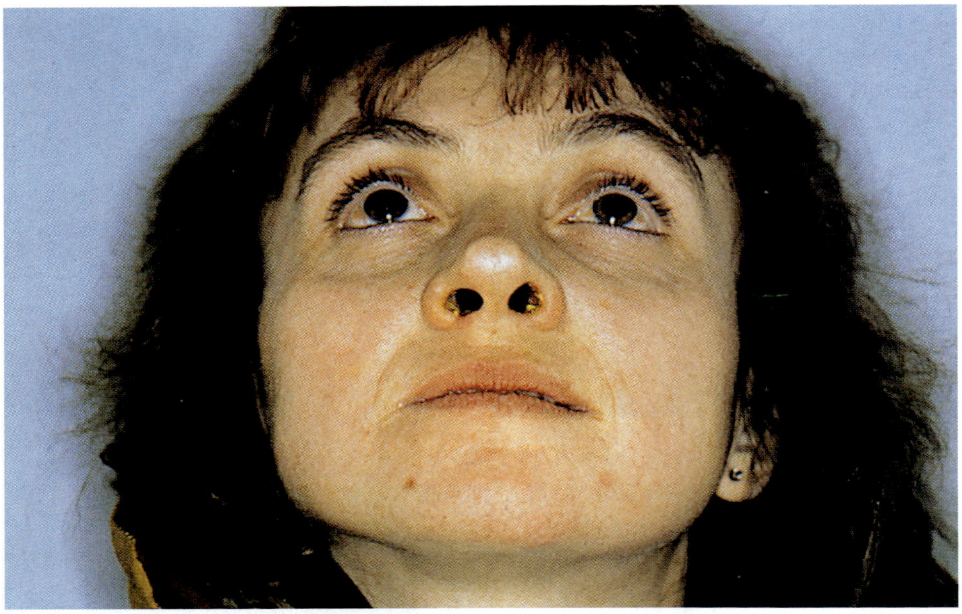

e

Fig. 5e. Postoperative basal view.

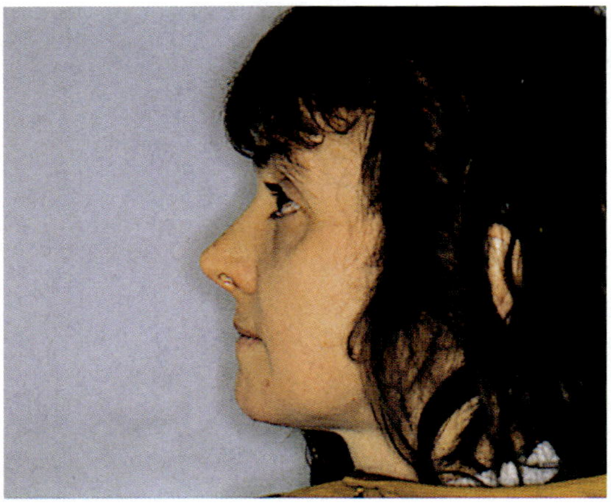

f

Fig. 5f. Postoperative lateral view.

the septum, vomer, perpendicular plate of the ethmoid, or from the auricle or rib (Fig. 5a-f). Tissue glue is often helpful for placing the graft directly into the midline and keeping it fixed during the healing period.

Our first recommendation is: keep the pocket small. Secondly: choose the right material for augmentation. Our first choice is autogenous cartilage, bone and perhaps alloplastic material, *e.g.,* goretex, for smaller defects.

In many cases of secondary deformities, the surgeon did not obtain a proper alignment of nasal bones. There could have been insufficient osteotomies or bony or cartilaginous breakdowns into the nasal passage way, leaving indentations or widening of the nasal pyramid.

Re-osteotomies

In almost all these cases, re-osteotomies have to be performed. We prefer the grooved chisel, depending on the thickness of the bone (3–5 cm width). Because of the laws of mechanics, it is possible to direct the bone cut by turning the chisel in whatever direction necessary. In secondary rhinoplasties, it is often overlooked that more than two osteotomies (medial and lateral) are needed to narrow the bony pyramid sufficiently.

Many years ago, we advocated triple

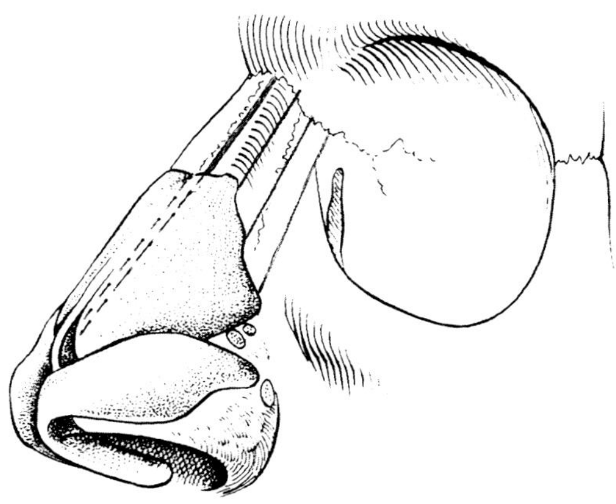

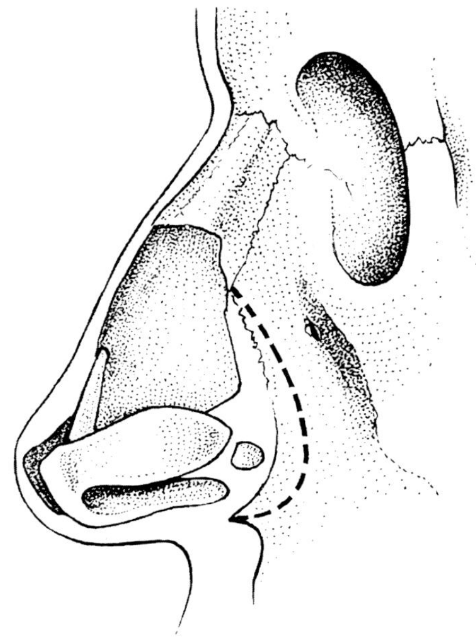

Fig. 6. Multiple osteotomies to narrow the nasal vault.

Fig. 7. Excision of bone at the piriform aperture to enlarge the nasal inlet and reduce the width of the bony vault.

and quadruple osteotomies in order to narrow nasal bones (Fig. 6). A long time ago, Baud and Eckel recommended (*cit.* Walter, Aesthetische Nasenchirurgie) that, in cases of periosteal thickening and bony growth, a partial bony resection of the ascending ramus of the maxilla (the frontal process) is more helpful than osteotomies to reduce the width of the nose (Fig. 7). In addition, over-excision of the bone should be avoided. Using very small chisels helps to avoid traumatizing the periosteum too much, and we feel that periosteal elevation should not be carried out prior to osteotomy as that would provoke collapse of the nasal bones. Without periosteal elevation, the nasal fragments are suspended like fingers in a glove.

Dorsum, columella and tip grafts

It is very difficult to reposition infractured bone and cartilage pieces and attempts to out-fracture these parts with consequent repositioning by intranasal packing have proved fruitless. In those cases, it is better to augment the defect either by some auricular, septal, or rib cartilage, or by small pieces of goretex, which we have been using in such cases for the past three years with good results. Such cases require only very circumspect tissue elevation to enable the surgeon to fit a piece of material of relevant size snugly into the pocket. The residual bony and cartilaginous open roof should be covered by a properly shaved piece of septal cartilage, bone, auricular or rib cartilage.

Correction of the lower third of the nose is a totally different entity. The basis for the correction of the ala, tip and columella is the nasolabial angle. Depending on ethnic characteristics, age and sex, the degree varies from 70° to 120°. After septal resection, we often see an acute angle, due to tissue and scar retraction around the nasal spine, or bowed over-shortened noses which are generally the result of over-resection and shortening of the septum and the ala cartilage.

The retracted columella is corrected using hemitransfixion with augmentation of the caudal portion of the membranous septum, or using a sublabial approach through an oral mucosal incision, elevating both halves of the membranous septum and inserting a strut. It is better to over-correct slightly, relying on tissue

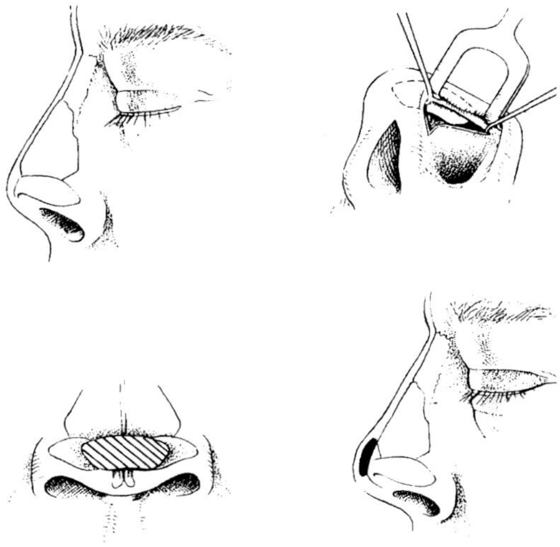

Fig. 8. Tip augmentation using rim incision.

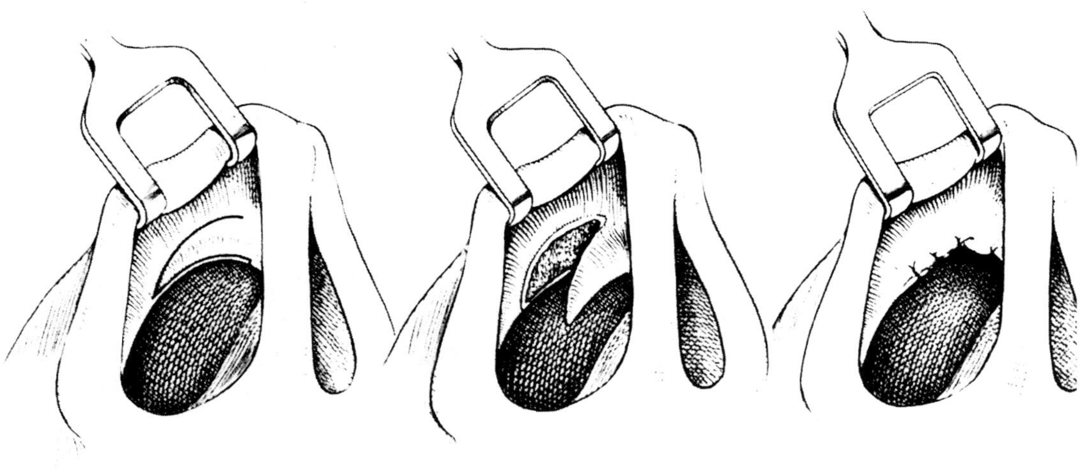

a b c

Fig. 9a,b,c. Reconstruction of the inner valve by a lower lateral flap containing skin and cartilage from its cephalic border.

retraction and the absorption of cartilage, rather than implanting too little cartilage which leads to taking more tissue and more augmentation at a later date. It is always easier to trim the cartilage slightly after six to 12 months.

Lost tip support due to over-resection of the alar cartilage demands augmentation. The cartilage needed for this can be taken from the concha or the rib. We do not favor homogenous material or artificial implants, especially in a region which is continuously being touched and moved.

If loss of center tip support is the only deformity diagnosed preoperatively, it is sufficient to make a rim incision unilaterally, undermine the tip region and insert a piece of sculptured autogenous cartilage (Fig. 8). We do not see the need for the open technique because we find we are better able to stretch the skin and augment the nasal tip with cartilage which has an intact columella skin strip. In our opinion, all other nasal tip deformities require total exposure of the lower lateral cartilages, preferably carried out from a rim incision. This gives the surgeon a clear view of the deformity. It is not possible to find the proper remedy for each nasal tip deformity, but it should be stated that, according to individual needs,

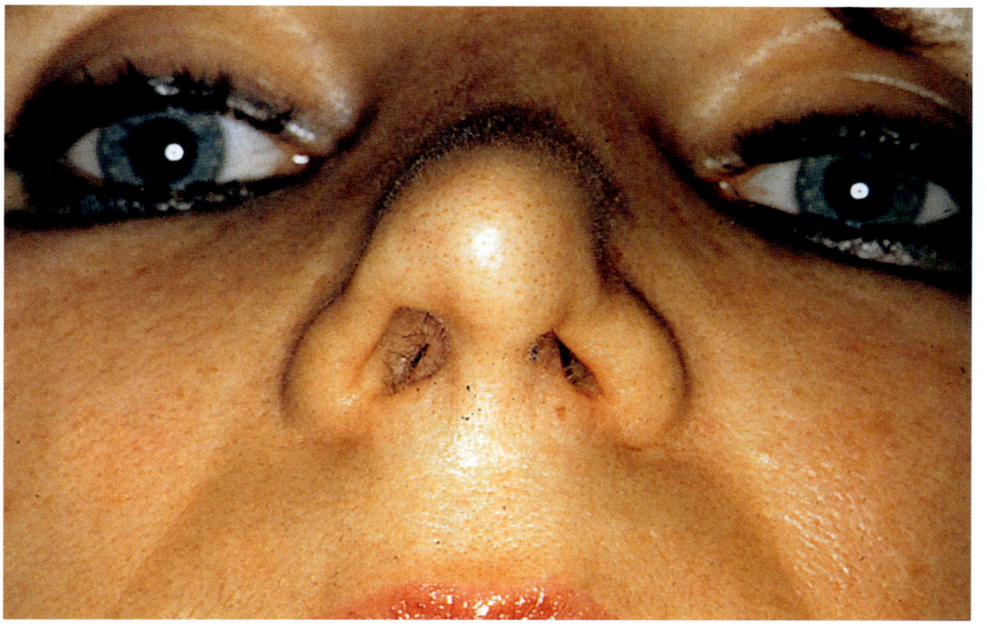

Fig. 10a. Basal view revealing severe bilateral vestibular stenosis.

a

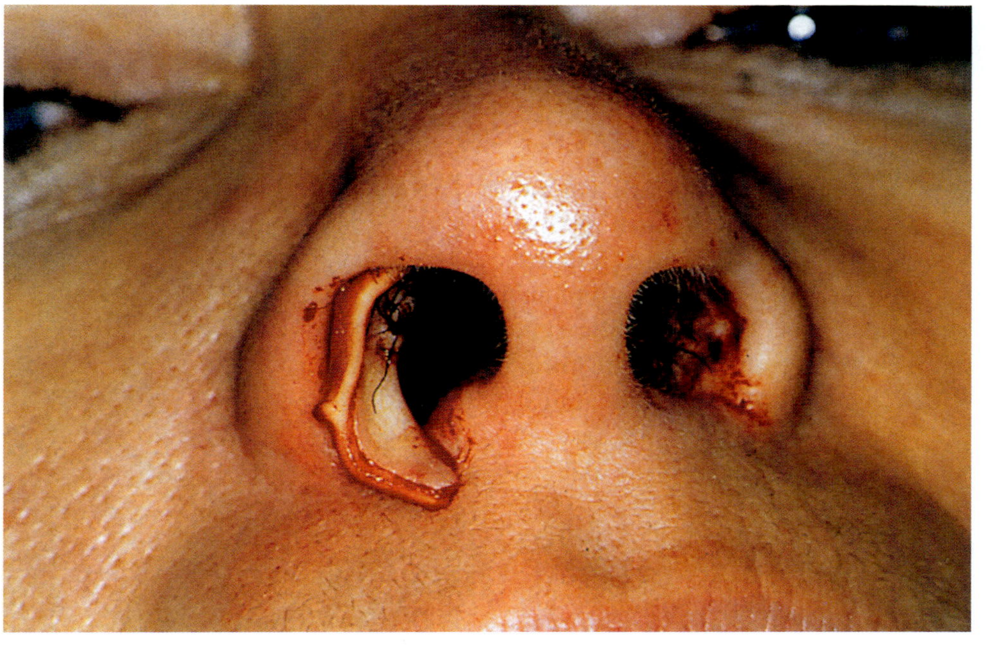

Fig. 10b. Insertion of a composite graft after scar excision.

b

there either has to be some cartilage resection or augmentation, occasionally using cutaway parts for the augmentation in other areas of the nasal tip. If enough skin is available, only cartilage onlay grafts are used which are secured by percutaneously placed sutures of 4.0 catgut over small bolsters in order to prevent stitch marks.

Endonasal passage way stenoses

The situation is quite different when, as a result of previous operations, cicatrization of the nasal entrance has occurred. So-called endonasal passageway stenoses can be confined to the region of the inner valve, the floor of the nasal entrance or the entire circumference.

Only the inner valve stenosis can be treated successfully by local flaps when

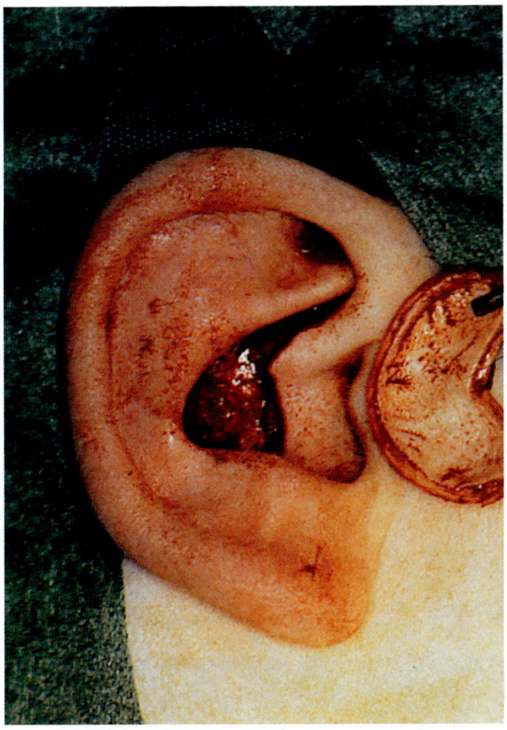

a

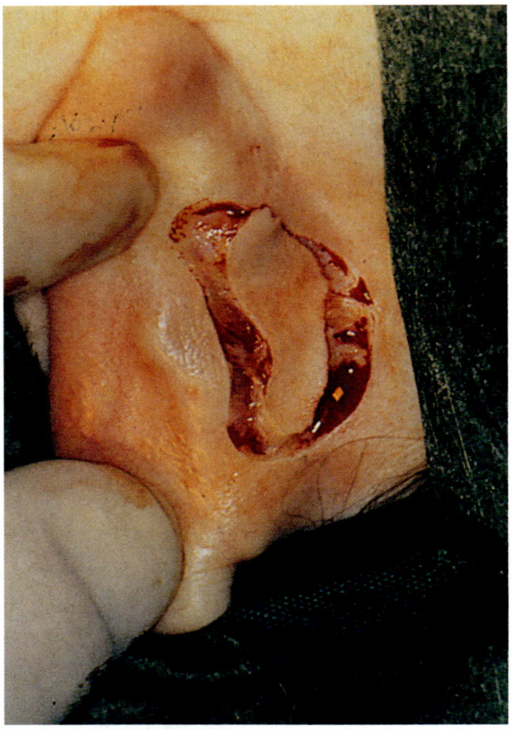

b

Fig. 11a. Excision of a composite graft from the concha.

Fig. 11b. Island flap circumcised on the postauricular side.

sufficient vestibular skin and cartilage are present laterally (Walter). In such a case, we divide the triangular cartilage from the septum, cut a medially-based flap from the cephalic border containing vestibular skin and cartilage of the right size, of the lower lateral cartilage and turn this flap almost 90° into the defect (Fig. 9). In case of endonasal passage way stenosis due to extensive scarring of the vestibular skin, composite grafts from the auricle are used to restore the nasal airway (Fig. 10a-b).

Composite grafts

We can use these grafts on the sidewall, in the superior or inferior portions of the nasal passageway. To ascertain a firm grip, it is important to let the cartilage overlap the skin portion to allow the surgeon to place the cartilage edges under the patient's own skin, after small tissue undermining. The area of skin contact and direct vascularization to revitalize the skin

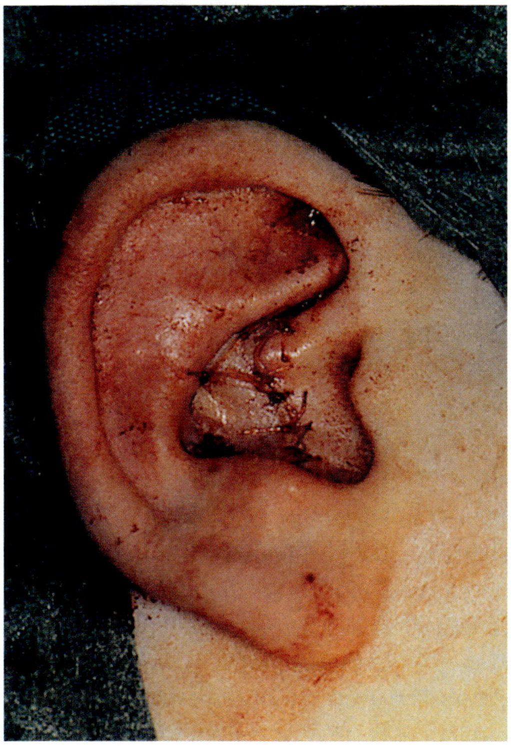

c

Fig. 11c. The flap sutured in place anteriorly. Catgut is used to avoid suture removal.

and cartilage is achieved faster in that way.

We prefer the concha part or the inner aspect of the helix for internal nasal

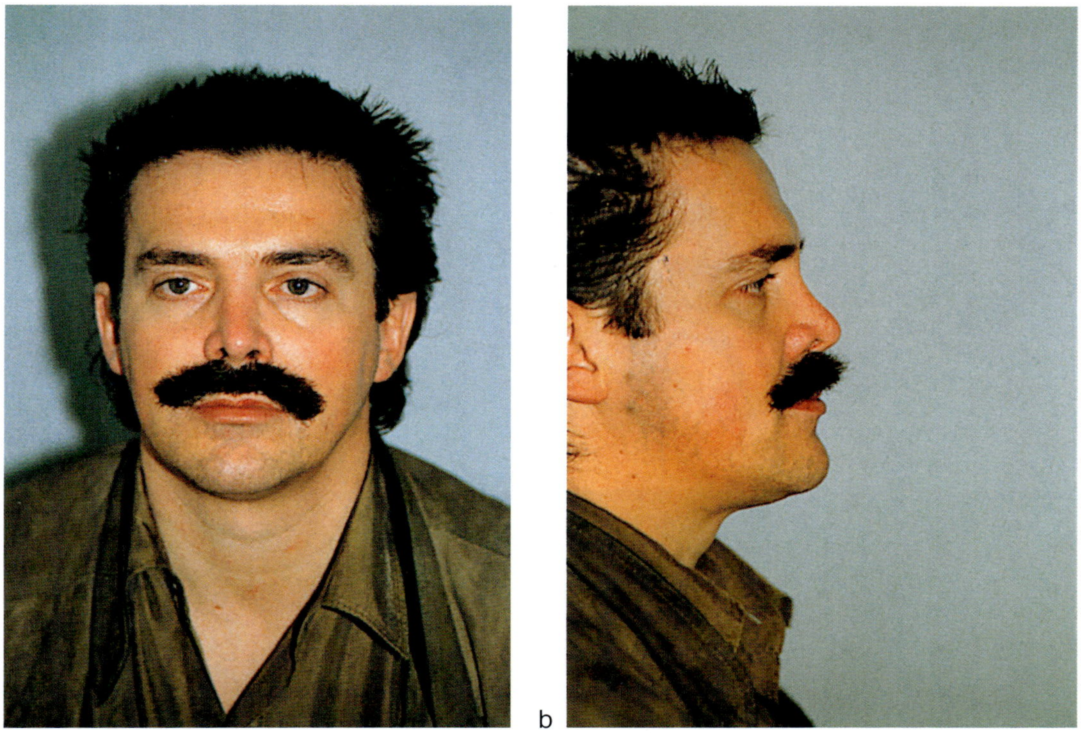

Fig. 12a,b. Patient after 3 rhinoplasties resulting in an overshortened nose.

a b

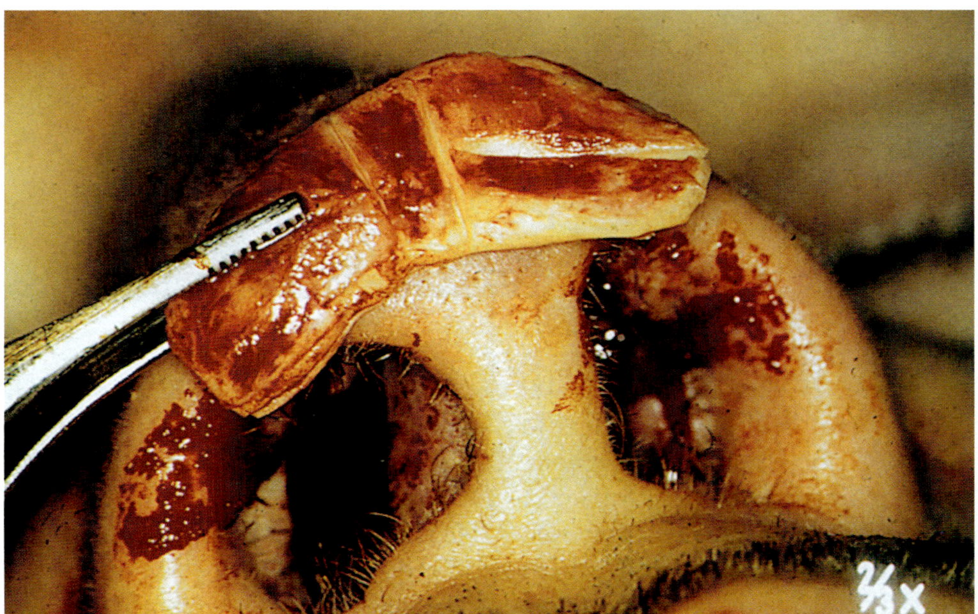

Fig. 12c. Composite graft prior to insertion after extensive skin undermining and scar excision.

c

coverage, due to the configuration of the cartilage and the tightly adherent skin. The donor site is closed by a postauricular island flap or (if not too large) left alone to granulate (Fig. 11a-c).

Only a few sutures, 2 mm apart, should be used for tissue fixation. In cases of extreme external or internal tissue loss, these grafts can be used as a two-layer graft, or as triple-layer grafts or saddle grafts going over the cephalic border of the septum if bilateral stenosis has occurred. We divide the skin portion in the midline to allow ourselves to suture the

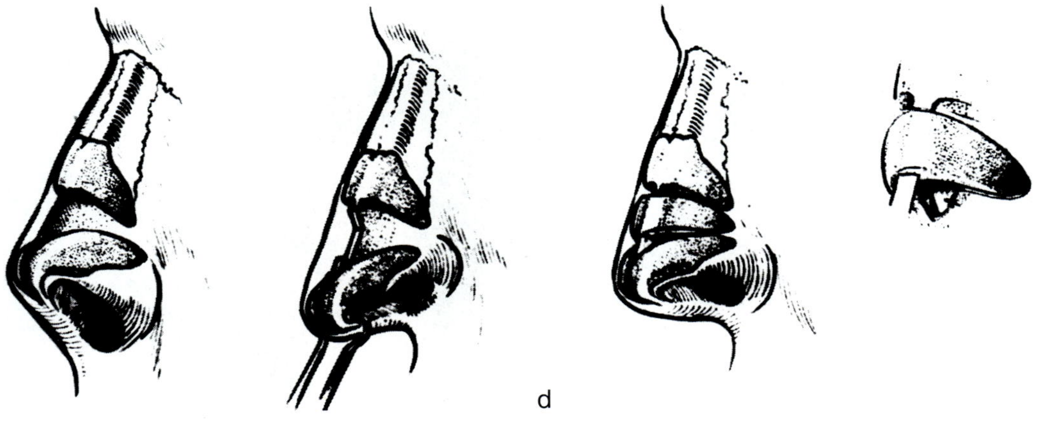

Fig. 12d. Operative procedure with small rectangular excision of cartilage to prevent pollybeak and sliding of the graft.

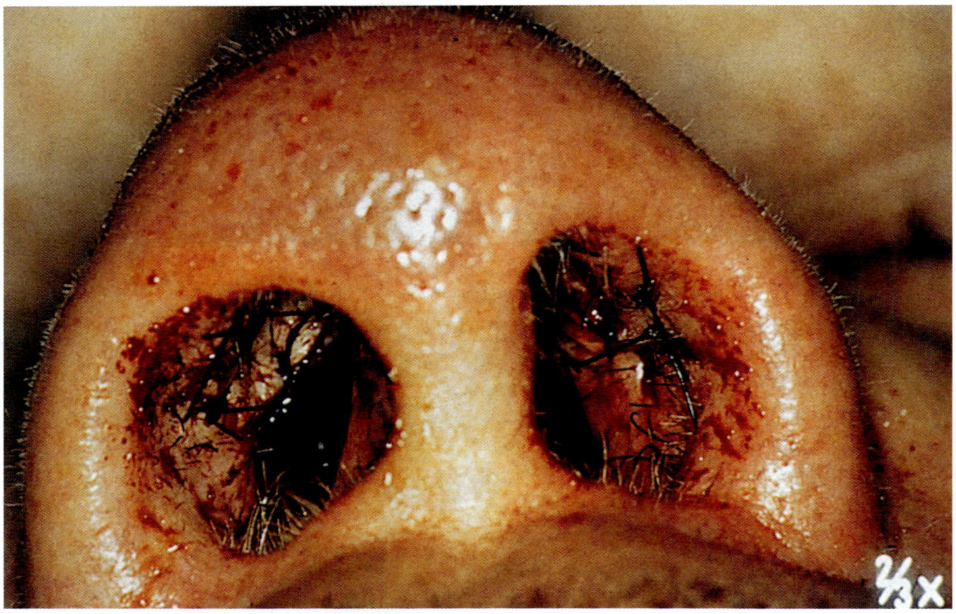

Fig. 12e. Graft sutured in place.

skin and mucosa on each side of the nasal passage, leaving only the cartilage to bridge the cephalic border of the septum. Small rectangular excisions of cartilage at the side of the insertion of the composite graft cartilage on the septum will help to prevent a pollybeak and the sliding of the cephalic border of the graft upwards to an unwanted position (Fig. 12a-g).

A hidden columella is corrected by inserting a composite graft preferably taken from the inferior antihelical crus, because this already contains a bent cartilage and skin duplicating the columella. By vertical incision of the skin of the graft and total transfixion, this graft can be inserted like a wedge, bringing the columella forward (Fig. 13).

This technique should only be used if, due to scar formation, there is no possibility of stretching the mucosa of the caudal portion of the septum for implanting grafts. We like to leave the nasal packing in place for five days and advise the patient to use oily nasal ointment in order to keep the grafts constantly moist and lubricated. In some cases, it is very advantageous to take an impression and mold an acrylic nasal obturator.

The patient should wear these per-

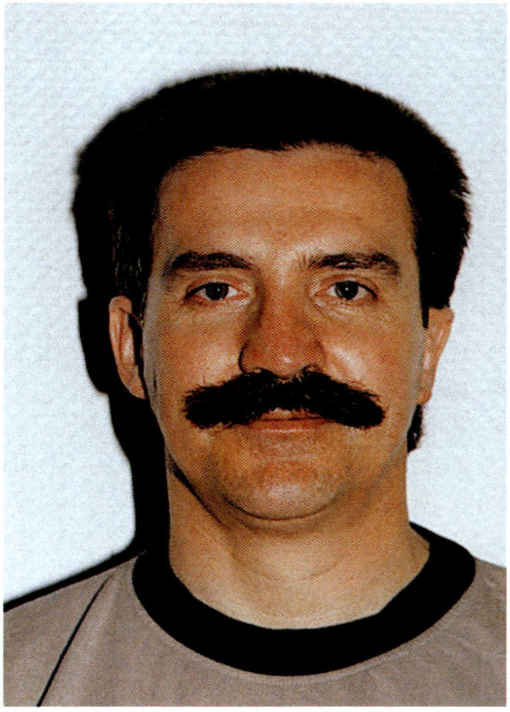
f

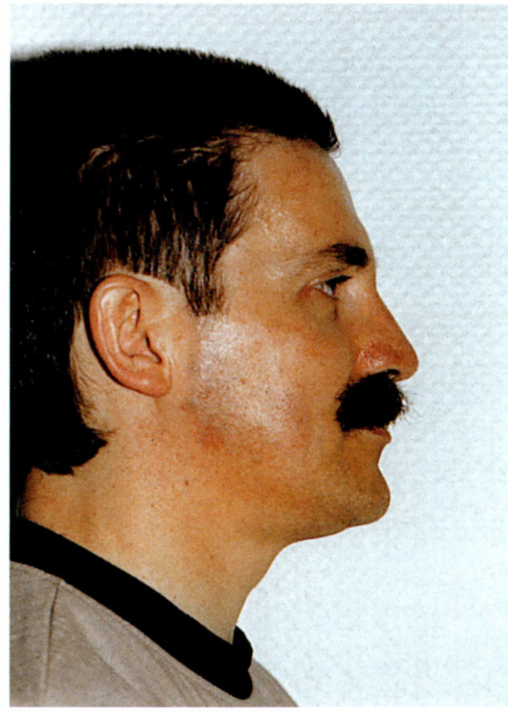
g

Fig. 12f,g. Postoperative frontal and lateral view 8 months after rhinoplasty with insertion of a composite graft.

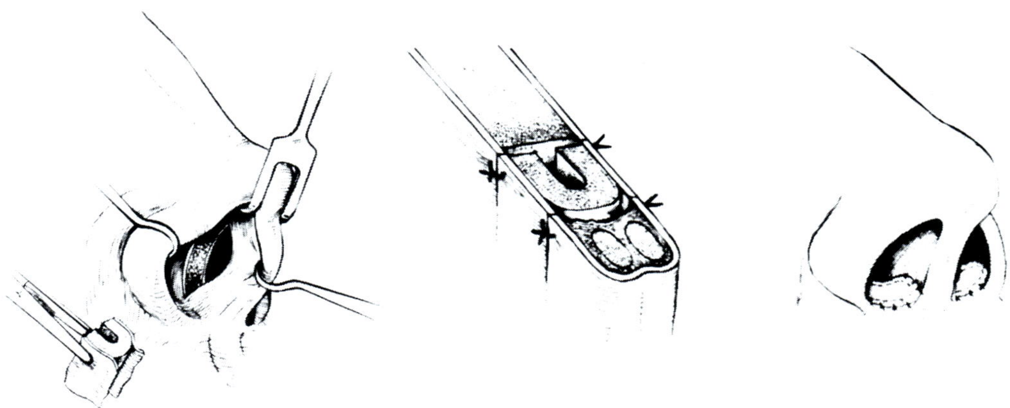

Fig. 13. Correction of a hidden columella with a composite graft of the inferior anthelical crus.

forated obturators for three to four months to enable him to breathe. This is an efficient manner to overcome any residual scar tendencies from contraction. Antibiotics and cortisone (Ultralan 60, 40, 20 mg daily) given systemically are very helpful in increasing the percentage of take.

22: NASAL VESTIBULAR STENOSIS

G.J. Nolst Trenité

Introduction

Impaired nasal breathing due to iatrogenic or congenital narrowing of the nasal vestibule is a difficult problem which, in most cases, needs surgical treatment. A thorough analysis of the pathological anatomical findings causing vestibular malformation and impaired nasal breathing is a prerequisite for successful surgical treatment[1]. The pathology can be situated in the nasal valve area (caudal end of the upper/ lateral, septum, head of the inferior turbinate and piriform aperture), in the external valve area (skeletal and soft tissue structure of the ala, columella and soft tissue of the vestibular floor), or in both valves (internal and external valve).

If the narrowing of the vestibule is caused by pathology of the anatomical structures surrounding the vestibule (caudal septal deviation, a collapsed upper lateral, protruding lateral crus and a too broad columella), surgical correction should not be too difficult[2,3]. In more severe cases in which a collapsed ala is caused by over-resection of the lateral crus and stenosing scar tissue, a more complicated surgical procedure, with the use of composite grafts, is indicated. Also, the (secondary) congenital vestibular stenosis in the unilateral cleft lip patient is difficult to correct. The results of the surgical treatment of the above-mentioned iatrogenic and congenital vestibular stenosis are often disappointing. What seems a good result in the immediate postoperative period will diminish in the first postoperative months due to scar tissue retraction during the process of healing.

The surgical treatment is complicated and demands a rational approach:

- a thorough analysis of the pathological anatomical findings
- meticulous planning of the operative procedure
- special prolonged postoperative care with the use of a vestibulum device (nostril splint) to prevent scar tissue retraction

Analysis and documentation

To analyze the local pathology of the vestibulum, it is important to examine the nose during quiet and forced nasal breathing in order to determine possible alar collapse (Figs. 1a,b) and to inspect the nose without disturbing the anatomy by using a speculum (Fig. 2). A speculum will distort the nasal valve angle. Palpation should not be forgotten when determining the pathology or the absence (partial or total) of the caudal cartilaginous septum, the alar cartilage, and when determining the tip recoil. When analyzing iatrogenic and/or congenital vestibular stenosis, it is important to assess the following:

- whether the stenosis is caused by an aberrant anatomical structure, such as a caudal septal deviation, a protruding lateral crus, or too broad a columella, which can be corrected by reallocation and resection of redundant tissue (Fig. 3)
- whether the stenosis is caused by malformation of cartilaginous structures which can be reshaped, or by malformation of the skin by scarring which can be resected and replaced by full thickness skin or composite grafts (Figs. 4a-g)
- whether there is a shortage of tissue (skin and/or cartilage) which can be replaced by local flaps, free transplants

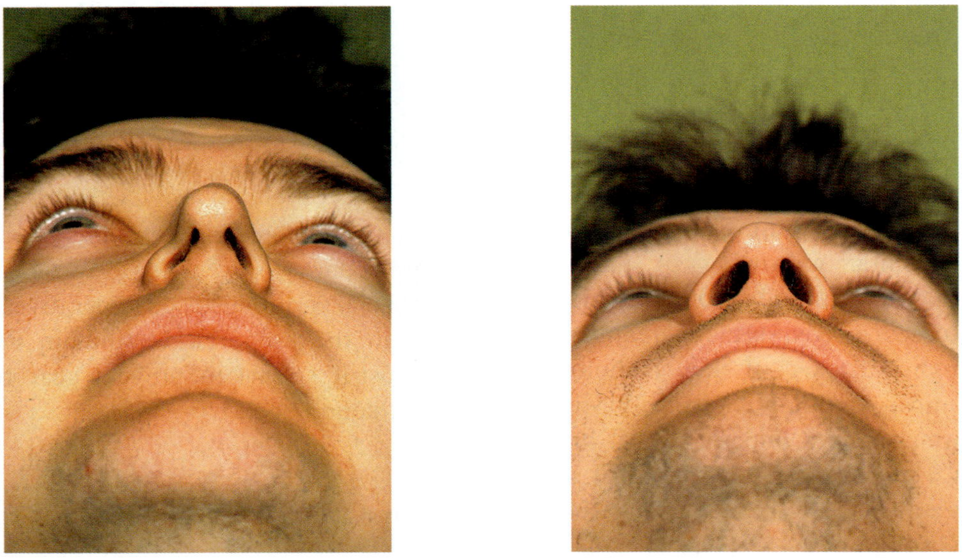

a

b

Fig. 1a. Alar collapse during forced nasal breathing due to too narrow a nasal valve angle. *b.* Postoperative view after external rhinoplasty to correct too narrow a internal valve angle with spreader grafts combined with narrowing of the columella base.

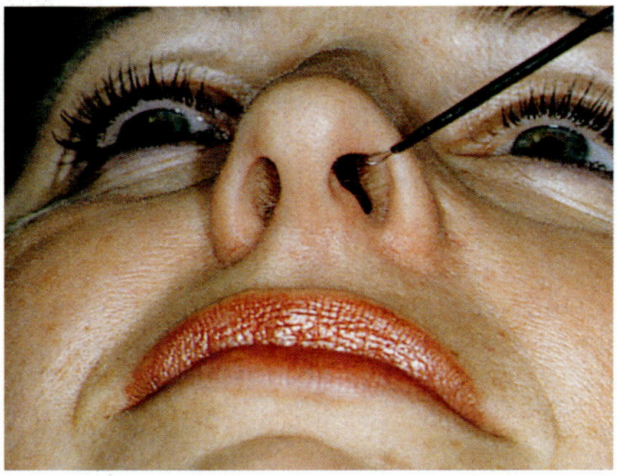

Fig. 2. Inspection of the vestibulum and the nasal valve area.

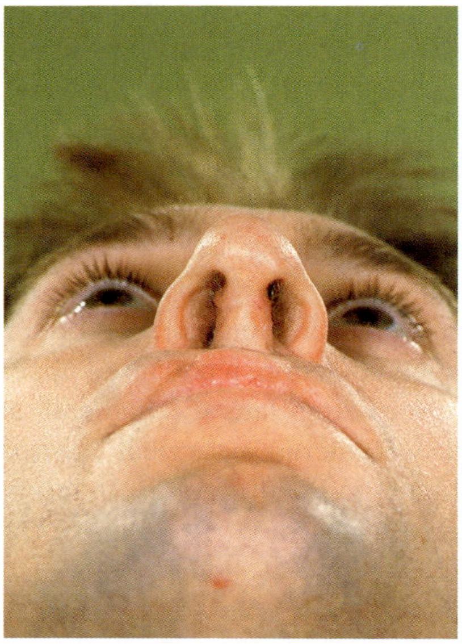

Fig. 3. Vestibular stenoses due to a broad columella and a caudal nasal septal deviation in a cleft lip patient.

of skin, cartilage and/or composite grafts (Figs. 5a-f).

After thorough analysis of the pathology, a rational step-by-step operative procedure should be planned. Furthermore, standard pre- and postoperative photographic documentation (frontal, lateral, oblique and basic view) is obligatory in order to evaluate the postoperative results, and, if possible, pre- and postoperative rhinomanometry and/or acoustic rhinometry tests should be performed to determine the functional result.

Operative techniques

The diverse etiology of vestibular stenosis demands a large spectrum of operative procedures. In the following discussion, we will only consider the more complicated surgical procedures, such as those in unilateral cleft noses and severe iatrogenic vestibular stenosis which require composite grafts.

Composite graft harvesting procedure

The auricle is a very appropriate donor site for composite grafts in nasal surgery. A careful operative procedure will not leave an obvious postoperative deformity of the auricle. Depending on the amount of composite graft needed for the recon-

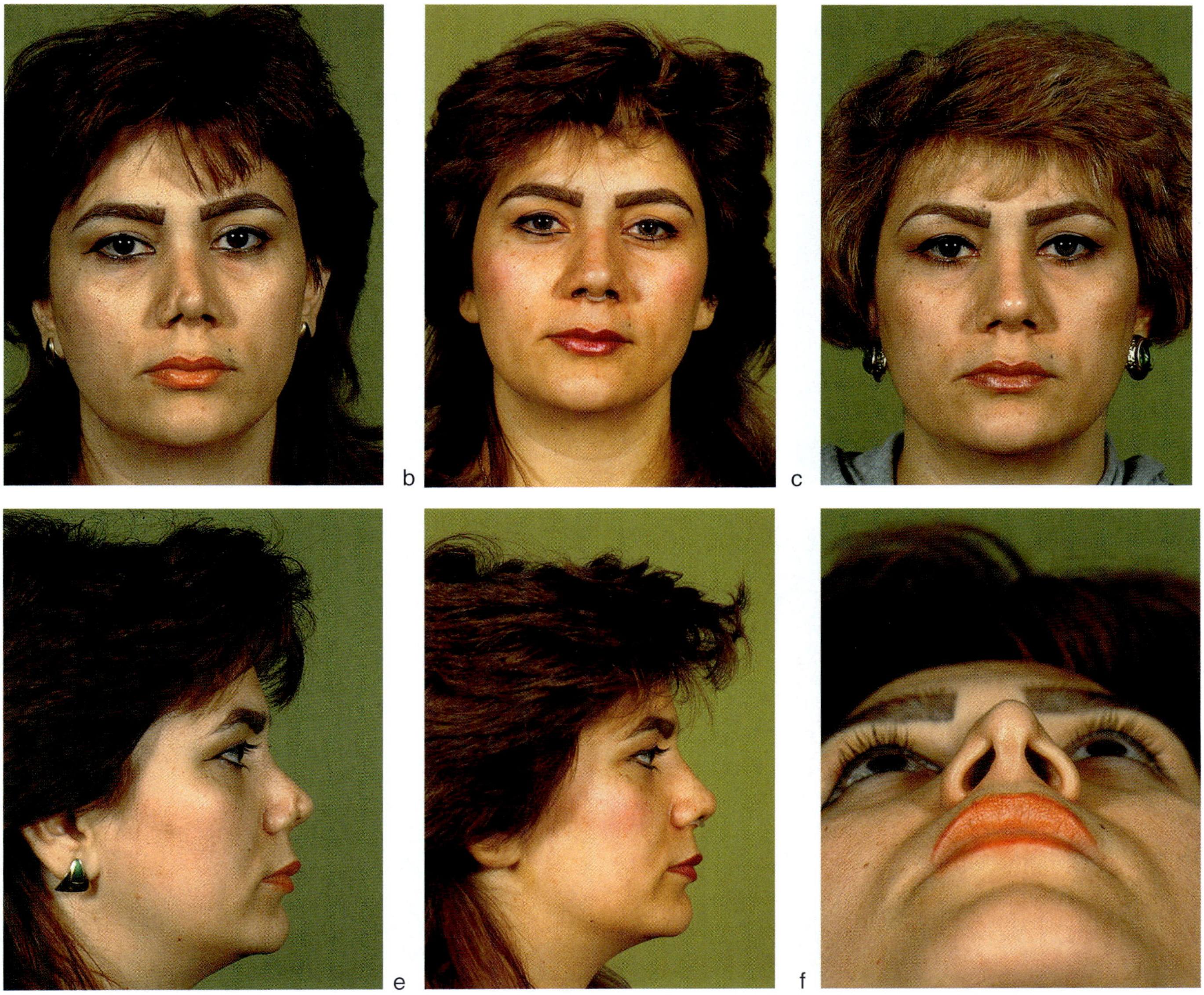

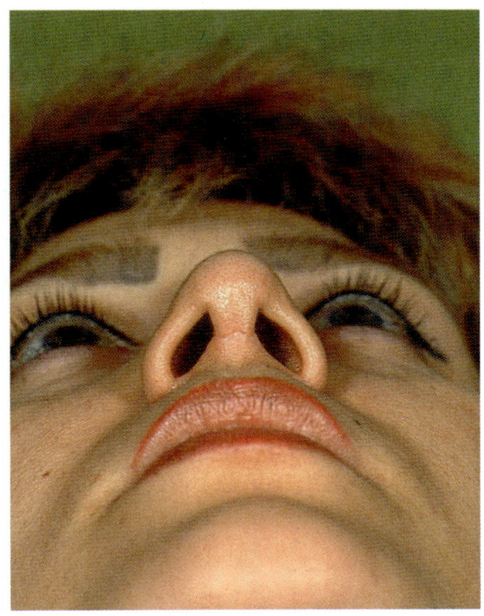

Fig. 4a. Preoperative view of a patient with vestibular stenosis on the right side due to over-resection of the lateral crus and scar tissue retraction. *b.* Frontal view in the early postoperative period with a custom-made vestibulum device in situ to prevent scar tissue retraction. *c.* Frontal view of the final result. *d.* Preoperative lateral view of the right side. *e.* Lateral view of the right side in the early postoperative period with the custom-made vestibulum device in situ. *f.* Preoperative basal view. *g.* Postoperative view with the broken columella incision scar, which is only slightly visible due to little inversion of the wound edges.

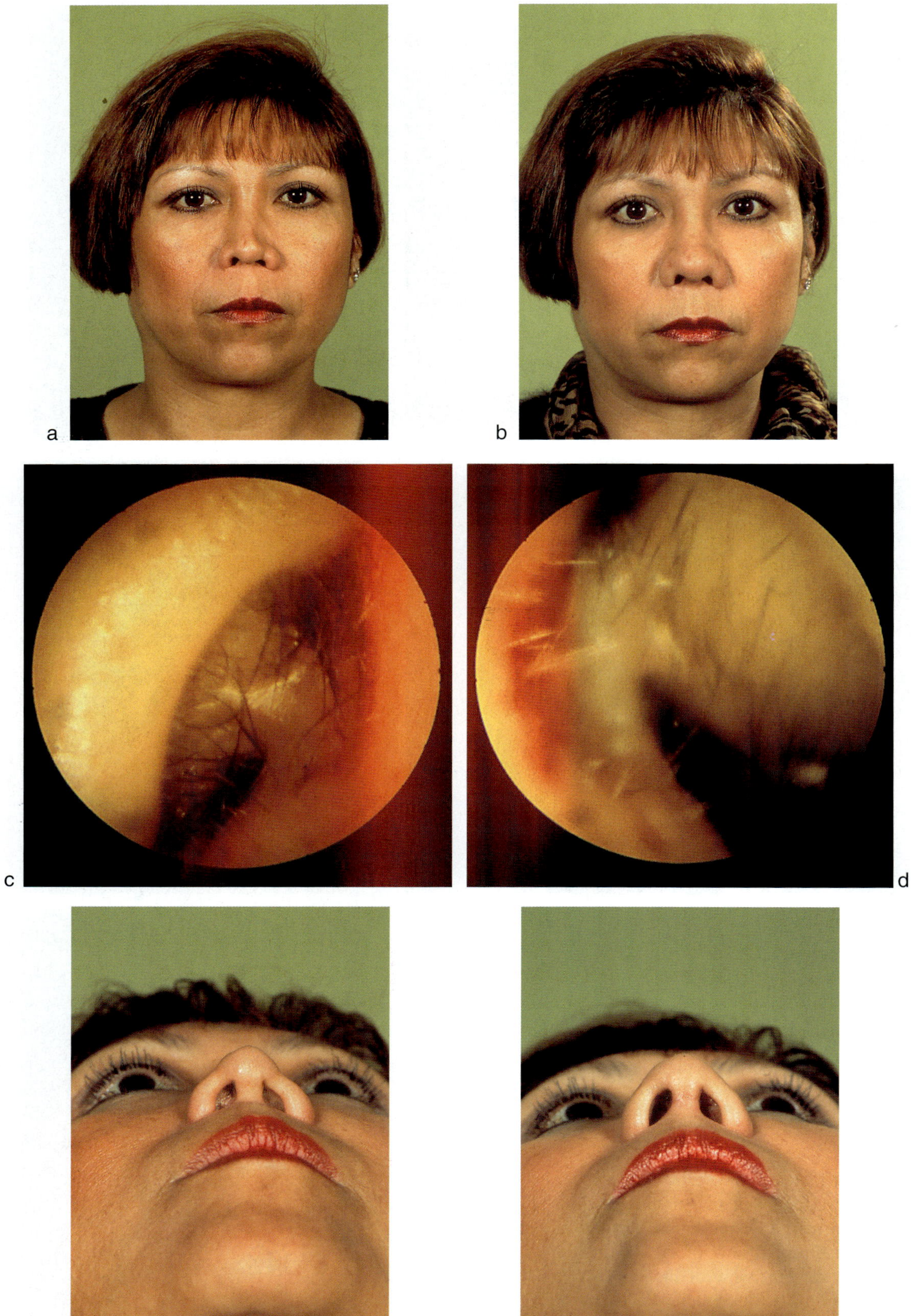

Fig. 5a. Preoperative view of a patient with severe vestibular stenosis, malformation of the tip and the dorsum due to over-resection of the nasal skeleton and soft tissue. *b.* Early postoperative result. *c.* Preoperative endoscopic view of the vestibular stenosis at the right side. *d.* Preoperative endoscopic view of the vestibular stenosis at the left side. *e.* Preoperative basal view. *f.* Early postoperative basal view after reconstruction of the nasal skeleton with the use of composite grafts to restore the nasal airway.

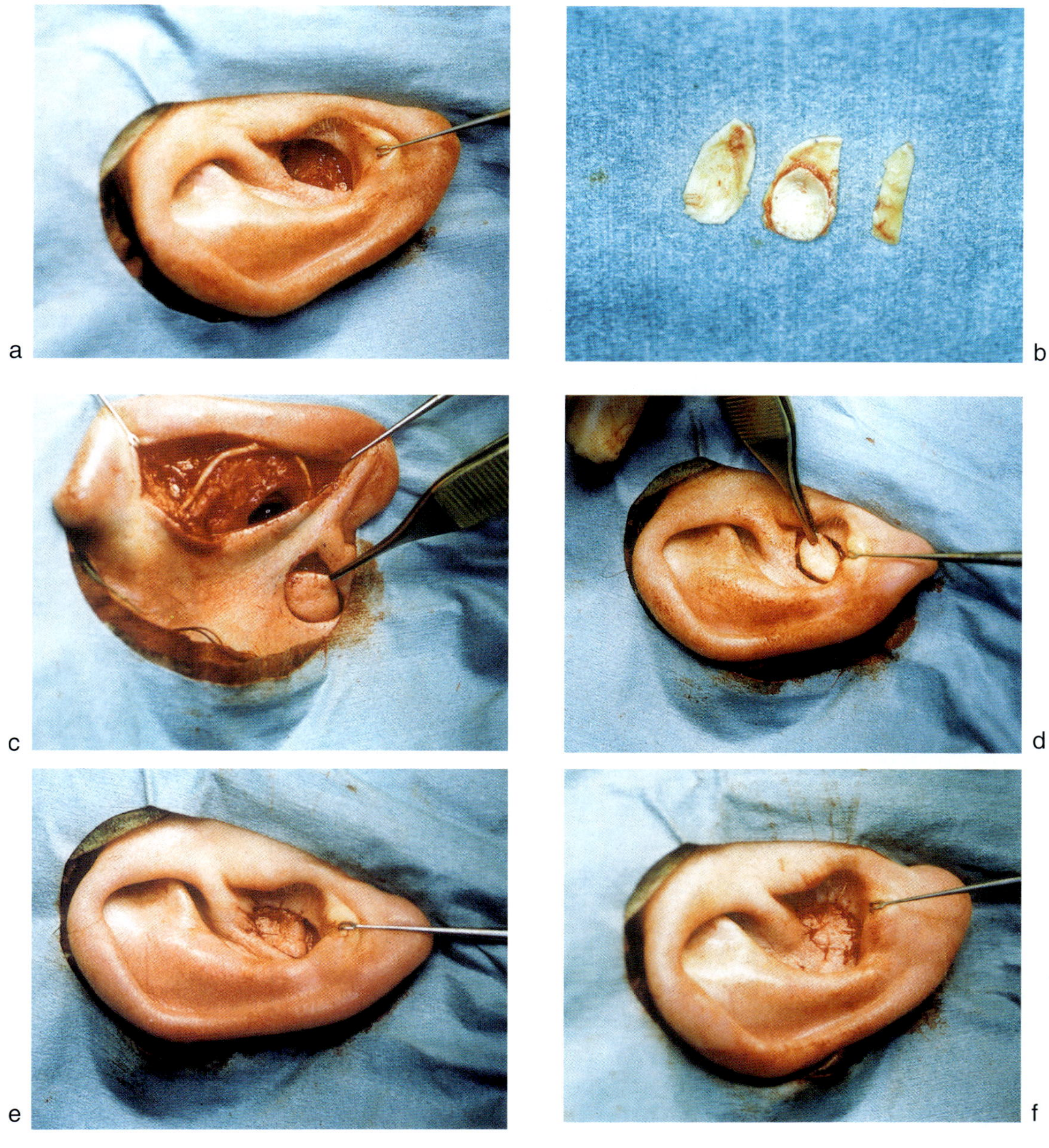

Fig. 6a-f. Surgical procedure to harvest a partial composite graft and cartilage grafts from the concha. The skin defect at the donor site is closed with an island skin flap

struction of the nasal vestibule, a *partial* or *complete* conchal composite graft can be harvested. To harvest a *partial* conchal composite graft, first mark the skin to be used for the composite graft on the anterior side of the concha and then use the postauricular approach to prevent a visible scar on the anterior side of the auricle. The harvesting procedure should start with isolation of the composite part of the graft. A circumferential skin incision extending to the cartilage (and including perichondrium) is made of the marked anterior auricular skin which is to form the composite part of the graft. Care must be taken to protect this part whilst the remainder of the anterior dissection is carried out in the subperichondrial plane. Posterior dissection is then performed in the supraperichondrial plane via a postauricular approach. The donor defect can either be repaired by an island skin flap of the appropriate size marked on the area medial to the auricular sulcus, so that it can be mobilized via a subcutaneous tunnel to the donor site, or by a free full thickness

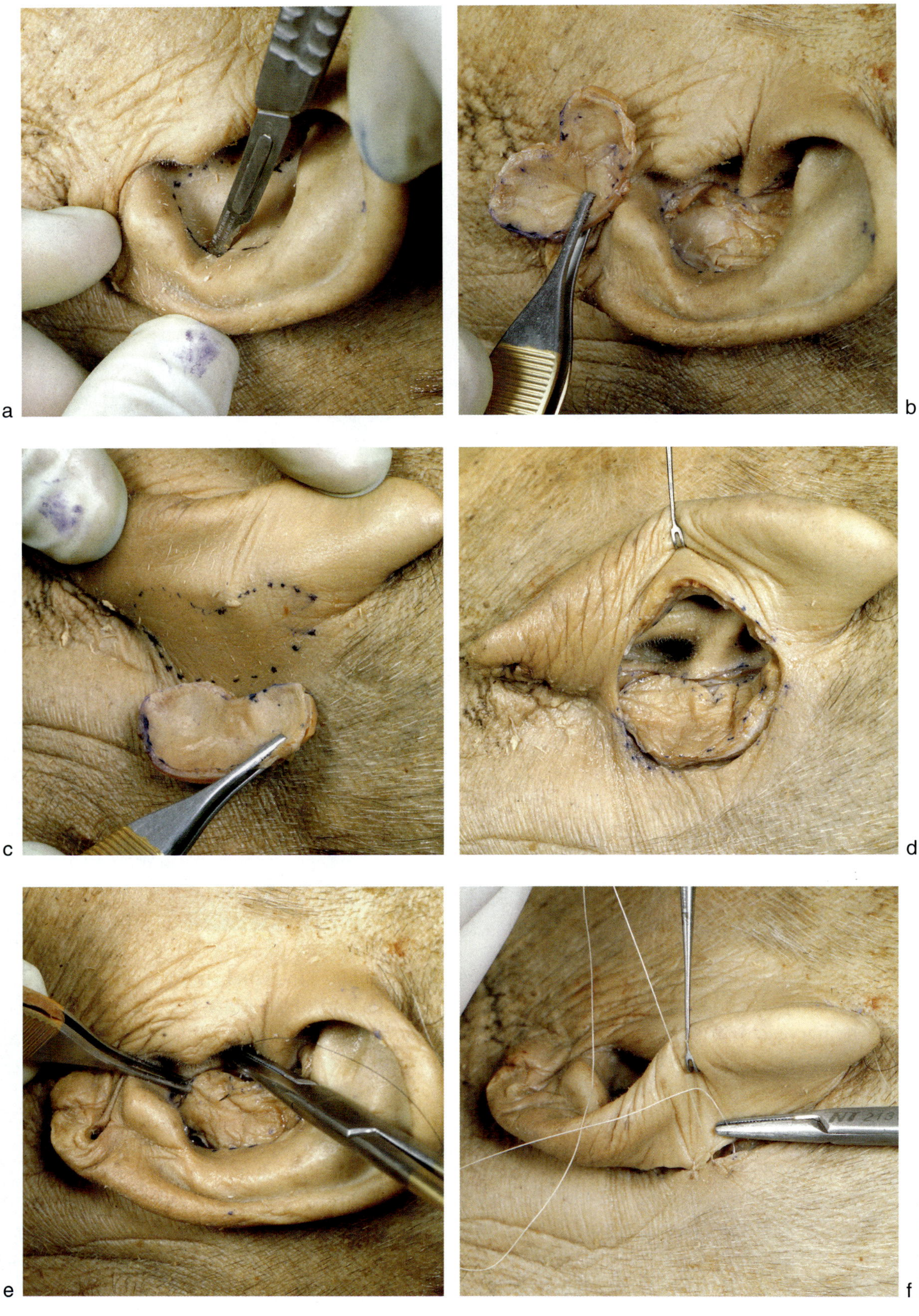

Fig. 7a-f. Cadaver dissection pictures of a complete conchal composit graft harvesting procedure.

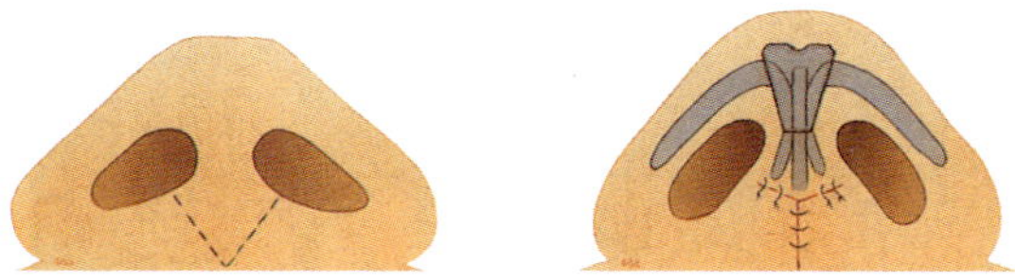

Fig. 8a,b. Illustration of a V-Y procedure to lengthen the columella.

a b

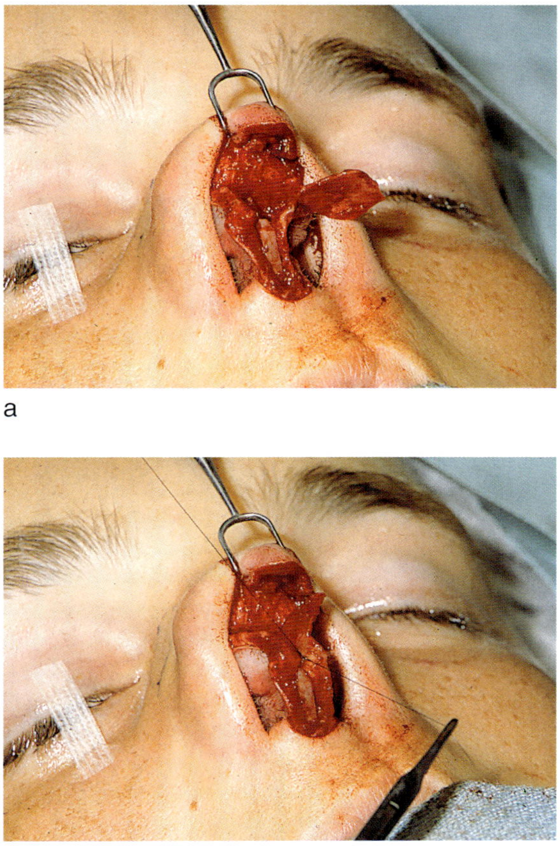

a

b

Fig. 9a,b. Dissection of the lateral crus at the cleft side followed by repositioning over a columella strut in a more antero/medial position with mattress sutures.

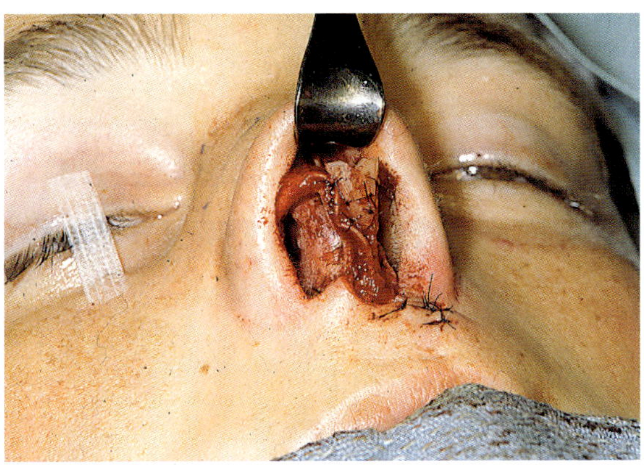

Fig. 10. Medialization and endorotation of the alar base at the cleft side with a modified Z plasty. To improve tip definition, a shield graft is sutured in place.

skin graft. The island skin flap or full-thickness skin graft is sutured *in situ* and the donor site is closed with 6/O ethylene (Figs. 6a-f).

When a *complete* conchal composite graft is needed, an anterior approach should be used. Prepare an island flap on the postauricular side in the auricular sulcus region. The island flap must not be too far from the postauricular area laterally, in order to prevent a postoperative glued-on appearance of the auricle (Figs. 7a-f).

Surgical correction of vestibular stenosis in the unilateral cleft patient

For the surgical correction of vestibular stenosis in the unilateral cleft patient, an external approach is very appropriate. However, instead of the usual broken columella incision, a V incision at the base of the columella is often preferred before finally performing a V-Y procedure to lengthen the columella (Figs. 8a,b). After developing the columella skin flap, the cartilaginous vault is dissected in a surgical plane directly supra-, or even sub-, perichondrially to prevent disturbance of the overlying SMAS (superficial musculoaponeurotic system). With this approach, direct binocular analysis of the pathology is possible, and reconstruction can be carried out under direct vision. The lateral crus at the cleft site should be dissected free, reallocated in a more anterior and symmetric position, and fixed in this position with the use of a columella strut with mattress sutures (Fig. 9a,b). As in most cases, the alar base is exorotated and, in retroposition, maxillary augmentation and medialization and rotation of the alar base with a modified Z-plasty will improve the aesthetic appearance (Fig. 10). In many cases there is still functional impairment due to an oblique skin band in the dome area and a subcutaneous bulk in the ala. This can be corrected by a vestibular Z plasty, in combination with subcutaneous debulking and fixation of vestibular skin with a transcutaneous mattress suture over a silastic button. Depending on the type of lip closure technique, there can also be narrowing of the vestibular floor by scar tissue in which case an auricular composite graft is appropriate to widen the vestibule. In case of primary congenital stenosis of the vestibule, often combined with hypoplasia of the corresponding ala, a double-cross plasty as described by Naasan and Page[4], or a vestibular labial mucosa flap as described by Blandini *et al.*[5], combined with a composite graft and an exchange plasty of alar base of the opposite site, are indicated.

Iatrogenic vestibular stenosis due to previous rhinoplastic surgery

Although there are many etiological factors resulting in iatrogenic vestibular stenosis, for example, surgical excision of vestibular skin tumors, electro coagulation, chemical cauterization, prolonged nasal packing, or nasal airway tube, a frequent sequela is a reduction rhinoplasty with abundant reduction of the vestibular skin and cartilaginous nasal skeleton, resulting in a functional aesthetic disaster (see Figs. 4 and 5). Surgical treatment consists of reconstruction of the nasal cartilaginous skeleton with autogenous cartilage grafts and rebuilding of the inner vestibular lining, in which case an auricular composite graft is very appropriate, especially in those cases in which there is scar tissue in the dome area and overzealous resection of the lateral crus. Either an endonasal or an external approach can be used, depending on the overall pathology and the reconstruction needs. In case of an endonasal approach, the cartilaginous part of the composite graft should be placed in a pocket made through a rim incision after resection of the scar tissue in the dome area, the composite part is placed in the anterior site, and the cartilaginous part is fixed

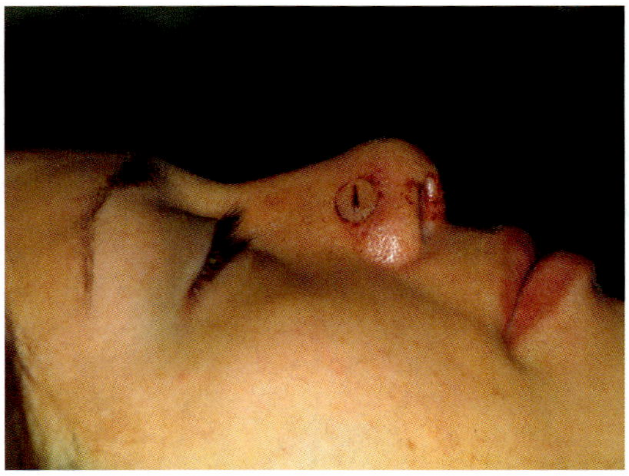

Fig. 11. Fixation of a vestibular composite graft with transcutaneous mattress sutures over a silastic button.

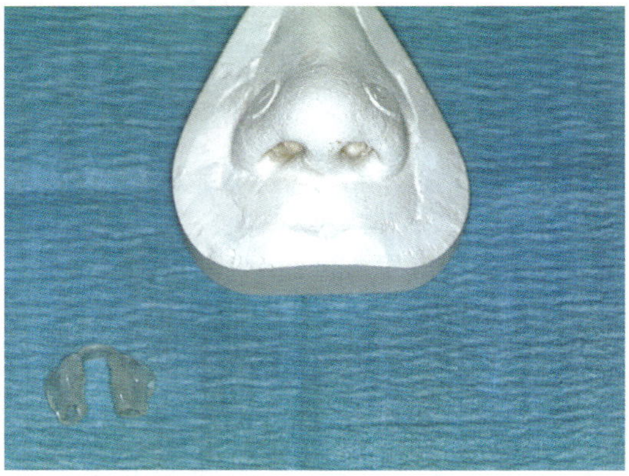

Fig. 12. Plaster of Paris cast of the nose, including the nasal vestibulum. A custom-made vestibulum device is fabricated from this case.

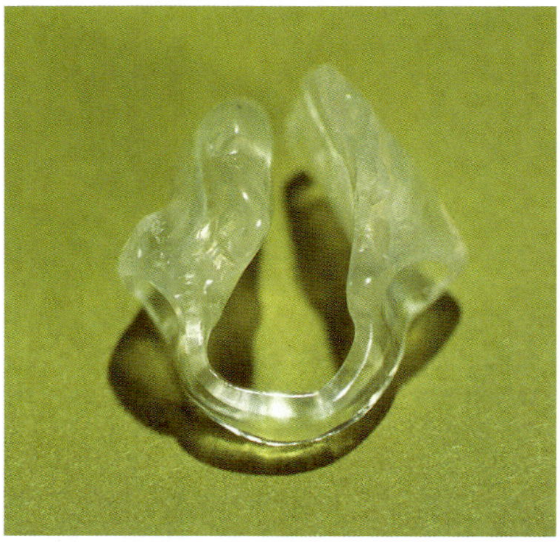

Fig. 13. A custom-made vestibulum device made of thermoplastic acrylic material.

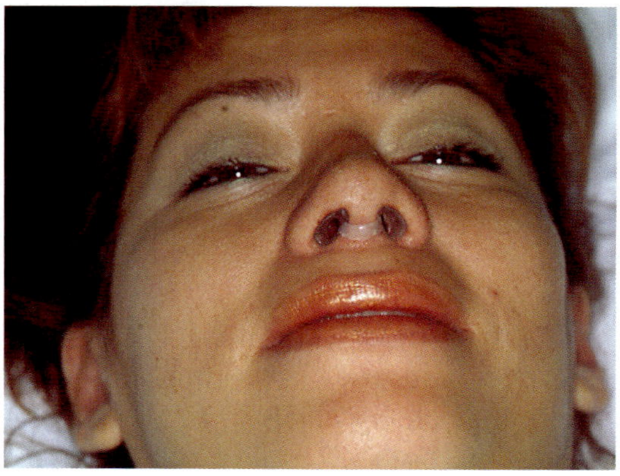

Fig. 14. Custom-made vestibulum device in situ.

posteriorly and more caudally than the natural site of the lower lateral in order to give extra strength to the alar rim. Fixation of the composite graft can be accomplished by transcutaneous mattress sutures over silastic buttons (Fig. 11). If the nasal valve is to be reconstructed, an external approach is more appropriate.

Special postoperative care with a custom-made device

A retrospective study of 52 rhinoplasties in cleft lip patients with a follow-up of one to six years showed, in 10% of the cases, worse re-stenosis than in the preoperative situation caused by postoperative scar tissue retraction[6]. To prevent this scar tissue retraction and to ensure good form and function, a special custom-made device was developed[6-9], based on the nostril splint described by Nakajima *et al.*[10].

One week postoperatively, immediately after removal of the nasal packing and dressing, a cast of the nose including the nasal vestibulum is made (Fig. 12). From this cast, a precisely fitting vestibulum device is fabricated from thermoplastic acrylic material (Fig. 13). Both vestibulum parts of the device are connected through a thin transparent band of the same acrylic material. Fixation in the nose is guaranteed by the precise fit (Fig. 14). The patient has to wear this vestibulum device day and night for the first six postoperative weeks and then, in the following six weeks, only at night. Thereafter, once a week, the patient should check whether it is easy to place the device, if not he should wear the device again, only at night, for several weeks. All patients (n=36, 20 unilateral clefts, four bilateral clefts, eight iatrogenic) with a follow-up of six months to three years, endured their device very well. There was no local reaction by the vestibulum skin. The preliminary results are encouraging, and so far, none of the patients has redeveloped stenosis of the vestibule (Figs. 15 and 16).

Conclusions

Surgical treatment of iatrogenic and congenital vestibular stenosis, due to insufficient support of the cartilaginous skeleton of the tip and vestibular soft tissue scarring, is a complicated matter, demanding (composite) grafting procedures. The auricle is an ideal donor site (for single and composite grafts) due to the natural concavity of the conchal cartilage and easy technical closure of the surgical defect with an island skin flap.

An immediate satisfactory postoperative functional and aesthetic result will often diminish in the first postoperative months due to scar tissue retraction. To prevent scar tissue retraction, a custom-made vestibulum device (nostril splint) proved to be of great value in 36 patients, none of whom developed re-stenosis of the nasal vestibule.

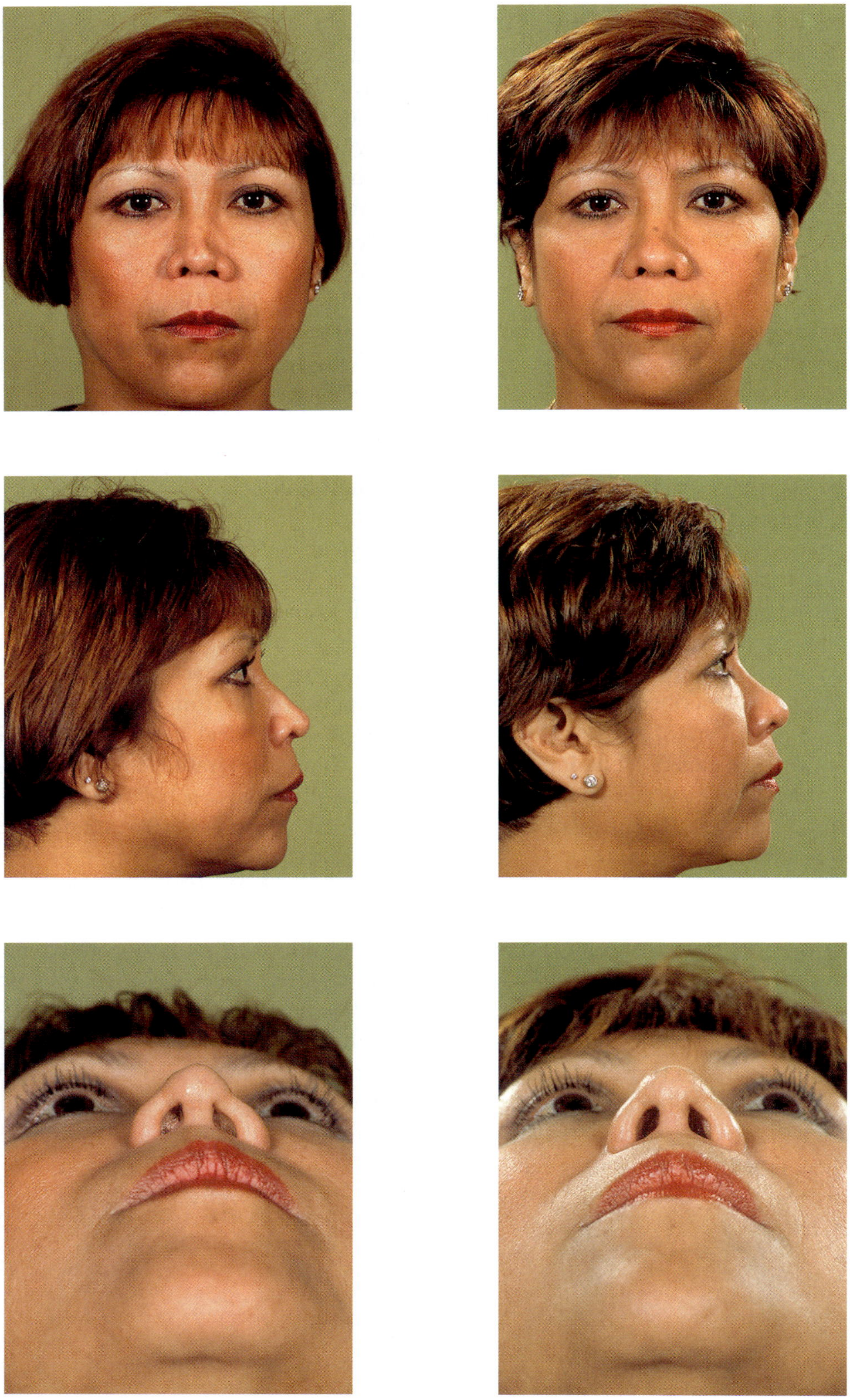

a b c d e f

Fig. 15a-f. Pre- and long-term postoperative views of a patient with severe vestibular stenosis, corrected using the external approach with composite grafts and dorsal onlay grafts of the concha of both ears.

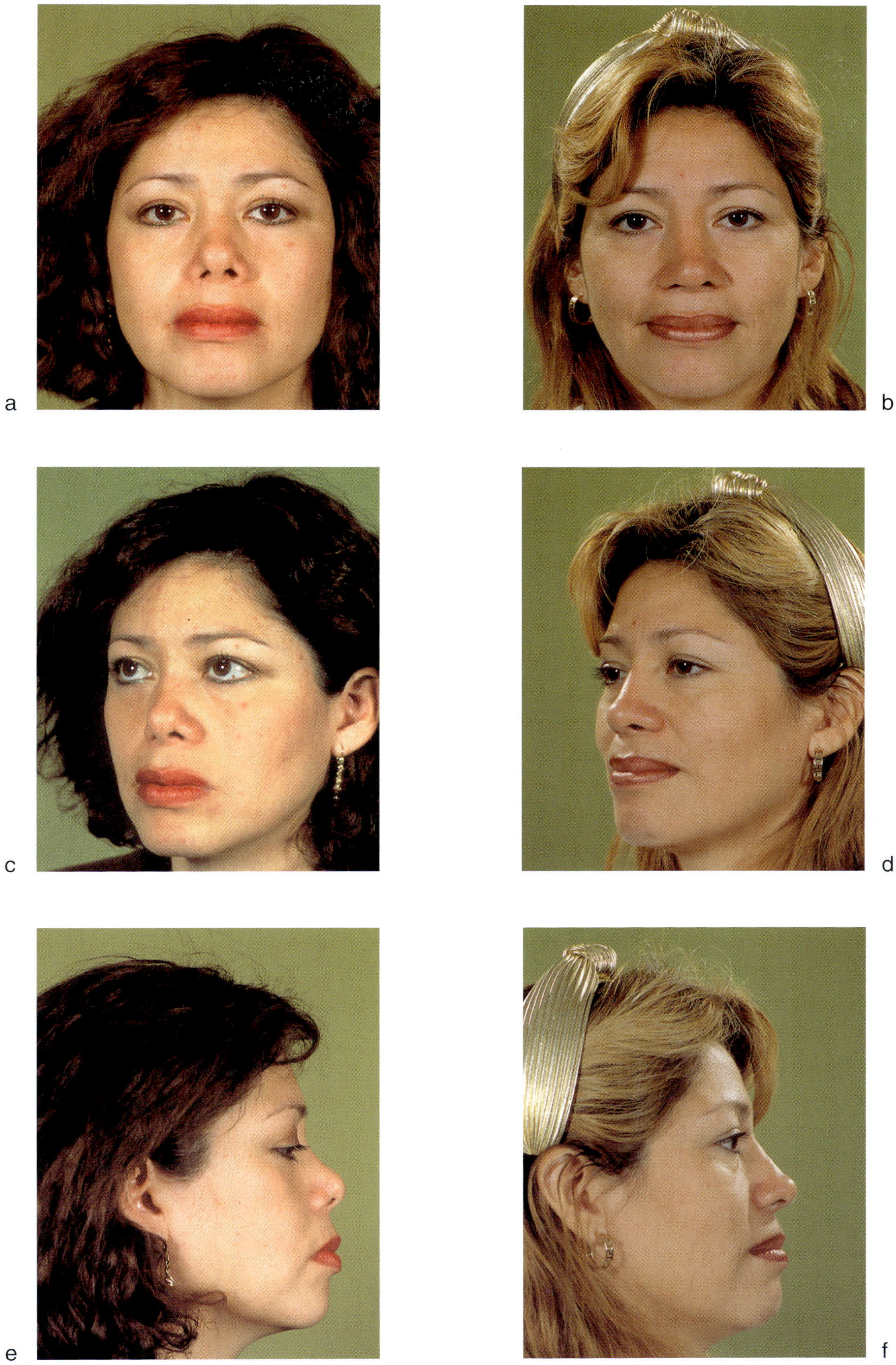

Fig. 16a-h. Pre- and long-term postoperative views of a patient with vestibular stenosis on the right side and over-resection of the nasal dorsum, corrected using the external approach with the use of a composite graft on the right side and dorsal onlay conchal cartilage grafts.

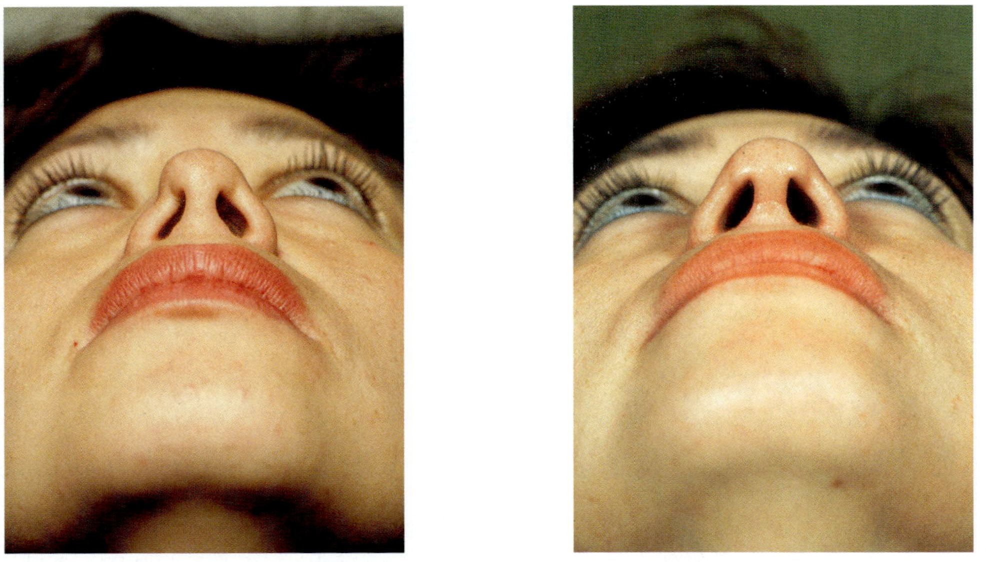

g h

Fig. 16g-h.

23: GUIDELINES FOR CADAVER DISSECTION

G.J. Nolst Trenité

Introduction

Cadaver dissection is an important teaching tool for acquiring knowledge of the surgical anatomy and for practising surgical procedures. In the past, inexperienced rhinoplastic surgeons had to follow a long and arduous path of trial and error in order to improve their skills in what is one of the most challenging areas of facial plastic surgery.

Nowadays, due to the common use of video presentations of the different surgical procedures, together with popularization of the external approach, which allows the preoperative assessment of the pathology to be verified by direct vision of the underlying anatomical substrate, this process of learning is considerably shorter. Although a growing number of rhinoplasty courses are combined with cadaver dissection, the majority of neophyte surgeons still begin septo-rhinoplasty procedures without having carried out cadaver dissections. In all teaching hospitals, cadaver dissection should be obligatory before starting live surgery, and this is a good reason to incorporate the dissection manual from my international course on modern rhinoplasty techniques, with accompanying illustrations, in this second edition of 'Rhinoplasty, A Practical Guide to Functional and Aesthetic Surgery of the Nose'.

The various approaches (non-delivery, delivery and external approach), tip sculpturing techniques, hump resection, micro-osteotomies and harvesting procedures of autogenous material have all been covered. For each surgical procedure, there is a list of the necessary instruments. To facilitate these guidelines, there are photographic illustrations of each surgical step. As cadavers are a precious commodity, I have developed a sequence of surgical procedures (first, on one side, the non-delivery approach, then, on the opposite side, the delivery approach, followed by the external approach to check the results of the former approaches '*in situ*'), which can all be performed on one specimen. The reason for starting with conchal graft harvesting is to obtain the correct soft tissue feeling of the cadaver specimen. This 'dissection guide' consists of a basic and an advanced part, each of which takes two to three hours of practice. In order to be able to perform all the procedures as described, it is important to follow the sequence of the surgical exercises closely. Apart from the specific NT instruments (see page 259), which are used in addition to the general septoplasty instruments, a pair of gloves, head light, marking and fixation needles, skin marker and suture material (as described), are obligatory.

Cadaver dissection

Basic part

Operative techniques

Conchal graft harvesting
Approaches to the tip
- non-delivery
- delivery
- external

Osseocartilaginous vault surgery
- hump resection
- micro-osteotomy

Advanced part

Operative techniques

Septal cartilage harvesting
- spreader grafts

- columella strut
- shield graft

Alar base wedge resection
- alar flair reduction
- nostril size reduction
- a combination of both

Tip suturing techniques
- interdomal suturing
- transdomal suturing
- lateral crural steal suture technique

Composite graft harvesting
- partial
- complete

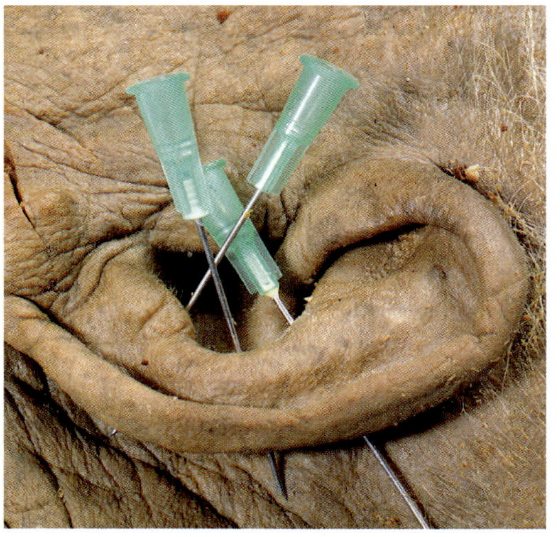

Fig. 1. Marking of the skin and cartilage incision.

Conchal graft harvesting

Instruments: No. 15 blade; rhinoplasty scissors, curved, sharp and Killner type; micro skin hooks; Adson Brown tissue forceps (side grasping teeth)

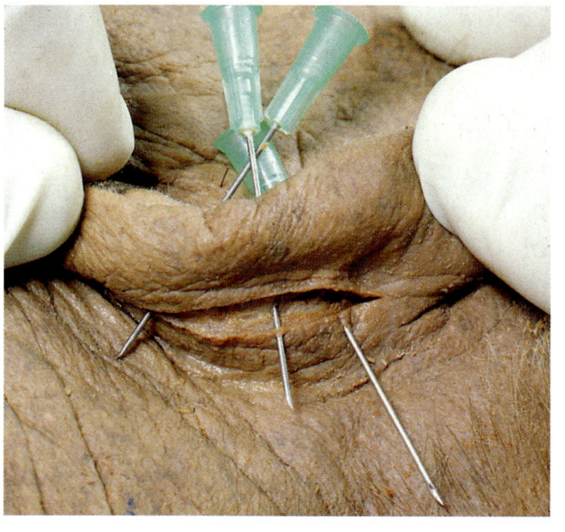

Fig. 2. Skin incision along the needle.

To harvest a large piece of conchal cartilage, the preauricular approach is technically easier than the postauricular approach, but it is less elegant since it leaves a preauricular scar. To outline the postauricular skin and cartilage incision, three needles are used, stabbed through the auricle from the anterior side just medial to the antihelix, following the lateral border of the cavum and cymba conchae.

After incising the skin along the line indicated by the needles, the postauricular perichondrium and conchal cartilage are incised, leaving the perichondrium intact on the anterior side. With a pair of sharp pointed, curved scissors, subperichondrial tunnelling is then carried out over the cavum and cymba conchae. The next step is to free the cartilage at the posterior side by blunt dissection in a supraperichondrial plane with Killner-type scissors. The cartilage is now incised just lateral of the ear canal (a 2-mm strip of cartilage is left) and around the radix helicis, which should be left intact for structural support, and finally resected. The skin incision is closed with a 5/0 atraumatic running suture.

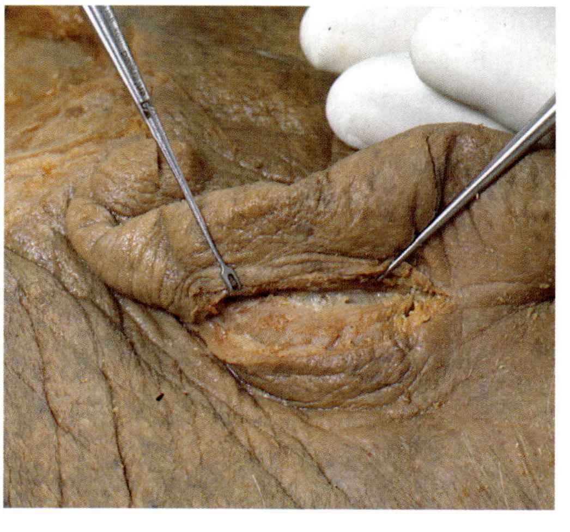

Fig. 3. Completed perichondrium and cartilage incision (posterior side).

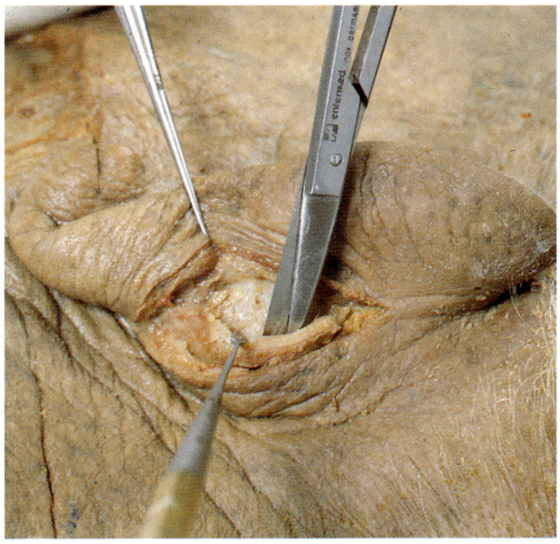

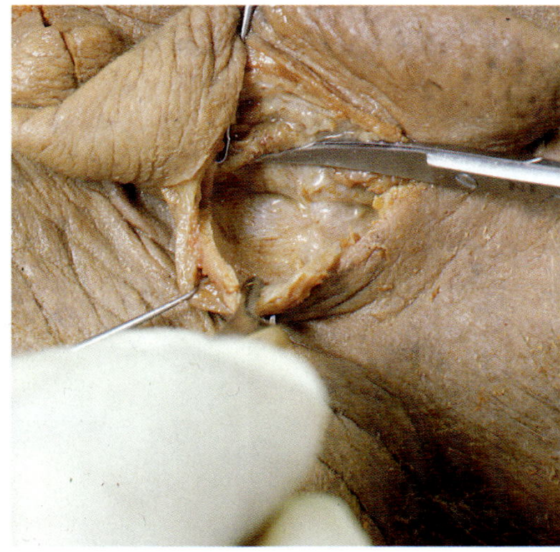

Fig. 4. Subperichondrial dissection at the anterior side.

Fig. 5. Completed subperichondrial dissection.

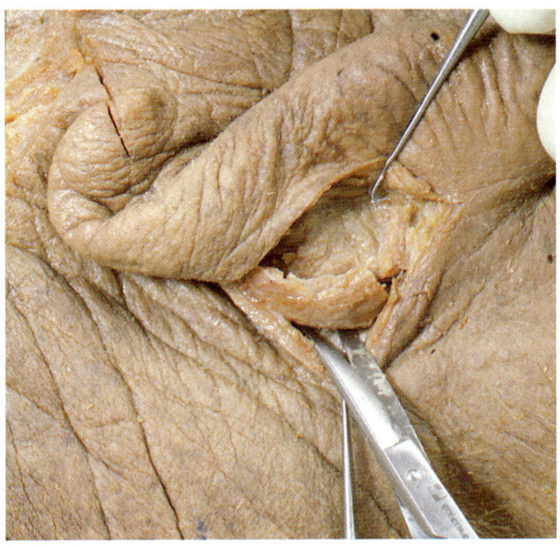

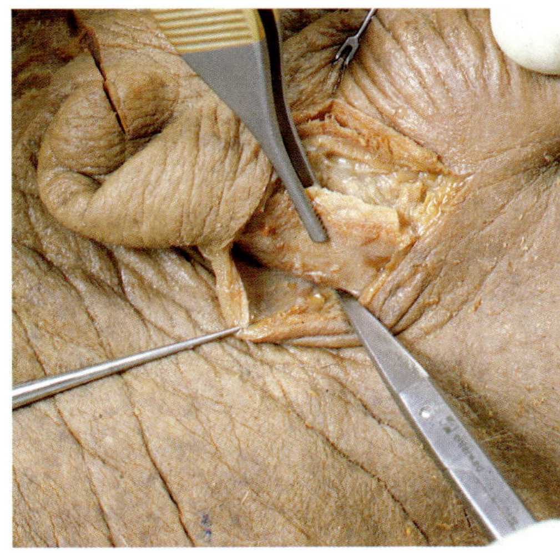

Fig. 6. Supraperichondrial dissection at the posterior side.

Fig. 7. Completed supraperichondrial dissection.

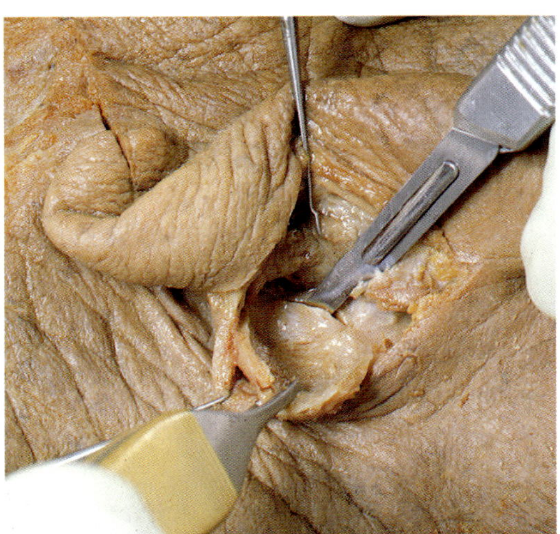

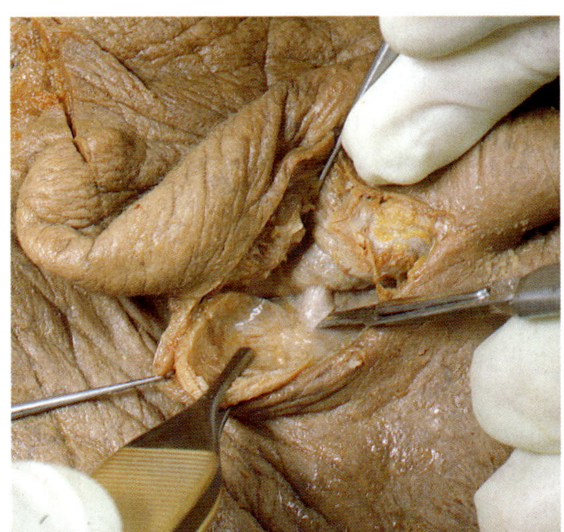

Figs. 8 and 9. Resection of the cartilage around the helical crus.

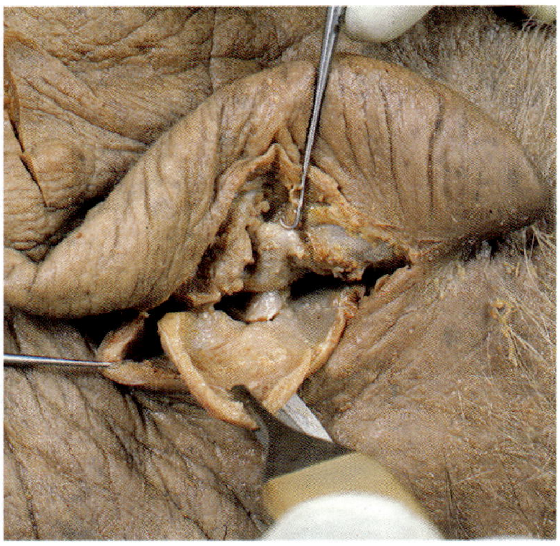

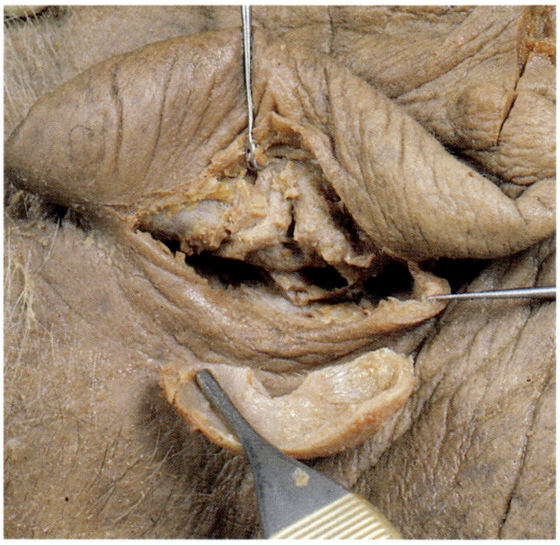

Figs. 10 and 11. Removal of the conchal cartilage graft.

Non-delivery approach

Instruments: No. 15 blade; micro skin hooks; double-hooked ala retractor; rhinoplasty scissors, curved, sharp (10 cm); Adson Brown tissue forceps (side grasping teeth)

The operative procedure for the cartilage splitting non-delivery approach is as follows: After drawing the skeletal landmarks and boundaries on the skin of the nose, the most cephalic part of the lateral crus to be resected is outlined with a marking pen on the external skin. It is helpful to indicate on the vestibular skin where the transcartilaginous incision should be made. This can be done either by a through-and-through needle from the outside or, more elegantly, by using the imprint of a surgical instrument on the vestibular skin.

Care should be taken to preserve at least 5 mm of uninterrupted cartilage (in a vertical dimension) of the lateral crus. Although many surgeons make their incisions through the vestibular skin and cartilage at the same time, it facilitates the dissection of the vestibular skin to perform this in two stages. A vestibular skin incision with a No. 15 blade is followed by dissecting the vestibular skin free of the proposed resection of the cephalic part of the lower lateral cartilage with a pair of sharp pointed, curved scissors. After splitting the cartilage, the non-vestibular side of the cephalic part to be resected is dissected free of the overlying soft tissue, and removed. Pressure of the middle finger of the operator's hand (holding the double-hooked ala retractor) on the lateral crus will give excellent exposure and control during surgery. After sufficient and symmetric volume reduction, the vestibular skin should be sutured carefully with 5/0 atraumatic absorbable suture material. This simple tip refinement procedure gives minimal surgical trauma, and leaves the integrity of the lower lateral crus intact to ensure the best chance of an uncomplicated healing process.

Delivery approach

Instruments: No. 15 blade; micro skin hooks; double-hooked ala retractor; rhinoplasty scissors, curved, sharp (10 cm); Adson Brown tissue forceps (side grasping teeth); small hemostats

The surgical procedure to deliver the alar cartilages starts with an intercatilaginous incision with a No. 15 blade. It is important to make this incision 1-2 mm from the internal valve, in order to prevent

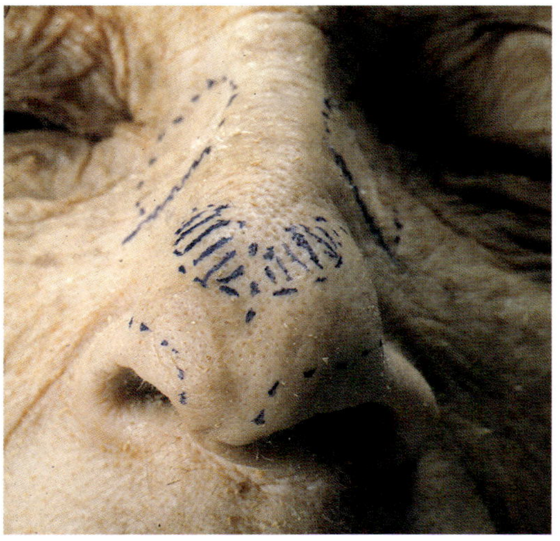
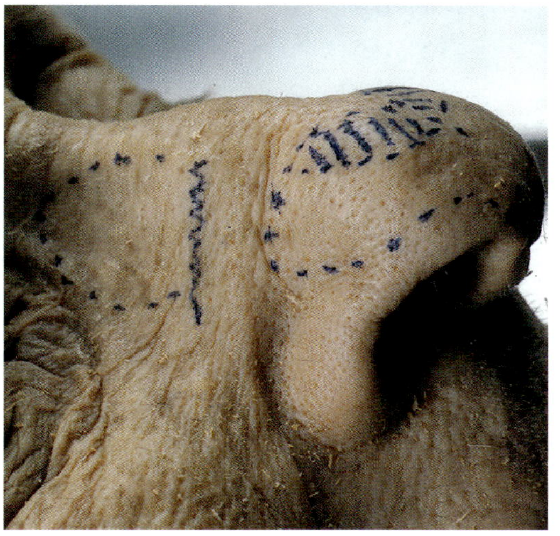

Figs. 12 and 13. Marking of the skeletal boundaries and the cephalic parts of the lateral crura to be resected.

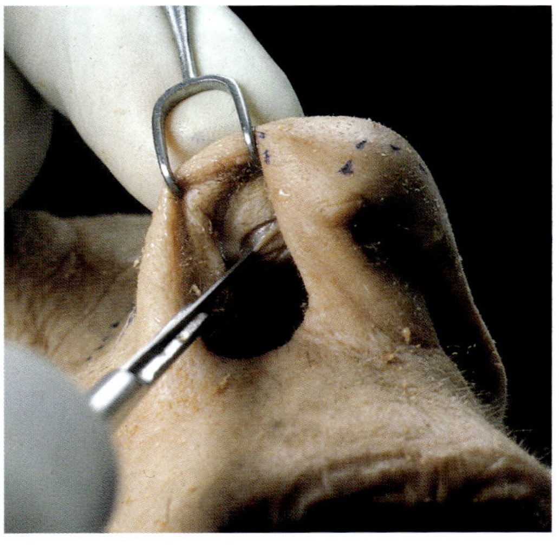
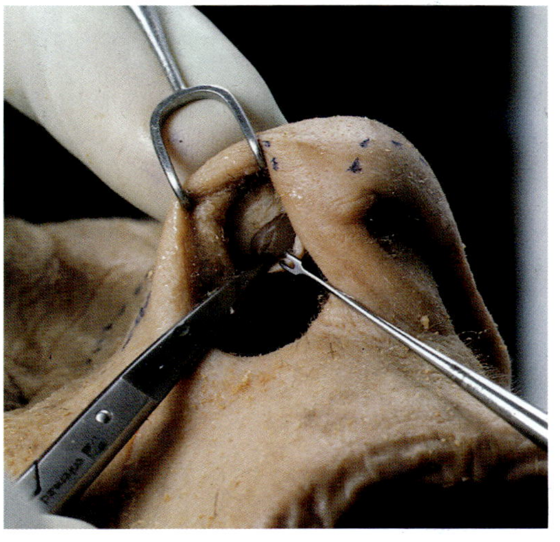

Fig. 14. Vestibular skin incision.

Fig. 15. Dissection of vestibular skin and perichondrium (subperichondrially).

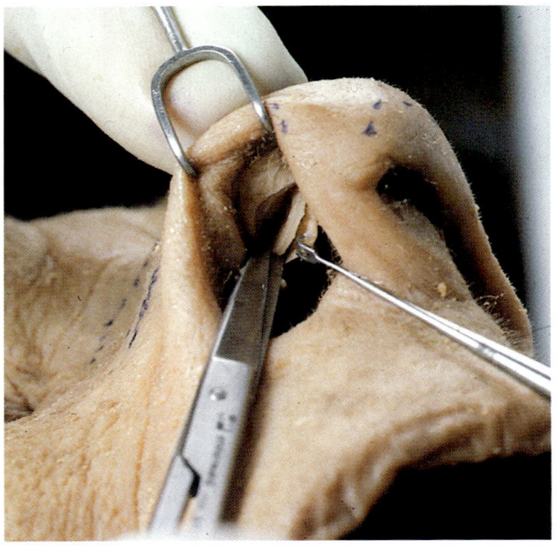

Fig. 16. Dissection at the non-vestibular side, *i.e.*, the supraperichondrial plane.

unnecessary scarring in the valve area. This intercartilaginous incision should be carried well around the anterior septal angle. If not, delivery could be stagnated.

The next step is to make a marginal incision (No. 15 blade), hugging the caudal rim of the lower lateral crus to prevent surgical damage to the soft triangle on Converse. The incision starts at the caudal rim of the lateral crus, goes around the dome, and follows the caudal rim of the medial crus as far as necessary. After these two incisions, the non-vestibular side of the lateral crus, dome and intermediate crus is freed from the soft tissue by dissection with a pair of sharp pointed, curved scissors in a

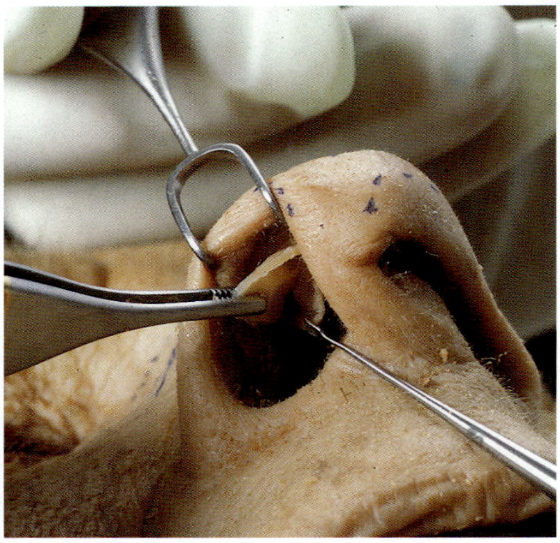

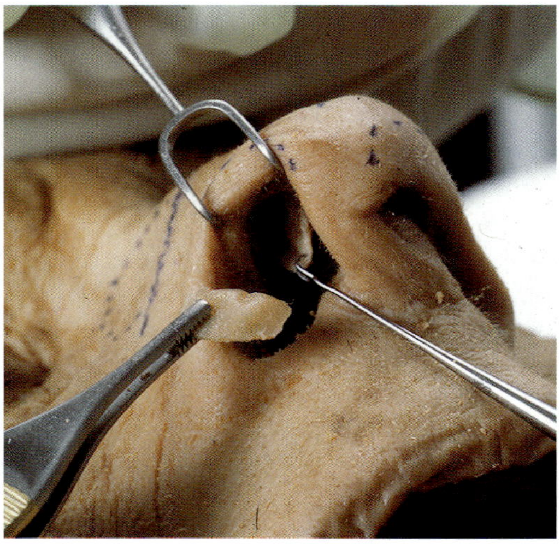

Figs. 17 and 18. Resection of the chosen cephalic part of the lateral crus.

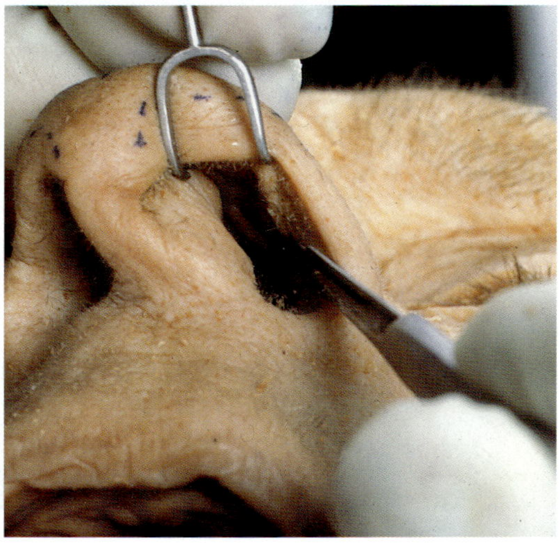

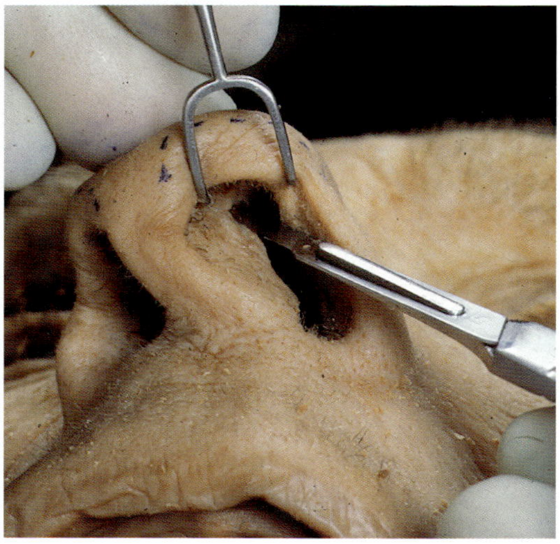

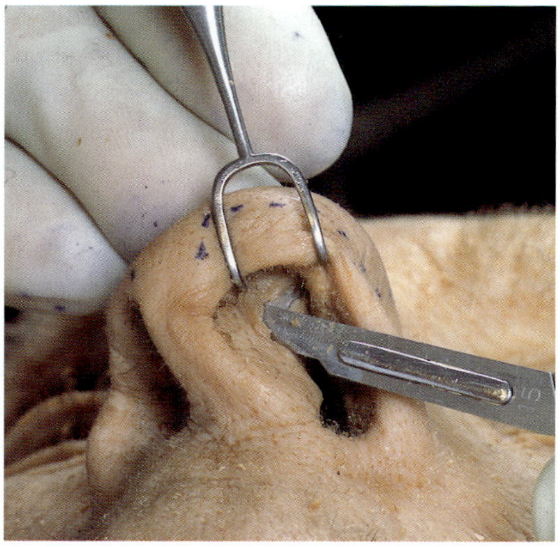

Figs. 19, 20 and 21. Intercartilaginous incision starting (1-2 mm) laterally to the internal valve, then medially and caudally well around the anterior septal angle.

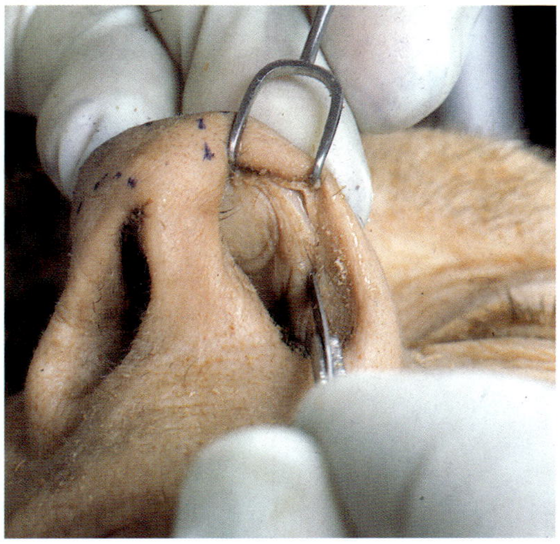

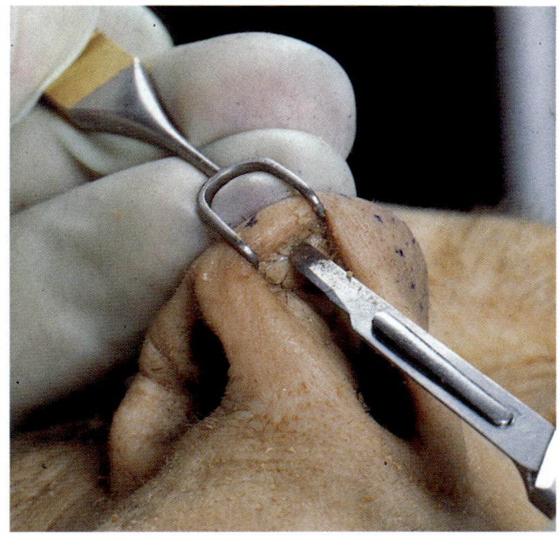

Figs. 22 and 23. Marginal incision in a lateral to medial direction along the caudal rim of the lower lateral crus.

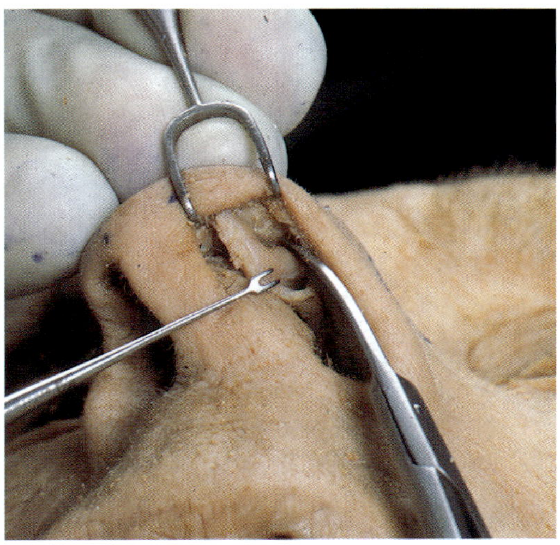

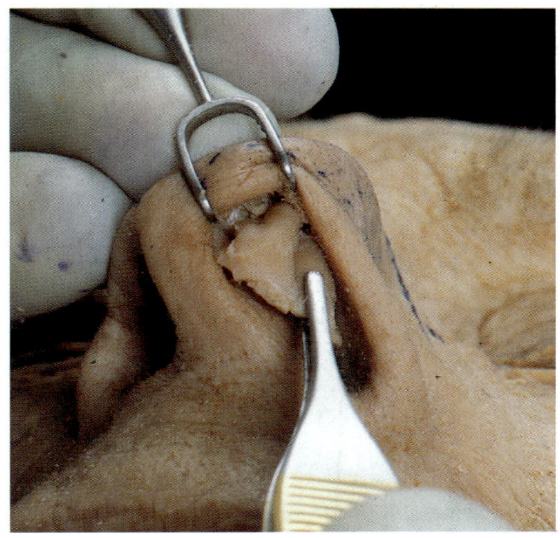

Fig. 24. Dissection of the lateral crus, dome and intermediate crus in a subperichondrial plane (on the non-vestibular side).

Fig. 25. Checking with a tissue forceps with side grasping teeth whether the bipedicle flaps can now be delivered.

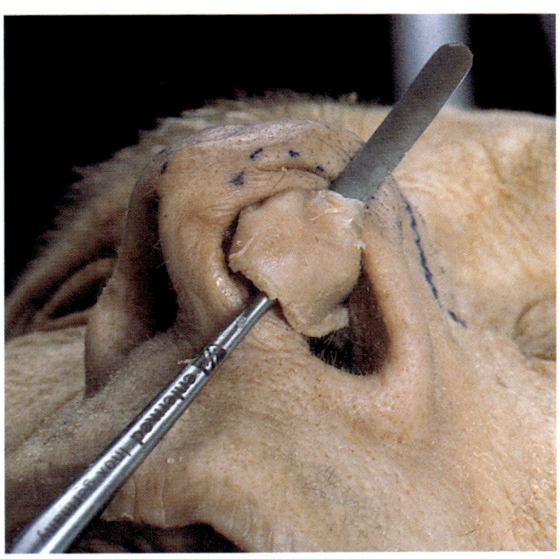

Fig. 26. The bipedicle chondrocutaneous flap is delivered.

subperichondrial surgical plane. Small curved hemostats are very handy for delivering the bipedicle chondrocutaneous flaps. Precise excision of cartilage is now possible under direct vision. When the lateral crus bulges, a weakening procedure (scoring or morselization) is performed, if necessary in combination with resection of a cephalic portion of the lateral crus.

External approach

Instruments: blade No. 11/15, micro skin hooks, a pair of sharp pointed curved rhinoplasty scissors and angled scissors (Walter or Converse type), double hooked

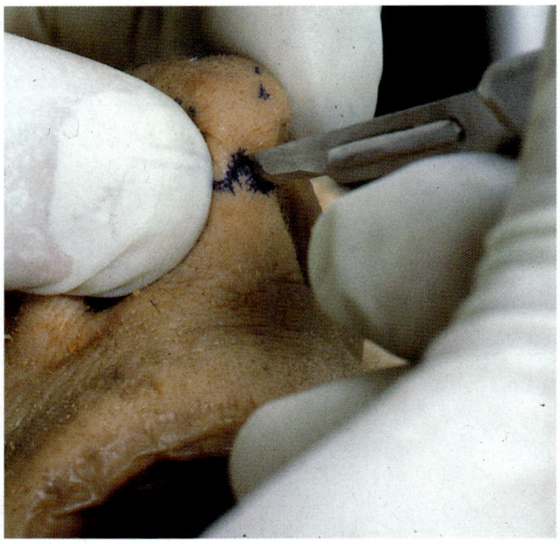

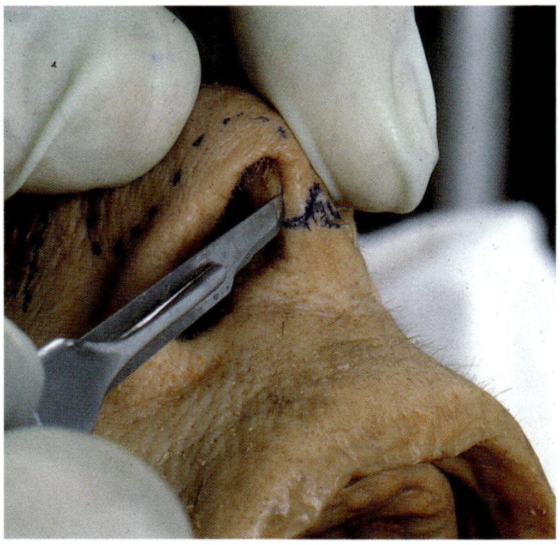

Figs. 27 and 28. Broken columella incision extended with a vertical columella incision 1.5–2 mm iside the vestibulum.

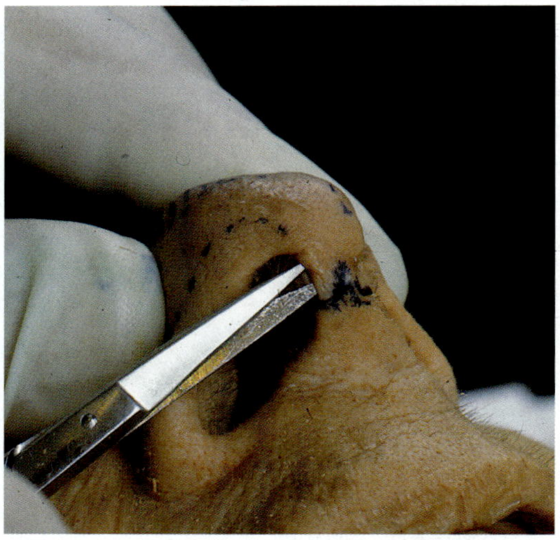

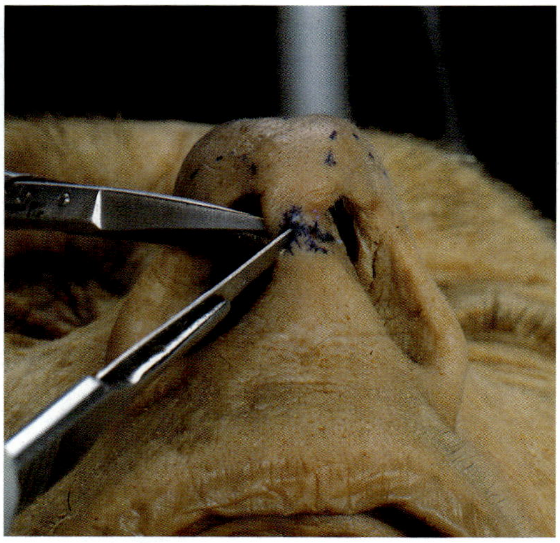

Fig. 29. Subcutaneous columella pocket with a pair of curved sharp pointed scissors.

Fig. 30. Completing the skin incision while the medial crura are guided by the scissors.

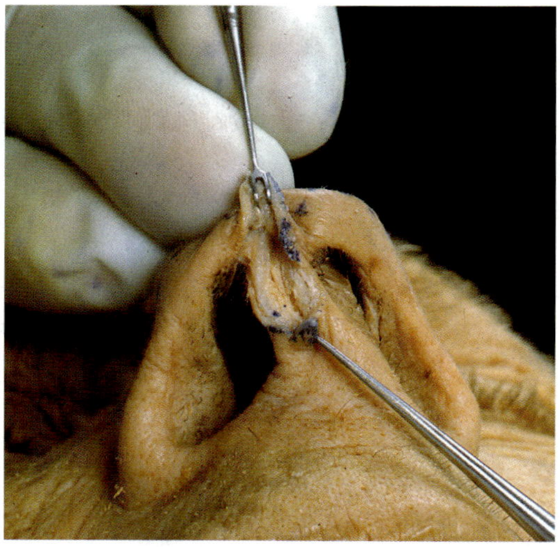

Fig. 31. Development of the columella skin flaps.

ala retractor, Aufricht nasal retractor, Adson Brown tissue forceps, Cottle elevator.

The nasal skeleton is exposed using a mid-columellar incision. The ultimate scar in the middle columellar region is supported by the intact medial crura, which diminishes scar contraction. Therefore care should be taken not to injure the medial crura. For the same purpose (to achieve a more or less invisible scar), the incision (No. 11/15 blade) is not straight over the columella, but broken using an inverted V. The mid-columellar incision is extended with marginal incisions. The columellar part with a No. 15 blade, the vestibular part with angled scissors, Walter or Converse type. After the vertical (marginal) incision in the columella, subcutaneous pockets (left and right connected) are made cephalic of the broken columella

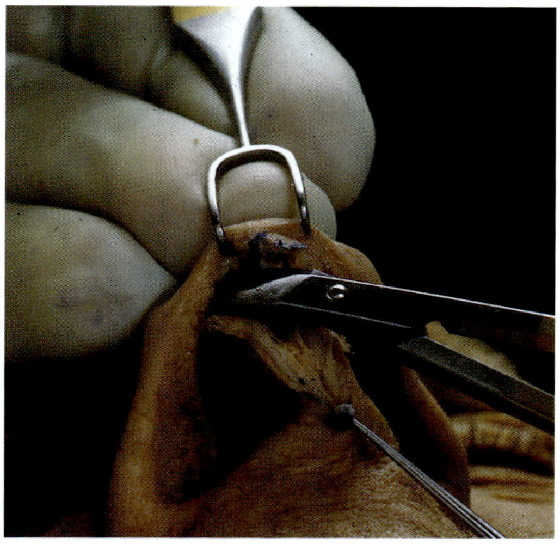

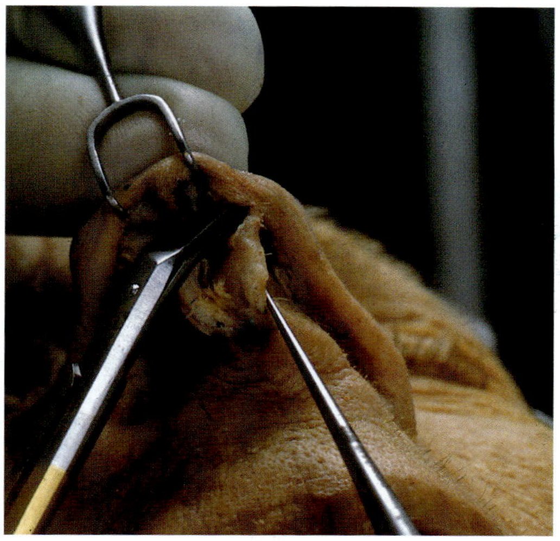

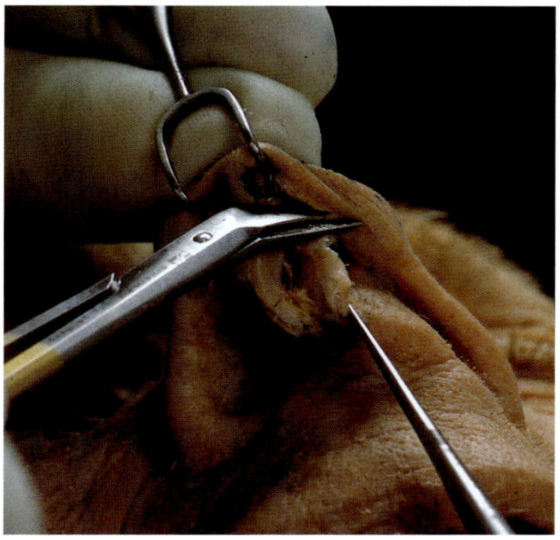

Figs. 32, 33 and 34. Denuding of the domes and lateral crura with hooked (Walter or Converse) scissors using the caudal rim of the lower laterals as a guide line.

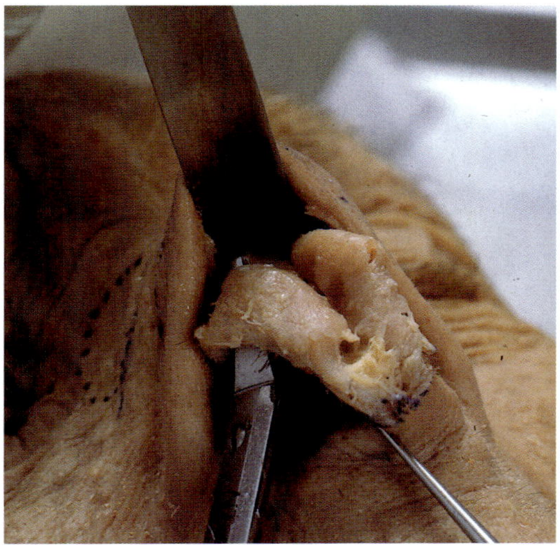

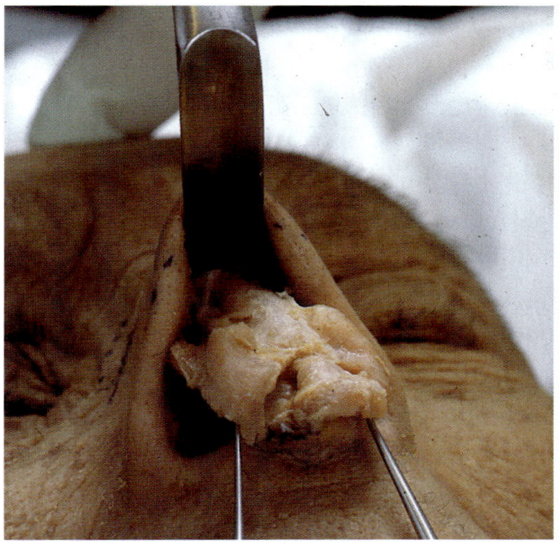

Figs. 35 and 36. Lower laterals and cartilagenous vault freed from the soft tissue envelope.

incision and extended caudally of the skin incision with a pair of sharp pointed curved scissors. This pair of scissors can now act as a guarding device for the medial crura, while completing the columellar skin incision. The columellar skin flap is elevated superficially to the medial crura with blunt dissection, leaving as much soft tissue as possible on the skin flap. This enhances the viability of the columellar skin flap, while the surgical plane is relatively bloodless. The vestibular part of the marginal incision can be completed with the angled scissors (Walter or Converse type) following the caudal margin of the lateral crus. The upper lateral cartilages, lower lateral cartilages and nasal dorsum up to the nasal frontal angle, can now be exposed in their undisturbed positions. To dissect the cartilaginous vault in a surgical plane it is important to dissect Sub SMAS from medial to lateral.

Further dissection of the bony vault will be described on page 247 (hump resection).

Hump resection

Instruments: No. 15 blade; double hooked ala retractor; micro skin hooks; rhinoplasty scissors, curved, sharp (10 cm) and Killner-type dissection scissors; Adson Brown tissue forceps; Blakesley (small) Joseph periosteal elevator; hump osteotome (10-14 mm); Cottle hammer; nasal rasp (tungsten carbide)

The nasal hump consists of a cartilaginous part and a bony part. In most cases, the bony part is much smaller than the cartilaginous part. With the *endonasal* approach, intercartilaginous incisions are connected by a transfixion incision in order to obtain ample access to the hump. It is important to dissect carefully between the upper and lower lateral cartilage in order to prevent postoperative irregularities of the lateral nasal wall. The inter-

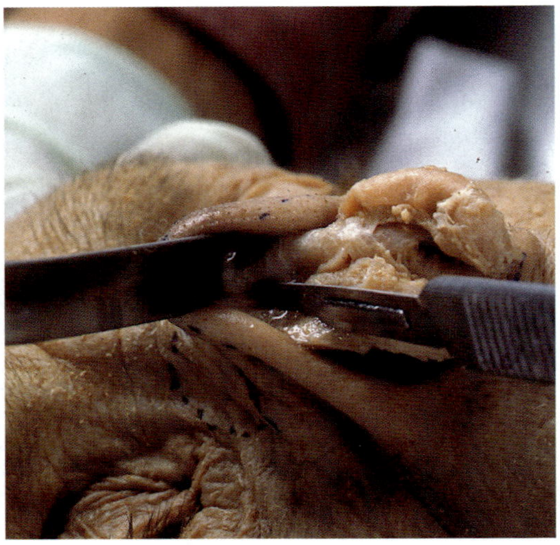

Fig. 37. Incising the periosteum at the caudal end of the nasal bone.

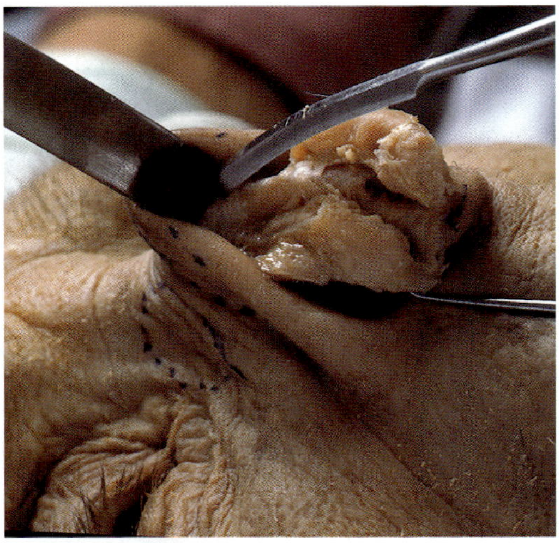

Fig. 38. Elevation of the periosteum with a Joseph elevator.

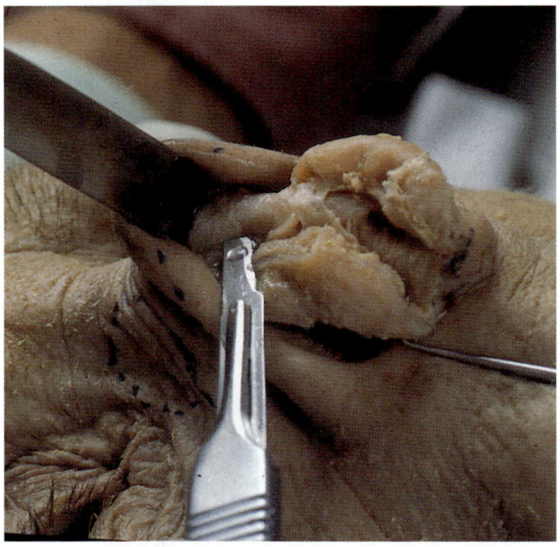

Fig. 39. Incising the cartilaginous vault (three cartilaginous 'layers') from the cephalic to caudal end.

cartilaginous incision in a lateral to medial direction, just caudal of the nasal valve, must be continued around the anterior sep-

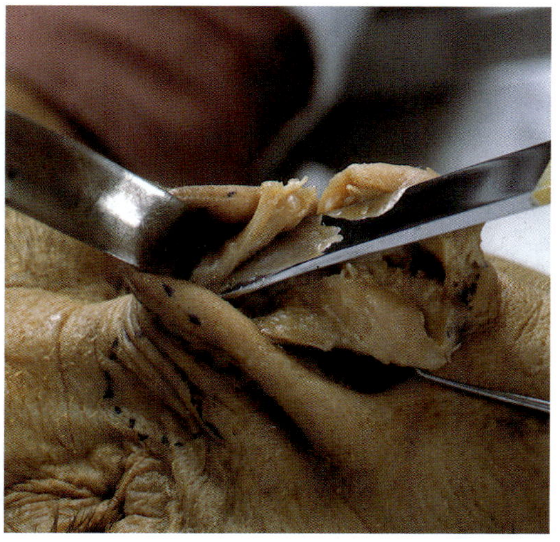

Fig. 40. Introduction of a 14-mm hump osteotome.

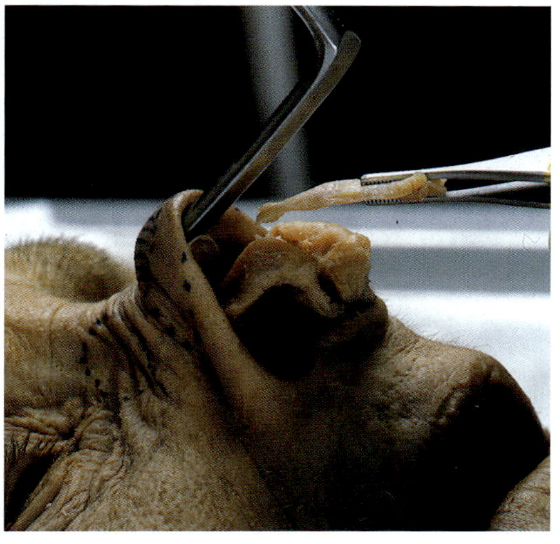

Fig. 41. Removal of the bony cartilaginous hump.

tal angle. The two intercartilaginous incisions should then be connected by a partial transfixion incision, unless there is specific indication for a complete transfixion incision. With a complete transfixion incision, an important support of the tip in its connection between the medial crura and the caudal rim of the nasal septum will be disturbed. The next step is to free the cartilaginous part of the hump from the overlying soft tissues. With careful and sharp dissection (No. 15 blade) in the supraperichondrial surgical plane, damage to the musculus trasversus nasi, as well as unnecessary scarring and bleeding, will be prevented. In this cadaver dissection, the hump resection technique is performed through an external approach.

After freeing the cartilaginous vault from the overlying soft tissues, the periosteum is incised at the caudal end of the nasal bone, and elevated with a Joseph elevator. There is no need to elevate the periosteum very far laterally. The procedure should be limited to the area of the hump to be resected. The periosteum attached to the sutura intranasalis can simply be cut from the bony vault with a pair of long scissors (i.e. Killner-type). With an 'Aufricht' retractor in place, the cartilaginous vault can now be incised by a through-and-through incision (No. 15 blade) from the cephalic to the caudal end at the 'planned' resection line. Using this cartilaginous cutting face as a guideline, the hump osteotome is introduced to loosen the bony part at the hump, followed by removal of the osseocartilaginous hump *en bloc*. A (medium-fine) tungsten-carbine or diamond rasp is now used to smoothen the bony surface and, if necessary, some extra shaving of the cartilaginous dorsum is carried out in order to obtain the desired supratip-tip relation. In the case of a small hump, it is easier to start shaving off small pieces of the cartilaginous hump to the desired level, and then to use a rasp to lower the bony dorsum.

Osteotomies

Instruments: No. 15 blade; micro-osteotomes (2 and 3 mm); Cottle hammer; double-hooked ala retractor

Osteotomies are required to mobilize the bony pyramid for in-fracture, out-fracture, or realignment. With the micro-osteotome, if necessary sharpened during surgery, it is not necessary to elevate the periosteum. This gives less surgical trauma and leaves the periosteum to a large extent intact, so that it can act as an internal splint. When a *medial-oblique osteotomy* is combined with a slightly curved lateral osteotomy,

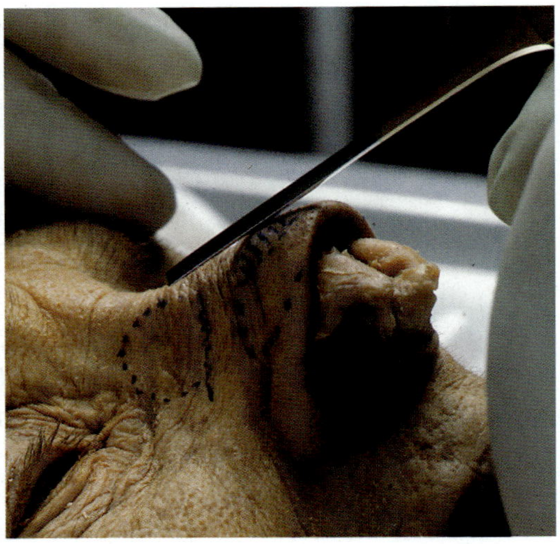

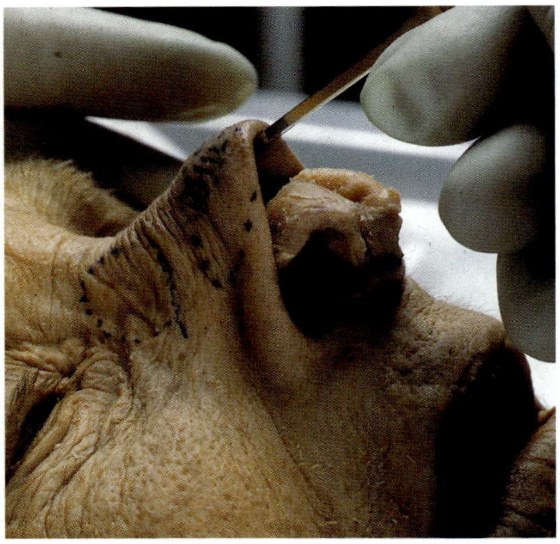

Figs. 42 and 43. Medial-oblique osteotomy with a 3-mm micro-osteotome.

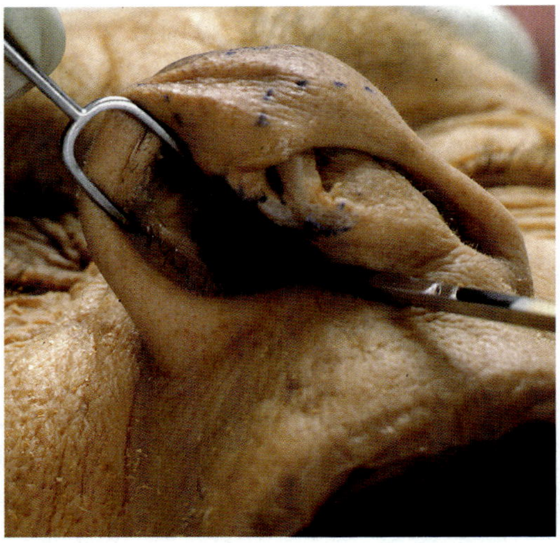

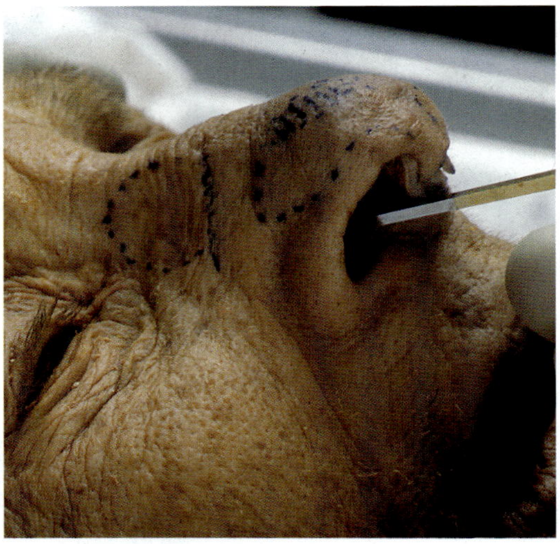

Figs. 44 and 45. Endonasal curved lateral osteotomy with a 2-mm micro-osteotome.

there is no need for a traditional transverse osteotomy. The crossover point of both osteotomies should not be (and aesthetically there is no need) more cephalic than the intercanthal line, thereby avoiding the thick bone of the radix nasi. It is important to leave the (external) periosteal and (internal) mucoperiosteal lining as far as possible intact.

Lateral osteotomies can be performed *percutaneously* as well as *intranasally*. Using the intranasal pathway, the micro-osteotome is inserted through the soft tissue of the lateral wall of the piriform aperture, starting at the ascending process of the maxilla at the superior margin of the inferior turbinate. For a low lateral osteotomy, it should then proceed laterally, preserving a bony ridge at the base of the lateral wall of the piriform aperture. In this way, any possible narrowing of the airway by in-fracture of the os nasale can be prevented. It should then proceed, slowly bending in a lateral to a medial direction, as far as the intercanthal line at the most cephalic point of the medial-oblique osteotomy. Readjustment of the osteotome after sliding off the bone, prevents unnecessary lesions of the periosteum. A 2-mm osteotome is often sufficient. When the bone is thicker than normal, a 3-mm osteotome is necessary.

In percutaneous lateral osteotomy, a 2-mm skin incision is made halfway along the planned osteotomy line, after which small point-osteotomies with a 2-mm os-

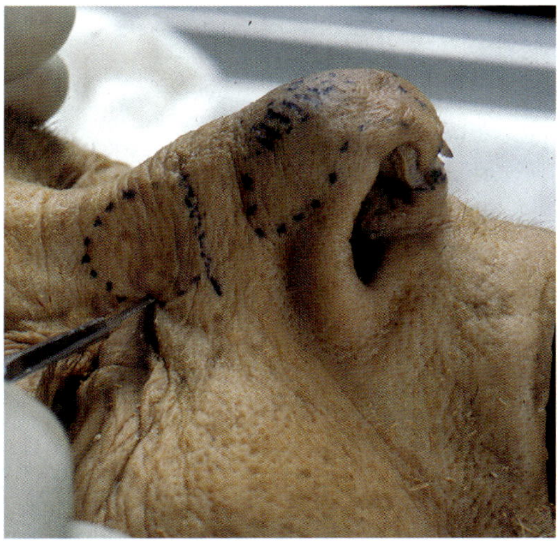

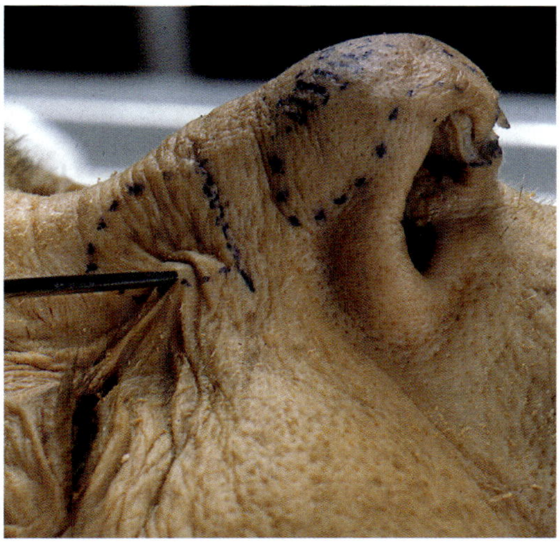

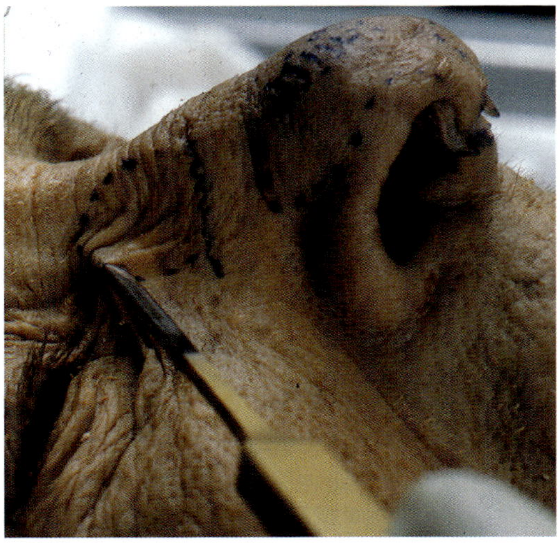

Figs. 46, 47 and 48. Percutaneous lateral point osteotomies with a 2-mm micro-osteotome following the marked osteotomy pathway.

teotome are made cephalically and caudally along the marked osteotomy line.

Septal cartilage harvesting (spreader grafts, columella strut and shield grafts)

Instruments: No. 15 blade; micro skin hooks; rhinoplasty scissors, curved, sharp (10 cm); nose speculum (Kilian type) and elevator (Cottle type); Adson Brown forceps (side grasping teeth); needle holder

Division of the medial inter-crural fibrous tissue offers wide exposure of the caudal septal angle down to the premaxillary spine. With a Cottle elevator, subperichondrial tunnels are made to expose the cartilaginous septum in order to harvest graft material (columella strut, spreader grafts, and a shield graft). Care should be taken not to disturb the continuity of that part of the quadrangular cartilage anterior to the imaginary line between the most caudal part of the nasal bone (rhinion) and the anterior nasal spine, in order to prevent sagging of the cartilaginous nasal dorsum.

The graft is best taken from the thick areas of the septum lying at the junction of the perpendicular plate and the vomer, using a nose speculum for optimal exposure. The average size of the spreader graft is: 15 × 1.5 × 3 mm; shield graft: length 10-12 mm, base width 3-4 mm, top

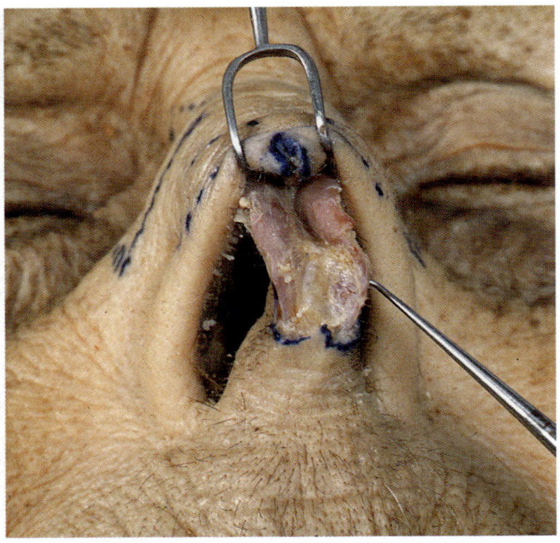

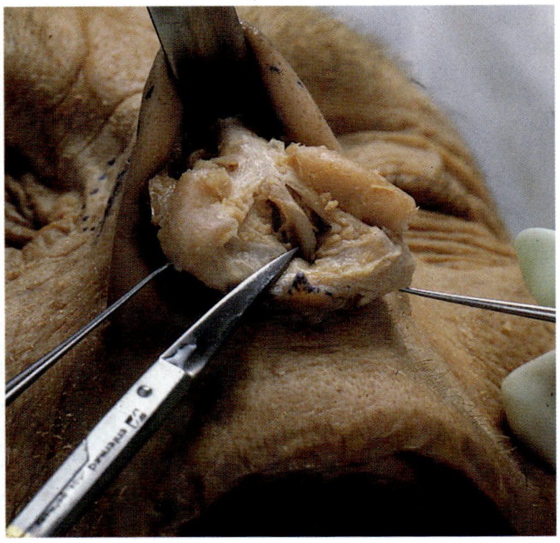

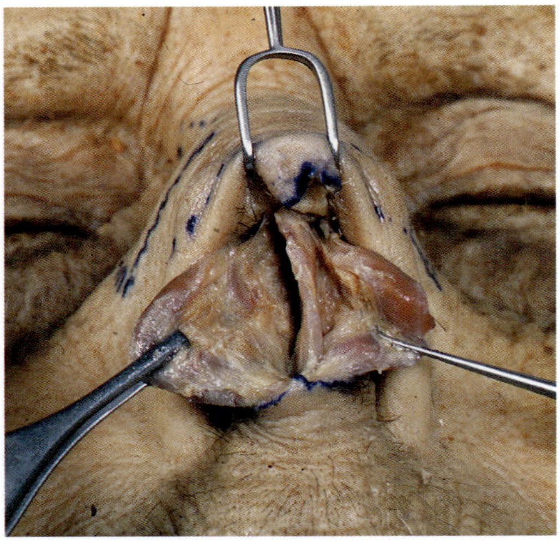

Figs. 49, 50 and 51. External approach to the cartilaginous septum followed by submucoperichondrial tunnelling on both sides.

width 6-10 mm; columella strut: average size 15 × 1.5 × 3 mm. The leftover cartilage should be crushed and replaced at the donor site (not necessary in cadaver dissection).

Spreader graft

After separating the upper laterals from the septum with a sharp dissection, the length of the graft is measured, and the adapted grafts will be placed between the septum and the anterior border of the upper lateral cartilage on both sides. Fixation with mattress sutures (5/0 vicryl with a P-3 needle, or 6/0 ethilon with a P-1 needle).

Columella strut

The columella strut will be adapted in length from 1-2 mm above the nasal spine to the level of the angle just below the domes of the alar cartilages. This sandwich construction is fixed to the septum with 4/0 vicryl mattress-type sutures (straight needle 5C-1).

Shield graft

Sculpting of the shield graft: the graft narrows away from the tip so that the width at the base is 3-4 mm (top approximately 6-8 mm; length 10-12 mm). The most inferior portion of the graft is thinned

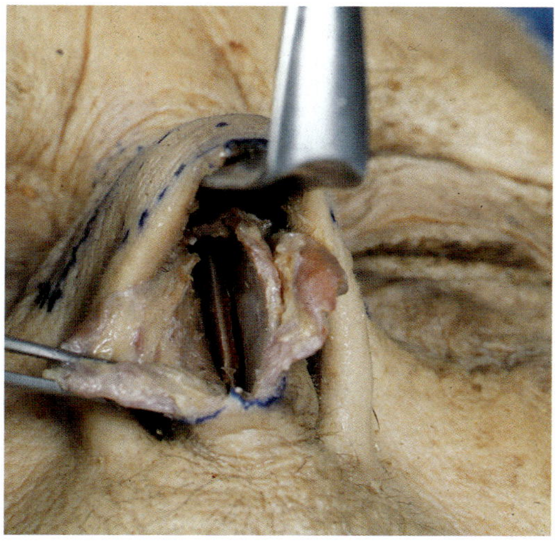

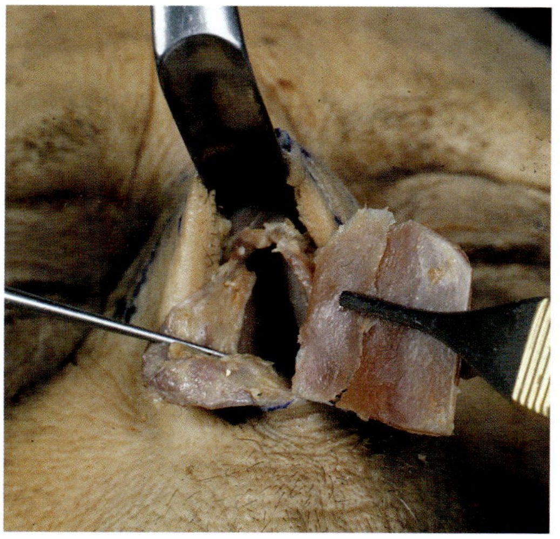

Figs. 52 and 53. Harvesting of septal cartilage behind an imaginary line between the rhinion and the anterior nasal spine.

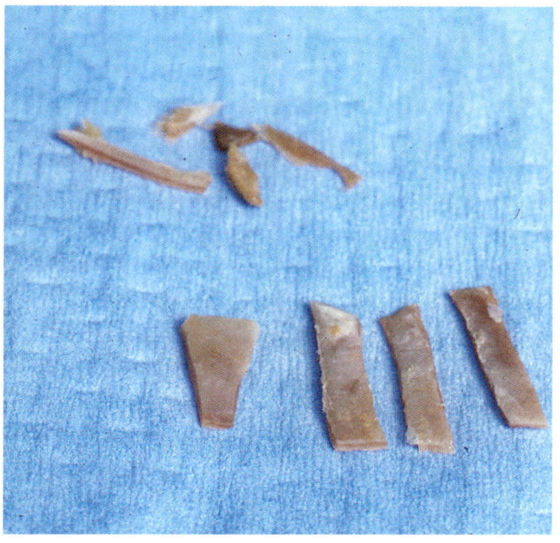

Fig. 54. Sculpted graft material (shield graft, columella and spreader grafts).

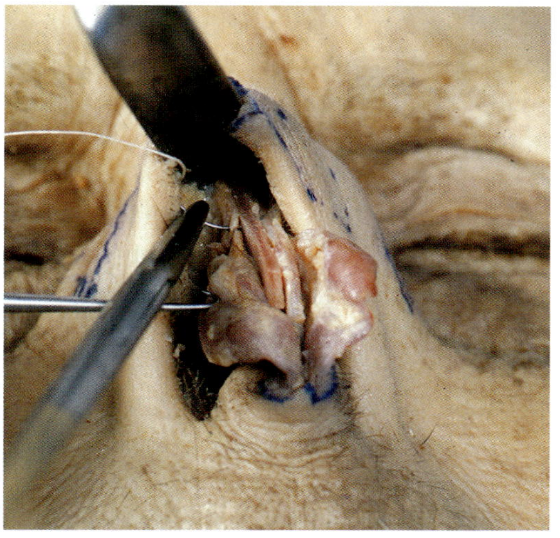

Fig. 55. Suturing a spreader graft strut in place between the septum and upper lateral.

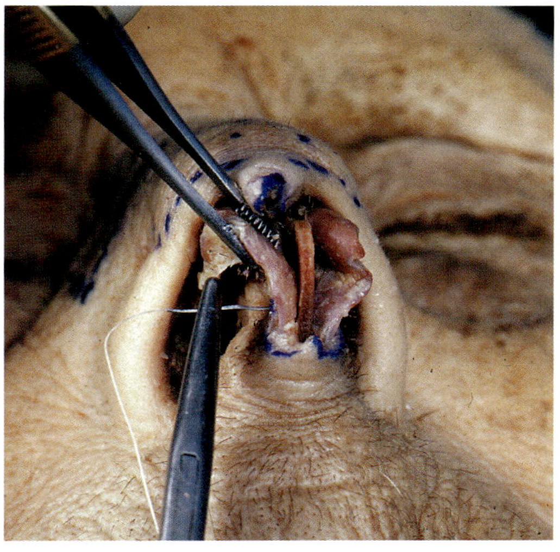

Fig. 56. Fixation of the columella strut with a mattress suture.

and the edges are baffled. Fixation of the shield graft to the medial crura is carried out with 6/0 ethilon using a P-1 needle, with two or three sutures on each side.

Tip suturing techniques

Instruments: Needle holder, 6/0 ethilon P-1 needle; rhinoplasty scissors, curved, sharp, pointed; micro skin hooks; Adson Brown tissue forceps (side grasping teeth)

Tip suturing techniques can be performed after a delivery or an external approach.

Interdomal suturing is indicated for a bulbous tip caused by a wide interdomal distance caused by an excess of interdomal

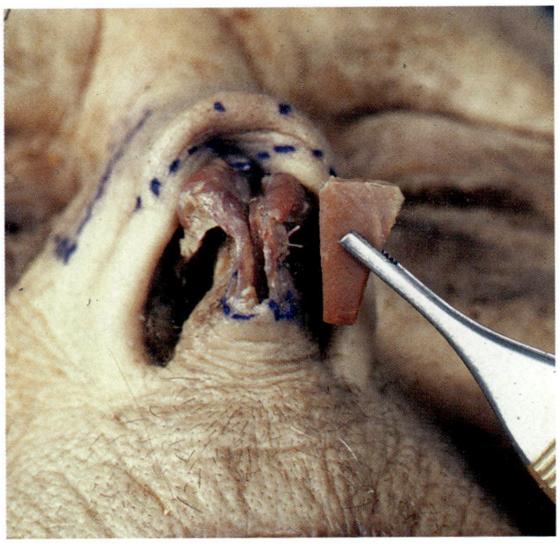

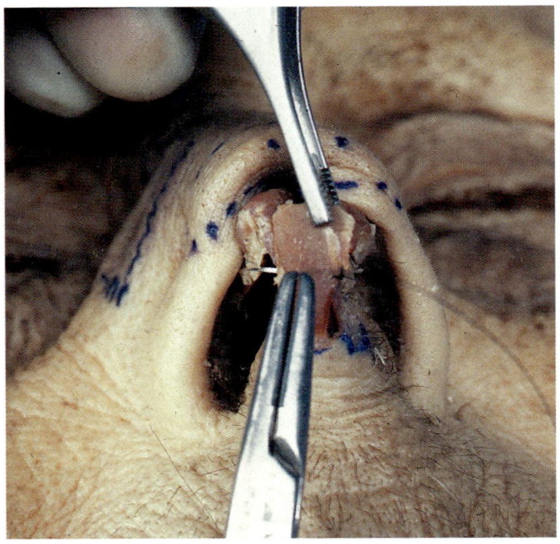

Figs. 57 and 58. Positioning and fixation of a shield graft.

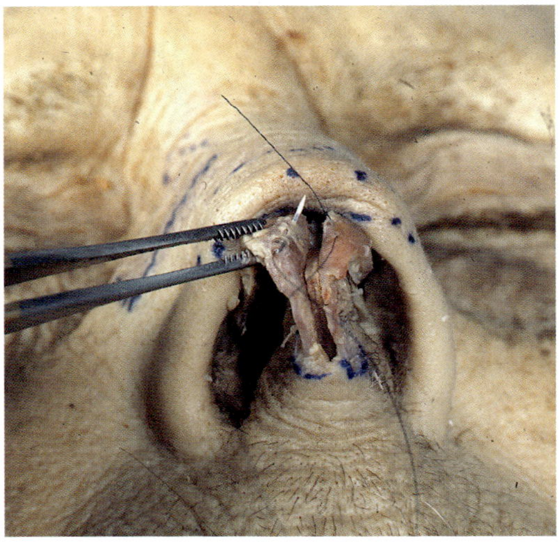

Fig. 59. Interdomal suture.

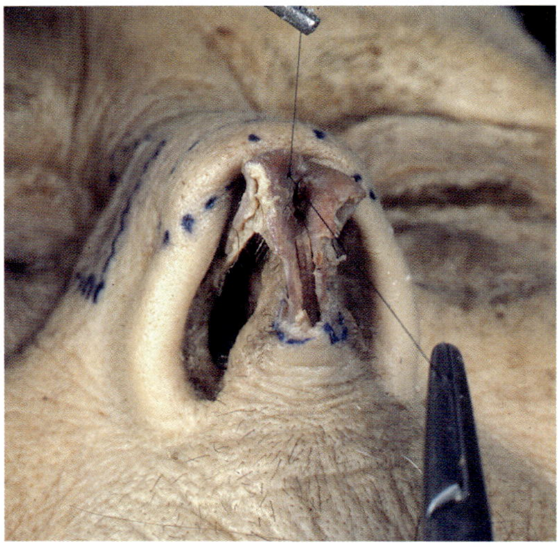

Fig. 60. Transdomal suture with lateral crural steal to enhance tip projection.

soft tissue, a broad middle crus and/or a large angle of domal divergence. Technique: remove the interdomal soft tissue and perform one or two mattress sutures with 6/0 ethilon and a P-1 needle.

Transdomal suturing is indicated for a bifid tip with broad angled domes. Technique: perform a horizontal mattress suture incorporating a middle and lateral crural part of the dome, and bury the knot between the two domes (5/0, P-1 needle).

The *lateral crural steal suture technique* is indicated for an amorphous and underprojected tip. Technique: dissection of the vestibular skin from the cartilage. Place a horizontal mattress suture just medial to or at the dome and reaching out laterally into the lateral crura. Both sides are performed separately (5/0, P-1 needle).

After the tip suturing technique, the broken columella incision should be meticulously closed with a 6/0 ethilon suture using a P-1 needle, followed by 5/0 vicryl (P-3 needle) adaptation sutures of the marginal incision.

Alar base wedge resection

Instruments: No. 15 blade; micro skin hooks; Adson Brown tissue forceps; needle holder

The large variety of alar base configurations demands differentiation in the shape, type and position of the wedge to be re-

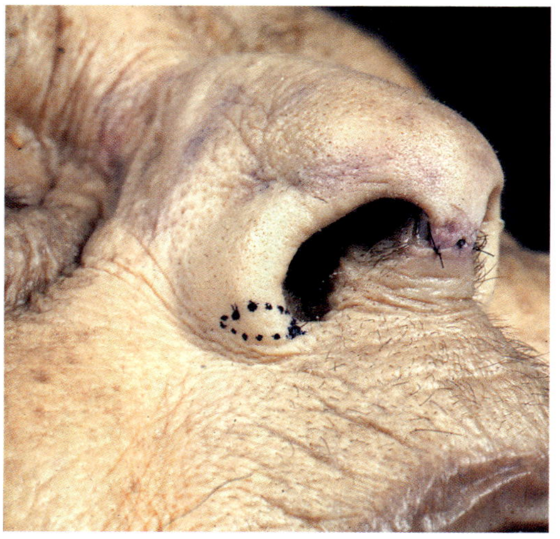

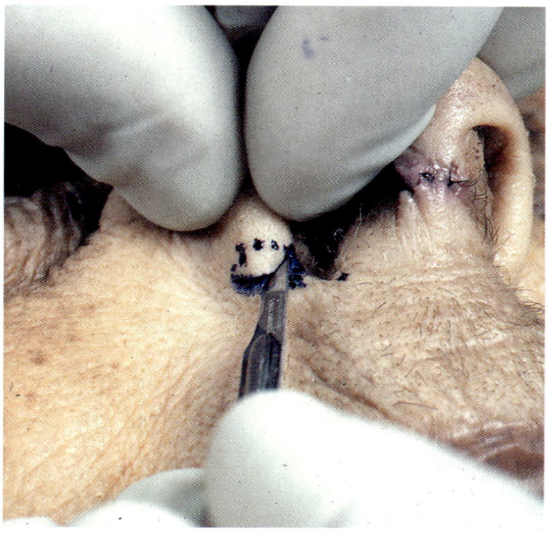

Fig. 61. Marking the wedge (alar flair reduction) to be resected on the alar skin.

Fig. 62. The first skin incision at the base approximately 2 mm from the alar groove.

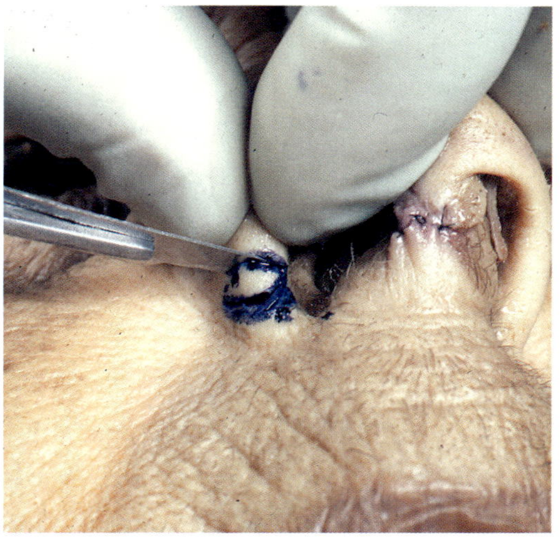

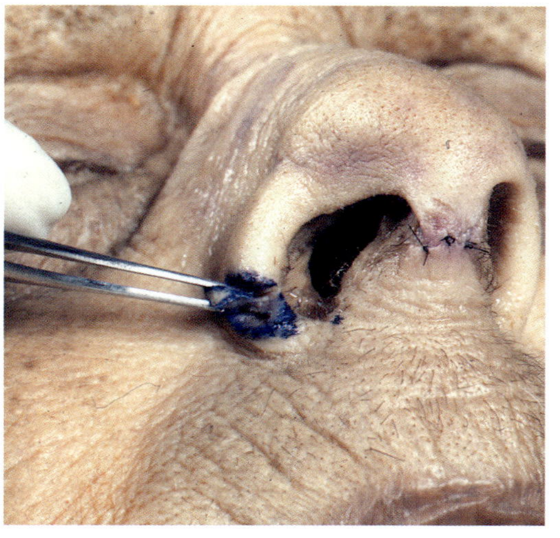

Figs. 63 and 64. The second skin incision followed by resection of the wedge.

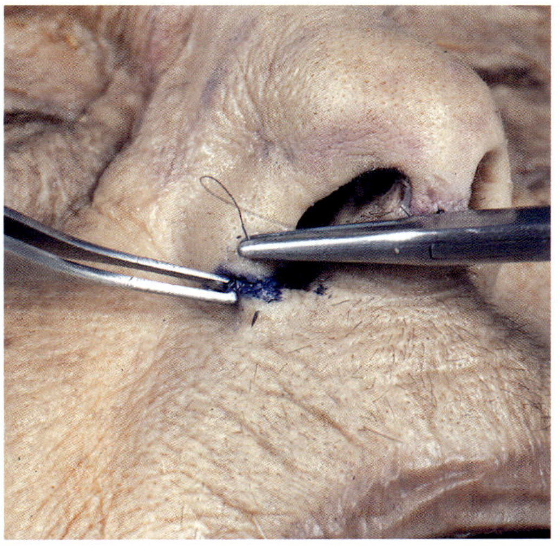

Fig. 65. Suturing the skin incision with 6/0 ethilon.

sected. The wedge can be V-shaped, inverted V-shaped, or rectangularly shaped.

There are three basic types of reduction:

– alar flair reduction
– nostril size reduction
– a combination of both

Choose your own type of alar base reduction. Outline the wedge to be resected on the skin. The skin incisions are made holding the alar lobule with the thumb and forefinger. The posterior skin incision (No. 15 blade) in the alar base should be approximately 2 mm on the lobular side and not in the alar groove, followed by the anterior skin incision. In case of resection of the vestibular skin,

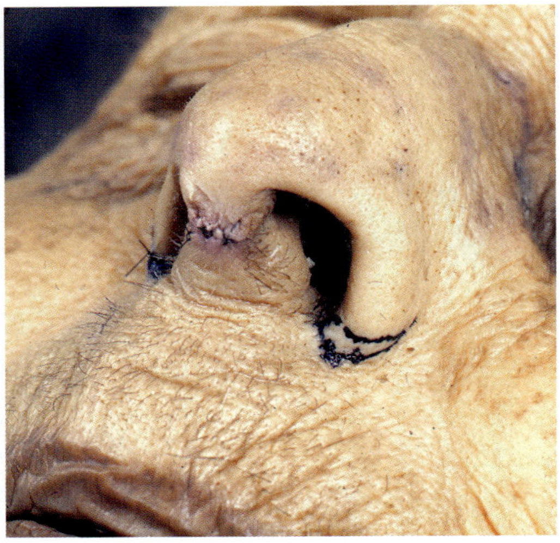

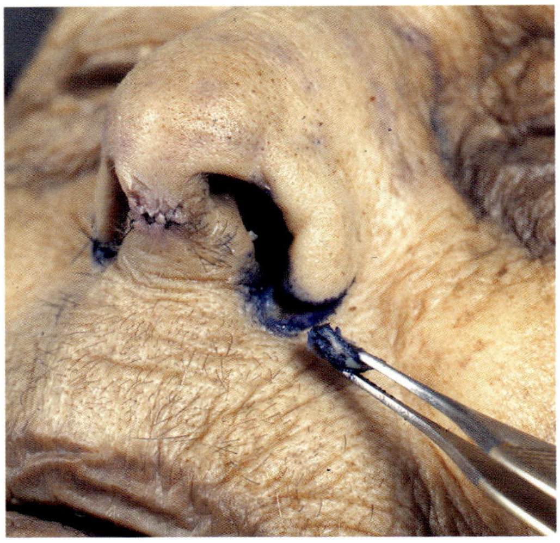

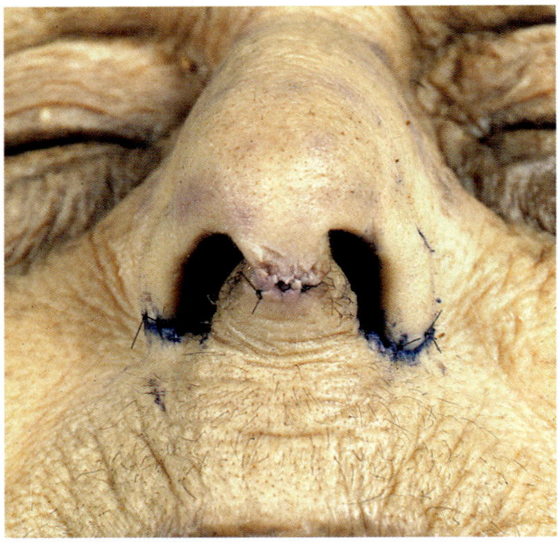

Figs. 66, 67 and 68. Marking a wedge for nostril size reduction, followed by resection and suturing. Note the difference in nostril size.

the skin margin in the nostril should be slightly baffled in order to prevent inversion of the skin after suturing. Break the straight line of the incision at the nostril sill with a 'hockey-stick' type incision in order to conserve the natural rounding of the nostril sill). Skin closure with 6/0 ethilon (P-1 needle).

Auricular composite graft and island flap

Instruments: No. 15 blade; rhinoplasty scissors, curve, sharp, and Killner-type scissors; micro skin hooks; Adson Brown tissue forceps (side grasping teeth); needle holder

Partial conchal composite graft

Mark the skin to be used for a composite graft at the anterior side of the concha. Use the postauricular approach (for the conchal graft harvesting technique, see page 238). Before starting the harvesting procedure postauricularly, circumcise the skin area and perichondrium anteriorly up to the conchal cartilage. Dissect the cartilage together with the marked and circumcised skin area by a postauricular approach. Prepare an island flap by cir-

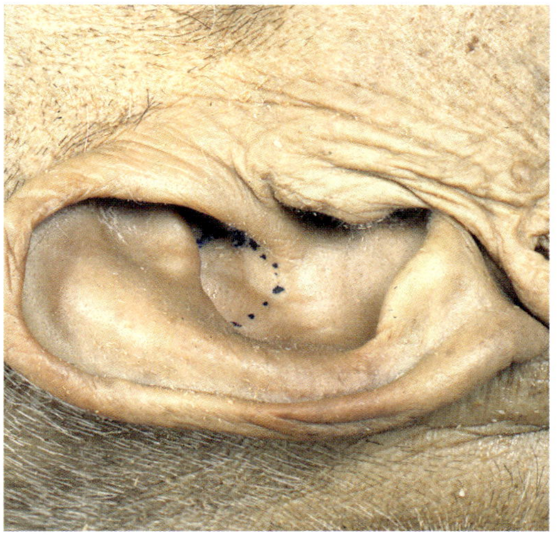

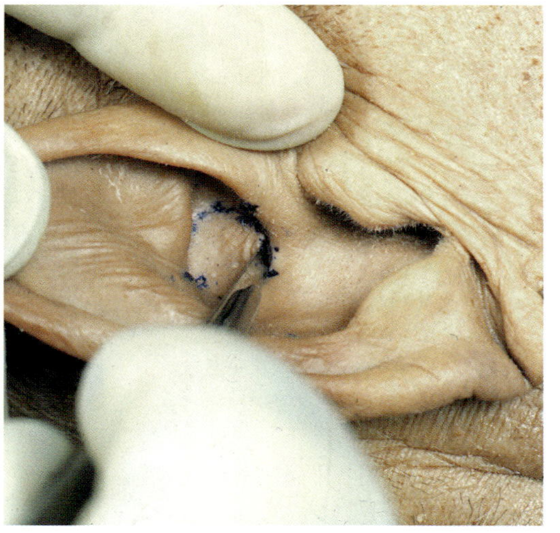

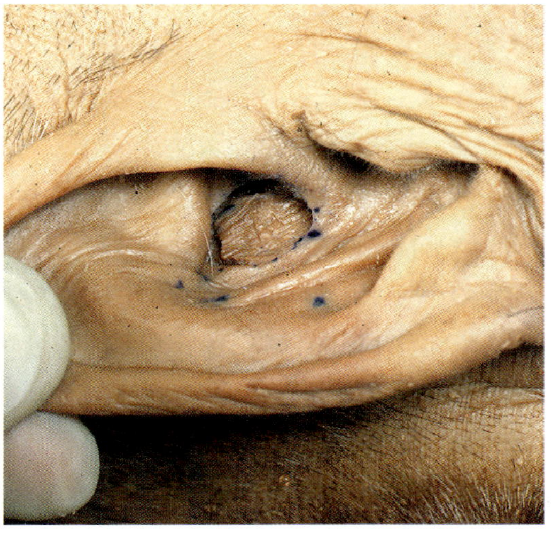

Figs. 69, 70 and 71. Marking and circumcising the chosen skin area of the partial conchal composite graft.

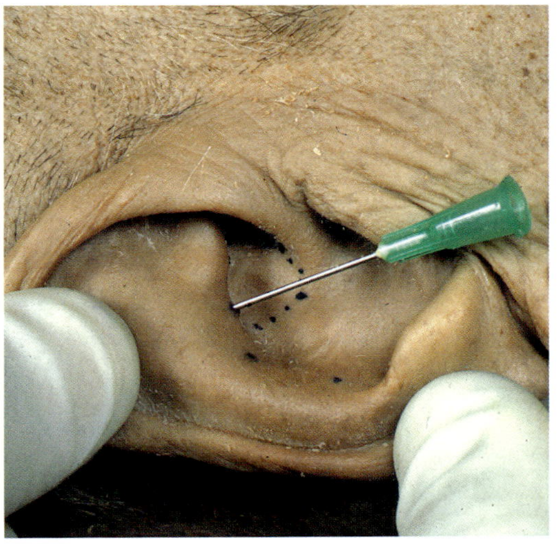

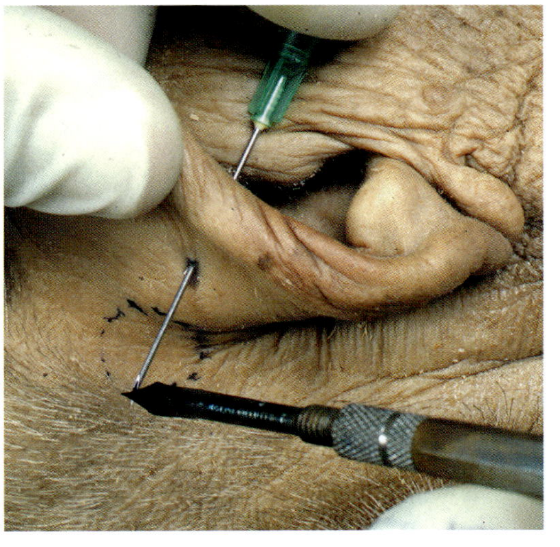

Figs. 72 and 73. Marking the skin and cartilage incision.

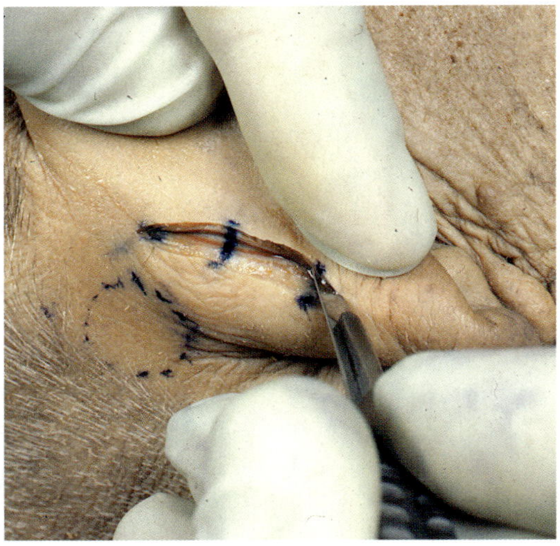

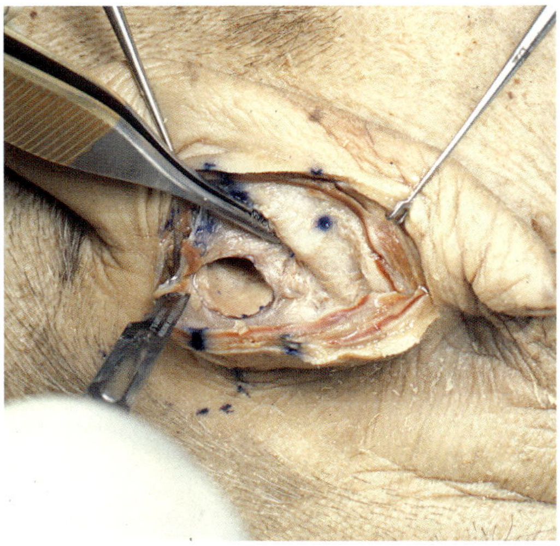

Figs. 74 and 75. Skin and cartilage incision along the marking points, followed by subperichondrial dissection at the anterior side up to the composite area, and supraperichondrial dissection on the posterior side.

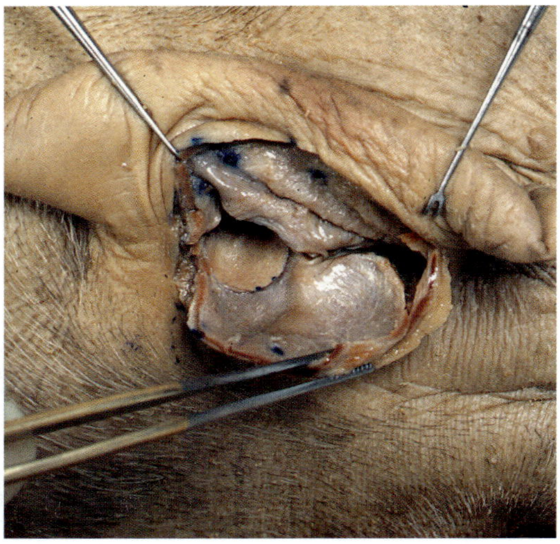

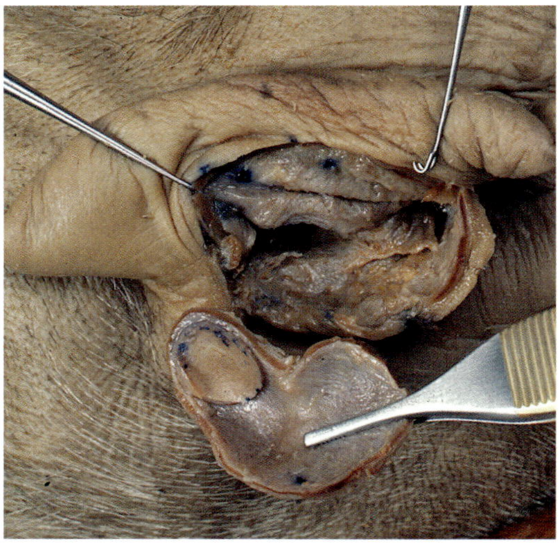

Figs. 76 and 77. Harvesting the 'partial' composite graft.

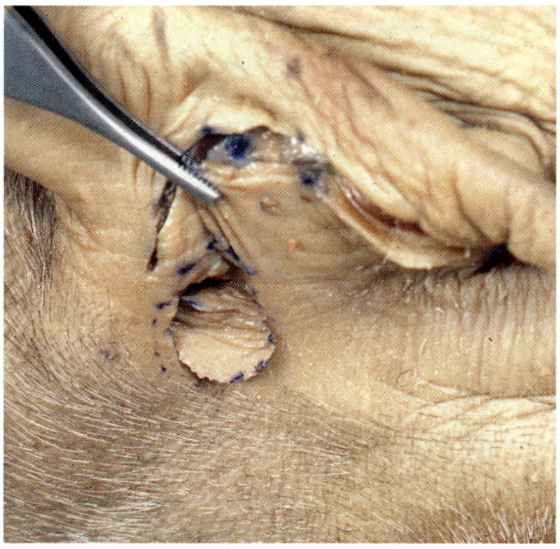

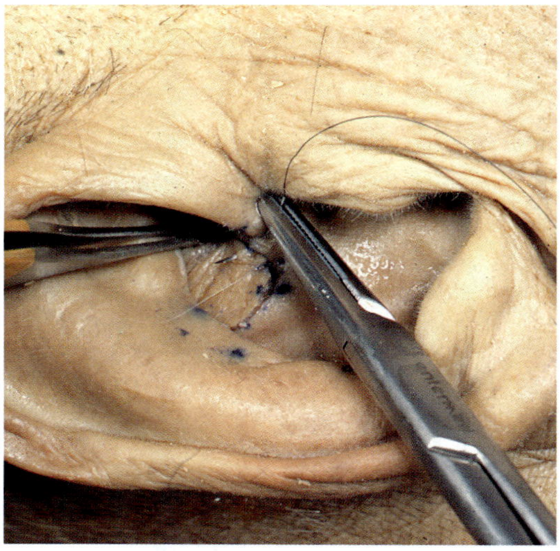

Figs. 78 and 79. Preparing the island flap, followed by suturing the flap *in situ* at the donor site.

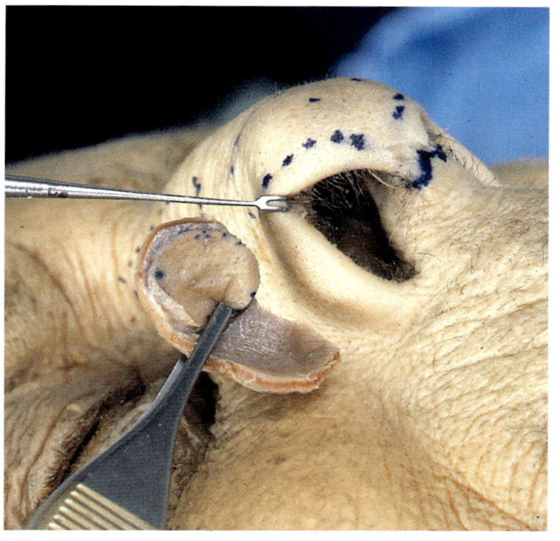

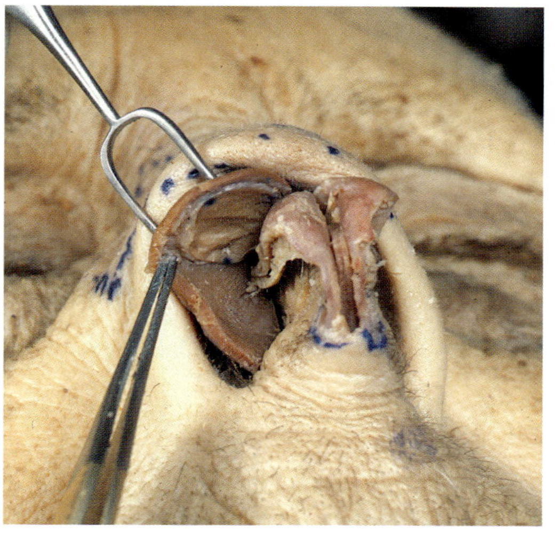

Figs. 80 and 81. Composite graft as used in cases of anterior vestibular stenosis.

cumcising the appropriate amount of skin retro-auricularly and medially to the auricular sulcus, followed by subcutaneous dissection. The next step is to bring the mobilized skin flap through a subcutaneous tunnel to the conchal donor site. Suture the island flap *in situ* and close the island donor site with 5/0 ethilon and a P-1 needle. An alternative is to use a full-thickness skin graft from the same postauricular region.

Complete conchal composite graft

Circumcise the skin and corresponding conchal cartilage (anterior side inside the antihelix, inferior crus and helical crus). Dissect posteriorly in a supraperichondrial plane and harvest the large composite conchal graft. Prepare an island flap on the postauricular side of the auricular sulcus region not too far laterally, in order to prevent a postoperative 'glued-on' aspect of the auricle. Skin closure with 5/0 ethilon. For the accompanying illustrations, see Chapter 22, pages 230 and 231.

List of instruments

Blade holder
Cottle hammer
Nose speculum (half Killian)
Micro-osteotome (2 and 3 mm)
Hump osteotome (10 and 14 mm)
Micro skin hooks, one and two prongs
Aufricht nasal retractor
Ala double-hooked retractor
Rhinoplasty scissors, curved, sharp, 10 cm
Angled scissors (Walter/Converse type)
Adson Brown forceps (tissue, dressing, side grasping teeth)
Blakesley, small
Dissection scissors, Killner type
Periosteal elevator, Joseph type
Elevator, Cottle type
Tungsten carbide nasal rasps (7/8)
Needle holder

Suture material

4/0 vicryl with straight needle (5C-1)
5/0 vicryl P-3 needle
5/0 ethilon P-1 needle
6/0 ethilon P-1 needle

24: SEPTOPLASTY – BASIC TECHNIQUES
The nasal septum in rhinoplasty

F.W.A. Otten

Introduction

Septal corrections form an important step in rhinoplastic surgery. Not only for functional, but also for aesthetic surgery the septum deserves attention. In the past the septum has been submitted to resection of bone and cartilage with sometimes even negative functional and cosmetic consequences. Nowadays, because of its supporting function, one tries in a septoplasty to operate as conservative as possible by preserving and reconstructing the septum.

The nasal septum consists of a posterior bony and an anterior cartilaginous part. Figure 1 shows a cadaver dissection specimen of the septum. The bony septum has two components: the vomer and the perpendicular plate. The anterior cartilaginous part, consisting of a quadrangular cartilage and two upper lateral cartilages, is a very important supporting structure of the nose (Fig. 2a,b). A straight and firm cartilaginous septum contributes to the contours of the external cartilaginous nose and an efficient airway (Fig. 3a,b). This means that anatomic malformations of the cartilaginous septum can cause functional and aesthetic complaints.

Functional complaints are often the result of cartilaginous septal deviations in the anterior nose. This area is the narrowest part of the nose (Fig. 3b). Small anatomical abnormalities give immediately rise to nasal airway obstruction.

Aesthetic complaints are seen in 'high' and anterior cartilaginous septal deviations resulting in a twisted cartilaginous nasal dorsum, an asymmetric columella or nasal tip (Figs.19a and 28a). A cartilaginous septal defect results in a depression of the nasal dorsum (Fig. 38a), while an overdeveloped dorsal or caudal part of the septum can result respectively in a cartilaginous dorsal hump, a blunt nasolabial angle or a 'hanging columella' (Figs 25a, 33a).

The bony septum has less supporting function than the cartilaginous septum and causes less functional problems as the nose is posteriorly much wider (Fig. 3b). As a

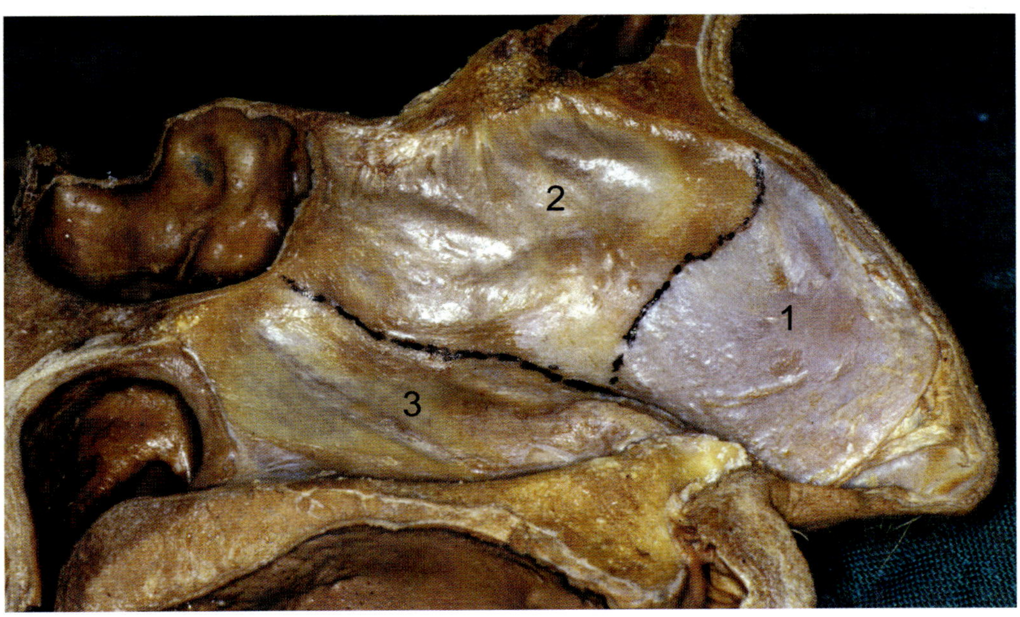

Fig. 1. The nasal septum exists of the quadrangular cartilage or the anterior cartilaginous septum (1), the perpendicular plate of the ethmoid (2) and the vomer (3).

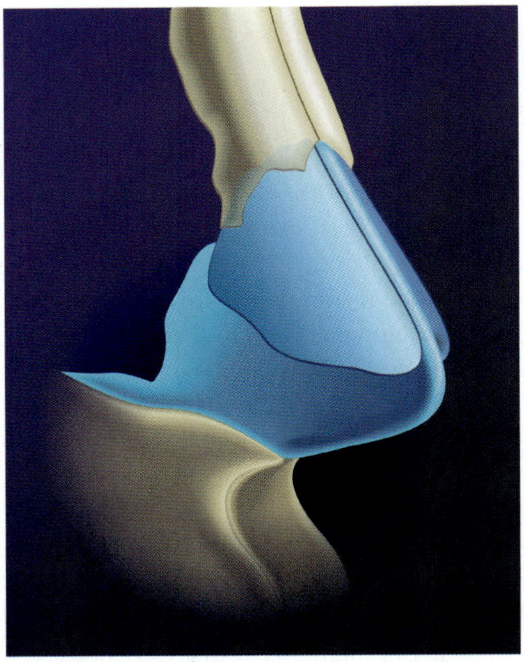
a

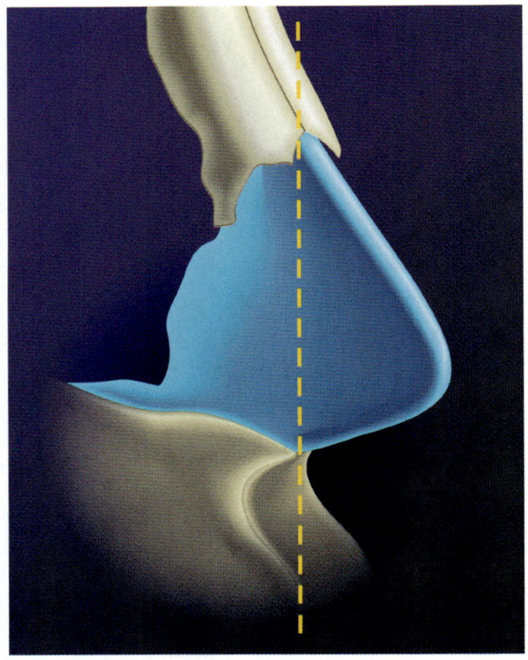
b

Fig. 2a. The cartilaginous septum and the upper laterals form one cartilaginous structure. *b.* The septal cartilage right of the dotted line forms the most important supporting component of the septum, determines the contours of the external cartilaginous nose and is important for a patent nasal airway.

result the bony septum is easier to handle.

Septoplasty frequently is the initial step in rhinoplasty because realignment of the septum, as the midline supporting structure of the nose, is essential for successful functional results, nasal tip and bony pyramid surgery.

The standard approach to the septum

As the cartilaginous septum is an important supporting structure, it has to be operated as conservatively as possible. By dissecting as little as possible, most of the mutual connections of this supporting structure can be left intact with the rest of the nasal skeleton. This goal can be achieved in the majority of the cases by tunneling the anterior septum only on one side, leaving the contralateral mucoperichondrium intact. The tunnel is made on the side where one has space for handling. If one has to deal with an inferior deviation of the septum a bottom tunnel is also created on the same side in order to visualize that part of the septum that has to be corrected. After dissecting the cross-fibers of the covering connective tissue at the base of the septum the anterior and bottom tunnel become one compartment, which gives a good view of the septum and its underlying premaxilla. The above mentioned procedure is schematically seen in Figures 4a-d. Subsequently the septal tunnel is enlarged in a posterior direction by elevating the mucoperiosteal flap of the bony septum on the same side. By blunt division of the junction between the carti-

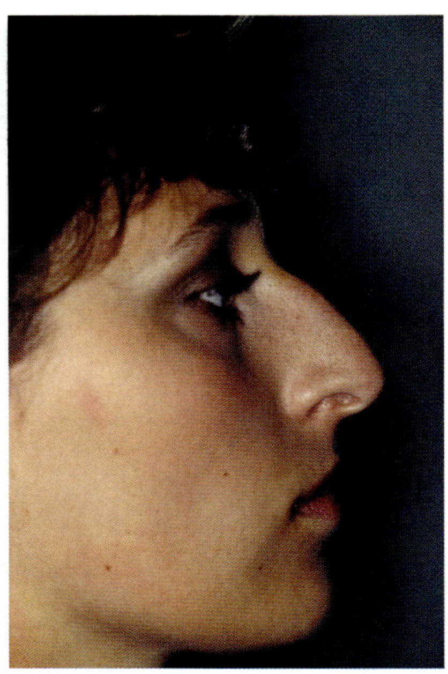
a

Fig 3a. Strong nasal profile because of a 'high' anterior cartilaginous septum.

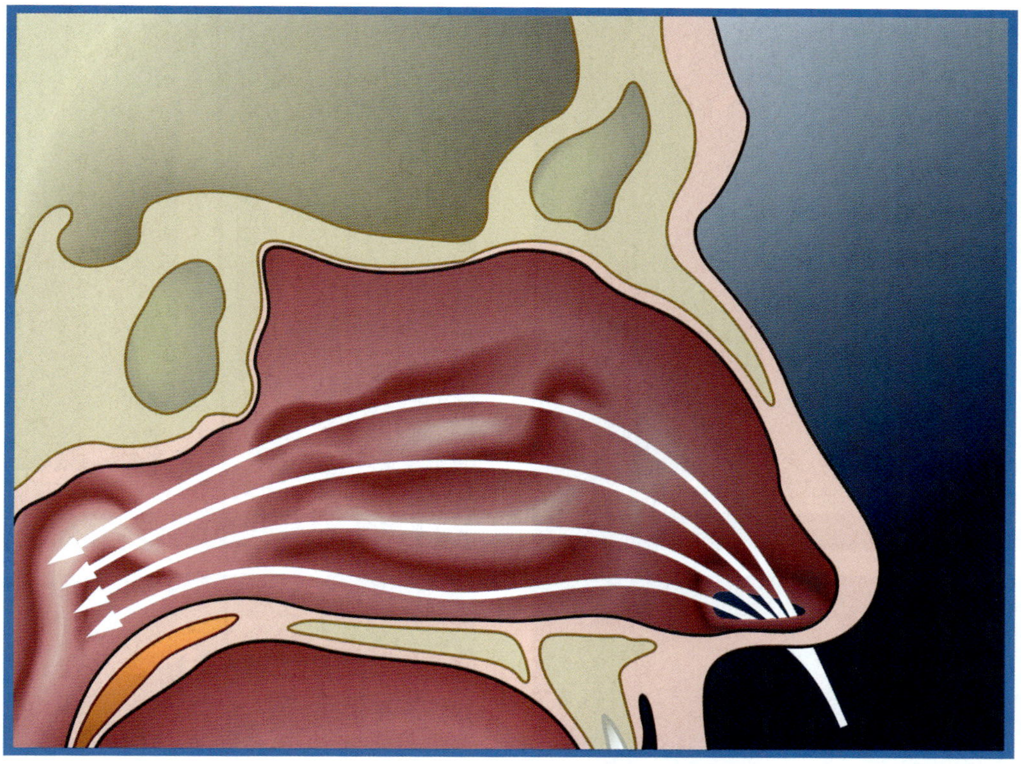

Fig 3b. Cross-section of the nasal cavity to indicate the narrowness of the anterior nose in relation to the posterior nose.

b

laginous and bony septum, the mucoperiosteal flap on the contralateral side of the bony septum can also be elevated (Fig. 4e). By this standard approach the whole septum can be reached.

Cadaver dissection illustrates this procedure in Figures 5a-c. Blunt division of the cartilaginous and bony septum ('posterior chondrotomy') must not be carried out too high because then the cartilaginous septum loses completely the support of the bony septum and pyramid in the important so-called 'K(eystone)-area', the highest point of connection between the bony and cartilaginous septum (Fig. 5c). This is especially the case when also a hump removal has to be done, as with this latter procedure the K-area is also weakened and reduced from above (Fig. 5d). If the K-area is destroyed it results in a so-called 'saddle nose' (see Fig. 38a). By leaving the mucoperichondrium on one side attached to the septum one creates in this situation more stability for this supporting structure.

After luxating the cartilaginous septum to one side, bony septal deviations can be taken out with a biting forceps, leaving the anterosuperior bony septum intact in order to preserve the K-area. Figure 5e shows this. The rest of the bony septum does not have an important supportive function. If necessary, crushed pieces of septal bone can be put back at the end of the operation, preventing eventual mucosal atrophy in the long run.

Before or after this correction of the bony septum, the cartilaginous septum can be realigned from the one-sided anterior tunnel in about 90% of the cases. Resect as conservatively as possible and reconstruct the cartilage in the midline in order to preserve its supportive function. See for an example Figures 5f,g.

Tunneling on both sides, with resection of bony and cartilaginous parts of the septum, creates the risk that the septum falls into the nose, pivoting around the K-area (Fig. 6a). This results in a less supporting function of the septum and consequently deprojection of the nasal tip (Figs. 6b,c).

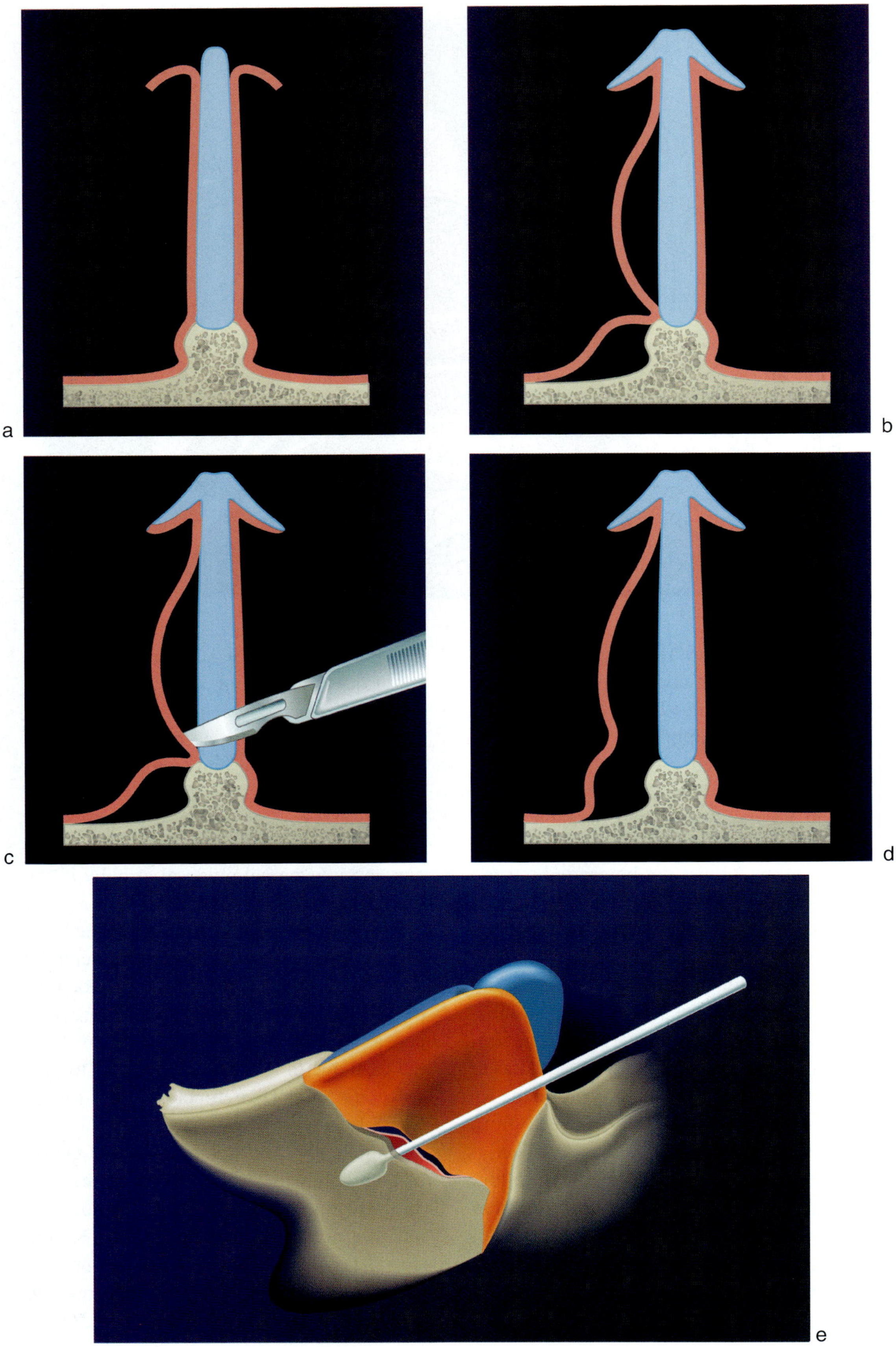

Fig. 4a-e. The standard approach to the septum: *a*. schematic cross-section of the anterior cartilaginous septum, *b*. anterior and bottom tunnel, *c*. dissection of the basal cross-fibers, *d*. anterior and bottom tunnel form one compartment for a better view of the nasal septum and supporting premaxilla, *e*. posterior chondrotomy with formation of the contralateral posterior septal tunnel along the bony septum. The contralateral anterior mucoperichondrium stays attached to the cartilaginous septum for a better stability.

Fig. 5a-g. Cadaver dissection of the septum. *a*. One-sided septum tunneling. *b*. Dissection of the basal cross-fibers.

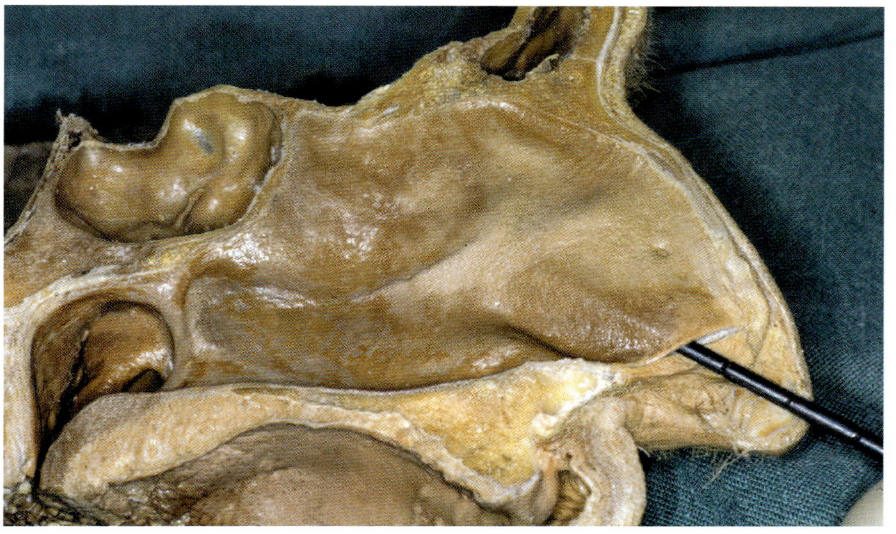

a

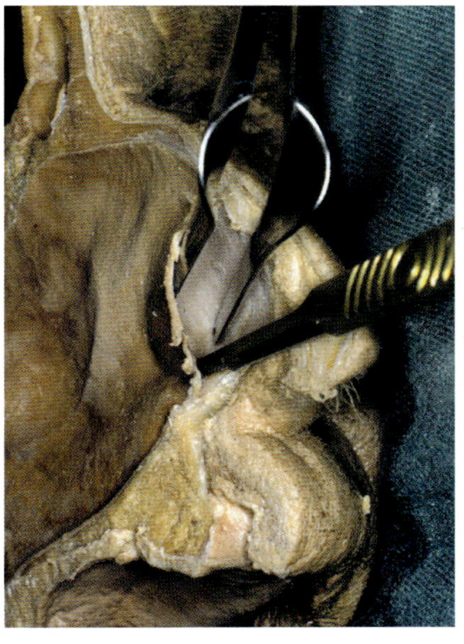

b

However, one could use this phenomenon in certain cases on purpose as a procedure to deproject the nose.

In general, a long hemitransfixion is made (Fig. 7a). In the subperichondrial plane an anterior tunnel is made on the same side (Fig. 7b). Spreading the mucoperichondrial flap of the anterior tunnel from the septum with a nasal speculum gives a good view of the cartilaginous septum. However, by subsequently pulling down the inferior corner of the long hemitransfixion incision with a small hook one creates in practice a much better exposure of the septum (Figs. 7c), particularly when the cross-fibers of the connective tissue between the anterior and bottom tunnel are also dissected with a knife under clear and direct vision (Fig. 7d,e).

The situations that can be encountered in practice are described below. For 'preoperative management and anesthesia' see elsewhere in this book.

Functional corrections of the septum

The convex deviated high anterior septum

In this case the too high septum is still in place on the maxillary crest. After creating an anterior septal tunnel with a blunt elevator on the concave side, the firm basal attachments of the mucosa to the caudal septum and maxillary crest are dissected with a knife. After freeing the caudal edge of the cartilaginous septum and the maxillary crest from their overlying mucosa, the two structures are separated bluntly from each other so that a caudal sliver can be resected from the oversized cartilaginous septum. The mucoperichondrium on the contralateral side of the septum is left in place. Care must be taken not to resect too

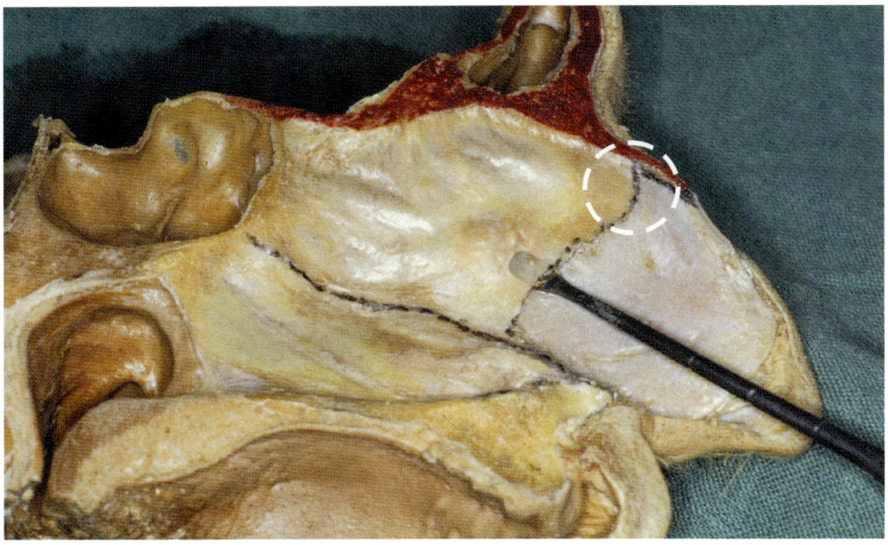

c

Fig. 5c. Posterior chondroto my; the white dotted circl indicates the K(stone)-area

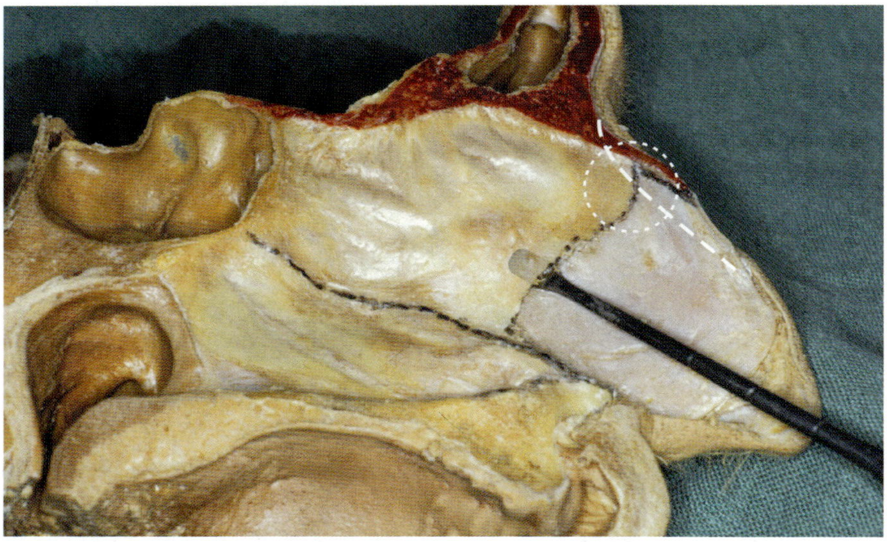

d

Fig. 5d. Relationship be tween K-area and dors hump resection.

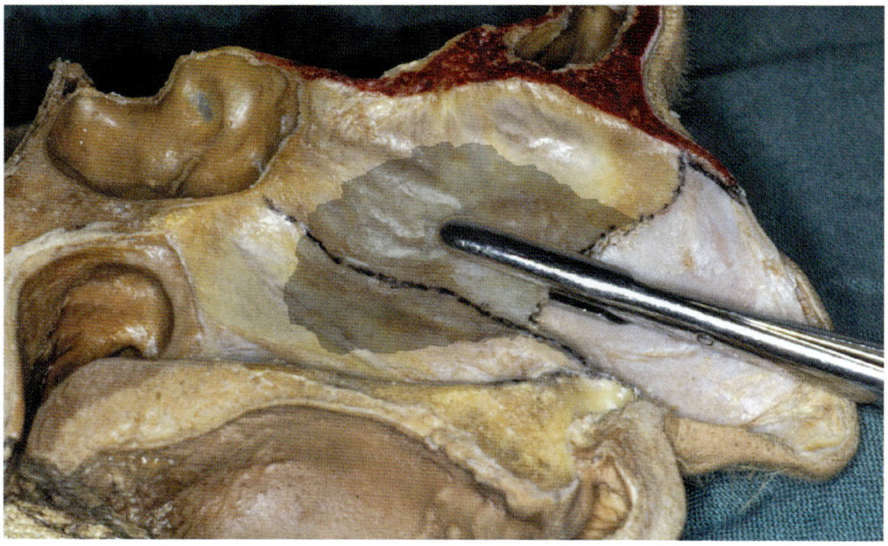

e

Fig. 5e. Area where normal deviated bony parts of th septum are removed.

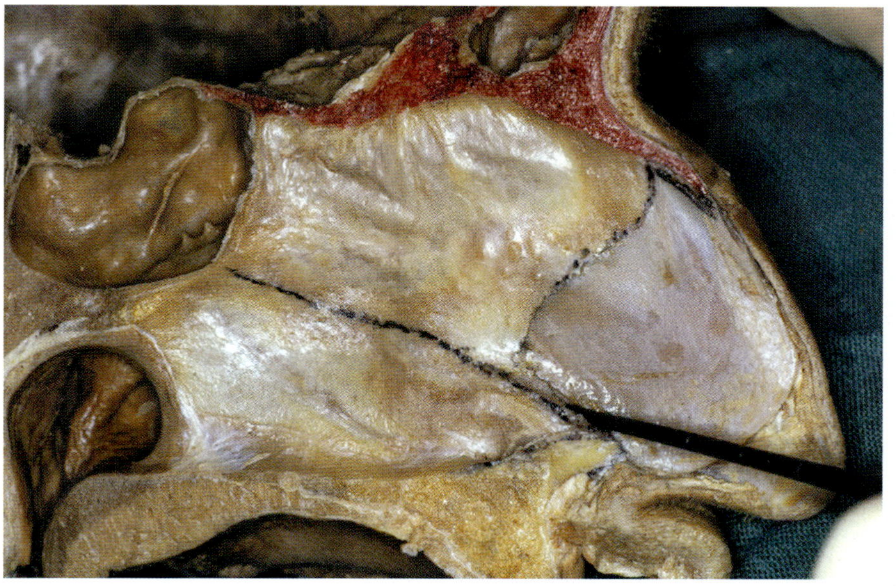

f

Fig. 5f. Luxation of the caudal border of the cartilaginous septum to the one-sided tunnel.

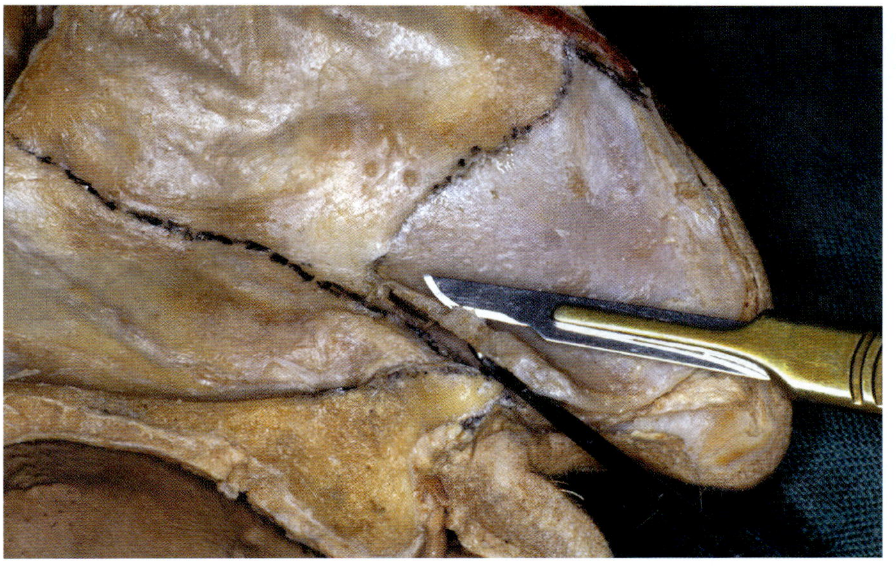

g

Fig. 5g. Resection of a basal strip in case of a too high and/or luxated septum.

much in order to preserve the supporting function of the septum (Figures 8a,b,c and 5f,g). The cartilaginous septum can now be realigned with the midline, stabilized by the attached contralateral mucoperichondrium.

There are situations where the septum will hold its curved position (Fig. 9a,b). In these cases one can straighten the cartilage by scoring on the concave side, breaking the interlocked stress of the cartilage. Simultaneously the elasticity of the contralateral mucoperichondrium helps to realign the septum (Fig. 9c,d). The attached mucoperichondrium on the convex side gives stability to the scored cartilaginous pieces, even if the cartilage has been cut through completely. This situation can be further strengthened by a 4x0 Vicryl through-and-through suture, situated above and beneath the deflection, whilst being knotted on the convex side (see Figure 9e).

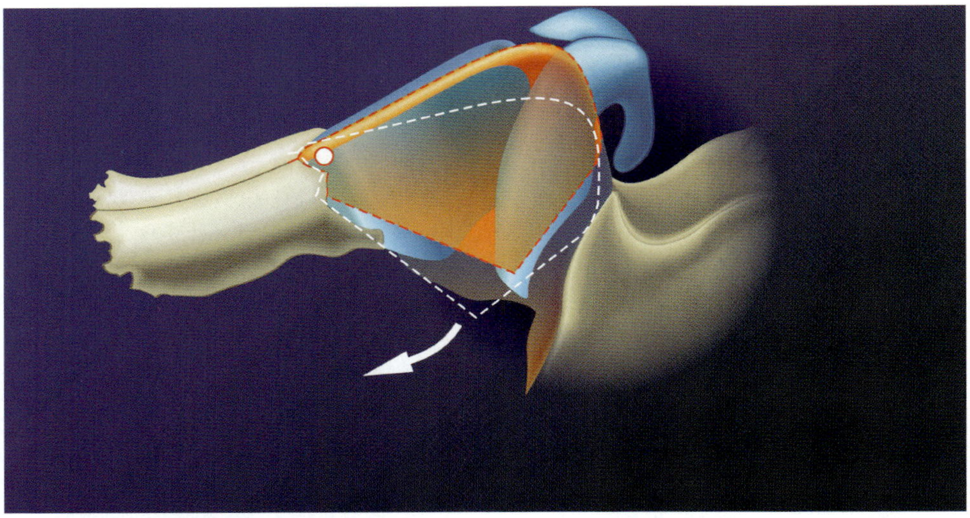

a

Fig. 6a. Schematic illustration of deprojection of the nose as a result of loss of septum support. This can happen after tunnelling the septum on both sides, resection of anterior parts of the bony septum and caudal parts of the cartilaginous septum.

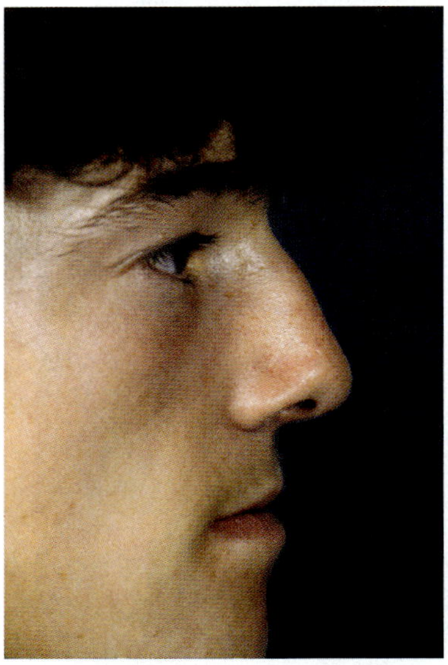

b

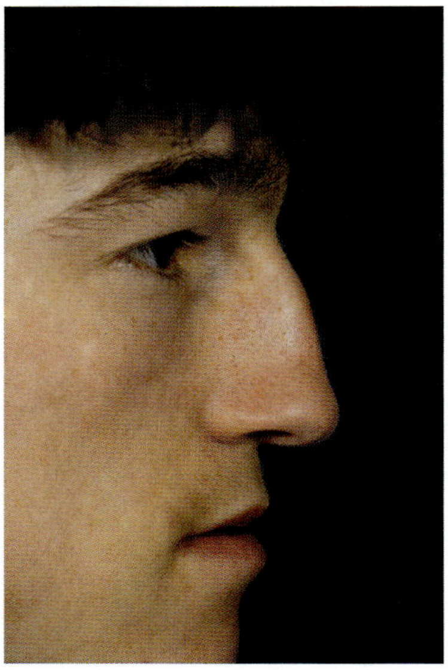

c

Fig. 6b. Patient before septum surgery. *c.* Postoperative view of the same patient: deprojection of the nose as a result of loss of septum support after septum surgery.

The luxated anterior septum

In this scenario the septum stands beside the maxillary crest (Fig. 10a). Consequently the anterior septal tunnel is for handling best when made on the contralateral side. Through the junction between the cartilaginous septum and the maxillary crest, the nasal floor on the other side of the nose can be reached by lifting the luxated septum (Fig. 5f and 10b,c). With this maneuver, the luxated septum is freed on the caudal side. After elevating the mucoperiosteum from a part of the contralateral nasal floor, the luxated septum can be pulled back and repositioned in the midline on the maxillary crest (Fig. 10d).

In case of an oversized luxated cartilaginous septum, the caudal border can be reduced in the same way as the previously mentioned resecting procedure, leaving the mucosa as a stabilizing factor on the contralateral side intact (Fig. 11a-d). The septum can be secured in the midline with a suture around the anterior nasal spine as illustrated in Figure 12.

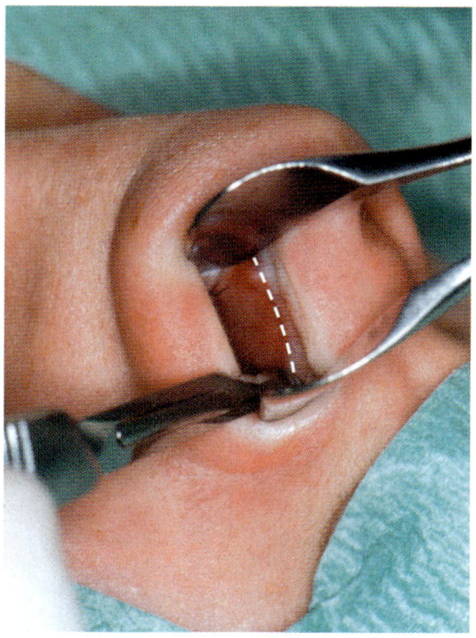

Fig. 7a. Hemitransfixion.

a

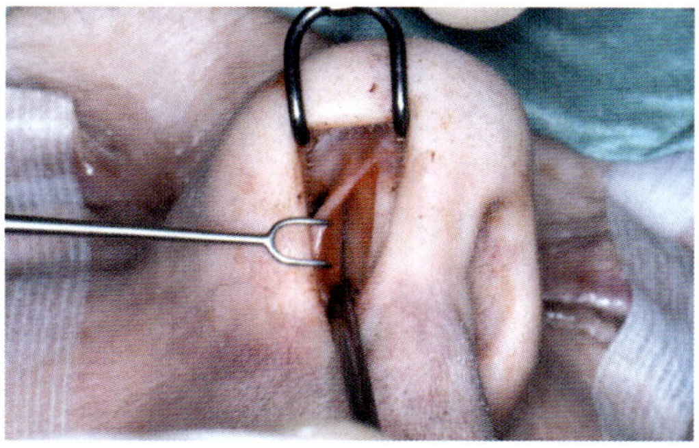

b

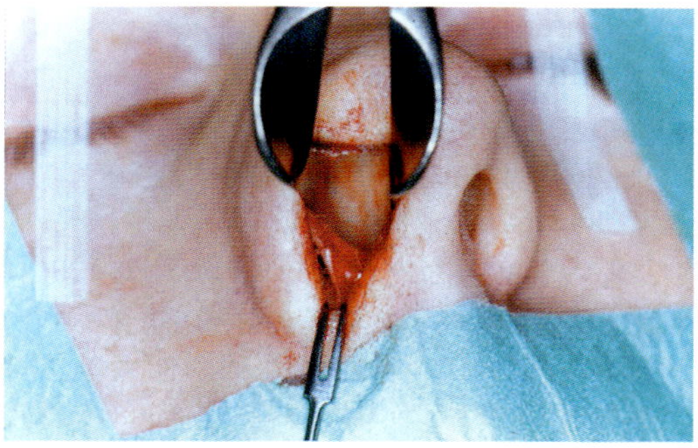

c

Fig. 7b. Anterior septum tunnel. *c.* Exposition of the caudal septum and premaxilla region by means of a small hook.

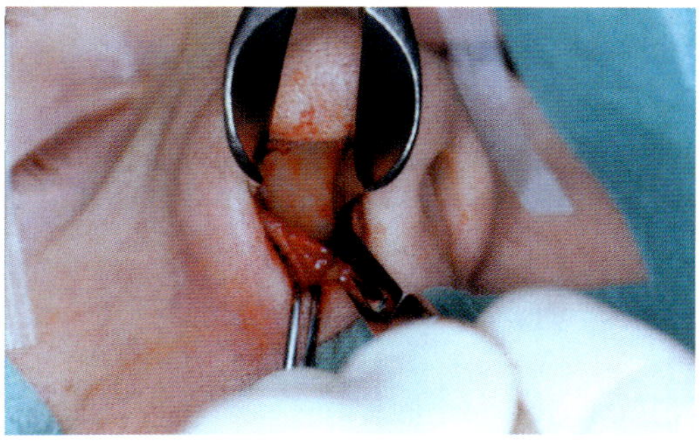

d

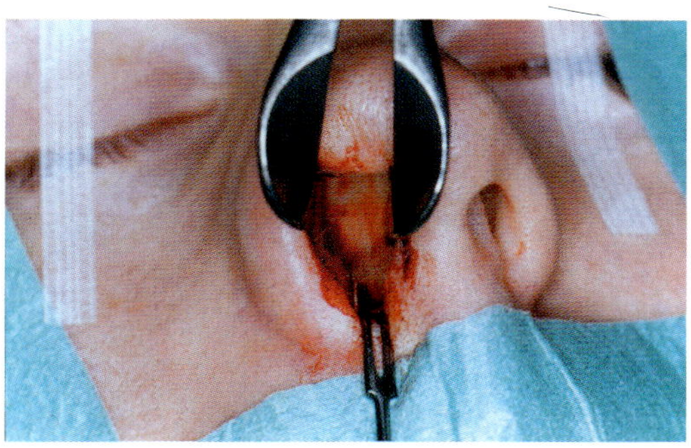

e

Fig. 7d. Dissection of the covering basal connective tissue. *e.* Exposition of anterior and bottom tunnel as one compartment.

The septal ridge and spur

Most of the time, a septal ridge is situated along the border of the cartilaginous septum and vomer. A ridge often tapers to a spur or spine. This malformation can best be reached and corrected from the contralateral side like in the luxated septum. After resecting the deviated part of the cartilaginous septum, the bony part of the ridge and spur are freed from the mucosa on the contralateral side, according to the standard approach, and taken out with a biting forceps or fractured into the midline.

Fracture lines of the septum

Fracture lines in the cartilaginous septum can run horizontally or vertically. In most cases the surplus or overlap of cartilage around the fracture lines has to be resected to realize realignment of the septum. This

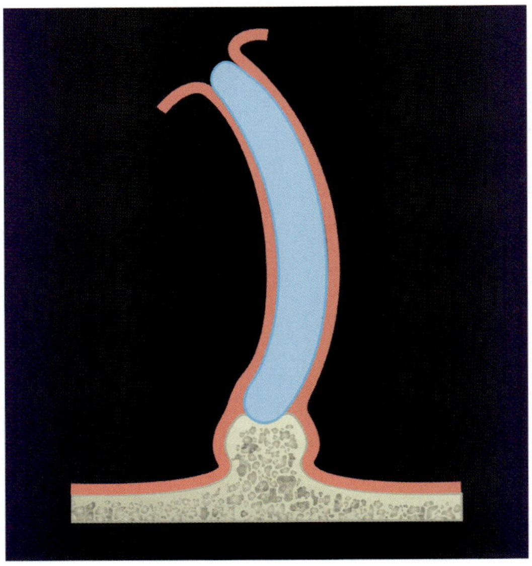
a

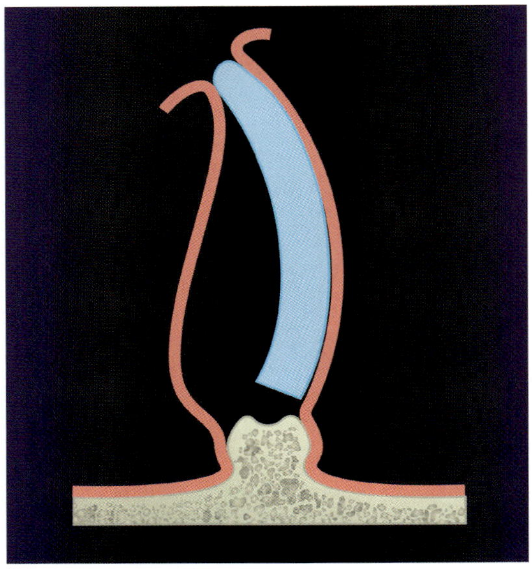
b

Fig. 8a. Convex deviated too high cartilaginous septum. *b.* Anterior septum-tunnel with resection of a basal strip of the too high anterior cartilaginous septum.

procedure is shown in a cadaver dissection in Figure 13. The resection can best be executed by using a hooked knife through a one-sided anterior septal tunnel, leaving the opposite mucosa intact to serve as a stabilizing structure (Fig. 14a). The new situation can be further fixed by putting mattress-sutures through the area of excision and the fractured pieces of the cartilaginous septum (Fig. 14b). In this situation the overlying contralateral mucosa is of great help in re-aligning this anterior septum and prevents overlap of the fractured pieces. An indication of what could occur after tunnelling on both sides is shown in Figures 14c and d.

The high septal deviations

Very high cartilaginous septal deviations are difficult to correct when they belong to the important supporting K-stone area of the septum (Fig. 5c). Resection of these malformations bear the risk of destroying this supporting area. A high deviation of the septum can be carefully realigned with a cartilage crusher (Fig. 15a,b). Crushing weakens and straightens the cartilage in this area, but leaves its supporting function intact.

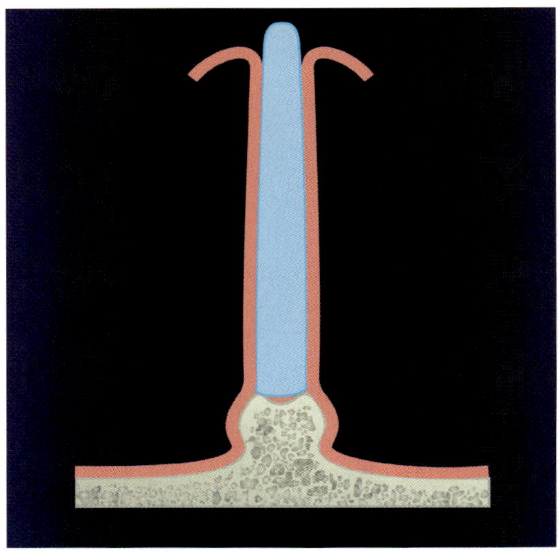
c

Fig. 8c. Spontaneous straightening of the cartilaginous septum after resection of the basal strip.

The anterior septal defect

An anterior cartilaginous septal defect (by trauma or previous surgery) results in loss of support of the cartilaginous nose. This results in functional and also cosmetic complaints. The septum has to be reconstructed by a columellar strut. Via a relatively posterior performed hemitransfixion incision a pocket is created in the membranous part of the septum and the columella, between the medial crura of the alar cartilages (Fig. 16). Be sure to cut all the bridges of scar tissue in this pocket in order to be able to introduce the new columellar strut properly. This

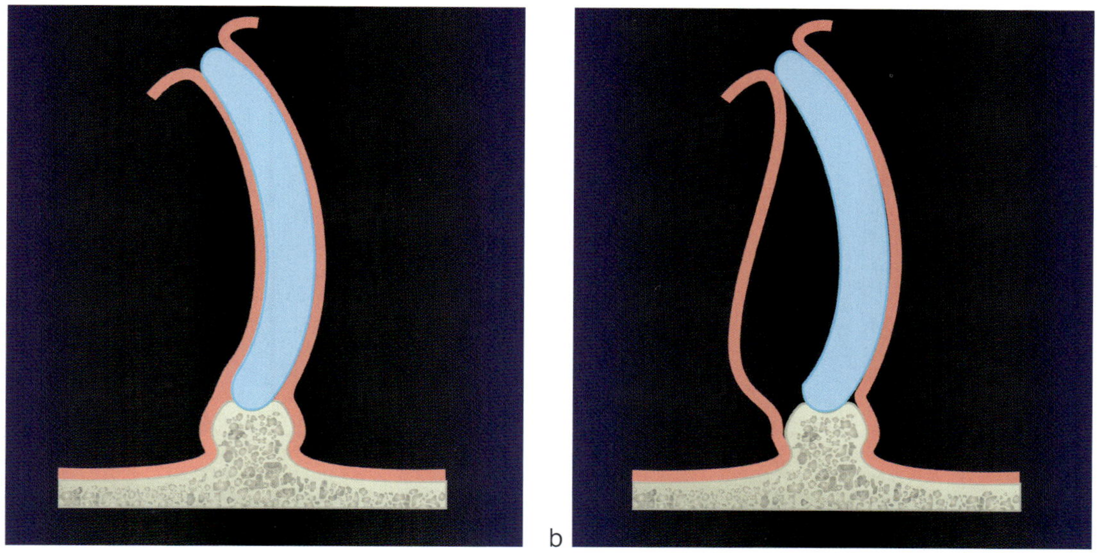
a b

Fig. 9a. Curved anterior cartilaginous septum.
b. Anterior septum tunnel without spontaneous straightening of the septum.

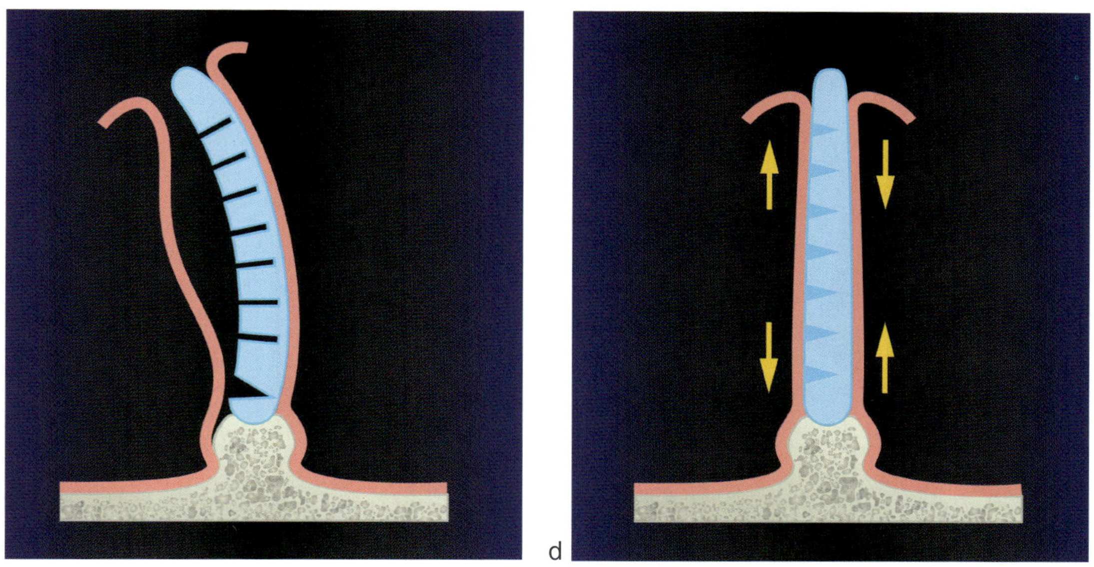
c d

Fig. 9c. Scoring of the concave side of the septum. *d.* Straightening of the septum as a result of (1) the broken interlocked stress in the cartilage, and (2) the elasticity of the contralateral mucoperichondrium.

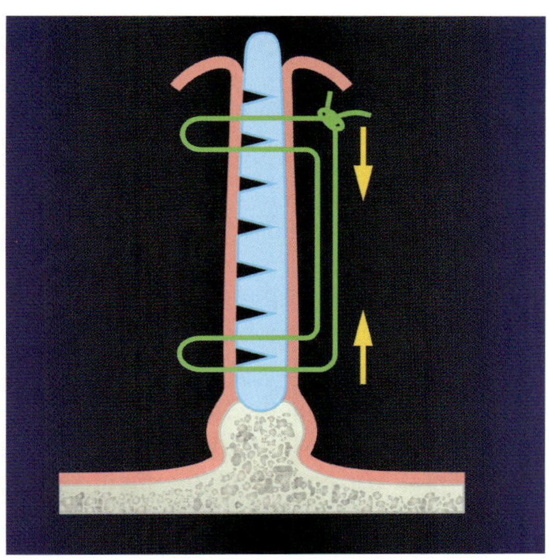
e

Fig. 9e. Stabilization of the new position of the septum with a through-and-through suture.

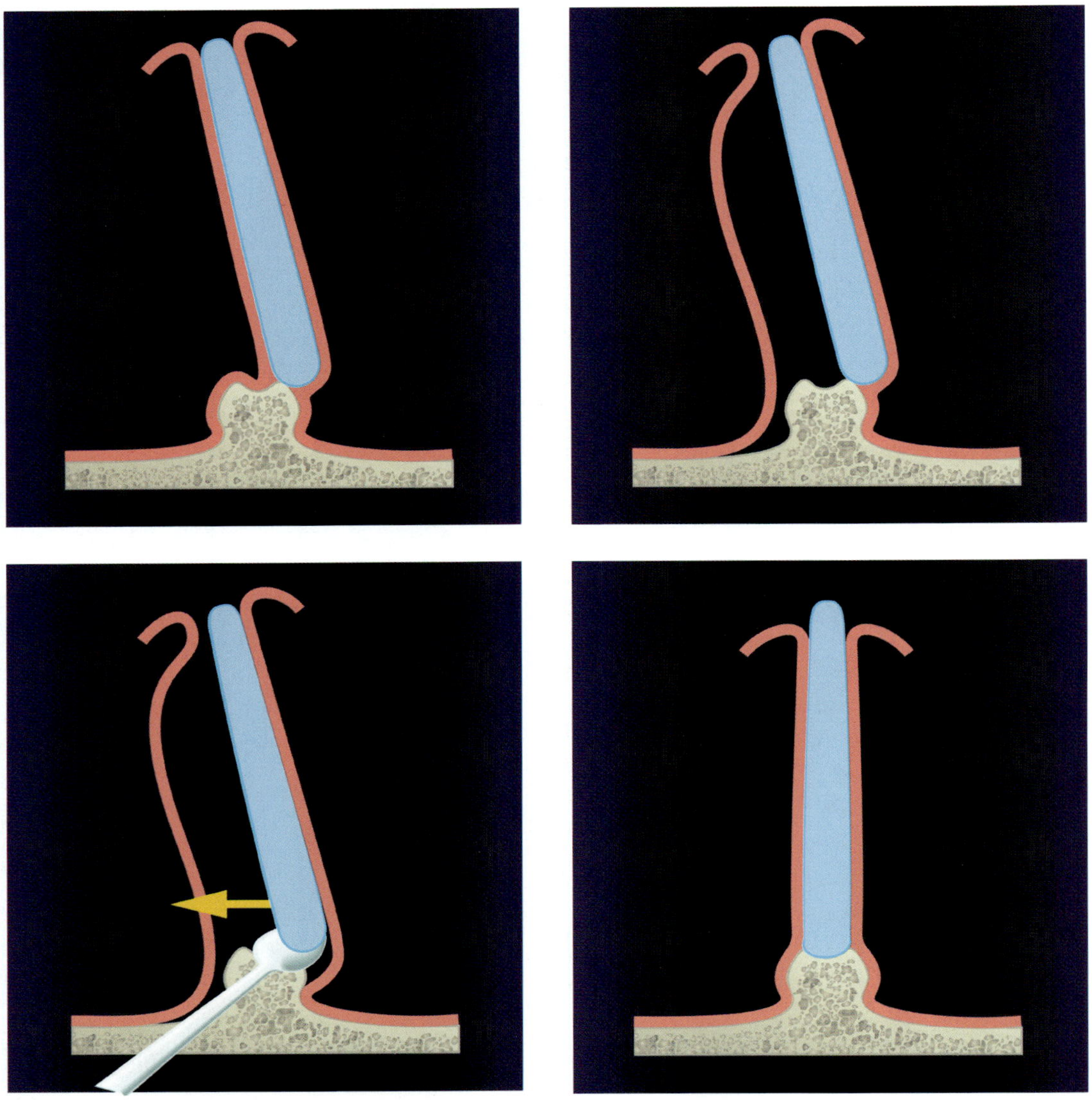

a b

Fig. 10a. Luxated anterior cartilaginous septum.
b. Anterior and bottom tunnel.

c d

Fig. 10c. Freeing and lifting of the anterior septum from the maxillary crest.
d. Repositioned septum in the midline.

strut is made of posterior septal or ear cartilage, placed on the anterior nasal spine and fixed with mattress-sutures upon introduction in the columellar pocket (Fig 17a,b.). The new support of the strut opens the anterior nose in the valve area. Figures 18a and b show the effect of this maneuver on the appearance of the external nose.

Aesthetic corrections of the septum

In rhinoplasty, cosmetic goals can regularly be reached by corrections of the nasal septum. By looking in greater detail at the septum, one can analyse which part has to be corrected in order to reach a certain aesthetic goal.

Some of these situations are described below.

The twisted cartilaginous nasal dorsum

A high deviation of the cartilaginous nasal septum can result in a twisted cartilaginous nasal dorsum on the outside (Fig. 19a). In these circumstances the upper lateral cartilages are often asymmetric. Besides a routine septal correction, realignment of the dorsal side of the septum can best be

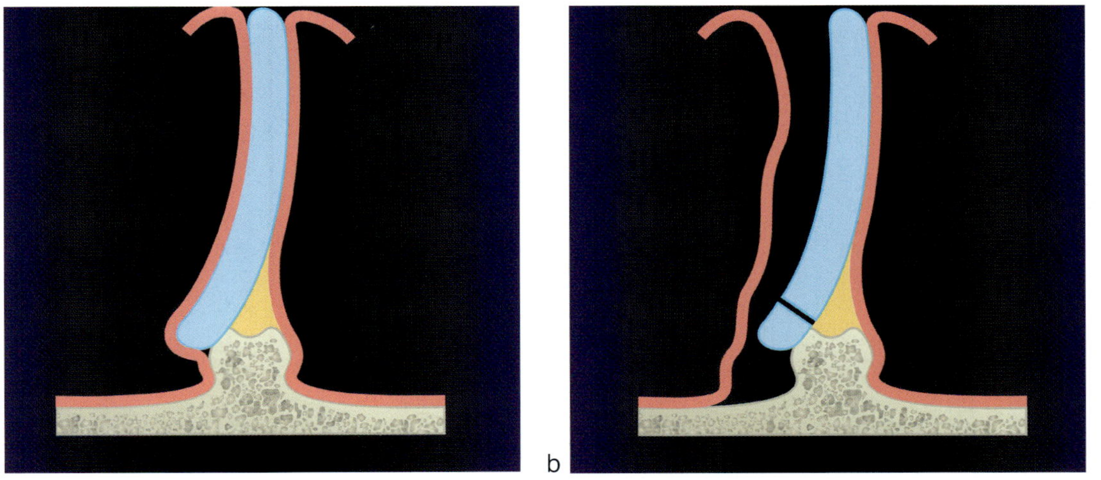

a b

Fig. 11a. Luxated too high anterior cartilaginous septum. *b.* Anterior and bottom tunnel.

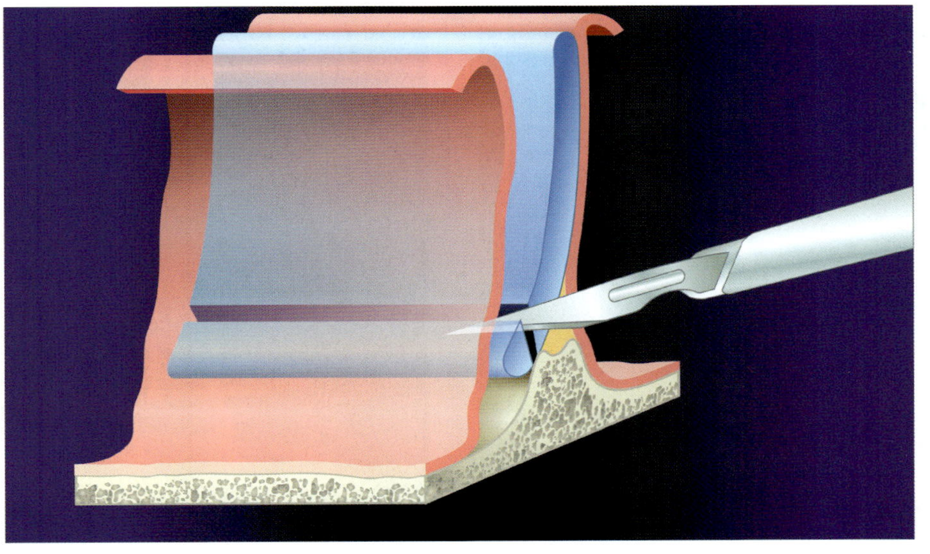

c

Fig. 11c. Dissection of a basal strip of the septum.

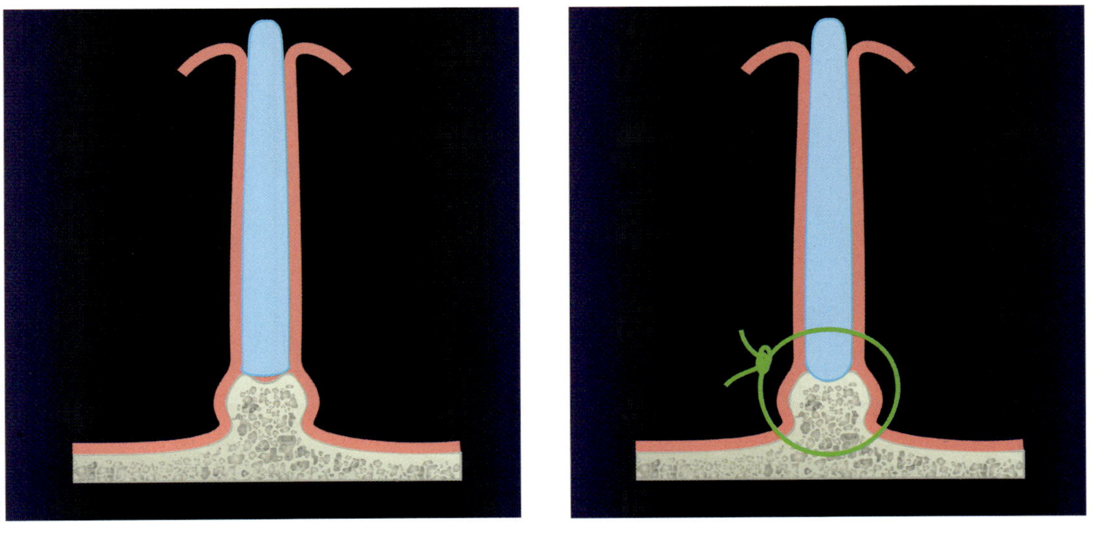

d

Fig. 11d. Realignment of the septum.

Fig. 12. Stabilization of the cartilaginous septum by suturing the basal septum to the nasal spine.

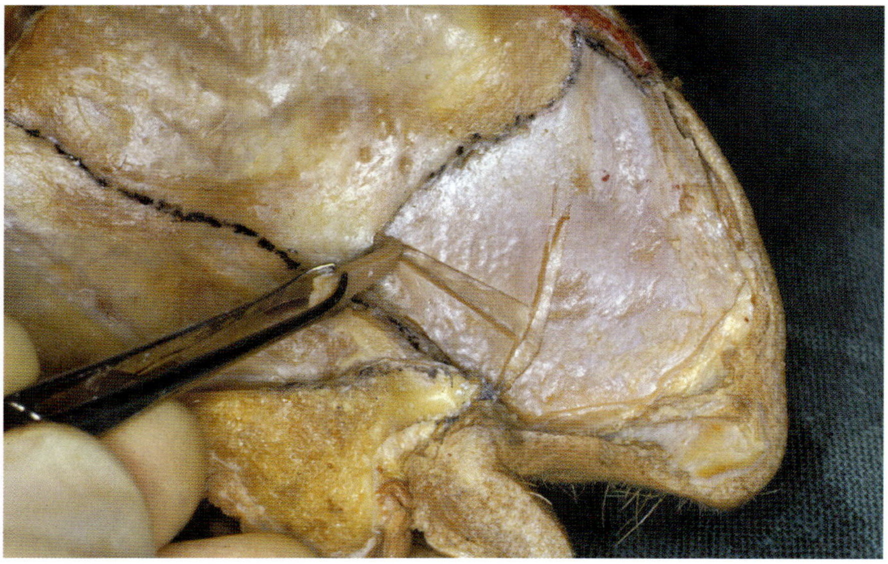

Fig. 13. Resection of the surplus of cartilage in a vertical and horizontal fracture line .

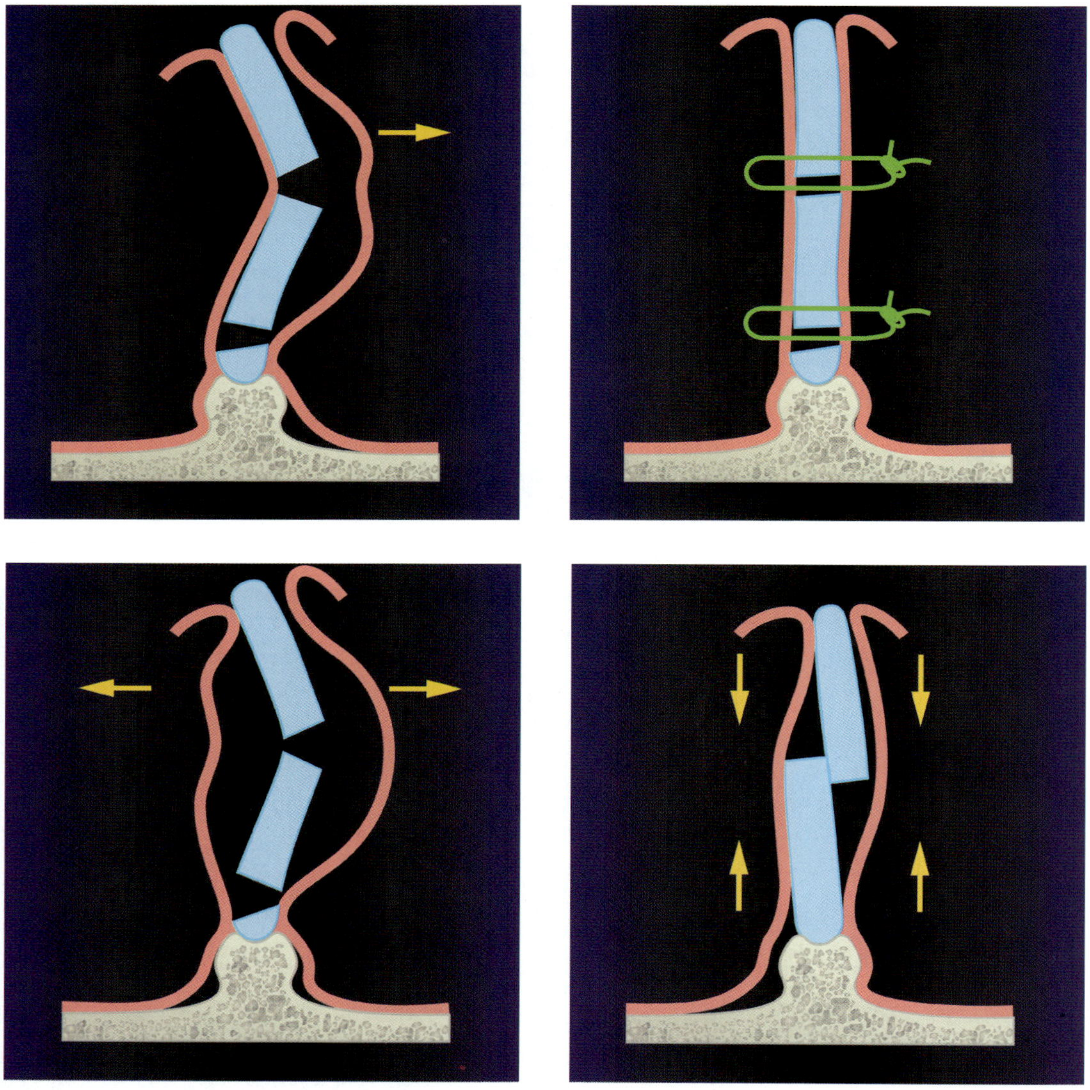

a b c d

Fig. 14a. Resection of fracture lines through a left-sided septum tunnel. Stabilization of the fracture pieces by means of the connected contralateral mucoperichondrium.
b. Realignment of the septum and fixation with through-and-through sutures.

Fig. 14c,d. Destabilization of the fractured cartilaginous septum after tunneling on both sides.

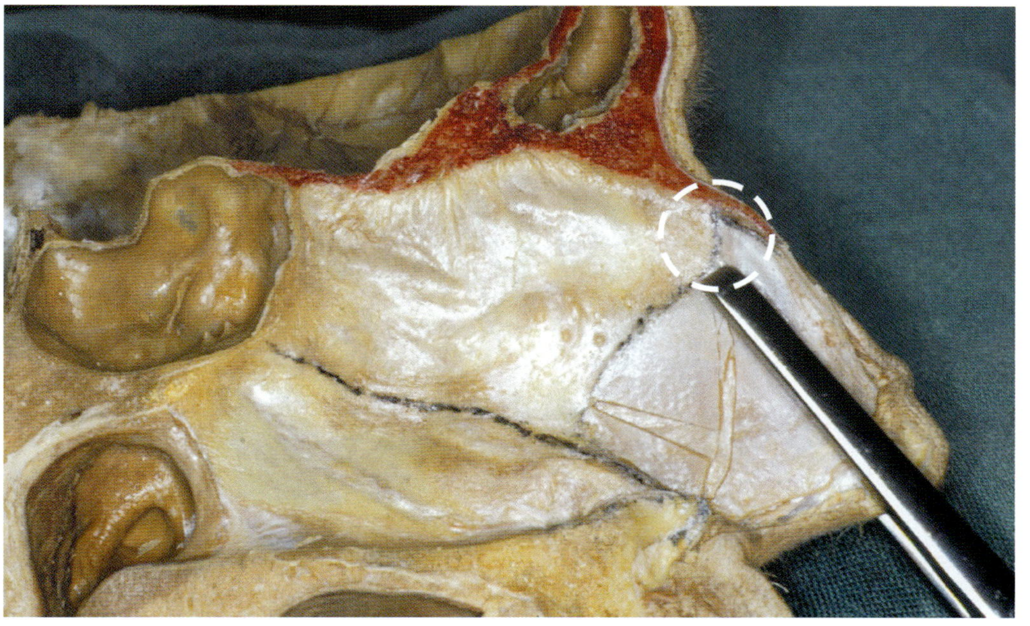

a

Fig. 15a. Crushing of a high septal deviation in the K-area.

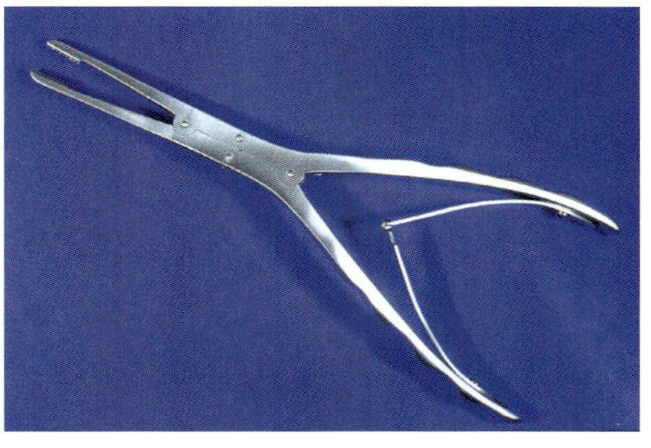

b

Fig. 15b. Cartilage crusher.

acquired after separating one (on the convex side of the septum) or both of the upper lateral cartilages from the nasal septum. This can carefully be done through the nasal cavity and cranial nasal mucosa with a knife (Fig. 20a). The nasal dorsum is palpated at the same time with a forefinger, feeling the knife coming through the cartilage underneath the nasal skin (Fig. 20b). The upper laterals realign automatically along the straightened septum. Suturing is not necessary.

The effect of this procedure is outlined in figures 21a-g. If necessary, the skin of the nasal dorsum can be elevated through the hemitransfixion incision (with scissors over the anterior septal angle) in order to free the dorsal side of the septum from its restrictive attachments to the skin (Fig. 22a, b). These maneuvers help to straighten the cartilaginous dorsum of the nose, as can be seen in Figure 19b. An alternative is introducing spreader grafts between the septum and the upper laterals by means of an open approach.

Nasal tip rotation

In case of downward rotation of the nasal tip, this is frequently the result of a too prominent anterior septal angle and adjacent caudal edge of the cartilaginous septum (Fig. 23a). Palpating with thumb and forefinger helps to diagnose this variation of septal anatomy. It can be corrected by merely resecting cartilage and overlying mucosa of the anterior septal angle and the adjacent caudal edge (Fig. 24a,b). After this simple procedure the nasal tip automatically rotates upwards as a result of the elasticity of the dorsal skin (Fig. 23b). Then the defect is closed primarily with resorbable sutures.

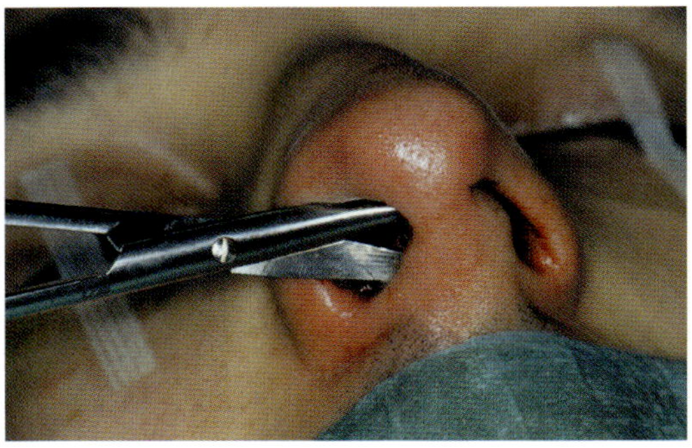

Fig. 16. Performing a columella pocket with curved scissors.

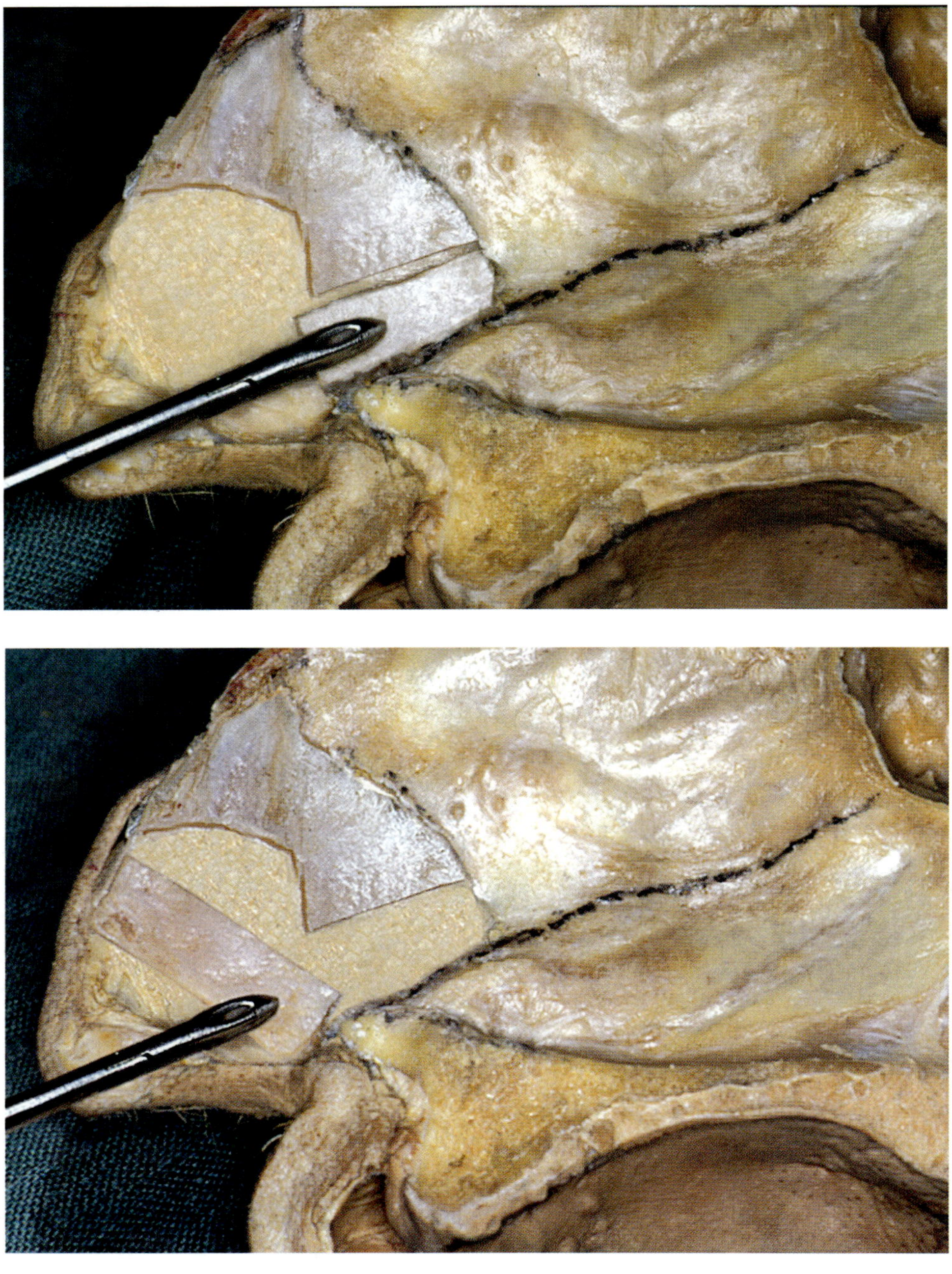

a

b

Fig. 17a. Harvesting cartilage from the posterior cartilaginous septum.
b. Reconstruction of the anterior cartilaginous septum with a columellar strut.

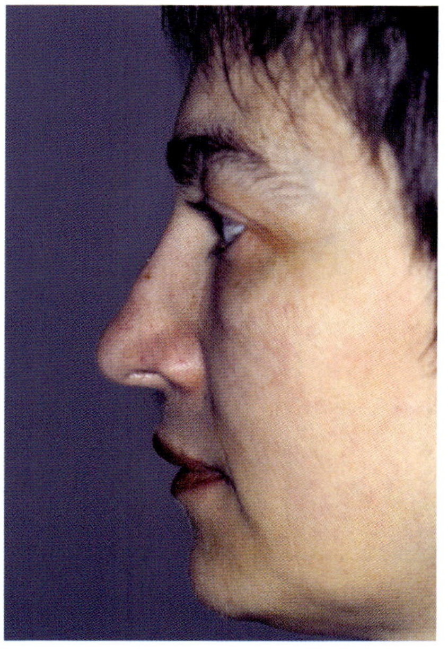

a

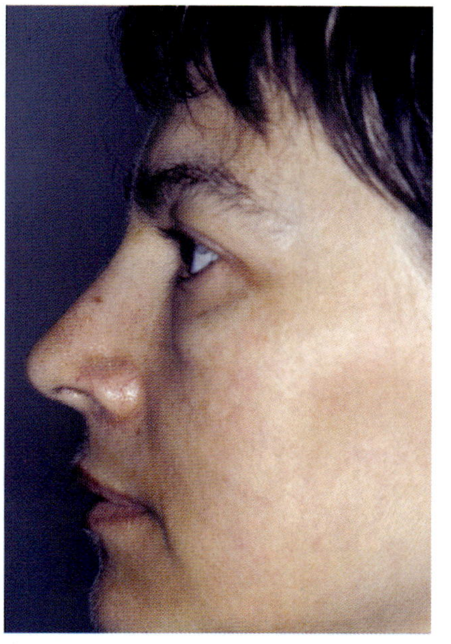

b

Fig. 18a. Preoperative view of a patient with loss of support of the septum as a result of an anterior cartilaginous septal defect. *b.* Postoperative view of the same patient after reconstruction of the septum, as illustrated in figure 17a,b.

Correction of the nasolabial angle

A prominent caudal border of the septum near the nasal spine often forms a blunt nasolabial angle (Fig. 25a). As above, palpation helps to discover the underlying anatomy. By resecting this part of the caudal border with the overlying mucosa, in combination with a nasal spine reduction (if necessary), the nasolabial angle can be reduced (Fig. 26a,b). Illustration 25b shows the result of this procedure.

The overdeveloped 'hanging' columella

In this situation (sometimes in combination with large medial crura of the alar cartilages) the whole caudal septal edge is often too prominent.

This malformation can be corrected by means of a complete transfixion incision. This way, the whole caudal edge of the cartilaginous septum can be trimmed together with the overlying mucoperichondrium (Fig. 27a,b). By suturing the defect primarily, the too prominent columella can retract in the desired position.

Deviation of the caudal edge of the septum

When a deviation of the caudal edge of the septum is present, the result is a distorted columella and occasionally an obstructed nostril on the deviated side (Fig. 28a). If the caudal septum is too long, the deviated rim is simply resected with its overlying mucosa (Fig. 29). Having a normal length, the septal cartilage will have to be scored on the concave side in order to reposition it in the midline, after creating a columellar pocket (Fig. 28b). See *The anterior septal defect* for creating a columellar pocket (Fig. 16).

In an exceptional situation even the nasal tip can be asymmetric as a result of a strong deviation of the caudal septum. In these circumstances the whole cartilaginous septum is freed from overlying mucosa *on both sides*, resected, reconstructed and put back, fixing it with mattress-sutures, in order to prevent columellar retraction (Fig. 30a,b).

Deviation of the nasal base.

When the septum is strongly deviated and luxated at its caudal edge, complete realignment of the septum is not always possible.

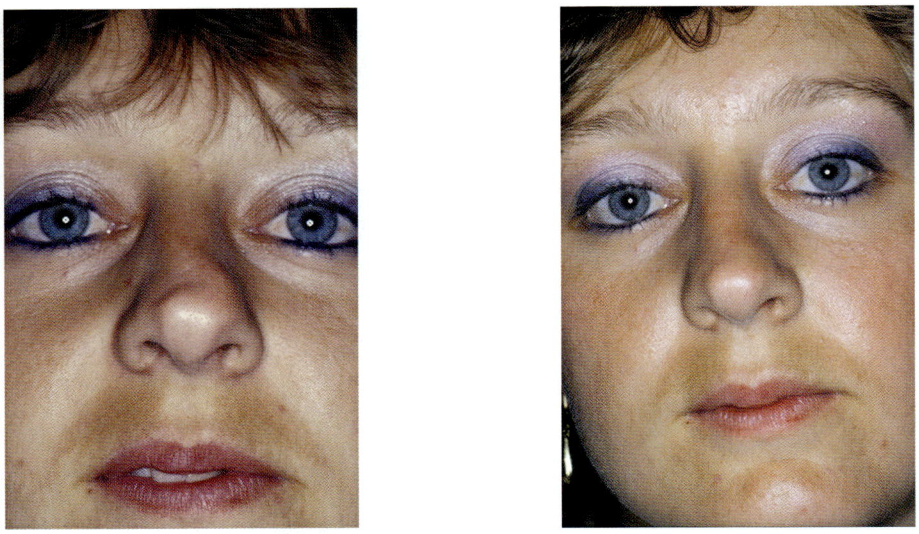

a b

Fig. 19a. Patient with a twisted cartilaginous dorsum as a result of a high cartilaginous septal deviation. *b.* Postoperative view after correction of the septum and the upper laterals.

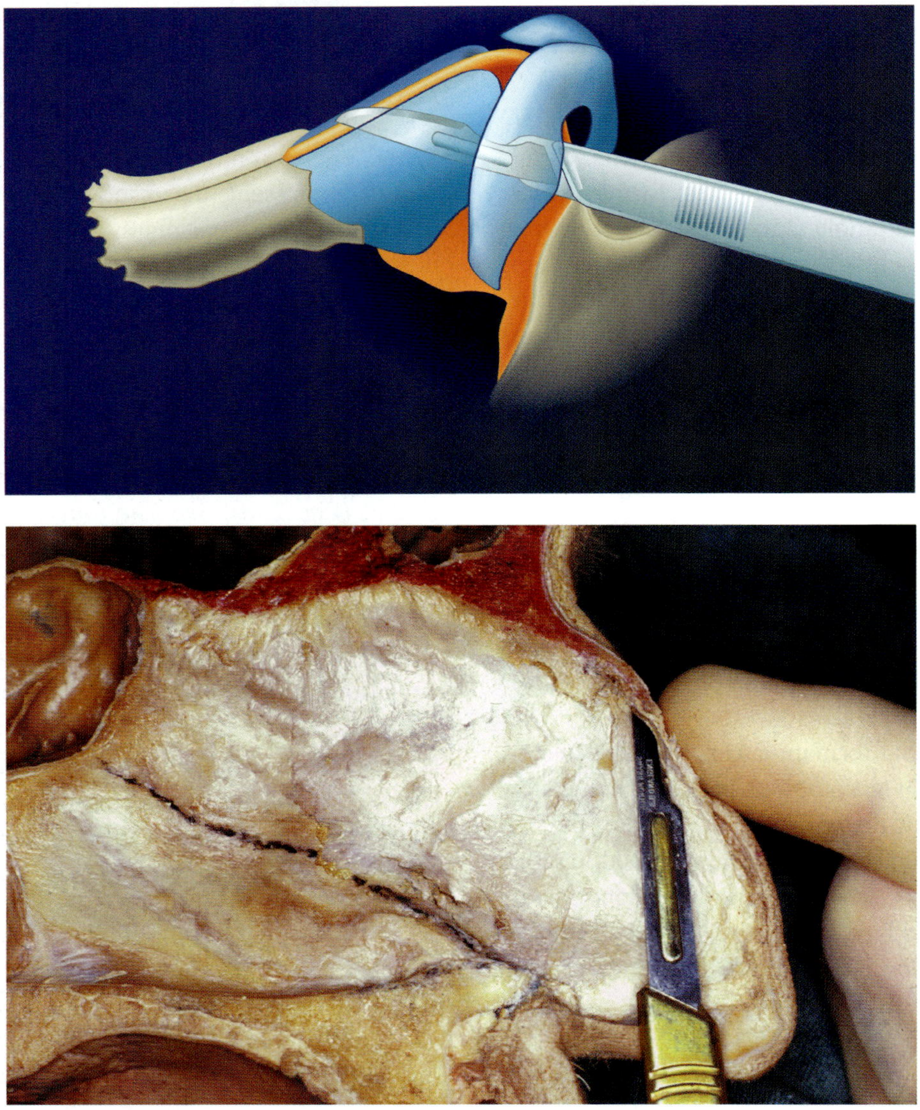

a b

Fig. 20a. Separation of the right upper lateral cartilage from the septum, directly through the nasal cavity.
b. Palpating finger on the dorsum of the nose to feel the knife coming through the upper lateral cartilage underneath the nasal skin.

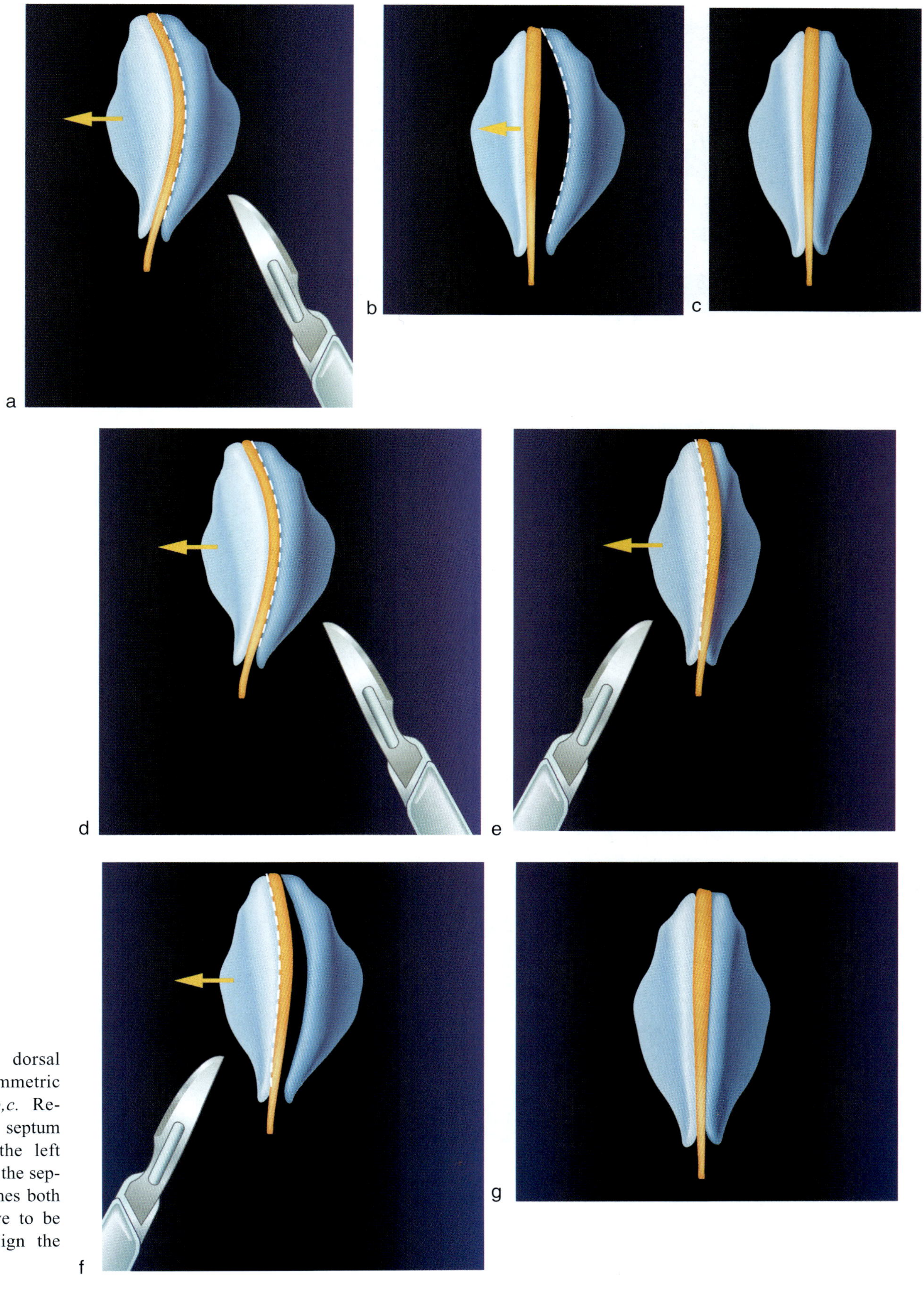

Fig. 21a. Twisted dorsal septum and asymmetric upper laterals. *b,c.* Realignment of the septum after separating the left upper lateral from the septum. *d-g.* Sometimes both upper laterals have to be separated to realign the dorsal septum.

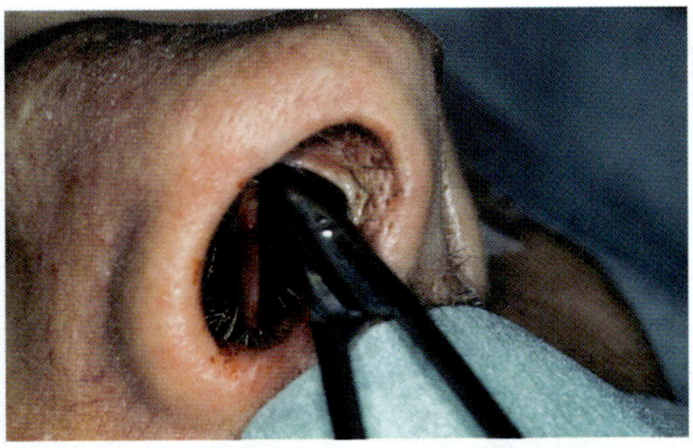

a

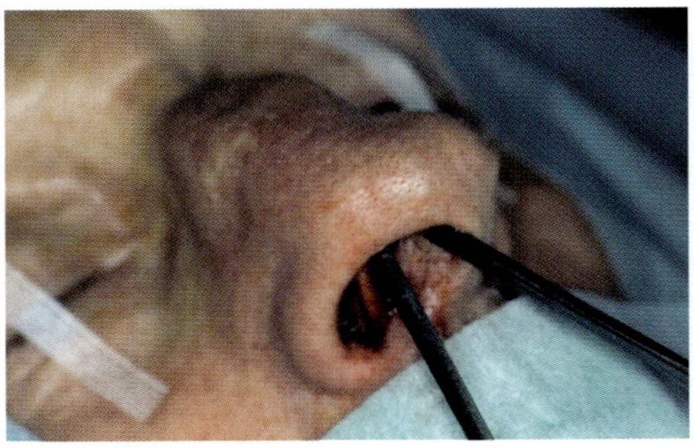

b

Fig. 22a,b. Undermining of the dorsal nasal skin through the hemitransfixion incision in order to straighten the dorsal septum.

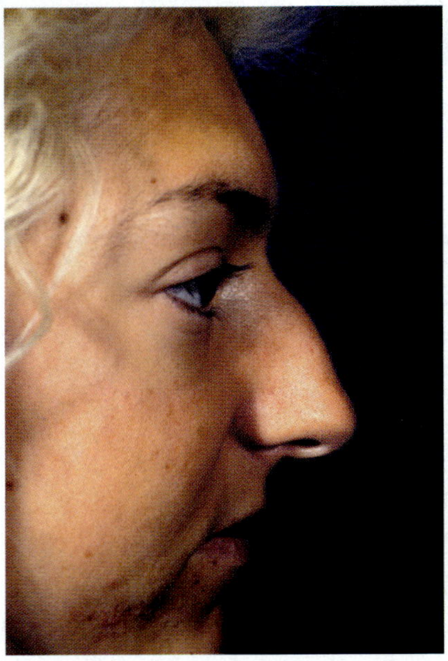

a

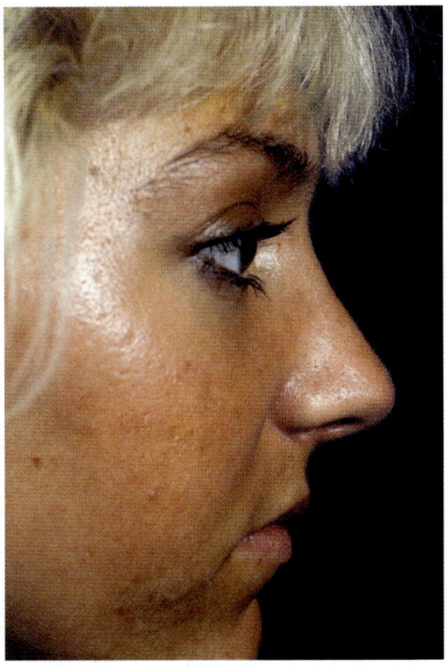

b

Fig. 23a. Patient with a too prominent anterior septal angle and adjacent caudal edge of the cartilaginous septum (and hump).
b. Postoperative view after resecting the anterior septal angle (and hump). Notice the upward rotation of the nasal tip by this procedure.

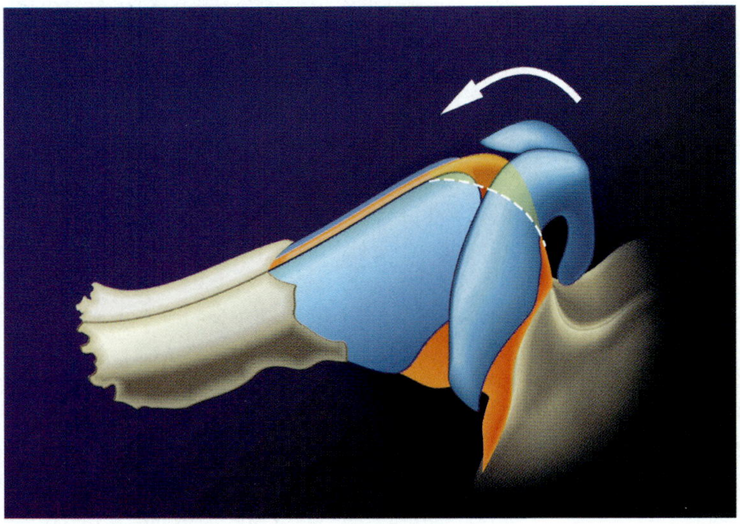

a

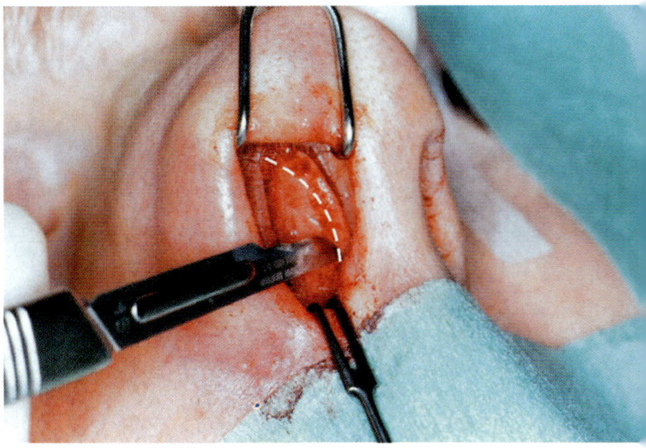

b

Fig. 24a. Area of anterior septal angle resection. This resection results in an upward rotation of the nasal tip. *b.* Resection of the anterior septal angle during surgery. The overlying mucosa is resected in the same amount as the cartilage.

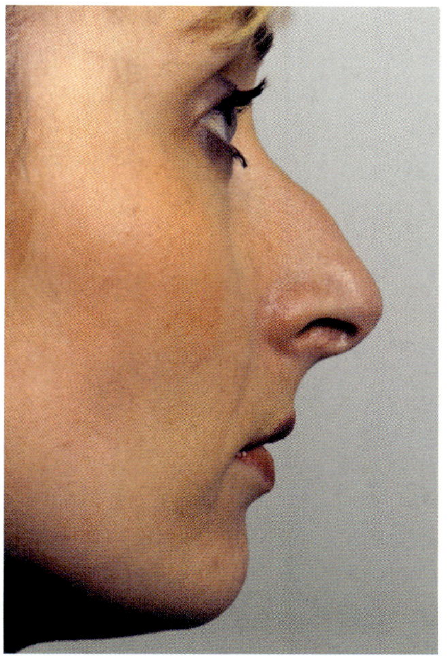

a

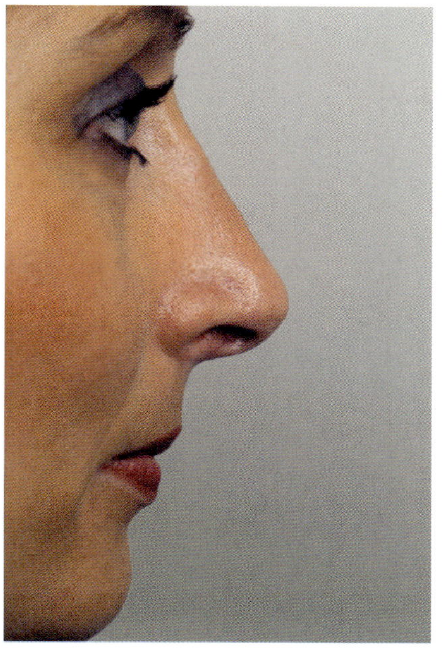

b

Fig. 25a. Preoperative view of a patient with a blunt nasolabial angle as a result of a too prominent caudal border of the septum (and nasal spine).
b. Postoperative view after resection of the caudal border of the septum and the nasal spine (as well as frontal angle re-construction).

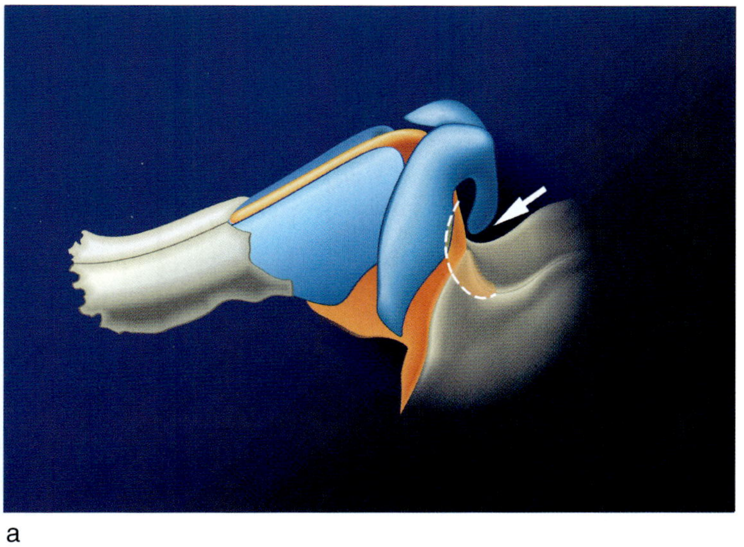

a

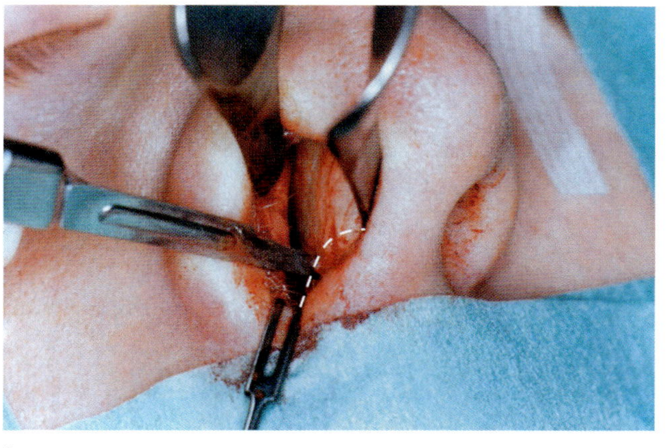

b

Fig. 26a. Area of septum and nasal spine resection for correction of a blunt nasolabial angle. *b.* Resection of septum, as illustrated in figure 26a, during surgery. The overlying mucosa is resected in the same amount as the cartilage.

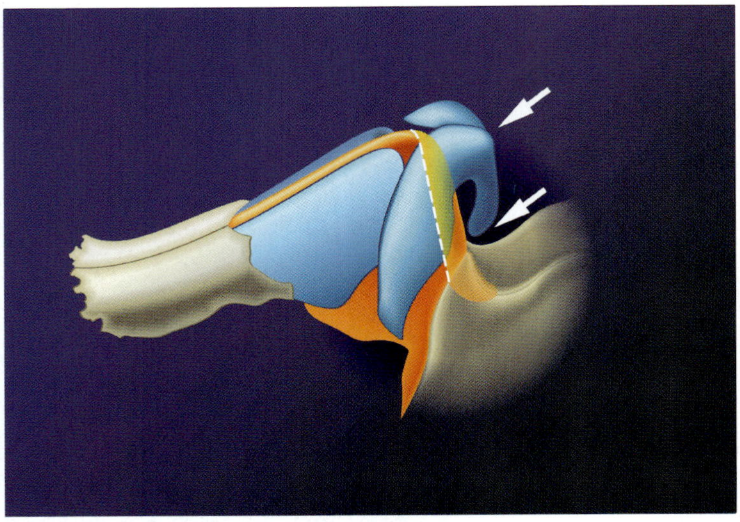

a

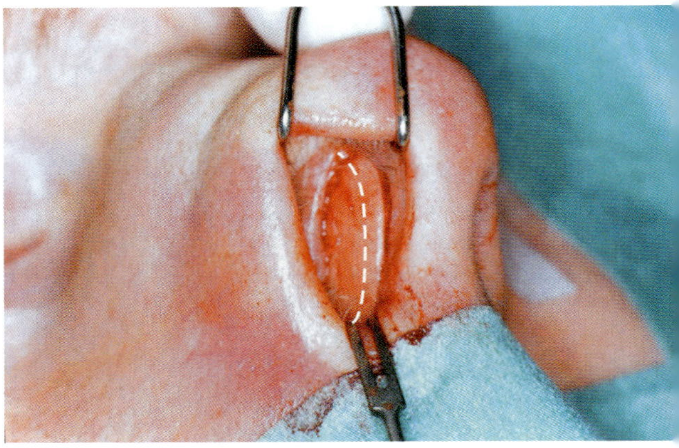

b

Fig. 27a. Resection of the total caudal edge of the septum in case of an overdeveloped 'hanging' columella. *b.* The same situation as in figure 27a during surgery. The overlying mucosa is resected in the same amount as the cartilage.

a

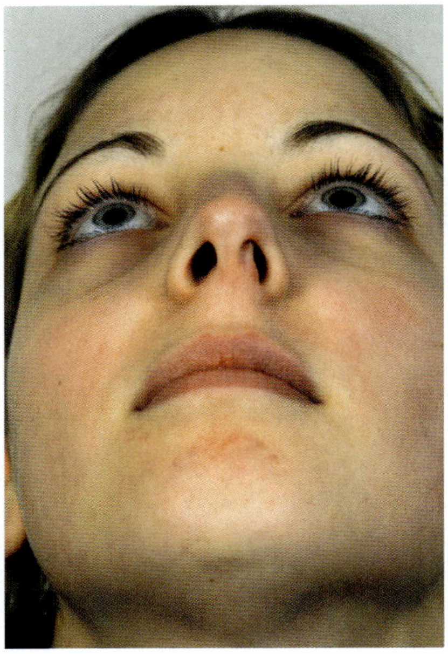

b

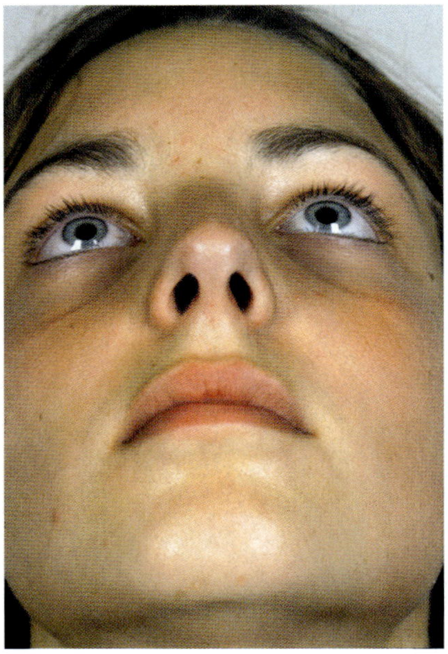

Fig. 28a. Preoperative view of a patient with a deviation of the caudal edge of the cartilaginous septum. Notice the partly obstructed left nostril.
b. Postoperative view of the same patient after correction of the caudal septum.

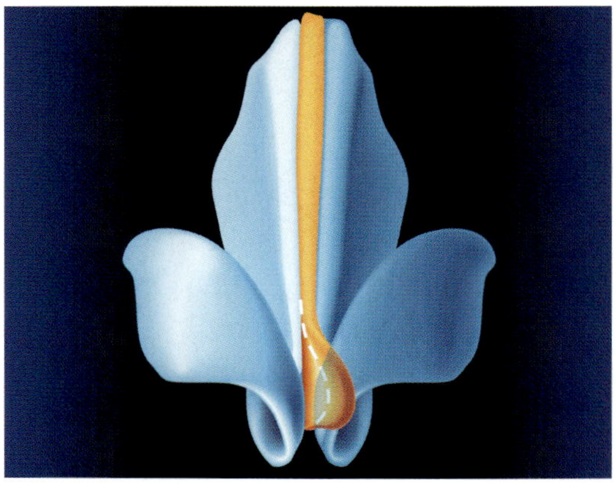

Fig. 29. Area of resection or scoring of the septum in case of a caudal septal deviation, as illustrated in figure 28a, b.

This because the whole nasal base is occasionally asymmetric (Fig. 31a). In these circumstances the area between the skin of the nasal base (and part of the upper lip) and the musculus orbicularis oris has to be undermined to completely straighten the septum and the base of the nose. Undermining of this so-called 'magic plain' is easily realized by spreading the tissue bluntly with slightly curved scissors through the hemitransfixion incision (see Figures 32a,b).

The result of this maneuver is illustrated in Figure 31b.

The cartilaginous nasal hump

A cartilaginous nasal hump is the result of an overdeveloped cartilaginous dorsal septum (Fig. 33a). To correct this situation the dorsal side of the quadrangular cartilage has to be resected (Fig. 34). This in itself is a correction of the septum. It is difficult to judge the precise amount and place of reduction. Frequently also the anterior septal angle has to be trimmed to prevent a so-called 'polly beak' (Fig. 33b). In an endonasal procedure the best approach to reach this goal is a transfixion incision in combination with an intercartilaginous incision on both sides. After freeing the anterior septal angle and cartilaginous dorsum the exact amount of dorsal cartilage that has to be reduced can be estimated (Fig. 35). This is essential for a good aesthetic result of the nasal profile (Fig. 36a,b).

The cartilaginous nasal dorsal defect, 'the saddle nose'

Small defects of the cartilaginous dorsum can be reconstructed with small layers of patients' own cartilage in the defect of the dorsum (Fig. 37a,b). Through an endonasal incision the graft is introduced in the area of the defect into a small pocket, to prevent displacement of the graft on the dorsum.

In case of a collapse of the cartilaginous nasal dorsum (Fig. 38a), the total septum has to be reconstructed. For this correction, an external approach is often indicated. The procedure is schematically seen in Figure 40a,b and is discussed elsewhere in this book. Posterior septal cartilage, bony septum, ear- or rib-cartilage are the materials one can choose from. Reconstruction gives a strong aesthetic change of the nose and face as a whole. Figures 38a,b and 39a,b show the result of this procedure in a patient's nose that has been reconstructed with cartilage taken from his protruding ears. In the same operation an otoplasty has been performed on both sides. This gives an extra change to his face.

Postoperative management

If necessary, after one of these procedures the anterior cartilaginous septum can be sutured to the nasal spine (Fig. 12) to accomplish secure realignment of the anterior septum. Optionally, the elevated mucoperichondrial flap can be reattached to the septum by through-and-through sutures in the cartilaginous septum. This prevents septal hematoma and creates stability.

Nasal tampons can stay *in situ* for 24 to 48 hours. Routine antibiotic treatment is not necessary. See also *Postoperative care and complications* elsewhere in this book.

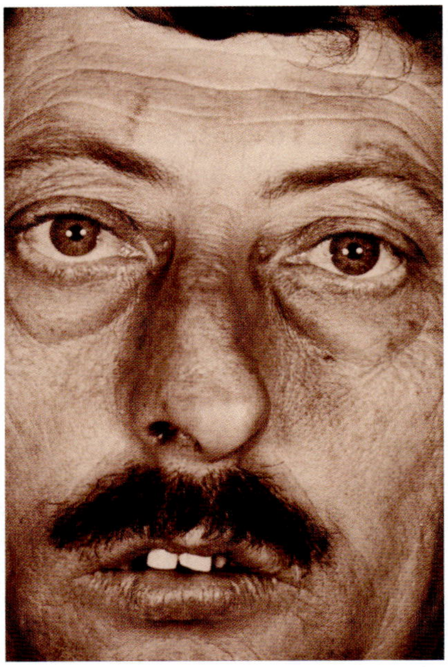
a

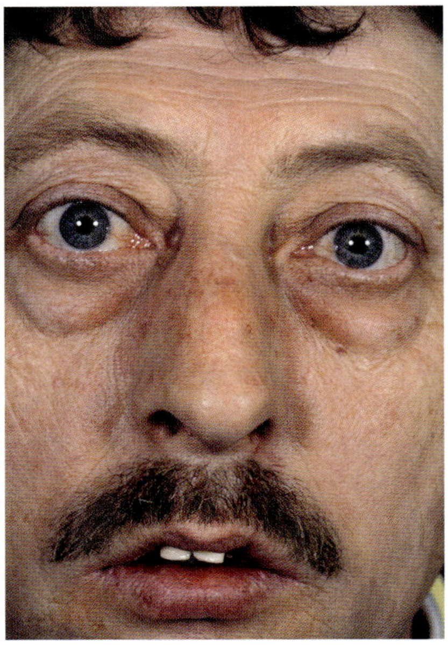
b

Fig. 30a. Preoperative view of a patient with a nasal tip asymmetry as a result of a severe deviation of the anterior cartilaginous septum. *b.* Postoperative view of the same patient after reconstruction of the septum. No nasal tip surgery was performed.

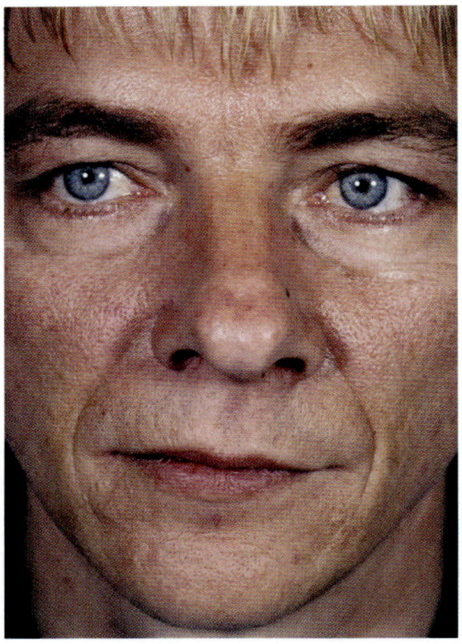
a

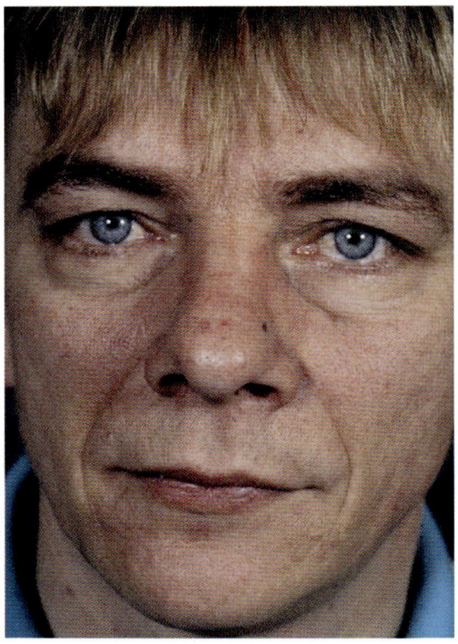
b

Fig. 31a. Patient with deviated caudal septum and an asymmetric nasal base. *b.* The same patient after septal correction and undermining of the nasal base or 'magic plane' (see fig. 32a, b).

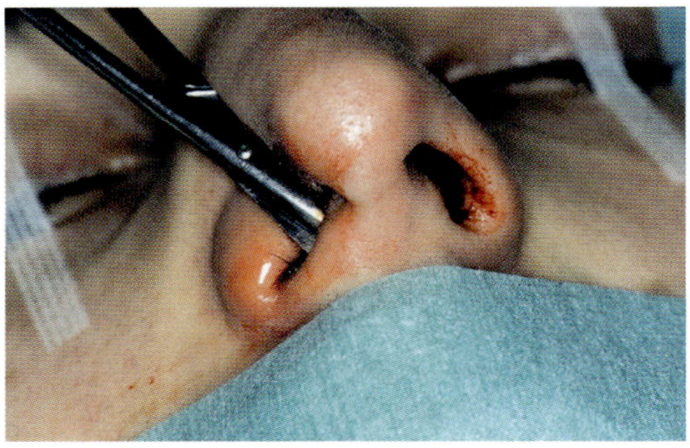
a

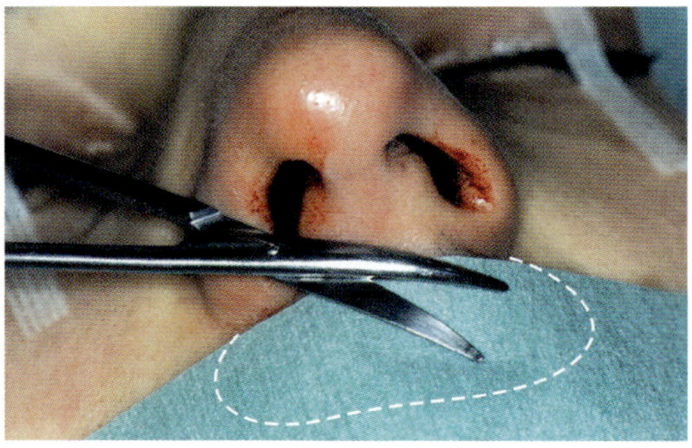
b

Fig. 32a. Introduction of scissors into the nasal base or 'magic plane' via the caudal part of the hemitransfixion. *b.* The dotted line indicates the 'magic plane'. This is the area that has to be undermined during a septum correction, to realign an asymmetric nasal base.

Fig. 33a. Preoperative view of a patient with a bony and cartilaginous hump. The cartilaginous part of the hump exists of septum cartilage. *b.* Postoperative polly beak (yellow arrow) after hump removal. This is the result of too less dorsal cartilaginous septum reduction.

a

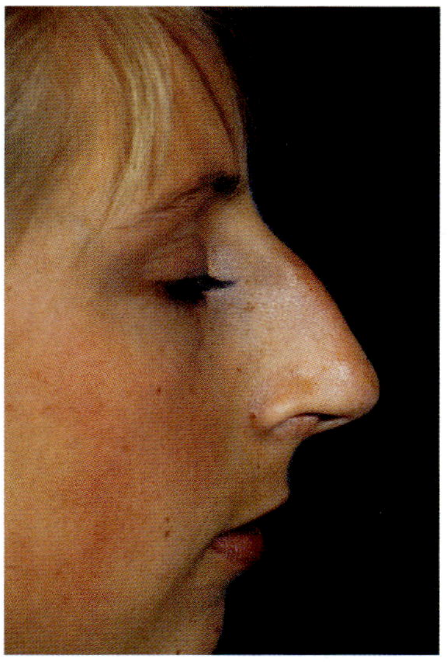

b

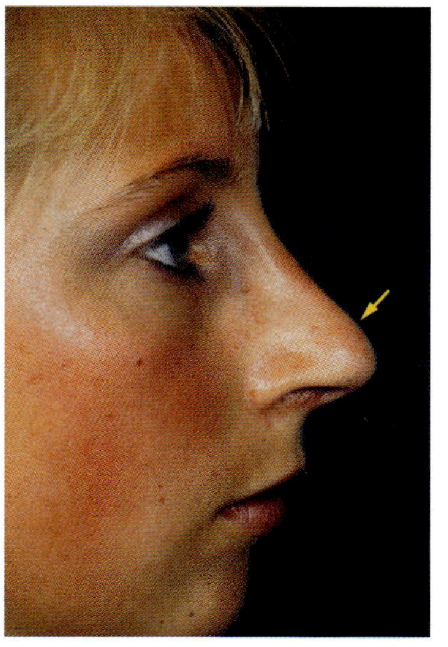

Fig. 34. The dotted line indicates the correct area of dorsal (cartilaginous septum) reduction that should have been done in the patient of Figure 33a. Notice that also the anterior septal angle has to be resected.

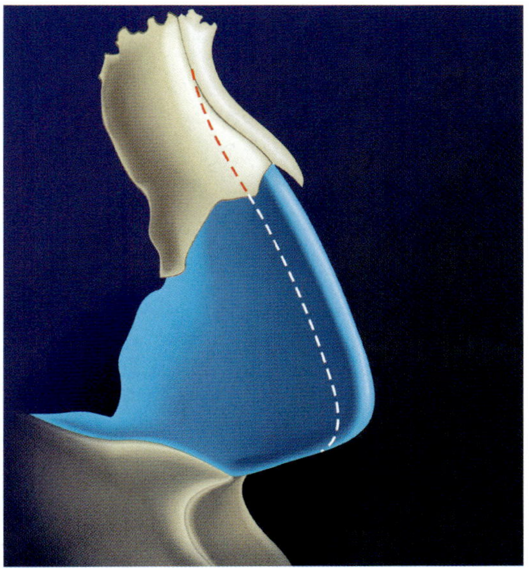

Fig. 35. Resection of the anterior septal angle in case of a cartilaginous hump removal during surgery. Precise judgement of cartilage resection is essential for a good result of hump removal.

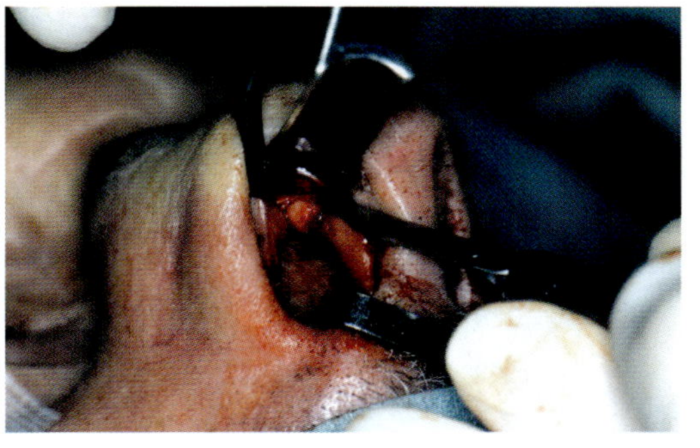

Fig. 36a. Preoperative view of a patient with a bony cartilaginous dorsal hump ('tension nose'). *b.* Postoperative view of the same patient of Figure 36a after correct resection of the hump (with the anterior septal angle). Note the indirect change of the ala, the nostril and the nasal tip (reduction) as a result of this maneuver.

a

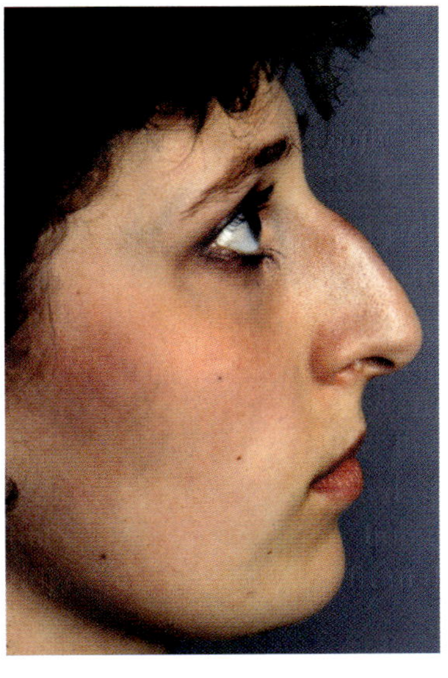

b

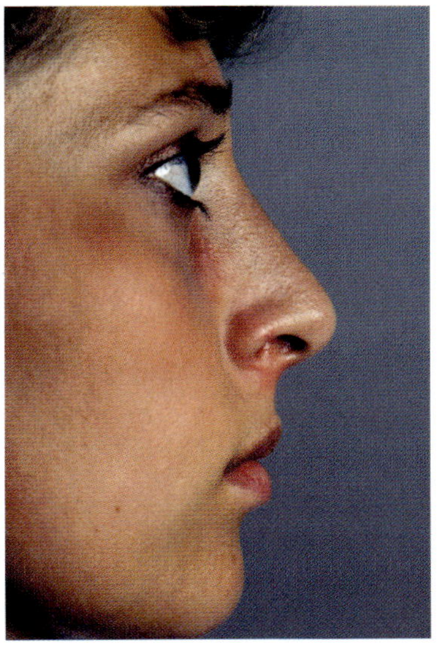

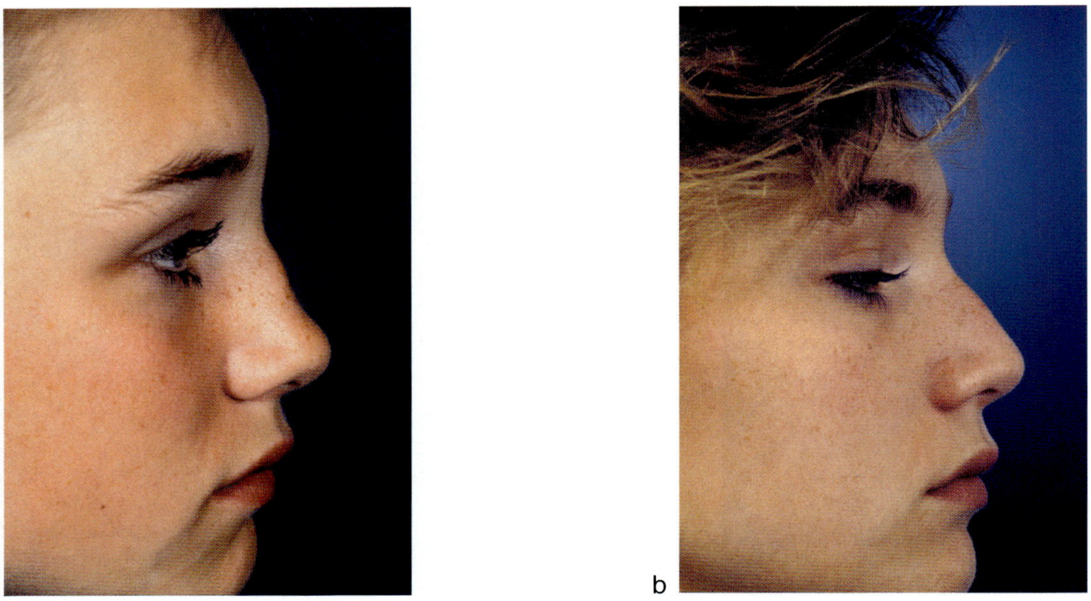

a b

Fig. 37a. Patient with a small defect of the dorsum of the cartilaginous septum. Preoperative view.
b. Postoperative view of the same patient after filling the defect with the patient's own cartilage.

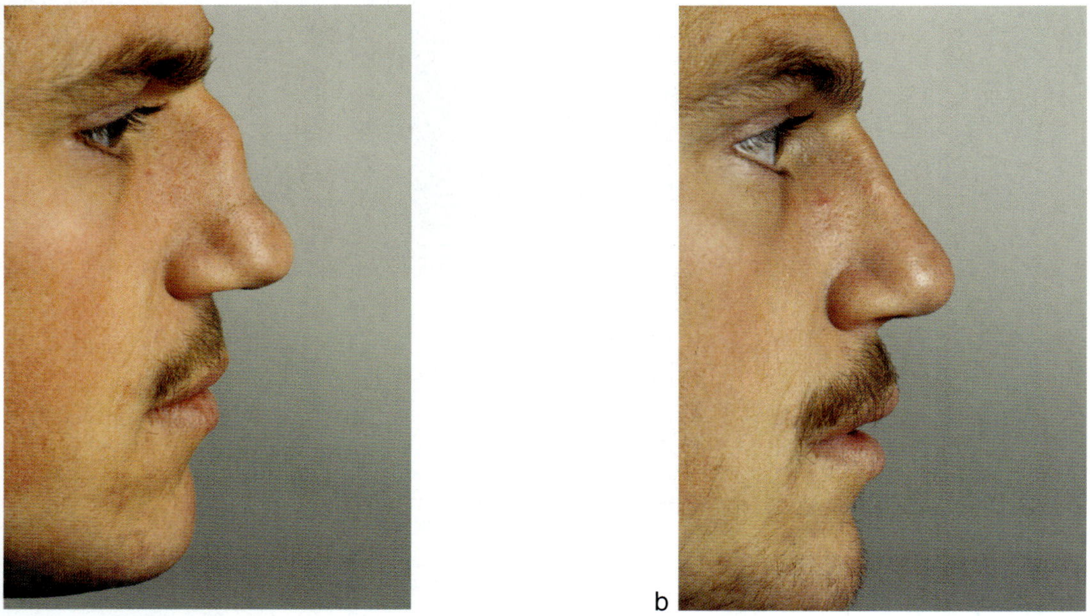

a b

Fig. 38a. Patient with a severe 'saddle nose' after over-resection of septum cartilage during surgery.
b. Postoperative view of the same patient after septum reconstruction with the patient's own ear cartilage.

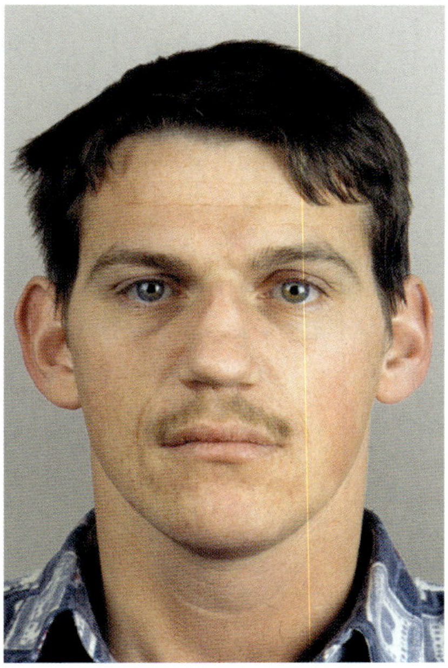

a

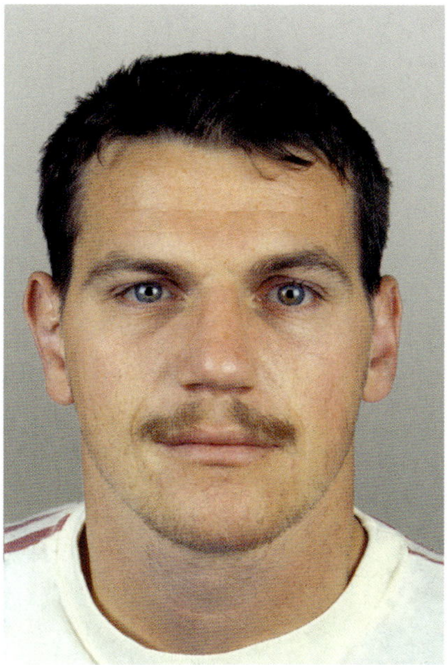

b

Fig. 39a. Preoperative anterior view of the patient in Figure 38a. Saddle nose and protruding ears.
b. Postoperative anterior view of the same patient after reconstruction of the septum with ear cartilage. Notice that also an otoplasty on both sides has been done.

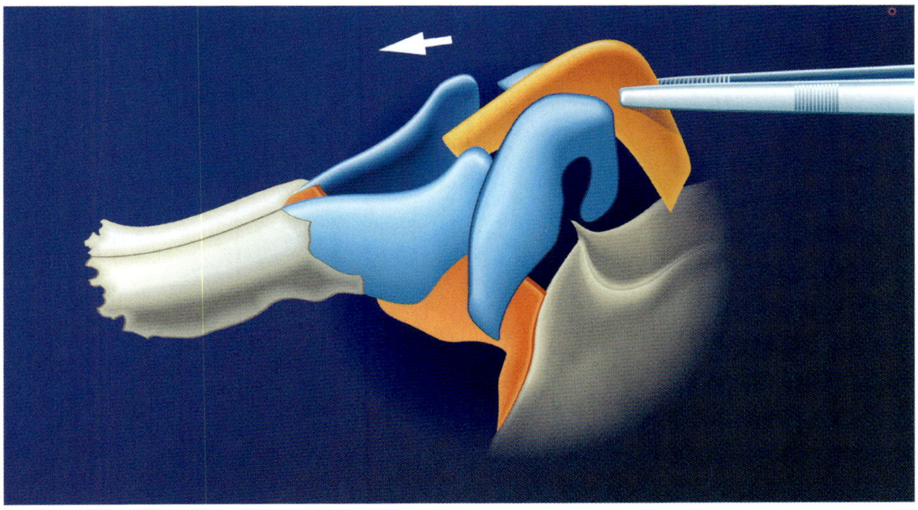

a

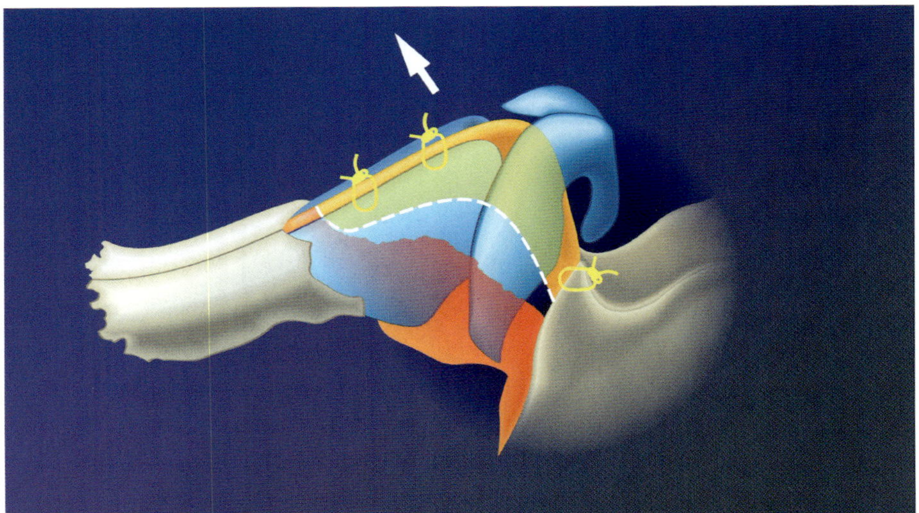

b

Fig. 40a. Schematic reconstruction of the anterior cartilaginous septum with a cartilage transplant.
b. Fixed cartilage transplant. Notice the change of the dorsal profile of the nose.

25: NEW CONCEPTS IN RECONSTRUCTIVE SEPTOPLASTY

M. Boenisch and G.J. Nolst Trenité

Introduction

The nasal septum, which is the main midline structure of the nose, should be flat, flexible, and solid at the same time, in order to fulfil its most important functions: to support the external nose, regulate air flow, and support the mucosa.

In pursuit of a straight septum, classic 'submucous resections' often lead to loss of stability with severe sequelae (*e.g.*, septal perforation and vibration of the septum during breathing).

Over the last 20 years, the principles of septal correction have evolved into more conservative and reconstructive procedures, consisting of atraumatic dissection and mobilization of the septal cartilage followed by realignment.[1]

The various methods of providing the cartilage with a new shape (cartilage incisions, dividing and thinning) may cause decreased stability, which particularly interferes with its supporting function. In order to avoid the complication of a saddle nose in such cases, surgeons are sometimes forced to compromise: a sufficiently broad strip of cartilage must remain untouched in the area of the nasal dorsum, regardless of any deformities.

An excellent, proven and well known technique for avoiding such a compromise when correcting severe especially posttraumatic deformities is extracorporal or external septoplasty.[2-4] This technique consists of dissecting the entire quadrangular cartilage free of the mucoperichondrium on both sides, detaching it from the perpendicular plate, vomer and maxillary crest, as well as from the upper laterals. Then the entire septal cartilage is removed in one piece. The excellent view outside the nose makes it easy to correct even extreme deviations, usually by dividing the cartilage into straight piec285es. Problems start with reconstruction of the septum. In order to avoid postoperative sequelae such as saddling, the pieces of cartilage must be reconnected meticulously to form a straight, and at the same time solid, plate. There are various techniques for connecting the pieces of cartilage to each other, *e.g.*, suturing them onto part of the removed perpendicular plate; however, these techniques are technically difficult and time-consuming.

Extracorporal septoplasty can be assisted by the use of a connecting material. A resorbent material would be particularly helpful since this will guarantee good support of the nasal dorsum and, since it will completely disappear, will also eliminate long-term complications. Since 1996, we have been using a PDS foil (Polydioxanone) as the resorbent supporting material for this purpose.[5] This polydioxanone plate (PDS foil, Ethicon Norderstedt, Germany) is well known and has been used successfully for many years in the restoration of bone discontinuities in, for example, orbital floor reconstruction. Polydioxanone is a resorbent material which is degradable by hydrolysis and is completely metabolized in the body. The foil is produced by the company in various sizes and gauges (0.15, 0.25, and 0.50 mm). The thinner gauges are also available with perforations. The general biological properties of the implant in combination with bone have been examined in numerous studies.[6] The thicker foils are resorbed within eight months.

However, we do not know much about the biological properties of the implant in combination with the cartilage. For example, does the foil have an influence on the cartilage itself, or does it cause any inflammatory responses or reactions in the perichondrium.

Experimental study (1)

In order to obtain histological information, PDS foil was implanted into the outer ears of young rabbits in combination with a cartilage defect.[7] On the dorsal side of the outer ear, after blunt division of the muscle under the perichondrium, a 0.5 x 0.5 cm cartilage defect was created and a 1.5 x 1.5 cm piece of PDS foil (ZX8, 0.15 mm thick) was implanted, covering both the defect and the cartilage. The incision was closed in one layer using catgut sutures. After two, five, ten, 15 and 25 weeks, the prepared region was examined histologically. Two weeks after implantation, the implant is completely unchanged and is surrounded by minimal reactive tissue, forming a thin capsule. There is no inflammatory infiltration or foreign body reaction and the cartilage also remains unchanged (Fig. 1).

Five weeks after implantation the situation is similar. The continuity of the implant is still the same. There are absolutely no inflammatory or foreign body reactions; the cartilage remains unchanged (Fig. 2).

Ten weeks after implantation, resorption of the implant has already begun and its continuity is interrupted. The implant is still surrounded by the thin layer of reactive tissue, which in addition is by now filling the perforations in the foil, guaranteeing good fixation. For the first time, chondroblasts can be seen on the border of the cartilage defect (Fig. 3).

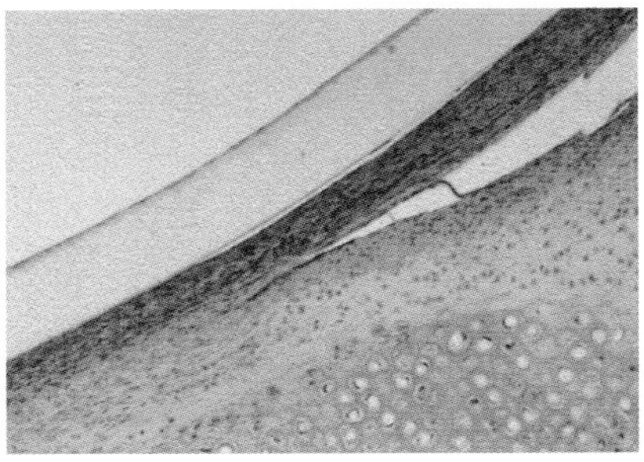

Fig. 1.

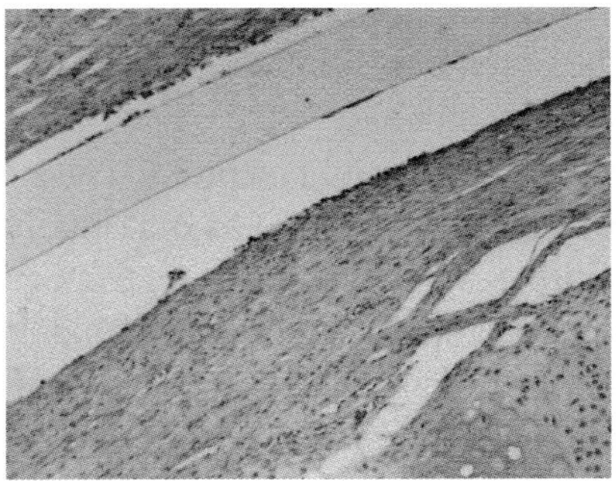

Fig. 2.

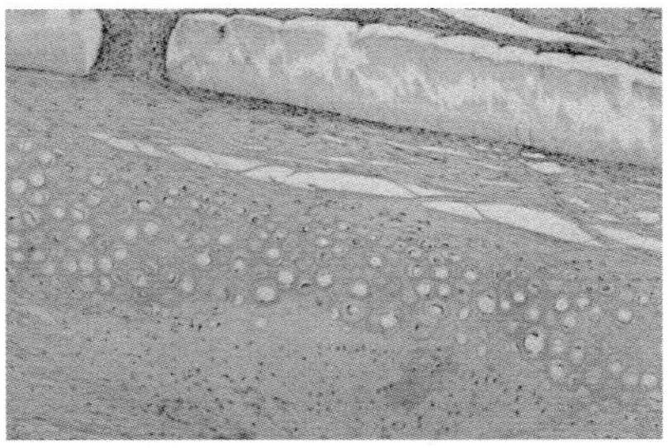

Fig. 3.

Fifteen weeks after implantation, the resorption procedure is progressing, the PDS particles are encapsulated by fibrous tissue. Any noticeable tissue reaction remains solely in the area of the implant (Fig. 4a). Newly formed cartilage is developing on the borders of the cartilage defect. The cartilage beneath the foil remains unchanged (Fig. 4b).

Twenty-five weeks after implantation, the implant has been completely resorbed.

a 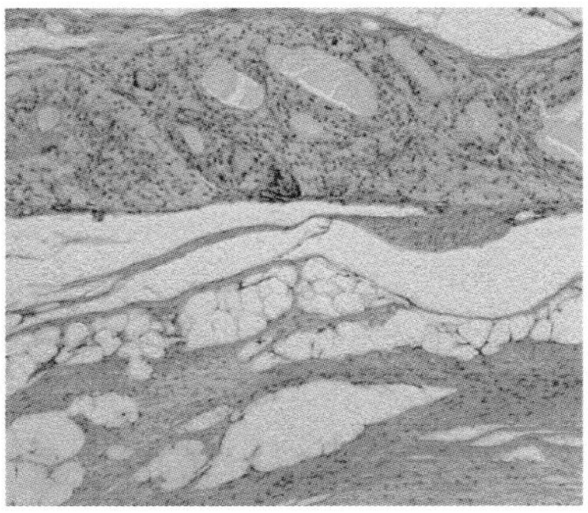

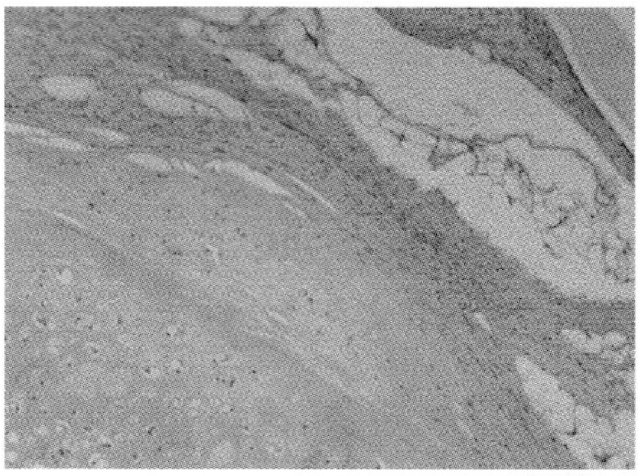 b

Fig. 4a,b.

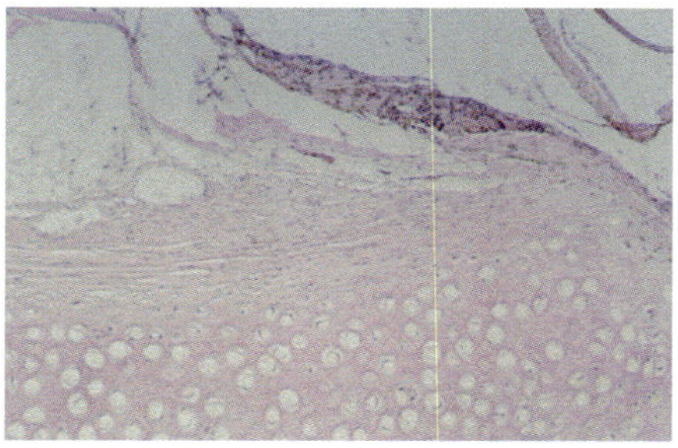

Fig. 5.

Even after examination of the entire specimen, no residues can be found. Only the minimal remains of fibrous scar tissue are evident (Fig. 5).

From these findings, the following conclusions can be drawn:

- using light microscopic examination, the implant remains unchanged for at least ten weeks;
- after 25 weeks the implant has been completely resorbed;
- only in the immediate vicinity of the implant does tissue reaction occur. The operation area remains free of inflammatory reactions and granulation tissue;
- the cartilage beneath the implant remains completely unchanged from a histological point of view. On the borders of the cartilage defect, first chondroblasts and later new formed cartilage appear;
- finally, after the conclusion of the resorption procedure, only minimal fibrous scar tissue remains.

Experimental study (2)

From the first histological study, we obtained information on the biological properties of the foil and its degradation products, which do not have a negative effect on the cartilage. However, we also wished to obtain more information on the situation within the nasal septum, where the surrounding cartilage tissues are different from those of the ear.

Therefore, in four-week-old New Zealand white rabbits, the nasal septum was approached via the nasal dorsum.[8] We performed cartilage work on the nasal septal cartilage in the same way as in normal septoplasty procedures (elevation of the mucoperichondrium, resection of a piece of cartilage, reimplantation of the resected cartilage with and without crushing). Observation time ranged between two and 25 weeks after surgery. Using light microscopic examination, we investigated the following two points with regard to the healing process:

- does PDS foil cause rejection or inflammatory infiltration in combination with the nasal septum?
- is there any effect on the histological properties of the new-formed cartilage and growing cartilage?

Similar to the study on ear cartilage, the specimen showed good tolerability of the PDS. There was no significant inflammatory reaction, no rejection of the foil, and no necrosis of the surrounding tissues. A further advantage seems to be that, after reimplantation of cartilage grafts in combination with PDS foil, there is significantly less overlapping of the cartilage fragments compared to earlier studies not using PDS.[9,10] The former investigations show that reimplanted cartilage grafts often develop an overlap in the area of the cut edges. However, the foil stabilizes the graft, reduces the overlap, and stimulates cartilaginous healing of the cut edges (Fig. 6).

This could be a similar reaction to the healing process of bone, where we know that the quality of the healing process

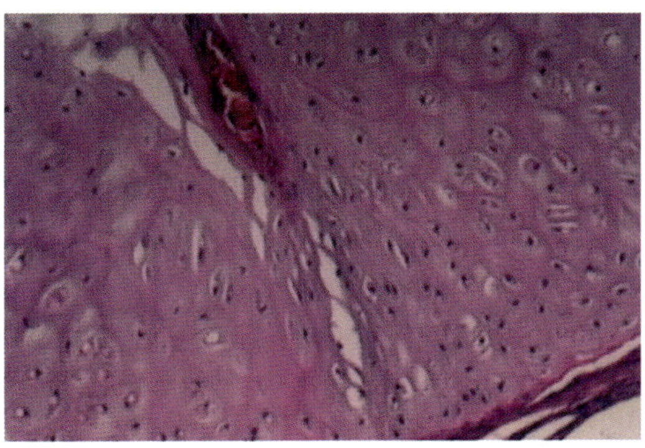

Fig. 6.

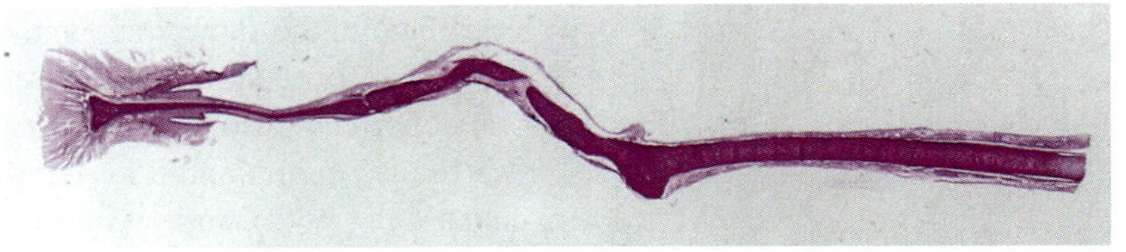

Fig. 7.

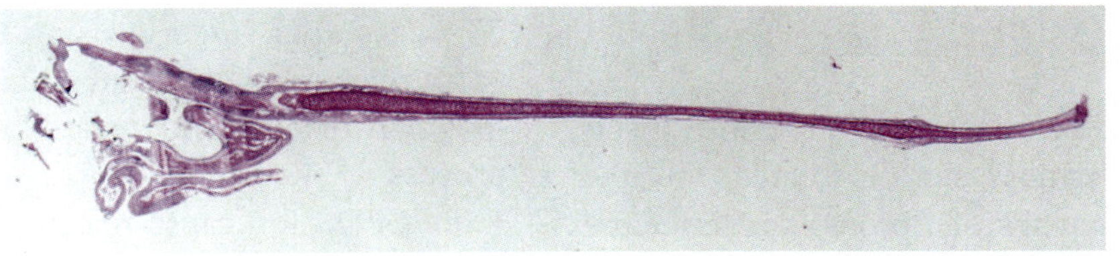

Fig. 8.

depends on the stable fixation of the fragments, as otherwise fibrous callus develops which interferes with a smooth healing process.

The exact fixation of the graft has the same positive effect with crushed cartilage. Earlier studies have shown that, after crushing, the contact between the original and the reimplanted cartilage is better, but that partial regeneration and resorption of the crushed cartilage graft causes varying degrees of secondary deviation (Fig. 7).[11]

In combination with PDS, secondary deviation of crushed cartilage grafts is significantly reduced (Fig. 8).

Operative technique

Surgery can be performed as a daycare or an inpatient procedure. Three days is recommended for perioperative antibiotic prophylaxis.

We usually start with an inverted V midcolumella incision intersecting the bilateral marginal incision and then the rhinoplasty begins. We usually feel that external septoplasty and the external approach should be performed together. This is true in most cases, because severe septal deformities, *e.g.*, posttraumatic ones, are often combined with severe deformities of the entire nasal pyramid, which require an external approach. However, this is not necessary because, as many surgeons have shown, it can also be performed with an endonasal approach, although this is slightly more difficult.

As is usual with an external approach, the next step is the separation of the skin and the soft tissue over the tip, cartilaginous and bony dorsum in the right surgical plane. After separation of the medial crura of the lower laterals, the caudal end of the septal cartilage is reached (Fig. 9). Starting from here, the mucoperichondrium is dissected free on both sides (Fig. 10).

After the posterior chondrotomia and separation from the upper laterals, the cartilaginous septum is detached from the vomer and maxillary crest (Fig. 11). The septal cartilage is now completely free and can be removed *in toto* (Fig. 12).

The cartilage thus removed is placed on the foil to act as a template for cutting the foil (Fig. 13). The outline of the removed cartilage can easily be copied onto the foil with a scalpel (Fig. 14), in order to determine the exact size of the septum to be reconstructed. Using scissors, the foil is cut along the marked lines. The deviating cartilage can now be seprated into straight pieces (Fig. 15).

These pieces are arranged on the foil, ideally covering most of it. Particular attention must be paid to those pieces of cartilages composing the dorsal and caudal septal borers. In each of these two cases, only one piece of cartilage should be used, regardless

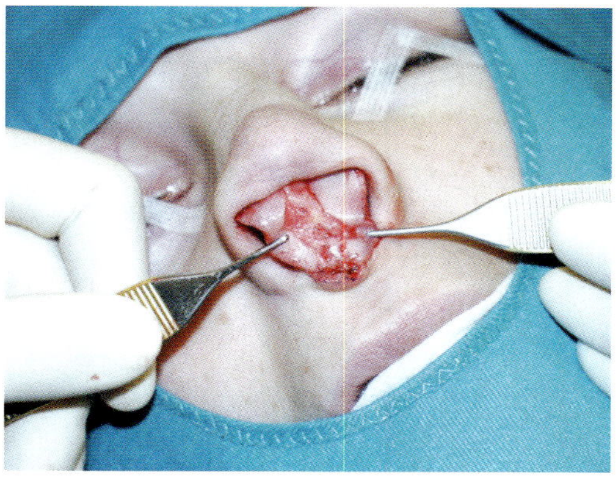
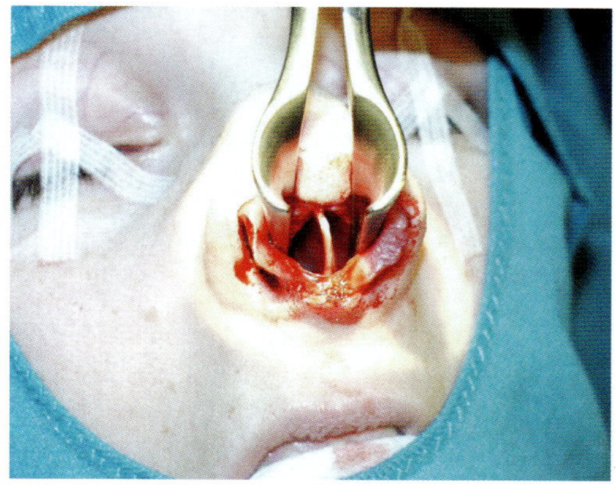

Fig. 9.

Fig. 10.

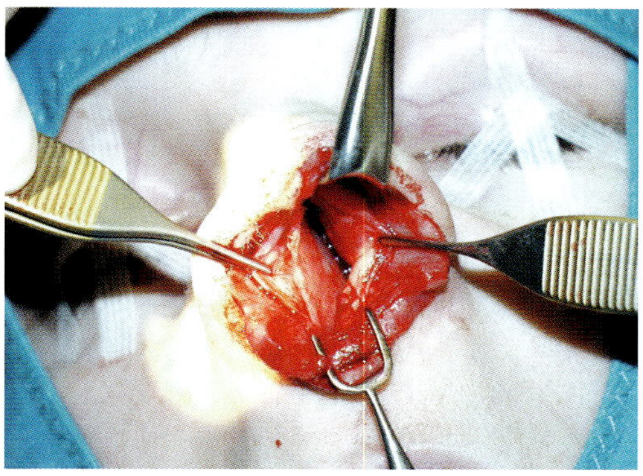
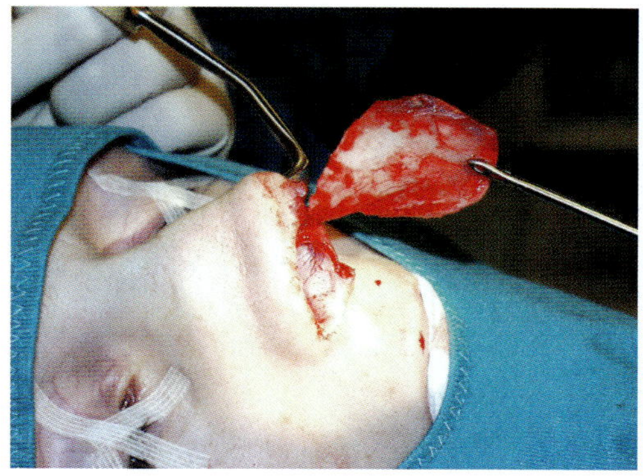

Fig. 11.

Fig. 12.

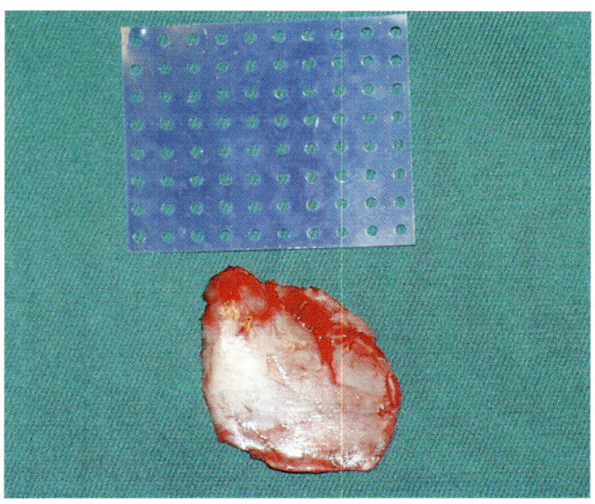
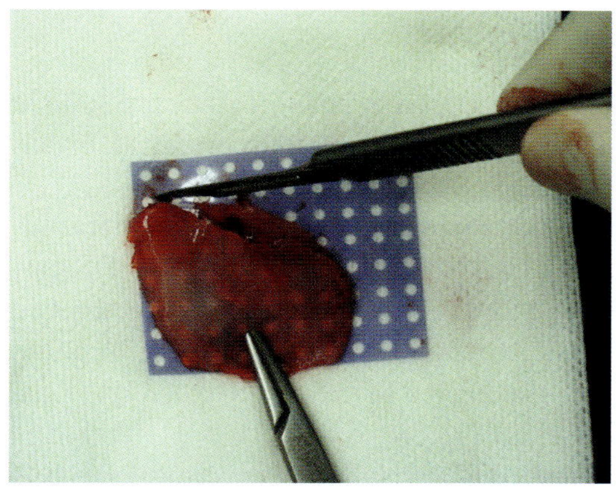

Fig. 13.

Fig. 14.

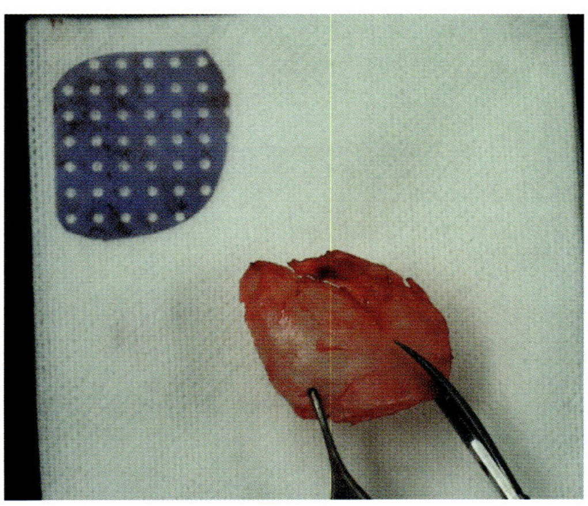
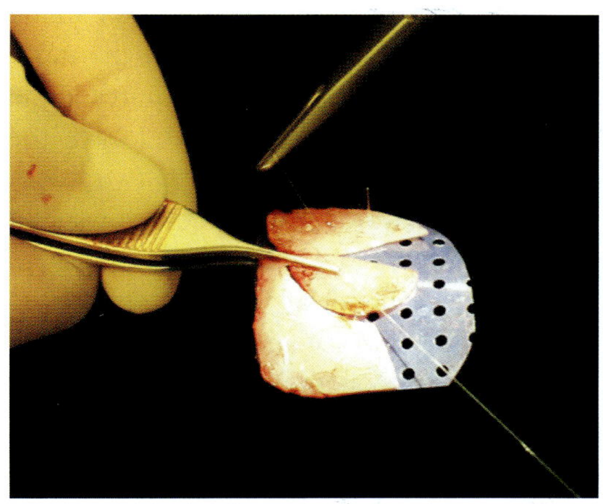

Fig. 15.

Fig. 16.

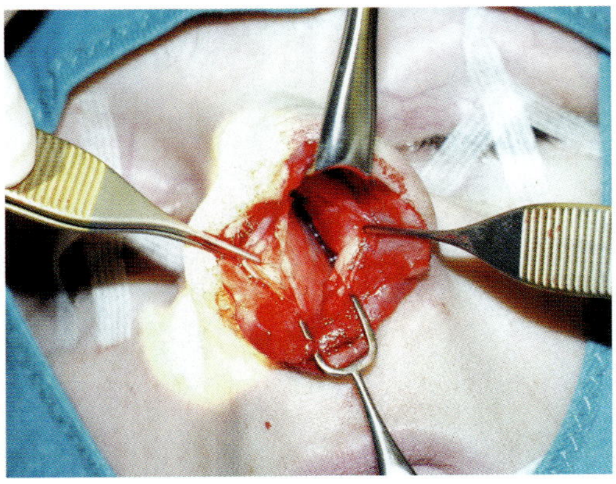

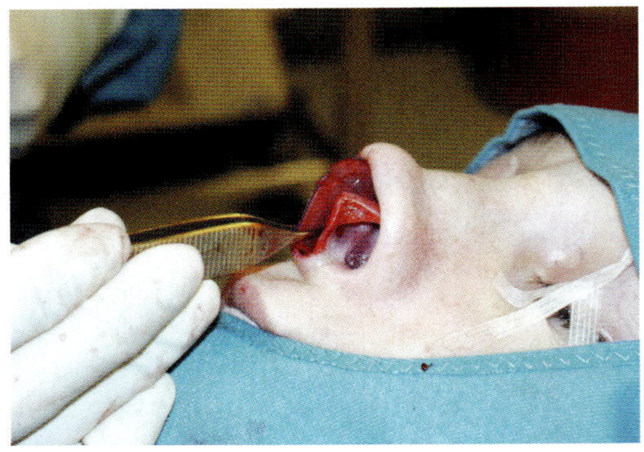

Fig. 17.

Fig. 18.

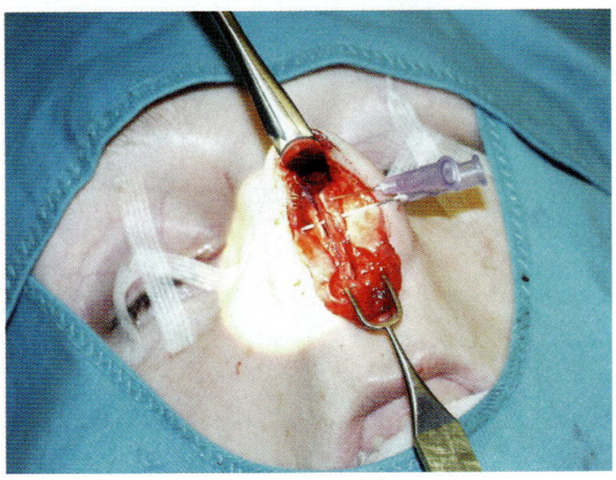

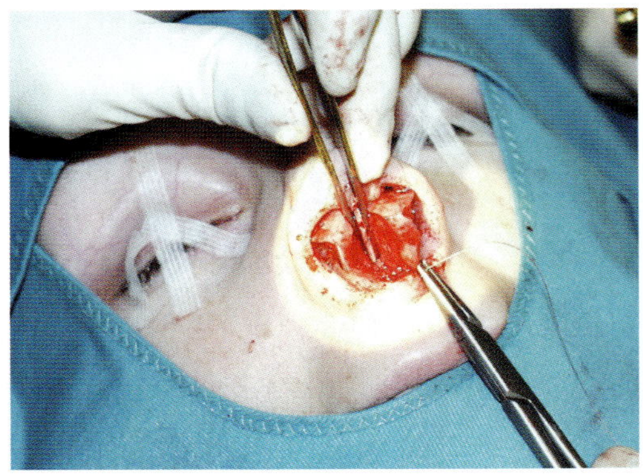

Fig. 19.

Fig. 20.

of its former position. After all these pieces have been put into position, they are sutured to the foil with PDS suture material, usually 4/0 (Fig. 16).

After correction of any possible deformities of the perpendicular plate, the PDS-cartilage graft is reimplanted between the two mucoperichondrial layers of the septum, and is adjusted to the correct position (Figs. 17 and 18).

In order to retain the graft in place, it is sutured to the upper laterals (Fig. 19), in the K area, and to the periosteum of the nasal spine (Fig. 20). To apply these sutures in the correct way, it is very helpful to fix the structures before suturing with two small needles. Afterwards, a series of transseptal mattress sutures are placed in order to fix the mucoperichondrial flaps, thereby closing all the dead space and firmly stabilizing the septal components. Finally, any deviations of the bony pyramid are corrected by osteotomies.

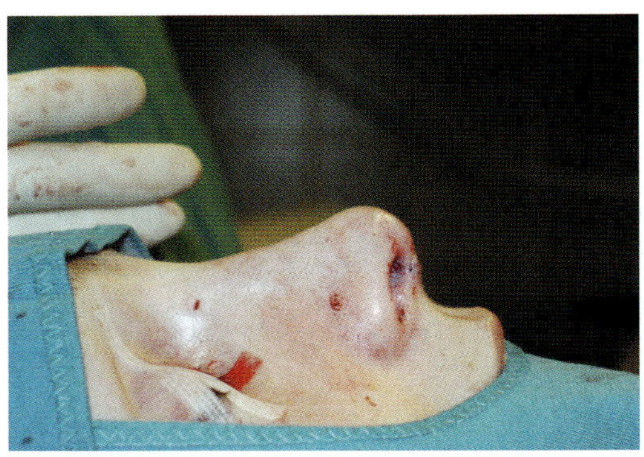

Fig. 21.

To finalize the operation, silicone splints are positioned in the airway until the following morning, instead of nasal packing. These even allow the patient slight breathing through the nose (Fig. 21). No further endonasal packing is used. After meticulous closure of the skin incision with nylon 6/0, the lateral view of the nose is fixed from outside with Denver splints or plaster of Paris.

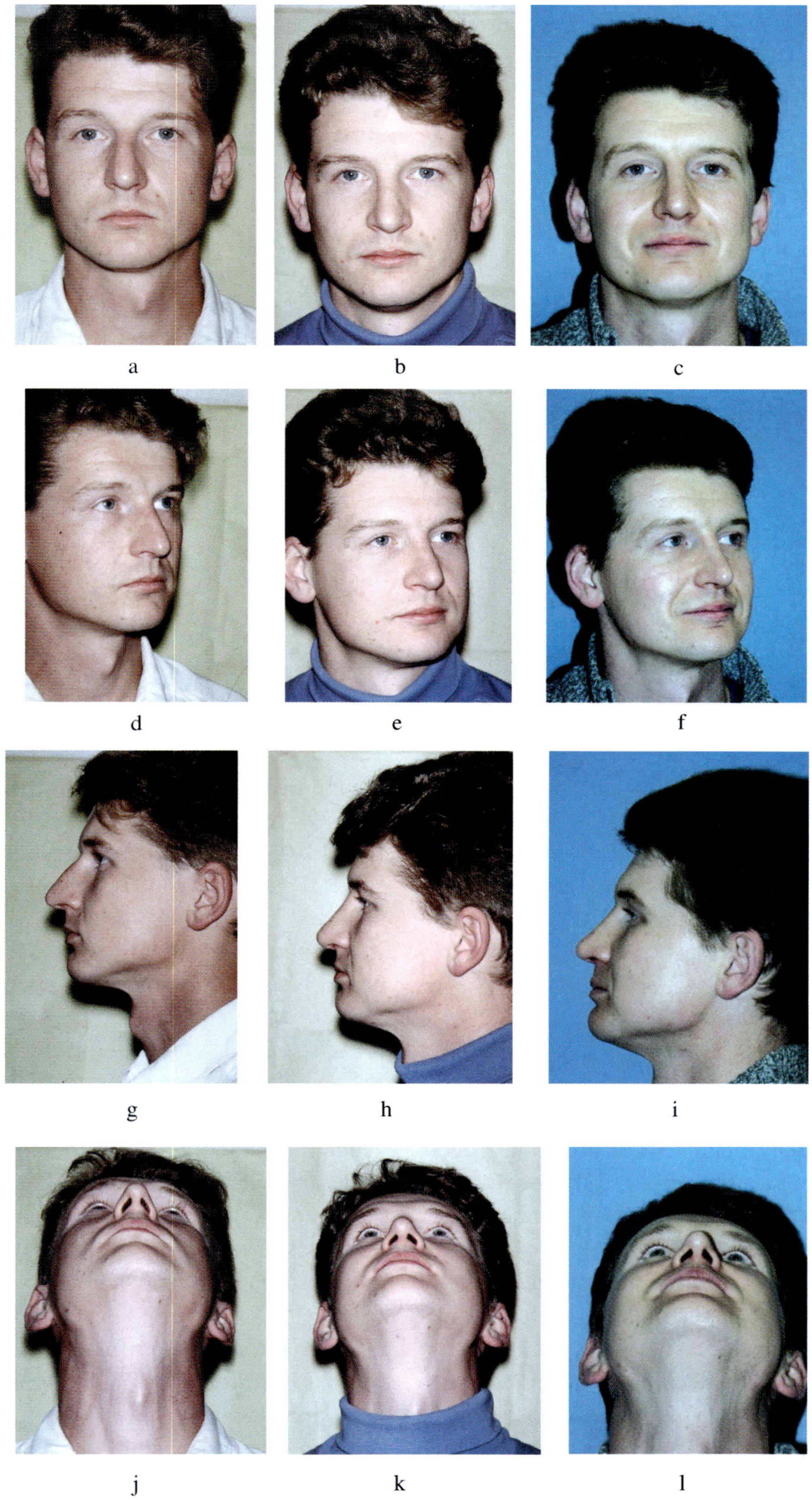

Fig. 22a-l. Pre- and post-operative anterior, oblique, lateral and basal views before (*a,d,g,j*), and three months (*b,e,h,k*), and five years (*c,f,i,l*) after external septal reconstruction with PDS foil.

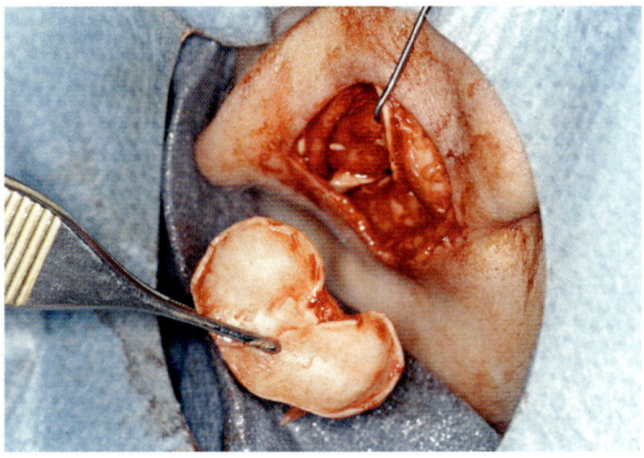

Fig. 23. Conchal cartilage for septal reconstruction, harvested by means of a retro-auricular approach.

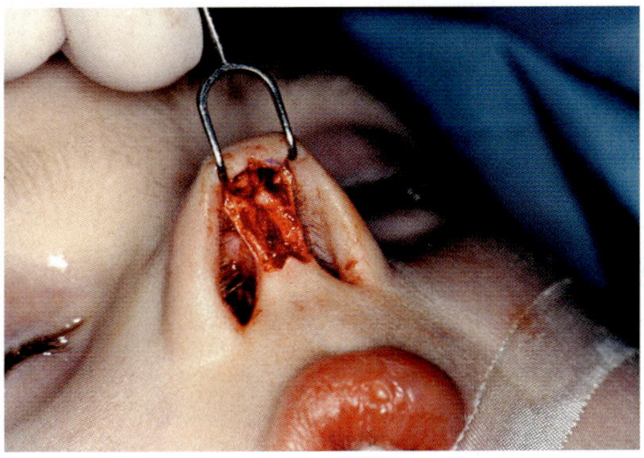

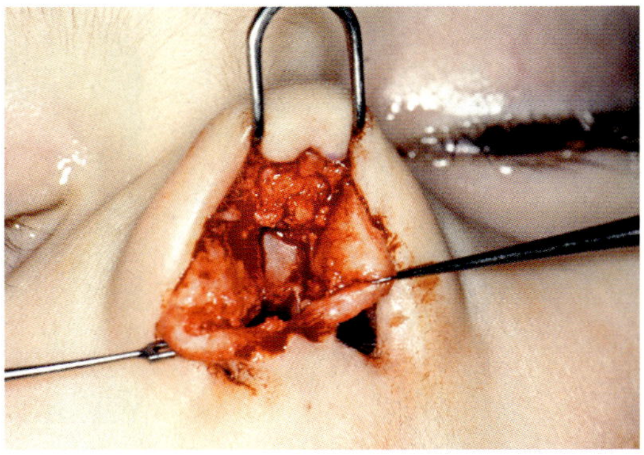

Fig. 24. External approach using a broken columella incision.

Fig. 25. Exposure of the skeleton after separating the medial crura.

Follow up

In the immediate postoperative follow-up period, the endonasal splints are removed the following morning, while the external fixation remains on the nose for five to eight days.

Comment

During operation and reconstruction of the nasal septum with PDS foil, the newly reconstructed septum appears to be relatively weak and is probably not stable enough. However, up to now sufficient stability has been maintained in each case in order to guarantee a straight septum.

So far with this technique, no immediate complications such as hematoma, inflammatory response or necroses have occurred.[12] Postoperatively, some patients have slight thickening of the septum for about three weeks, which disappears over the following two weeks. After a follow-up period of one year, the foil has already been resorbed, which ensures a long-lasting result. Postoperatively, a straight septum is achieved in 98%. In some cases, slight subluxation of the caudal septal border may occur. No late complications, such as atrophy of the septal mucosa, or cosmetic defects, such as saddle deformity or loss of tip support, have occurred so far. There were no cases of rejection of the foil. No septal perforation was encountered, even after intraoperative tearing of the mucosa. All patients had improved nasal airways, and even after severe postoperative nasal deformities, the cosmetic results were satisfactory.

A further indication for the use of PDS foil has been found by Nolst Trenité,[13] who has implanted PDS foil in the treatment of septal abscesses in children. The work on the management of septal abscesses in children can be summarized as follows: posttraumatic septal hematoma and abscesses in

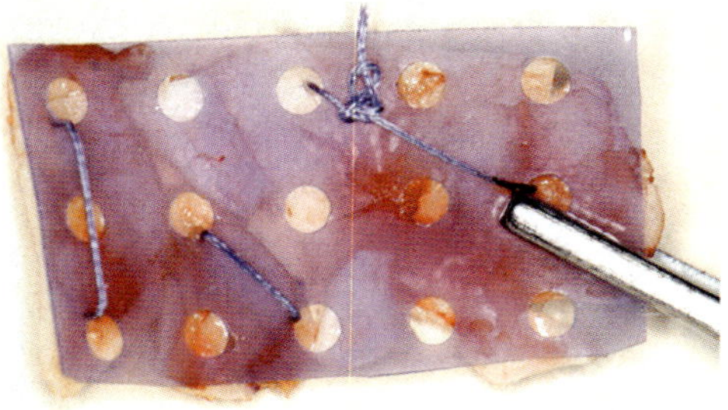

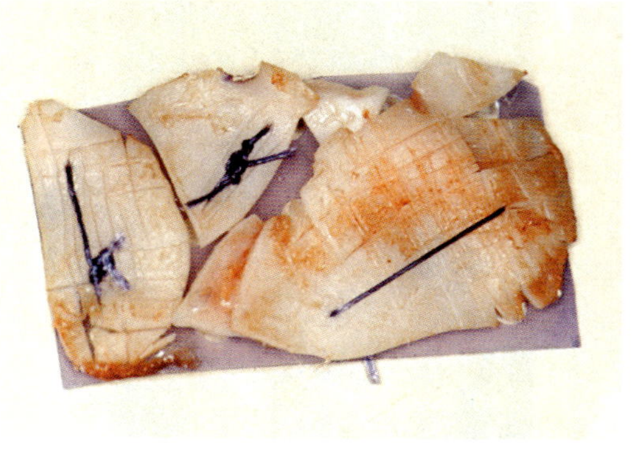

Fig. 26. PDS foil with ear cartilage sutured to it on the opposite side.

Fig. 27. Mosaic made up of pieces of conchal cartilage sutured to the PDS foil.

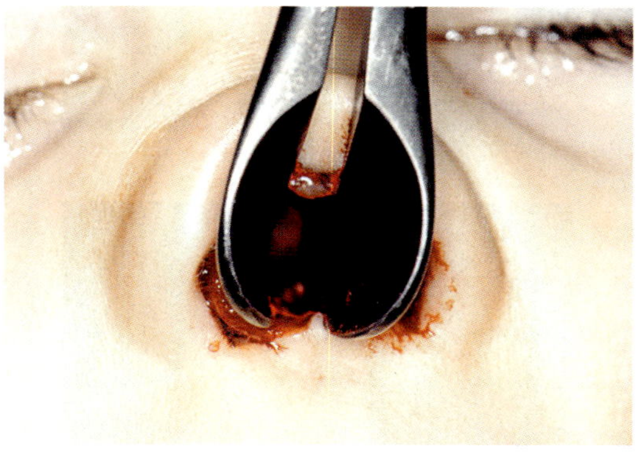

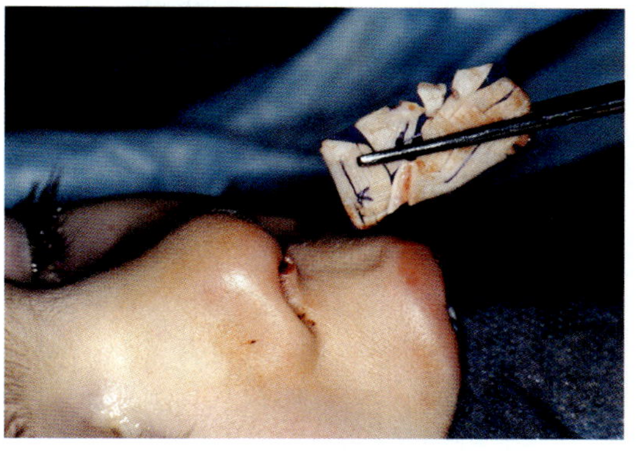

Fig. 28. Exposure of the space between the mucoperichondrial blades.

Fig. 29. Composite graft of PDS and cartilage ready for implantation.

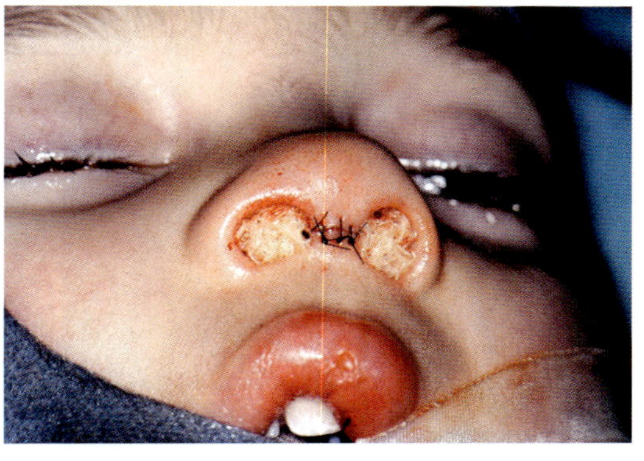

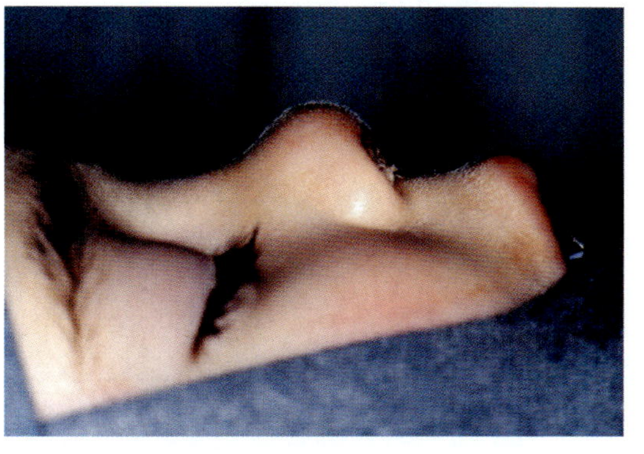

Fig. 30. Postoperative situation after closure of the broken columella incision (basal view).

Fig. 31. Direct postoperative lateral view with normal dorsal support.

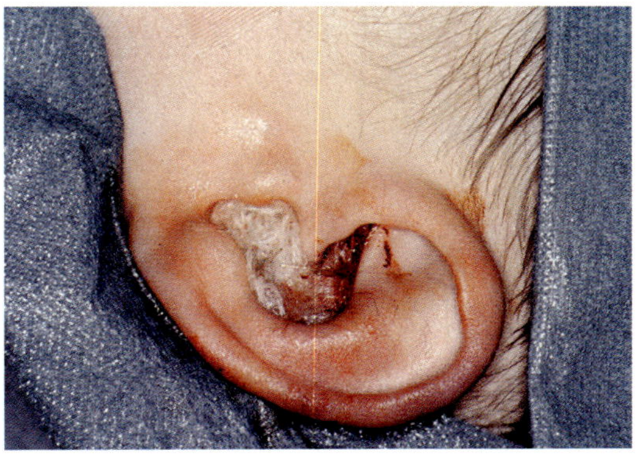

Fig. 32. Left auricle after harvesting conchal cartilage, with transcutaneously fixed packing to prevent hematoma.

children are an firm indication for surgical inspection under general anesthesia. Cartilage loss after a septal abscess requires reconstruction of the septum in order to prevent growth inhibition and nasal deformity. This reconstruction can be carried out either immediately or later on. In both cases, the use of PDS foil is recommended: in later reconstructions in order to prevent fibrous tissue between the mucoperichon-

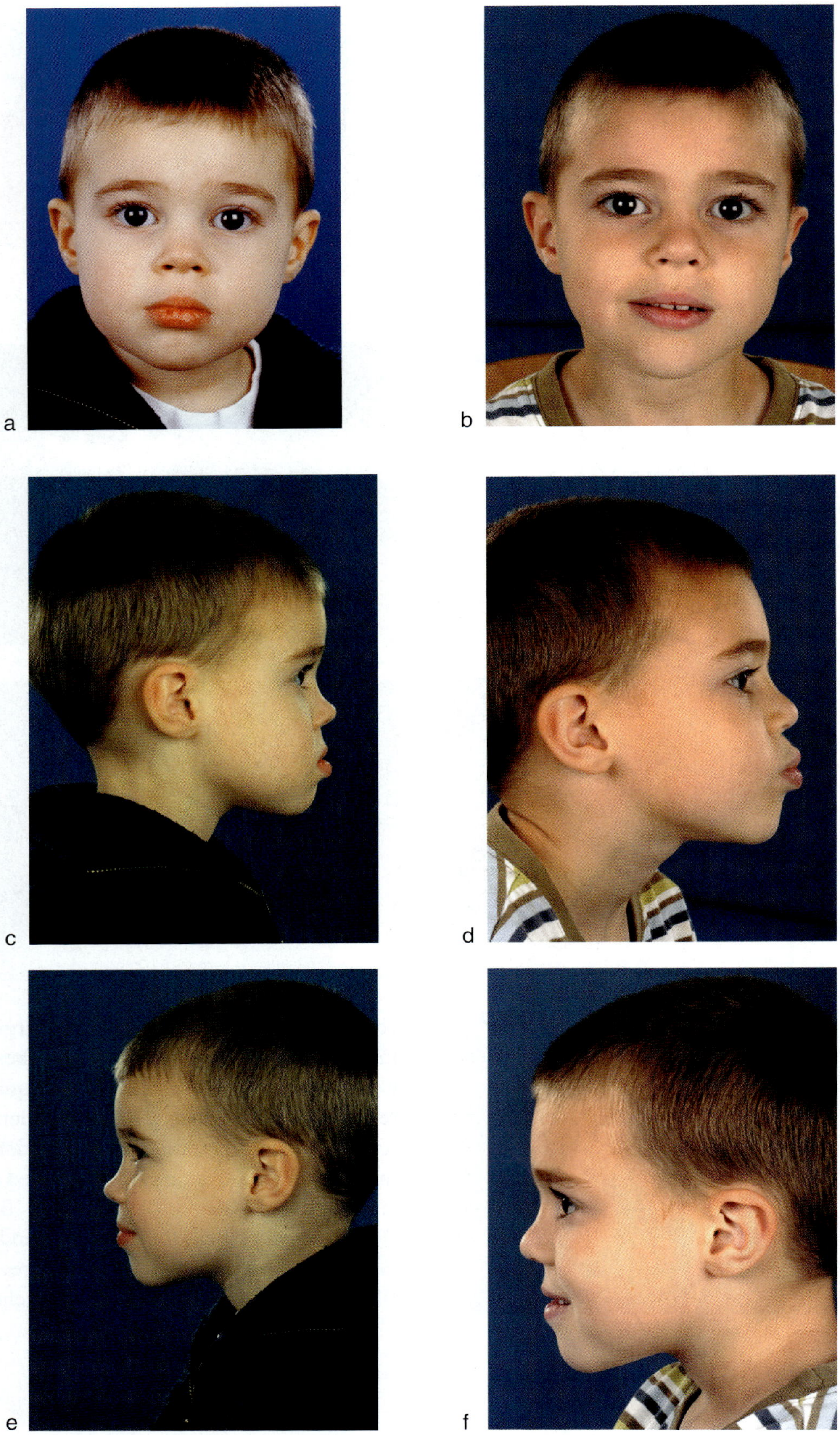

Fig. 33a-f. Preoperative views (*a,c,e,g,i*) of a four-year-old child one week after a septal abscess with destruction of the cartilaginous septum. Postoperative views (*b,d,f,h*) more than two years after septal reconstruction with a PDS-conchal cartilage graft and, up until now, normal growth and septal support of the nasal dorsum.

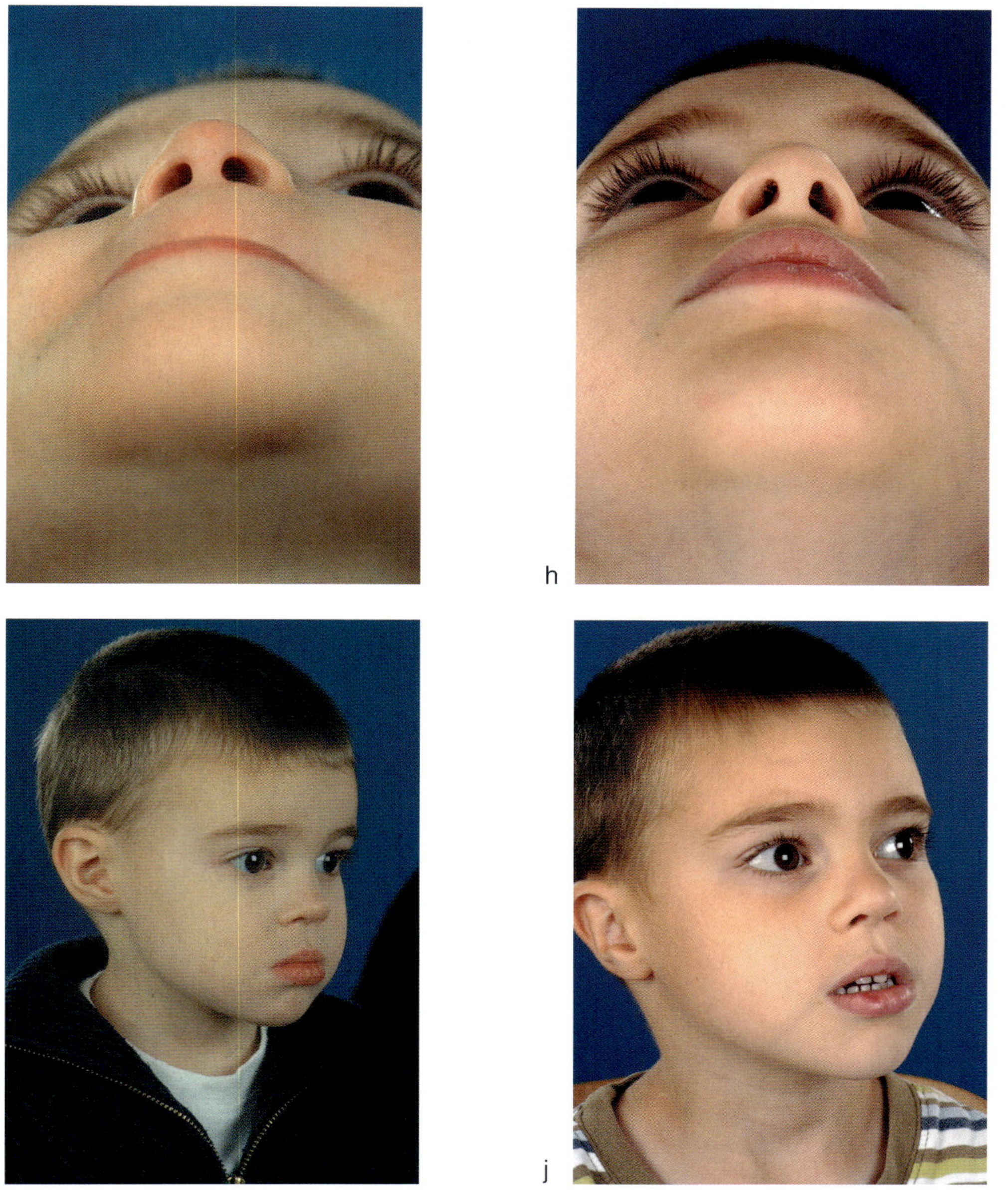

g h i j

Fig. 33g-j.

drium blades; in immediate reconstructions, the foil helps the surgeon to create a stable graft out of the autogenous cartilage (ear or rib) that is recommended for reconstruction. The surgical technique is shown in Figures 23 to 32 and the pre- and postoperative pictures of the same patient in figures 33a-j.

26: DEVELOPMENTS IN THE OPEN RHINOPLASTY APPROACH

R. Cobo

Introduction

External incisions have always been used in rhinoplasty and date back to about 600 BC when the Sushruta Ayurveda described an open approach to the nose in India.[1] In the early 1900s, Jacques Joseph, an orthopedic surgeon, described a reduction rhinoplasty by placing a midline incision over the length of the nose in order to resect skin and the underlying tissue.[1,2] In 1920, Gillies described an 'elephant trunk incision' placed low in the columella to approach the nasal tip.[3] The first complete description of an external approach to the nasal tip was published in 1934 by Rethi from Budapest, who used a transverse columellar incision to make changes to the nasal tip alone, because he did not believe this approach would allow adequate exposure of the nasal dorsum.[4] In 1958 in Zagreb, Sercer extended the operation to include the nasal pyramid and called his technique 'nasal decortication'.[5] Padovan, a disciple of Sercer, included the nasal septum in this open approach, and stated that this approach gave excellent access to the nose and allowed correction of external and internal problems. He presented his experience in New York during the First International Symposium of the American Academy of Facial Plastic and Reconstructive Surgery in 1970.[6] Goodman who was recognized as the first promoter of this technique in North America, developed the 'butterfly incision' in 1974. Much of his original descriptions are still used today.[7,8] In 1969, Jack Anderson, one of the main promoters of this approach, popularized the term 'open rhinoplasty approach'.[9] In the 1980s, Johnson and Toriumi introduced the term 'open structure rhinoplasty', which combined the open approach with a philosophy whereby the support structures of the nose were built up or maintained while changes to the nasal contour were performed.[10-12] Today, the terms 'open rhinoplasty' and 'external rhinoplasty' are used interchangeably and are considered to be an additional approach to the nose used by many surgeons worldwide.

When performing a rhinoplasty operation, the different structures of the nose (lower lateral cartilages, upper lateral cartilages, cartilaginous middle nasal third and septum, and bony structures of the nose and nasal base) must be approached by either the various closed approaches: non-delivery (cartilage splitting, retrograde), delivery approach; or by an external or open rhinoplasty approach.[13]

The approach to be used should be defined by the surgeon's personal ability to obtain the best possible results. The final surgical outcome does not exclusively depend on the approach used, it mainly depends on the surgeon's ability to make an accurate anatomical evaluation, perform the necessary corrective maneuvers, and modify the nasal structures in an adequate manner so as to provide the patient with, hopefully, a satisfactory long-term result.

'Open rhinoplasty' or 'external rhinoplasty' has become a widely used teaching tool in various residency programs throughout the world. It provides maximal exposure to the nasal tip, cartilaginous dorsum and bony nasal vault. The surgeon is able to diagnose in an accurate manner any existing deformities, asymmetries and structural alterations. The structures of the nose can be manipulated in a more precise manner, and sutures and grafts placed and fixed adequately. The general philosophy regarding rhinoplasty has changed over the years. There is a tendency to perform conservative resections and to reinforce the support structures of the nose, while changes in the nasal contour are achieved by reorienting the nasal structures with the use of sutures and grafts.[10,11]

Indications

The open rhinoplasty approach permits maximum exposure of the underlying nasal structures and permits exact placement of sutures and/or grafts. The various indications are:

- asymmetry of the alar cartilages or upper lateral cartilages (twisted tip)
- nasal tip with lack of support, projection or rotation
- over-projected nose
- crooked nose
- cleft-lip nose/saddle-nose deformities/other congenital nasal deformities
- septal perforations
- aging nose
- revision rhinoplasty
- teaching purposes

Disadvantages of open rhinoplasty

The disadvantages of the open approach are:

- increased operating time
- columellar scar
- compromise of the columellar flap with skin loss
- prolonged edema of the nasal tip

Of these disadvantages, the one that is probably cited most frequently by surgeons who do not use the open approach is the columellar scar. If proper closure techniques are used, this scar is rarely noticeable and generally disappears with time.[14] Compromise of the columellar flap with skin necrosis has been reported, but this is extremely rare. It is thought that it could be caused by elevation of the flap in a very superficial plane, very tight taping of the nasal tip, or aggressive resection of the subdermal nasal tip soft tissue. Prolonged edema of the nasal tip can be treated with subdermal injections of 1-2 mg tiamcinolone acetonide (Kenalog: 10 mg/ml) followed by taping of the nasal tip. These injections can be started one to three weeks after surgery and can be repeated every four weeks if required.[15]

Anatomy

When performing external rhinoplasty, it is important to have clear knowledge of the nasal vasculature in order to avoid any complications occurring on the cutaneous or musculo-aponeurotic flap that is being elevated.

The most important arteries, veins and lymphatics are located above the musculo-aponeurotic tissue of the nose. The arteries involved in the irrigation of the external nose are mainly branches of the facial artery, which comes from the external carotid system (Fig. 1):

- lateral nasal artery: a branch of the facial artery that follows the cephalic border of the lateral crura and unites in the midline with the columellar arteries
- angular artery: runs along the lateral nasal wall and unites with the dorsal nasal artery near the medial orbit
- dorsal nasal artery: a branch of the ophthalmic artery (branch of internal carotid artery)
- columellar arteries: branches of the superior labial artery

The lateral nasal artery and the columellar branches form a plexus which is responsible for irrigation of the nasal tip.

With the open approach, the columellar arteries are sectioned, but if the dissection is kept under the musculo-aponeurotic plane, vascular supply and lymphatic drainage are preserved, guaranteeing the

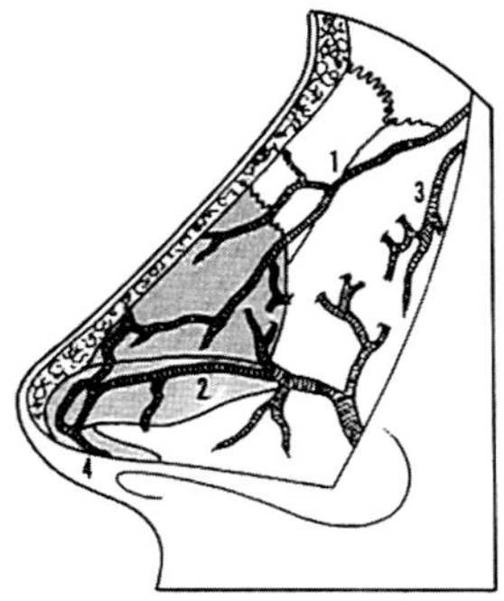

Fig. 1. Nasal vasculature: 1. dorsal nasal artery; 2. lateral nasal artery; 3. angular artery; 4. columellar artery.

survival of the flap and diminishing post-surgical edema of the nasal tip.[16]

Surgical technique

Approach to the nasal septum/graft harvesting

Cartilage for grafting can be harvested from many places, the most common ones being the septum and auricular concha. Septoplasty can be performed through several incisions: a hemitransfixion incision, a Killian incision, or through the same open approach. When using the open approach, the medial crura must be separated to reach the caudal septum. This approach is a very good choice in the management of tension noses, severe caudal deviations, and in patients with septal perforations. It is a more complicated approach and care must be taken to reconstruct the support structures of the nasal tip (columellar strut) in order to avoid loss of tip support.[16-19]

Cartilage is harvested depending on the patient's needs, always taking care to leave at least 1-1.5 cm of cartilage in the form of an inverted 'L' caudally and dorsally.[12] This will prevent collapse of the support structures of the nose with the passing of time. Any septal deviations should be corrected. If there is a need to perform turbinate surgery or functional endoscopic surgery of the paranasal sinuses, this is performed prior to management of the septum. Septal mucosa is sutured with a continuous 5-0 chromic or monocryl suture.

If the septum does not have enough cartilage for grafting, this can be obtained from the auricular concha. Auricular cartilage can be harvested by means of an anterior or posterior approach, taking special care not to tear the cartilage and performing careful hemostasia of underlying structures. Skin is sutured with 5-0 prolene, and conchal packing with gauze impregnated with antibiotic ointment is secured by a single through-and-through mattress suture in order to help prevent the formation of hematoma, possible skin necrosis, or deformity of the ear.

Transcolumellar incision/elevation of flap

An inverted 'V' incision is marked at the level of the mid-columella. The incision should be placed in the middle of the columella above the feet of the medial crura, in order to provide support for the scar. The incision is performed with a No. 15 blade, care being taken not to bevel the edges, and is connected to bilateral marginal incisions that are placed no more than 2 mm behind the caudal margin of the medial crura, and extended bilaterally following the caudal margin of the intermediate and lateral crura (Fig. 2).[10,12,16] It is important that the marginal incisions are not performed as 'rim incisions' since this can cause retracted scars after healing.

Elevation of the flap should be performed with angled Converse or Walter scissors, placed below the musculo-aponeurotic layer of the skin covering the medial crura. Using a spreading motion with the scissors, the correct tissue plane is identified, keeping the caudal margin of the medial crura below the scissors and dissecting medially. The midcolumellar incision is then completed with the angled scissors, again care being taken not to bevel the cut. The flap is elevated off the columella using small skin hooks, keeping as close as possible to the cartilaginous structure of the nose, special care being taken not to damage the caudal margin of the medial and intermediate crura, and dissecting laterally to the lateral crura. Once dissection of the nasal tip is complete, if the proper plane has been achieved, only a thin perichondrial layer is left on the cartilage. This is a relatively avascular approach where the only important vascular structures to be encountered are the columellar arteries that are transected when the midcolumellar incision is performed. This bleeding usually stops spontaneously, but if it persists, it can be cauterized with a bipolar cautery.

Once the flap has been elevated off the lateral crura, the dissection is shifted to the midline and the anterior septal angle is identified. Dissection of this areolar plane is performed in a blunt fashion with a cotton tip applicator. With this maneuver, the skin-soft tissue envelope can be dissected all the way up to the rhinion if necessary (Fig. 3).

If any work is going to be carried out on the dorsum, under direct vision using an Aufricht retractor, a Joseph periosteal elevator can be used to elevate periostium off the nasal dorsum and up to the nasion. The subperiosteal incision should be done 2 mm cephalad to the caudal margins of the nasal bones, care being taken not to disarticulate the upper lateral cartilages from the nasal bone. Subperiosteal dissection can be performed up to the nasion and laterally, care being taken not to extend dissection too far down to the bony nasal pyramid side walls. With this, the open approach is complete and the surgeon can then proceed with the rhinoplasty.

Approach to the osseocartilaginous dorsum

When using the open approach, the dorsum is first approached before proceeding to the middle third and tip of the nose.[11,20] When necessary, osteotomes and/or rasps are used under direct vision in order to lower and

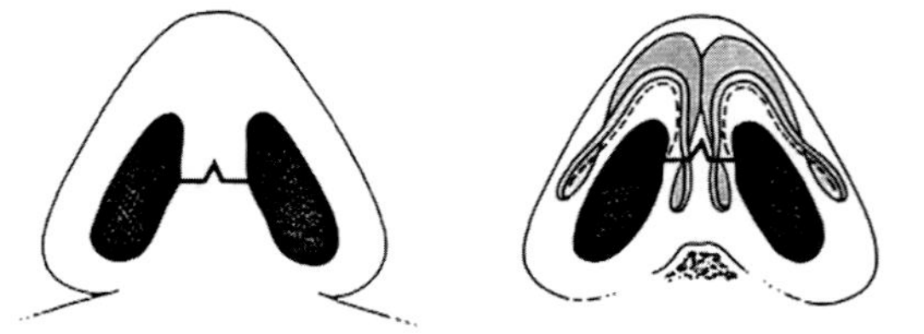

Fig. 2. Incision in open rhinoplasty: an inverted 'V' incision is marked at the level of the midcolumella and connected to bilateral marginal incisions which are placed no more than 2 mm behind the caudal margin of the medial crura. The incision is then completed following the caudal margin of the intermediate and lateral crura.

regularize the dorsum. The technique to be used really depends on the expertise of the surgeon. In selected cases when there is need to reduce the nasofrontal angle, this can be performed with a special guarded diamond burr to obtain satisfactory results. When planning a dorsal reduction, two points must always be borne in mind: the skin is thick at the nasofrontal angle and thin at the rhinion, if the surgeon wants a straight dorsum, his highest point should be the osseocartilaginous junction (rhinion) in order to avoid a slight dip in this area after edema resolves. When performing hump removal, this should be completed all the way up to the nasion (nasofrontal angle) and should always be done conservatively. If the dorsum is going to be approached using rasps, it is important to rasp angled away from the midline in order to avoid avulsing the upper lateral cartilages from the nasal bones. Any debris should be washed away with saline solution.

The cartilaginous dorsum is reduced *en bloc* or by performing multiple layered cuts, starting at the osseocartilaginous junction and moving down caudally to the anterior septal angle. It is important not to leave the anterior septal angle too high since this can create a supratip or 'polly beak' deformity. The final refinements to the cartilaginous dorsum should be performed after the tip procedures have been completed and osteotomies performed.

The open rhinoplasty approach is especially helpful in cases where the middle cartilaginous third of the nose has to be addressed. Bilateral or unilateral spreader grafts can be sutured in place between the

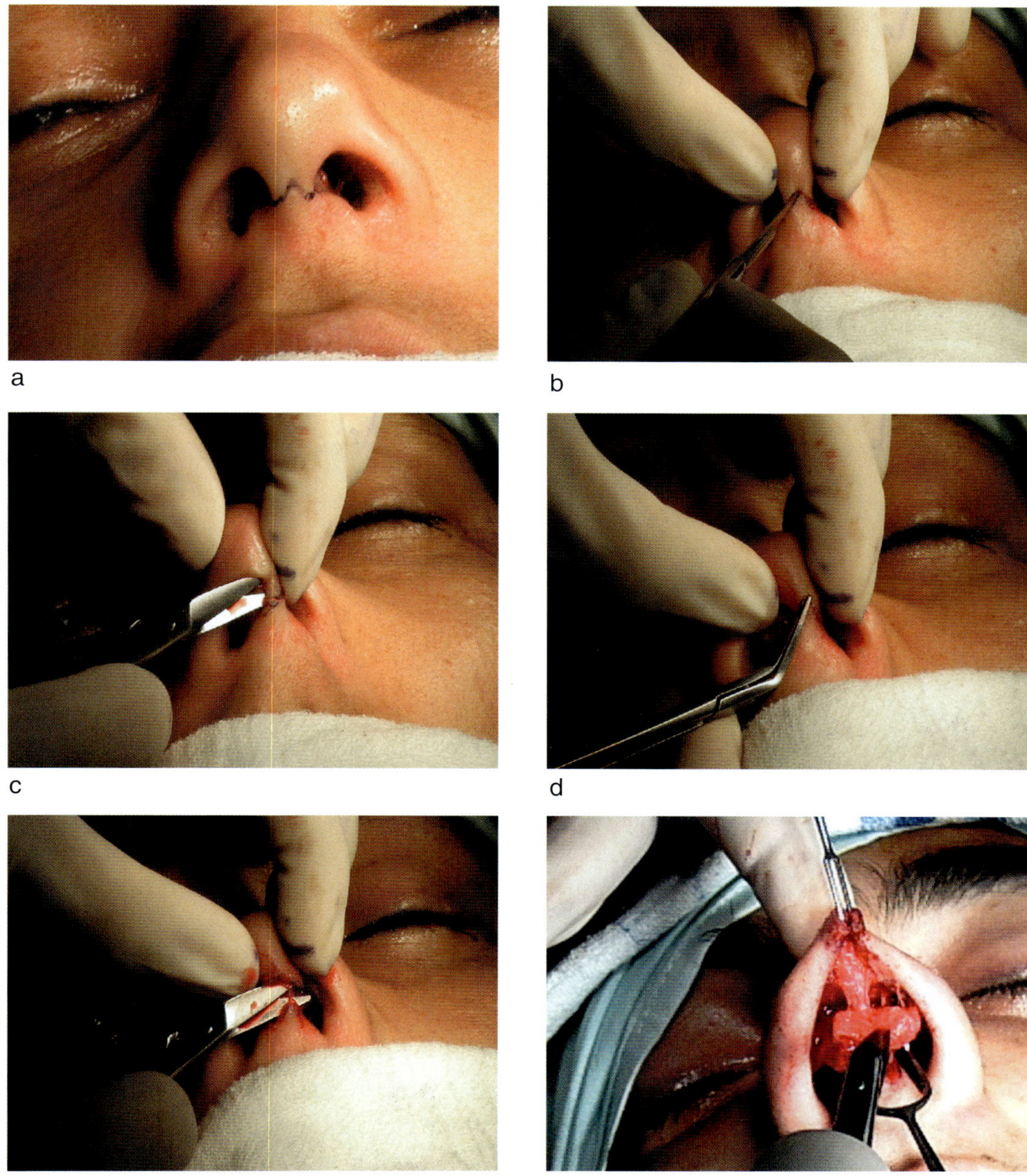

a b c d e f

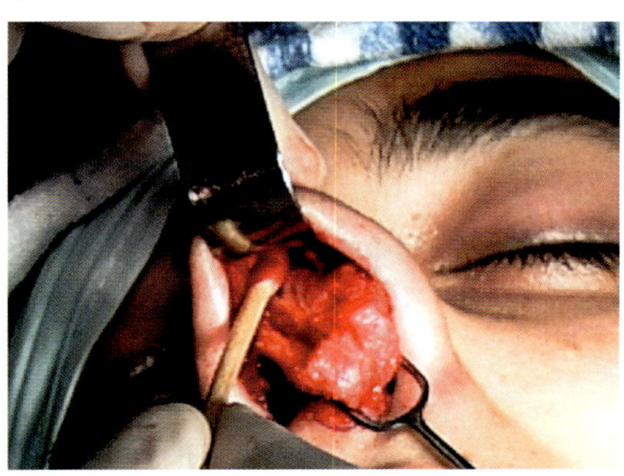

g

Fig. 3a-g. Flap elevation in open rhinoplasty: *a* and *b*. an inverted 'V' incision is marked at the level of the midcolumella and connected to bilateral marginal incisions using a #15 blade. It is important to keep the blade perpendicular to the skin edges, taking care not to section the medial crura. *c*, *d* and *e*. Once the incision is complete, converse scissors are inserted, using a spreading motion, under the musculoaponeurotic layer. If the columellar arteries are seen, they can be cut without compromising the flap. *f*. Using converse scissors and double hooks, the flap is dissected carefully off the lower lateral cartilages and the fibrous connections in the midline over the domal area are cut up to the cartilage of the middle third of the nose is identified. *g*. The dissection is continued up to the rhinion in a blunt fashion, using a cotton tip applicator.

upper later cartilages and septum in order to correct a narrow middle third of the nose, a crooked anterior (dorsal) septal border, or to manage nasal valve collapse (Fig. 4). In the cases where there is over-rotation of the nasal tip or an overly shortened nose, caudal extension grafts of the anterior nasal septum can be adequately placed through the open approach, since this permits exact fixation of these particular grafts.[21,22]

The grafts used in all these patients should ideally be harvested from the nasal

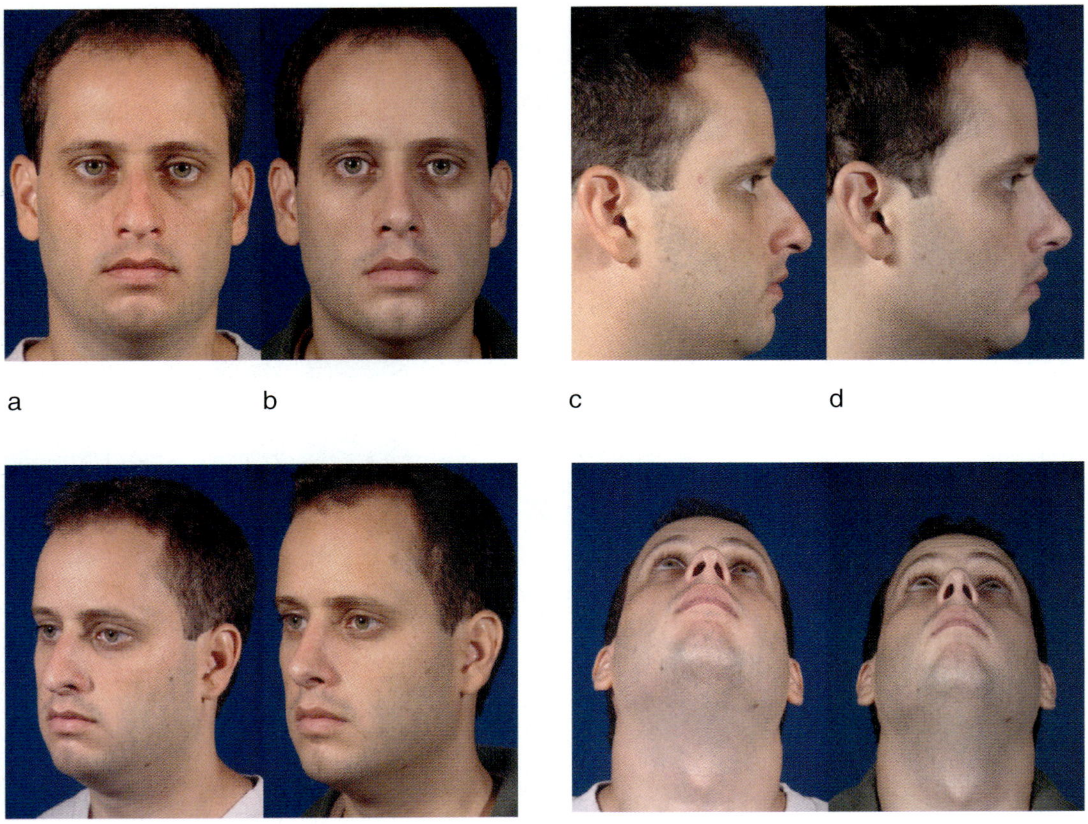

a b c d e f g h

Fig. 4a-h. a,c,e,g. Male patient with a small dorsal hump, a slightly droopy long nasal tip, and a narrow middle third of the nose. *b,d,f,h.* Post-operative images showing placement of bi-lateral spreader grafts, conservative hump removal, use of a columellar strut, and tip suturing techniques (lateral crural steal) to improve tip rotation and definition.

septum because it is straighter and firmer and tailored according to the patient's needs. The grafts are fixed with 4-0 or 5-0 vicryl or PDS horizontal mattress sutures, care being taken that the caudal edges of these grafts do not extend above the dorsal edge of the septum. Once the graft has been fixed, the upper lateral cartilages should be sutured to the graft and septum.

Columellar strut

In itself, the open approach produces disruption of the minor support structures of the nose that should be reconstructed with sutures or grafts in order to avoid post-surgical loss of tip projection.

This columellar strut (which is harvested from the septal or conchal cartilage) will provide additional support to the medial crura, help preserve rotation and projection of the nasal tip, correct buckling and asymmetries of the medial crura, and help create a stable base that can be used for the placement of tip grafts.

A small pocket should be dissected between the medial crura, care being taken not to go all the way down to the nasal spine (Fig. 5). The strut is placed in this pocket and sutured with a 5-0 vicryl mattress suture that should not be placed too near the domes or too close to the caudal margins of the intermediate crura. This can distort the normal divergence of the intermediate crura and produce loss of the double-break in the infratip lobule.[10-12] The superior portion of the strut should be cut 1-2 mm below the level of the final domes.

It is not unusual to see a hanging columella after placement of a columellar strut. For this reason, the caudal septum should be evaluated and, if it is long, conservative caudal resection should be performed before strut placement.

Approach to the nasal tip

One of the great advantages of the open rhinoplasty approach is the undistorted view it gives of the nasal tip structures and the opportunity to make an adequate evaluation of the various tip deformities. Changes carried out on the lower third of the nose should be performed keeping the tripod concept in mind. This tripod is formed by the conjoined medial crura and both lateral crura. Changes on any of the legs of the tripod will alter tip projection and rotation.[12] The open approach provides an ample surgical field, providing the surgeon with the possibility of performing exact changes that attempt to maintain symmetry as much as possible without compromising support structures. Surgical options should always be evaluated, starting with the simpler techniques and progressing to the more aggressive ones, depending on the individual patient's needs.

Intact strip procedures

In the majority of primary rhinoplasties, one of the main objectives is refinement of the nasal tip. Most techniques start with resection of the cephalic margin of the lateral crura, followed by different suture-narrowing techniques to help define the nasal lobule. Suture-narrowing and tip-defining techniques, such as the transdomal suture-narrowing technique, double-dome unit technique, and lateral crural steal, all have similar objectives: placement of sutures around the domal area in order to narrow the domes, define the nasal tip and increase tip rotation and projection.[23-25] When performing any of these techniques, the final cosmetic result will depend on how much cartilage is left behind and how symmetric the nasal tip looks after placement of sutures or scoring maneuvers. Aggressive cartilage excision will not additionally refine a nasal lobule, but instead with time will produce post-surgical nasal valve collapse, pinching, buckling, and bossae formation. This can be minimized by leaving approximately 8 mm of lateral crus and, if necessary, performing very conservative resections of the scroll area. Most refinement techniques can be adequately performed using an endonasal approach, but it is clear that, with the open approach, the surgical field is larger and cartilage incisions, excisions and suture placement can be carried out in an accurate manner (Fig. 6).

Incomplete strip procedures

Open rhinoplasty is especially helpful in cases where different vertical division techniques either of the medial or lateral crura are used. Overlapping techniques can be performed in a more precise manner using an open approach. What cartilage division technique is used, or where it is placed, really depends on the surgeon's preference and the patient's needs. Ideally, an intact strip should be reconstructed, bearing in mind that the tripod should not be weakened, in order to prevent asymmetries or buckling. Often when incomplete strip procedures are performed, grafts can be used for camouflage and to strengthen the tripod.[11,19]

Grafts

Grafts have always been used in primary and revision rhinoplasty. Some surgeons have the ability to place grafts through small pockets or by using an endonasal approach. However, it is clear that one of the great advantages of open rhinoplasty is graft and implant placement in the dorsum or graft placement in the nasal tip. Grafts and implants can often shift or migrate; the open approach helps to fix them in place with sutures.

The type of material used depends upon the surgical goal: if alar grafting is needed, conchal cartilage is the material of choice because of its natural convex shape. Tip grafts should ideally be carved from septal cartilage because it is stiff and gives support and definition to the nasal tip.

Grafts such as the shield graft in the infratip lobule can be very useful in patients needing additional tip defining procedures, or when the techniques used to refine the lobule do not completely satisfy the surgeon. The shield graft is a versatile tool that, if used properly, can increase tip projection, nasal length, columellar length, and define the nasal lobule (Fig. 7).

The shield graft is sutured to the caudal margins of the medial/intermediate crura-strut complex. It is important to have a stable, aligned tripod before placing a shield graft, since this additional structure can shift the tripod, resulting in an asymmetric or deviated tip. Shield grafts can be long, short, or multi-layered. They are ideal in thick-skinned patients, but can also be used in thin-skinned patients, care being taken to bevel the edges and not to leave any sharp angles. This graft is usually thicker at the tip and thinner in the inferior portion. The usual dimensions are 8-12 mm in width, 8-15 mm in length and 1-3 mm in thickness.[10,12] Placement of the graft is important, the upper leading edge should ideally be placed 1-2 mm above the domes and in thick-skinned patients, up to 3 mm above the domes (Fig. 8). Final carving of the graft can be performed after it has been fixed, in order to obtain a smooth contour. In cases where the graft is placed higher above the domes in order to give additional projection, a buttress graft can be placed behind the shield graft to avoid a dip and to create a smooth transition from the tip to the middle third of the nose. The buttress graft can be carved from septal or conchal cartilage, it is rectangular in shape and is sutured behind the shield graft.[10,11] Combination of these two grafts can help give additional support and definition to an underprojected, undefined, bulbous nasal tip.

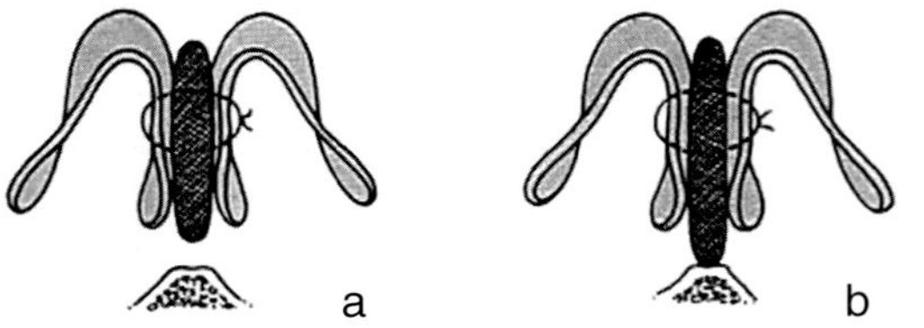

Fig. 5. Columellar strut: *a.* The strut is fixed with a 5-0 vicryl mattress suture, care being taken to correct any buckling or asymmetries of the medial crura. The suture should ideally be placed below the divergence of the intermediate crura in order to preserve the natural double break of the columella. *b.* The strut should not go all the way down to the nasal spine as it can shift to one side, creating asymmetries and caudal deviations; and it should not surpass the domal area as it can deform the nasal tip. When the suture is placed high near the domal area, the natural double break of the columella will be erased.

In patients with thin skin, in whom a shield graft is not the best option, but in whom there is a need for additional definition and projection, a 'cap graft' can be used. This graft is quadrangular in shape, with the narrower portion being sutured over the lower lateral crura and the wider border over the domes. If the graft is not carefully carved and appropriately fixed, it can become very noticeable over time. It is very important that all the edges are smoothed out so that it blends in well with the underlying cartilage (Fig. 9).[11]

In cases where slight additional support and augmentation are needed in a weak domal area, small rectangular cartilage wedges known as 'domal apex grafts' can be placed in a small pocket that is created between the vestibular skin and cartilage.[11] It is important to have symmetrical domes and grafts in order to avoid postsurgical tip asymmetry (Fig. 10).

Osteotomies

Osteotomies to narrow the upper third of the nose are not performed in all cases of rhinoplasty. When minimal or no resection is performed on the dorsum, and its width is in proportion with the nasal base, osteotomies are not necessary.

Medial oblique osteotomies are not carried out routinely, they are performed before lateral osteotomies, and are used when there is a very wide nasal dorsum with an appropriate profile, when minimal hump removal has been performed, or in a deviated nose. Lateral osteotomies are carried out at the end of surgery. An endonasal

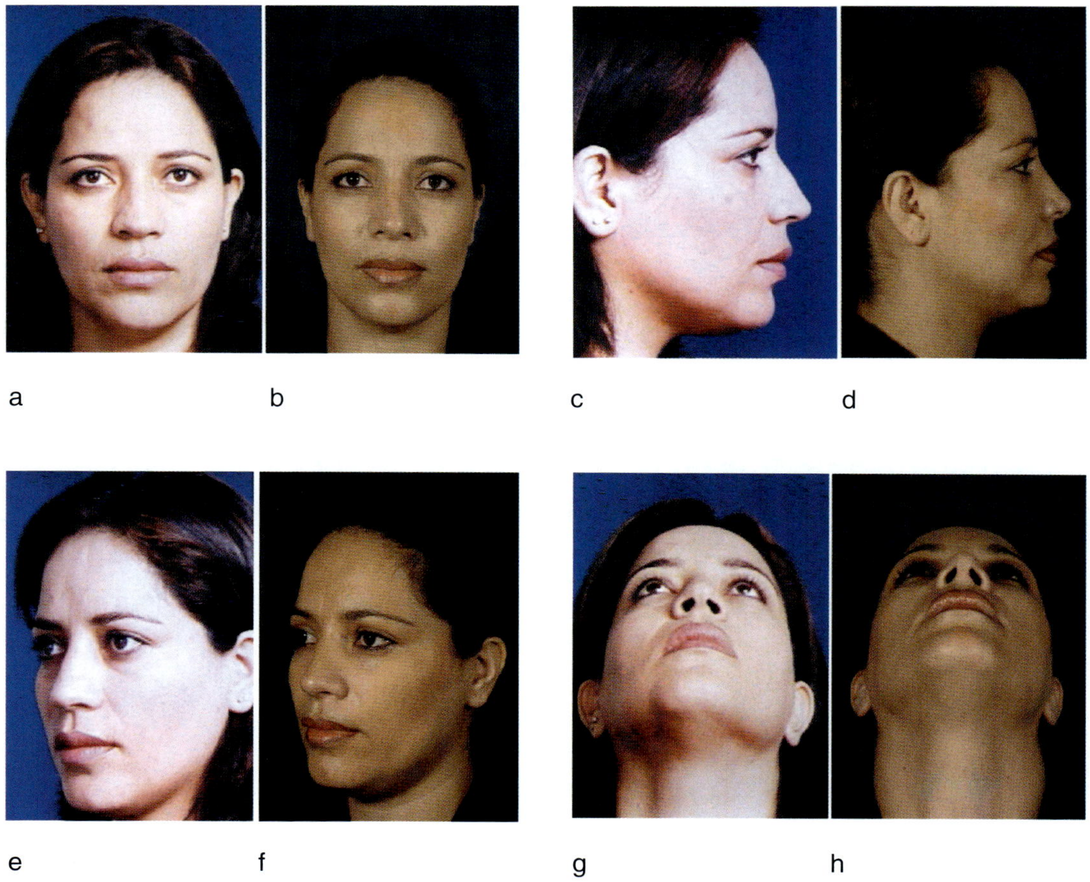

Fig. 6a-h. a,c,e,g. Female patient with a wide upper third of the nose, a small osseocartilaginous hump, and a slightly wide nasal tip. *b,d,f,h.* Post-operative images showing lateral osteo-tomies to narrow the upper third of the nose with rasping of the hump. The tip was narrowed and defined slightly by performing conservative cephalic trim of the alar cartilages. A columellar strut was inserted to preserve rotation of the nasal tip.

high-low-high technique is performed with a 2.2-mm guarded osteotome, finishing at the level of the medial canthus with back-fracture of the bone. Back-fracture of the bone can be carried out by rotating the osteotome inwards, percutaneously, with a 2-mm osteotome, or by means of digital pressure. If dorsal onlay grafts are going to be used, these are placed under direct vision and sutured in place with non-absorbable sutures after all the bony work has been completed.

Closure of a mid-columellar incision

Closure of the mid-columellar incision is very important in open rhinoplasty. If done correctly and the skin edges are everted and not closed under tension, there will be no scarring no matter what type of skin the patient has. The incision can be closed with 6-0 nylon or prolene and marginal incisions with catgut or vicryl. When wound closure is carried out under tension, a single subcutaneous absorbable 6-0 suture can be used to ease any tension on the skin suture. The first skin suture is always placed in the midline at the tip of the inverted V. Closure is continued with angled off-midline sutures, starting medially from the inferior flap and extending laterally to the superior flap. This helps recruit skin medially and prevents lateral notching of the columellar incision.[10,16] The vestibular skin of the columellar flap can be closed with 6-0 prolene or chromic catgut. Marginal incisions are closed with a single 5-0 chromic, monocryl or vicryl suture, which is placed slightly laterally to the domes, care being taken that there is no notching or distortion of the domes or the caudal extension of the ala.

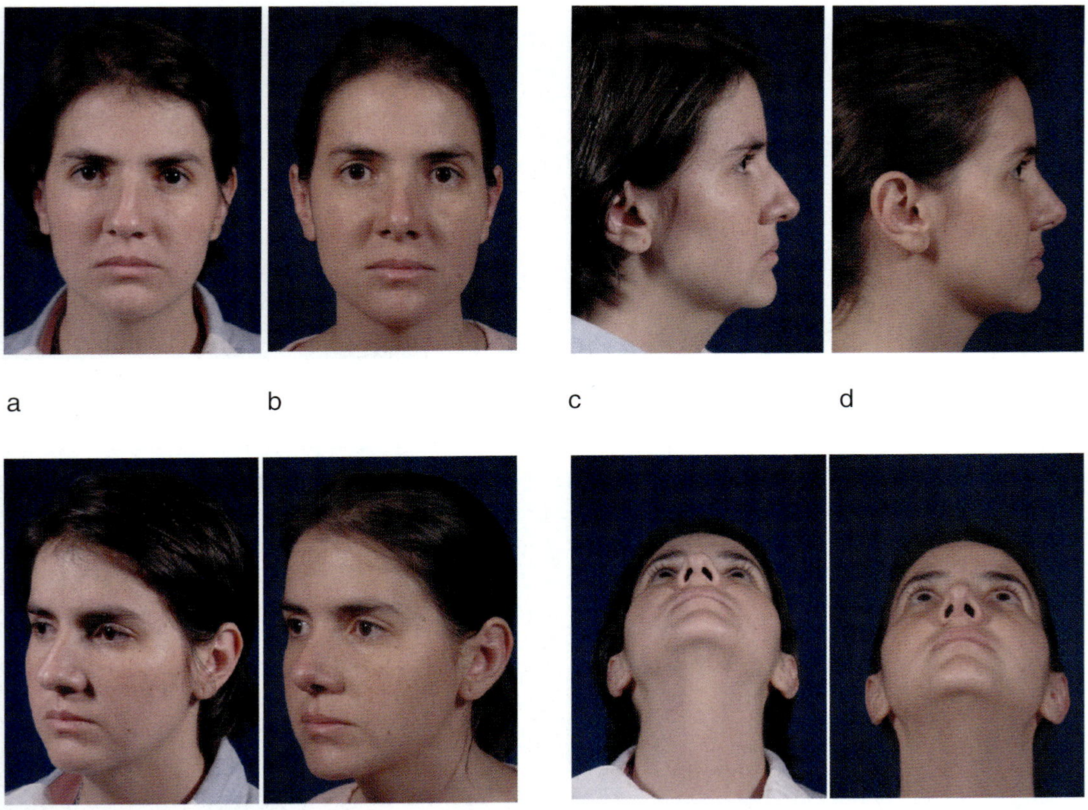

Fig. 7a-h. a,c,e,g. Female patient with a deviated nose, collapse of the right upper lateral cartilage and a wide bulbous boxy nasal tip. *b,d,f,h.* Post-operative views showing lateral osteotomies and placement of a right spreader graft to correct nasal deviation. The tip was approached by performing cephalic trim of the alar cartilages; placement of transdomal sutures to correct a boxy tip deformity, and placement of a columellar strut and shield graft to give final definition and symmetry to the nasal tip.

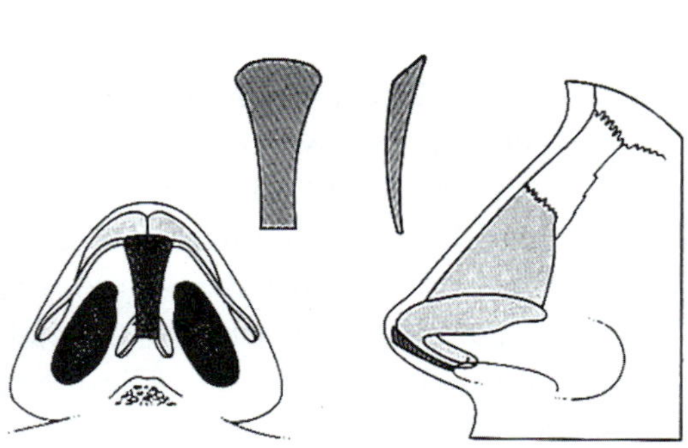

Fig. 8. (Left.) Shield graft: this graft is ideally harvested from septal cartilage, but auricular cartilage can also be used. It is wider and slightly thicker superiorly and thinner and narrower at its base. The graft is sutured to the caudal margins of the medial and intermediate crura. It is important to have a stable aligned nasal tripod and base before graft placement. Shield grafts increase tip projection and definition. They are ideal in thick-skinned patients.

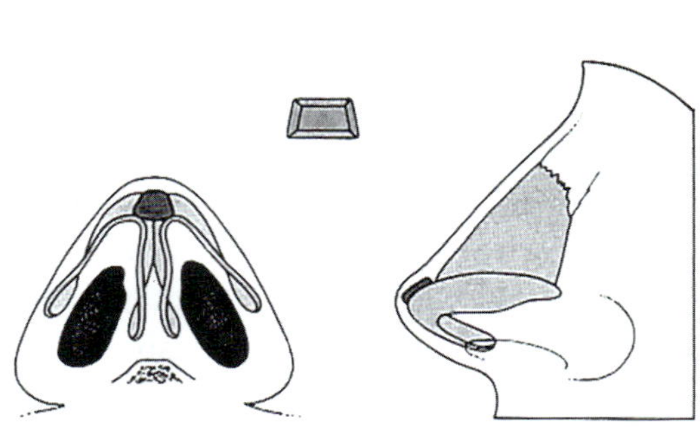

Fig. 9. (Right.) Cap graft: this is a quadrangular beveled piece of cartilage with its wider edge placed over the domal area and its narrower edge over the cephalic portion of the lateral crura. It gives additional projection and definition to the nasal tip.

Nasal packing/external splinting/post-operative care

How much and what packing is placed inside the nose will depend on the type of functional surgery being performed. In routine septal work, usually a 4-0 or 5-0 continuous horizontal mattress absorbable suture will be sufficient. When extensive septal work or additional endoscopic sinus surgery and turbinate surgery has been performed, some intranasal packing can be used to prevent any postsurgical bleeding, formation or hematoma or synechia. Packing is removed 24-48 hours later, and the nasal cavity is kept moist with saline solution sprays in order to prevent excessive crust formation.

Many different types of external splints can be used: plaster, metallic, or thermoplastic. The nasal dorsum and tip is taped, and the splint is applied covering upper and

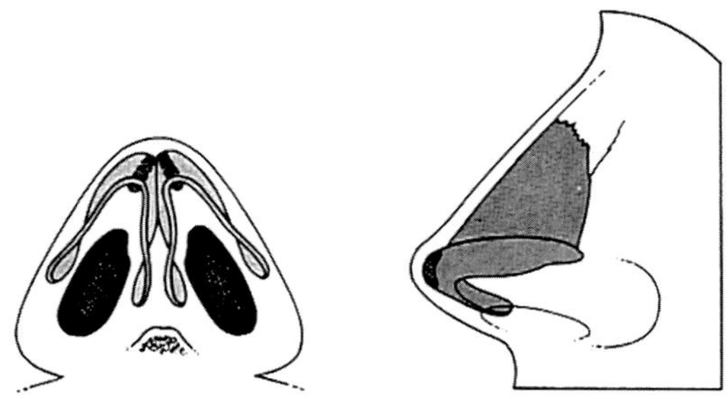

Fig. 10. Domal apex grafts: these are small rectangular wedges of cartilage (ideally harvested from the nasal septum) which are placed in an accurately-formed pocket under the domes. They augment support to the domal area. They should be placed symmetrically in order to avoid post-surgical tip irregularities.

middle third of the nose. Nasal tapes and external splints should not be too tight since this can compromise the vascularity of the nasal flap.

Columellar sutures are removed after four to six days, care being taken to tape the incision site posteriorly. External splints are removed after seven days, and the nose is taped for an additional three to seven days, depending on the formation of edema and type of skin.

Conclusions

The open rhinoplasty approach has evolved throughout the years and today is considered an additional approach in rhinoplasty. Its uses are not limited to difficult or revision noses. It gives an undistorted generous view of the surgical field, permitting adequate diagnosis of any deformity, exact placement of grafts and sutures, correction of asymmetries, and modification of the different nasal components without compromising the support structures of the nose. It is a versatile surgical approach which can be used for all rhinoplasty procedures, unless the surgeon feels he can obtain the same or better results by means of an endonasal approach. Rhinoplasty has always been a challenging operation where it is difficult to obtain consistent satisfactory results. What really counts in rhinoplasty is not the approach to be used, but rather the choice of surgical technique that can give pleasing, aesthetic and functional, consistent long-term results.

27: ETHNIC RHINOPLASTY

R. Cobo and G.J. Nolst Trenité

Introduction

Rhinoplasty is one of the most popular and frequently performed aesthetic surgical procedures, not only in the USA, but also in all other countries worldwide. The world is composed of hundreds of different ethnic groups with huge variations between them. Historically, through the ages, people of all races and ethnicities have always had an interest in looking attractive. Rhinoplasty has been growing in demand over the years, and every time people from different ethnic groups want to reshape their noses into what they consider to be more attractive.

The standards of beauty have changed through the ages, and each race possesses its own unique beautiful features that, as rhinoplasty surgeons, we cannot ignore. Each ethnic group has distinctive features that characterize it, and it is important to be able to identify these and to define which of these characteristics we want to preserve and which we want to modify. In our culture, communication media have spread and popularized the Caucasian or 'western' look as a world standard for beauty. And although, due to globalization, the world is evolving towards a mixture of races, this look still predominates in our society today.[1] The ideal Caucasian nose is defined as one with a slightly projecting and defined nasal tip, a strong bony and cartilaginous dorsum, moderately thin skin, and defined gentle angles. This is still considered the gold standard in rhinoplasty today.[2] When evaluating an 'ethnic patient', the modern rhinoplasty surgeon should try to define his or her ethnic background, evaluate and define the specific nasal anatomy, and be able to offer realistic surgical options.

The ethnic nose frequently has a more modest osseocartilaginous framework, the skin tends to be thicker, and the nasal tip has flimsy unsupportive alar cartilages that give a more undefined look and less defined angles.[1,3] There are hundreds of different ethnic groups throughout the world, which have tended to become more mixed due to globalization and modernization. A practical way of approaching the main different ethnic groups is to divide them into important geographical zones: African, Asian, Mediterranean, Middle Eastern, North European, and Latin American. Even though within these groups many different ethnical variations will always be found, there are some general characteristics that can help the surgeon in his surgical approach. With time, the ideal nose will become a 'blending' of different ethnicities, especially if we take into account the fact that, today, most of the world is non-Caucasian.

Preoperative evaluation

Consultation

It is very important to have the time and the ability to communicate with the patient. Knowledge of the ethnic background is important, not only in defining whether the patient wants to maintain his or her ethnicity, but also to be able come up with an adequate surgical plan. The patient's desires and expectations must be fully understood and, as surgeons, we must be able to decide whether we can comply with them. It is always important to be able to identify the patient who will never be satisfied with the way he looks and to define his psychological eligibility for surgery.

During the consultation, possible complications such as bleeding, hematoma formation and infections, must be mentioned, as well as limitations on physical exercise and exposure to the sun. Additionally, the patient must understand that this is not a magical operation, it is always hard to obtain a perfect result in rhinoplasty, and the patient must be aware of this. Written information explaining the surgical procedure, anesthesia, possible complications, postoperative care and general recommendations will help the patient during his consultation with the specialist.[4]

Physical examination

Once a complete medical history has been obtained, a detailed physical examination must be undertaken, with time being taken to show the patient any asymmetries or facial characteristics that might influence the final surgical result. A complete external and internal nasal examination must be performed, to evaluate the function of the nose. This examination is usually performed with a nasal speculum and can be complemented with rigid or flexible nasal endoscopy. It is important to evaluate alar collapse and to define whether there is compromise of the internal or external nasal valve, septal deviation, availability of septal cartilage for harvesting, turbinate hypertrophy, or sinus disease.

Cosmetically, several things must be kept in mind when evaluating patients for ethnic rhinoplasty (Table 1):

- skin type: is it thick or thin/ oily and sebaceous or dry/elasticity
- nasal dorsum: is it high or low; does it have a hump
- nasal bridge: is it too wide or too narrow
- nasal tip: quality of alar cartilages: are they strong or flimsy/ wide or thin
- nasolabial angle: is it acute or obtuse
- nasal base: is it wide/normal/narrow
- orientation of nostrils: are they vertical, horizontal, or oval shaped; flaring or non-flaring
- nasal tip support: is it weak or strong/evaluation of tip recoil

Photography

Once these questions have been answered and documented, it is important to obtain a set of standard rhinoplasty photographs and to sit down with the patient and show him/her what results can be obtained. Digital programs that can modify images are useful for showing patients what can be obtained with surgery. They also help the patient to understand the limitations of the procedure and to create realistic expectations.

Standard pre- and postoperative rhinoplasty photographs should be taken routinely. Their applications are not just limited to the pre-surgical consultation, they are also an invaluable tool for:

- reference during surgery
- analysis of the final outcome of surgery, and evaluation of the different surgical techniques used
- documentation for medico-legal purposes
- teaching

Nasal anatomy of the main ethnic groups

Ideally, a complete description should be made of all the possible different ethnic groups existing today. It is incredible to see how many different variations there are to be found within the same ethnic group. Many of these ethnic variations will depend upon the geographical area the patient is from. Since complete ethnic listing is not feasible, six main ethnic groups, classified according to their geographical distribution, will be analyzed globally: African, Asian, Mediterranean, Middle

Table 1. Aesthetic nasal evaluation chart

AESTHETIC NASAL EXAMINATION

1. Skin type:
normal ☐ thick ☐ thin ☐
sebaceous ☐ dry ☐

2. Nasal vale:
normal ☐ compromised: internal nasal valve: right ☐ left ☐
external nasal valve: right ☐ left ☐

3. Nasal septum:
straight ☐ deviated: right ☐ left ☐ area of cottle: caudal ______
basal ______
cephalic _____

4. Nasal dorsum:
height in mm: _____
normal ☐ low ☐ high ☐
hump ☐
deviated: right ☐ left ☐

5. Nasal bridge:
normal ☐ narrow ☐ wide ☐

6. Upper lateral cartilages:
normal ☐ altered: wide ☐
collapsed: right ☐ left ☐

7. Nasal tip:
alar cartilages: normal ☐ thin ☐ wide ☐ scar tissue ☐
pinched: right ☐ left ☐
strong ☐ flimsy ☐

8. Nasolabial angle:
degrees: _____ acute ☐ obtuse ☐

9. Nasal base:
normal ☐ narrow ☐ wide ☐
intercanthal distance: _____ mm nasal base distance: _____ mm

10. Nostril orientation:
oval ☐ vertical ☐ horizontal ☐
flaring ☐ non-flaring ☐

11. Nasal tip support:
weak ☐ strong ☐
nasal spine: normal ☐ prominent ☐ small ☐

12. Donor sites for cartilage grafts:
nasal septum ☐ auricle: right ☐ left ☐ rib ☐

Eastern, Northern European, and Latin American (mestizo). This will help the rhinoplasty surgeon to evaluate different ethnic groups and to define which anatomical characteristics should be borne in mind during surgery.

African nasal anatomy (black patient)

- thick, sebaceous skin
- low nasal dorsum
- wide nasal bridge
- undefined, underprojected nasal tip with wide flimsy alar cartilages and broad domes; short columella
- acute nasolabial angle
- wide nasal base
- horizontally, round-shaped nostrils with flaring
- poor tip support with little tip recoil

Asian nasal anatomy

- moderate to thick skin (skin is thinner in the nasion and dorsum and thicker in the nasal tip area)
- low shallow nasion
- wide nasal bridge
- underprojected, moderately undefined and sometimes ptotic; flimsy alar cartilages; short columella
- acute-to-normal nasolabial angle
- wide, flaring nasal base but narrower than the African patient
- oblique-shaped nostrils
- poor tip support

Mediterranean nasal anatomy[5]

- moderate-to-thick skin
- straight-to-convex nasal dorsum
- normal-to-narrow nasal bridge
- plunging tip with wide strong alar cartilages (long nose)
- acute-to-normal nasolabial angle
- normal-to-narrow nasal base
- vertically-shaped nostrils
- normal-to-weak tip support

Middle Eastern nasal anatomy

- moderate-to-thick skin
- high arched nasal dorsum often extending into the glabellar region
- high nasal bridge, sometimes wide
- underprojected tip with downward rotation; wide alar cartilages with undefined lobules
- acute-to-normal nasolabial angle
- normal nasal base
- oval-to-vertically-shaped nostrils
- normal-to-weak tip support

North European nasal anatomy

- normal-to-thin skin
- high dorsum
- high narrow nasal bridge
- overprojected tip with long strong alar cartilages, sometimes bifid tip
- normal-to-obtuse nasolabial angle
- narrow nasal base with very strong projecting anterior nasal spine
- oval-to-vertically-shaped nostrils
- normal-to-strong tip support

Mestizo nasal anatomy[6]

- moderate-to-thick, sometimes oily, bulky skin
- small-to-normal bony vault
- normal-to-wide nasal bridge
- underprojected nasal tip with wide undefined lobule; flimsy unsupportive alar cartilages; normal-to-short columella
- normal-to-acute nasolabial angle
- normal-to-wide nasal base with thick alar sidewalls
- normal-to-horizontally-shaped nostrils
- flimsy tip support with poor tip recoil

Surgical plan

Once a complete medical history and physical examination has been performed, and with a clear understanding of the patient's ethnic background and specific desires, the surgeon can make an accurate diagnosis of the nasal structure and can draw a realistic surgical plan. Elaborating a surgical plan prior to surgery can be of immense help. Often, more than one surgical technique is needed in order to be able to solve the problem of an existing alteration adequately (Table 2). It is always important to evaluate the nose in relation to the patient's face and general physical features (height, weight, age, sex). The final surgical outcome should create a balance, if possible always trying to avoid an 'operated look or artificial nose' that does not blend in with the patient's ethnic background or physical characteristics.

When planning surgery, it is important to bear in mind the following recommendations:

- do not perform aggressive reduction techniques
- do not overuse sutures and grafts
- start with simple procedures and progress to more complicated ones
- it is always easier to come back and take out more tissue than to have to come back and reconstruct

Approaches and basic surgical techniques

There are three basic approaches to the nose: the non-delivery approach (cartilage splitting, retrograde dissection); the delivery approach (intercartilaginous and marginal incisions); and the external (open) approach (marginal and transcolumellar incision).[7,8] The decision about which approach to use depends on the type of surgical goal to be achieved, and on the surgeon's expertise. In general, the delivery and external approaches are most frequently used in ethnic rhinoplasty.

In order to apply the basic rhinoplasty technique, it is helpful to divide the nose into three areas: dorsum, nasal tip, and nasal base.

Nasal dorsum

In a large percentage of ethnic patients, the nasal dorsum is low with a wide sometimes flat nasal bridge. It is important to assess the need for dorsal augmentation and to decide on what type of material will be used.

Grafts and implants have been used in nose surgery for many years, and the choice depends on many factors: the amount of material needed, the type of defect being corrected, whether the patient has any grafting material that can be used, and the surgeon's experience with the various types of grafts and implants. The materials commonly used in the nose can be divided into three categories: autografts, homografts (allografts), and alloplasts (Table 3). Autografts are those tissues obtained from one area of a patient and implanted in a different recipient area: septal cartilage, auricular cartilage, rib cartilage and calvarial bone. Homografts are tissues or materials obtained from a human donor and transplanted into a patient. In nasal surgery, the homograft most commonly used is irradiated rib cartilage. Alloplasts are synthetic implant materials which are biologically compatible, under ideal conditions produce minimal inflammatory reaction, and are well tolerated for indefinite periods of time: silicone implants, Gore-Tex, Medpore.[9-11]

The patient's own nasal cartilage is always the material of choice in rhinoplasty. If no septal cartilage is available, auricular cartilage is an excellent alternative. Autograft and homograft rib cartilage or calvarial bone can be used as an alternative when large quantities of grafting material are needed for dorsal augmentation.[12-14] When there is insufficient autogenous grafting material, synthetic implants can be used as an alternative, especially in dorsal augmentation. Implants do not cause any donor site complications, but they are not incorporated biologically into the nasal tissues, making them more prone to infection, mobility,

Table 2. Surgical planner sheet

SURGICAL PLANNER SHEET

1. **Functional procedures:**
   septoplasty ☐ turbinate surgery ☐ FESS: right ☐ left ☐

2. **Cartilage grafting/implants:**
   septum ☐ auricular ☐ rib ☐ calvarial bone ☐
   irradiated rib cartilage ☐
   implants: Gore-Tex ☐
   Medpore ☐
   silicone ☐
   other: ___________

3. **Nasal dorsum:**
   hump removal ☐ augmentation ☐ none ☐

4. **Nasal bridge:**
   narrowing: lateral osteotomies ☐ widening: ☐
   medial oblique osteotomies ☐
   intermediate osteotomies ☐

5. **Upper lateral cartilages:**
   hump removal ☐ augmentation ☐ none ☐
   narrowing ☐ widening: spreader grafts: right ☐ left ☐

6. **Nasal tip:**
   A. alar cartilages:
   - complete strip procedures
     cephalic trim: ☐
     double-dome technique ☐
     transdomal suture narrowing ☐
     lateral crural steal ☐
     other: ___________
   - incomplete strip procedures
     lateral crural overlay ☐ vertical dome division ☐
     other: ___________
   - no change ☐

   B. columella:
   - trimming caudal border
   - suture crural feet ☐
   - resection caudal septal border ☐
   - septocolumellar suture ☐
   - other: ___________ no change: ☐

7. **Nasal base:**
   - no change: ☐
   - alar wedge resection: ☐
   - other: ___________

8. **Grafts:**
   - columellar strut ☐ shield graft ☐ cap graft/tip onlay graft ☐
   - dorsal onlay graft ☐
   - spreader graft: right ☐ left ☐ alar batten: right ☐ left ☐
   - pre-maxilla plumping grafts : ☐
   - other: ___________

9. **Additional procedures:**

Table 3. Grafts and implants for augmentation in rhinoplasty

	Type of graft or implant	*Uses*
Autografts	• septal cartilage	dorsal augmentation dorsal onlay grafts collumellar struts tip grafts spreader grafts plumping grafts camouflage
	• auricular cartilage	dorsal augmentation dorsal onlay grafts reconstruction of alar cartilages alar batten grafts composite grafts for alar retraction or vestibular stenosis camouflage
	• rib cartilage	dorsal augmentation
	• calvarial bone	dorsal augmentation
Homografts	• irradiated rib cartilage	dorsal augmentation
Alloplasts	• silicone implants	dorsal augmentation pre-maxilla implants
	• Gore-Tex	dorsal augmentation
	• Medpore	dorsal augmentation pre-maxilla implants

inflammation, and extrusion. However, some authors feel that, if the right surgical procedure is performed and the implants are manipulated properly, they are an excellent alternative for augmentation with minimal complications (Fig. 1).

When a wide nasal bridge needs to be narrowed, lateral and, when necessary, medial oblique osteotomies are performed. These are preferably carried out at the end of surgery in order to avoid excessive swelling during the postoperative period.

Nasal tip

There is no standard procedure for approaches to the nasal tip in ethnic patients. The final objective is a more defined nasal tip which is in harmony and balance with the nasal dorsum and base. Surgery must be performed always maintaining, and if possible building up, the support structures of the nose. It is important to start with simple surgical options and to progress to more aggressive ones, depending on the patient's needs and what final result the surgeon wishes to achieve. Most procedures performed on the tip involve suturing techniques and placement of graft material to give additional support and definition (Figs. 2 and 3).[6,15] Depending on the size of the tip, procedures can be carried out using complete or incomplete strip techniques when deprojection is necessary (Table 4).

Nasal base

The width of the alar base should be similar to the intercanthal distance and to the width of the eyes when evaluated from a frontal view.[2] In ethnic rhinoplasty, alar base reduction is performed more frequently in noses that are platyrrhine or mesorrhine in order to decrease alar flare, alar base width,

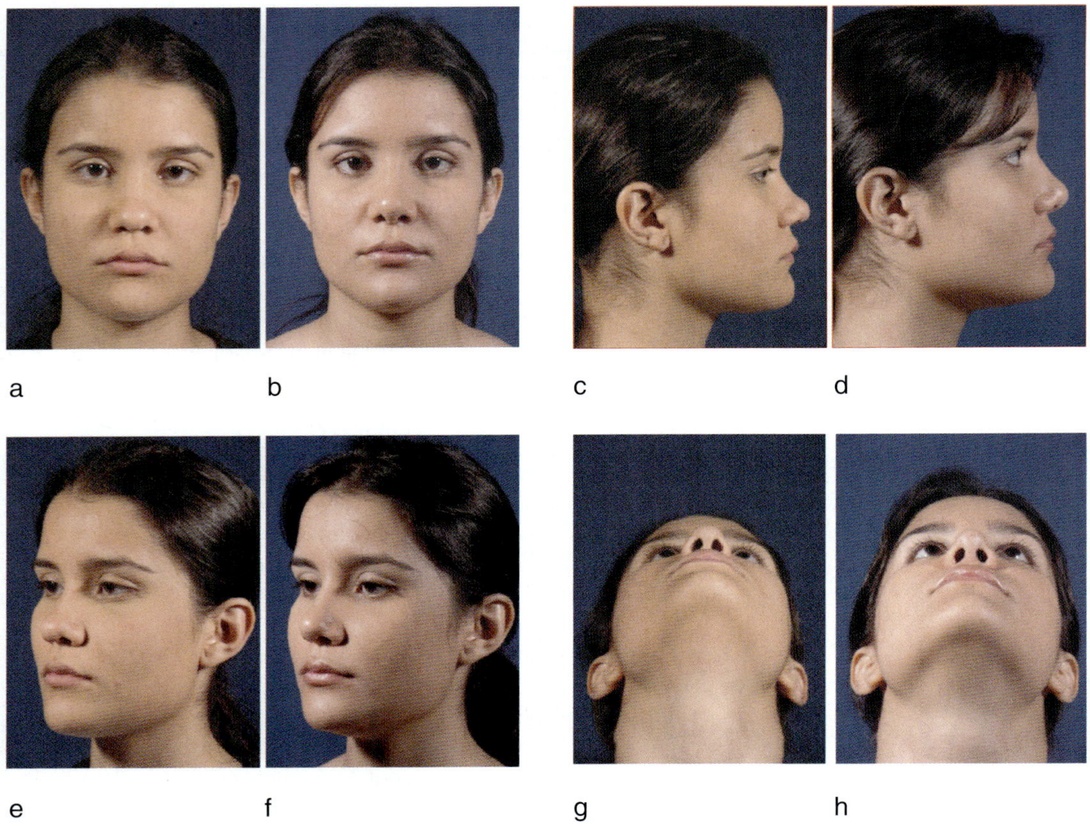

Fig. 1. Pre- (*a,c,e,g*) and post- (*b,d,f,h*) operative views of a patient with a bulbous tip without any support and a very low nasal bridge. Using an external rhinoplasty approach, a Gore-Tex implant was placed on the nasal dorsum. Tip rotation projection and definition was improved by using suturing techniques (lateral crural steal, double dome unit) and tip grafts (columellar strut and long shield graft).

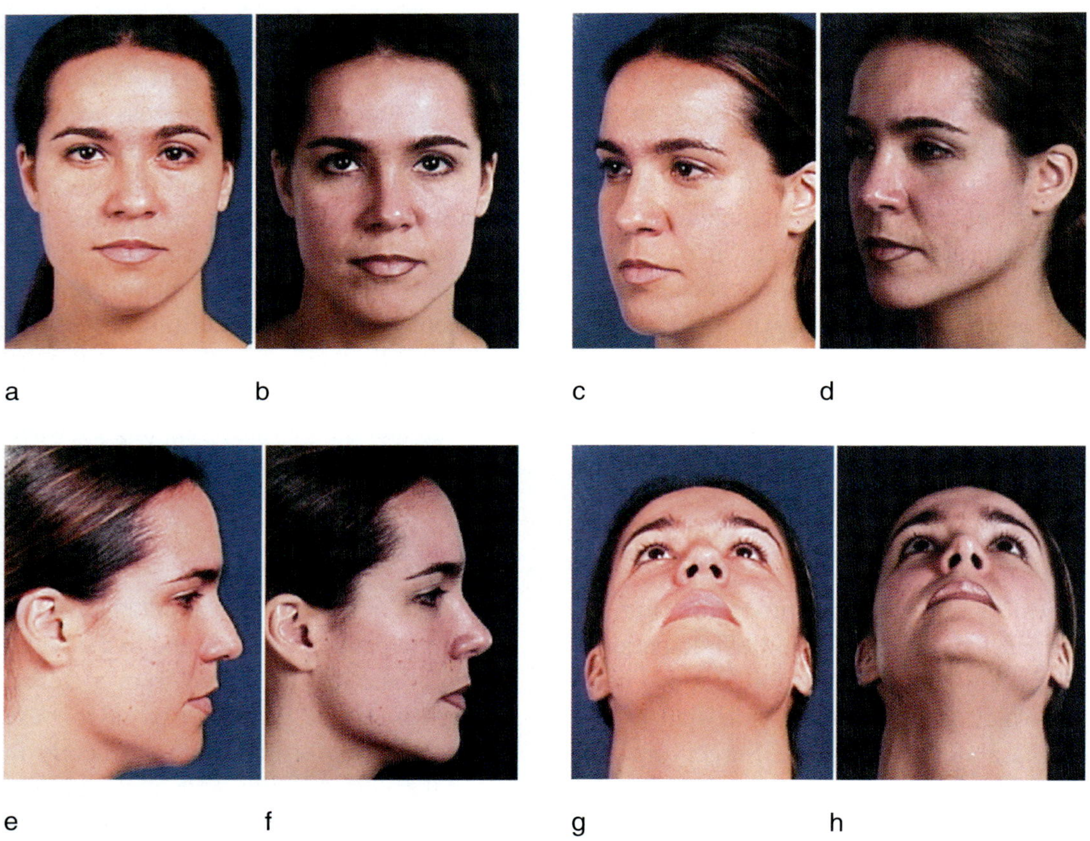

Fig. 2. Pre- (*a,c,e,g*) and post- (*b,d,f,h*) operative views of an ethnic patient with thick oily skin, an undefined bulbous nasal tip with little support, and a small osseocartilaginous hump. Conservative hump removal was performed and lateral osteotomies were carried out to narrow the upper third of the nose. Tip rotation and definition were improved by performing cephalic trim of the alar cartilages with a lateral crural steal, columellar strut, and placement of a shield graft.

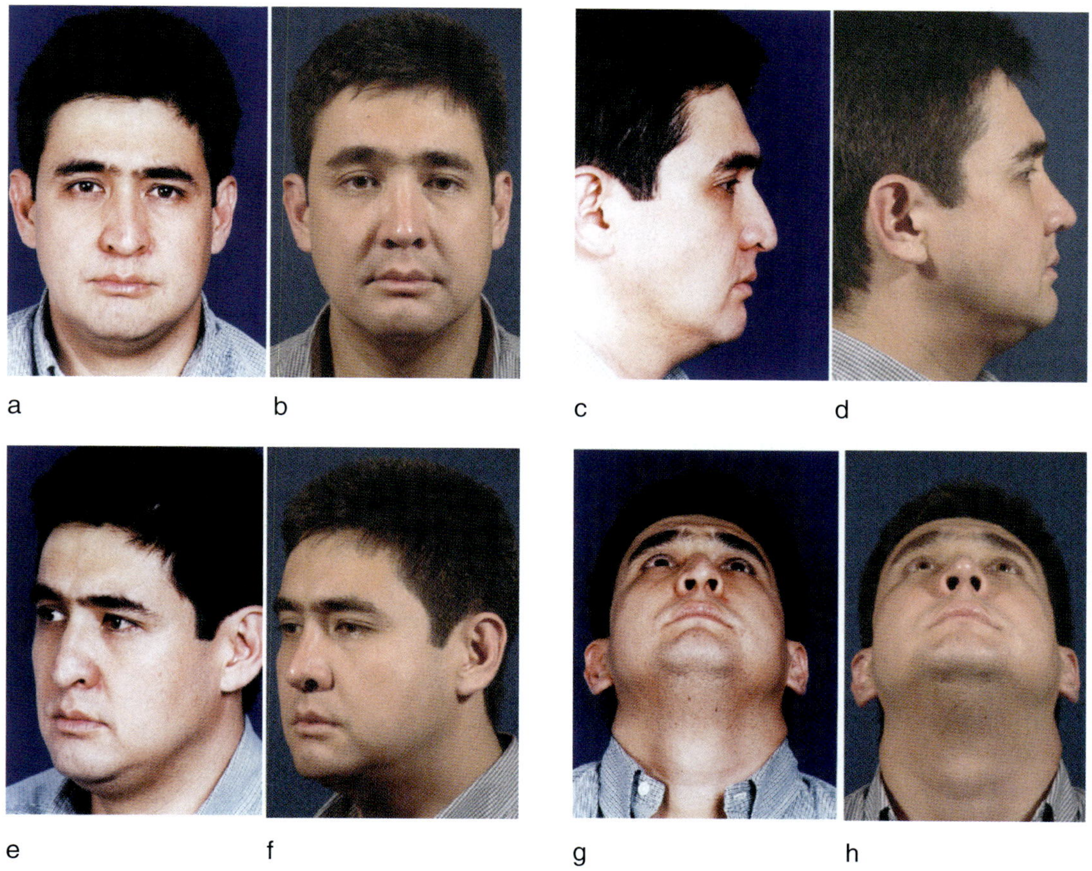

Fig. 3. Pre- (*a,c,e,g*) and post- (*b,d,f,h*) operative views of a male patient with traumatic collapse of the middle nasal vault, right internal nasal valve collapse, and tip asymmetry. Bilateral spreader grafts (double on the right side), right alar batten grafts, a columellar strut and shield graft were placed to improve asymmetry, nasal valve function, and tip projection and rotation.

or both. Various techniques can be used: alar base wedge resection to decrease nasal flare; excision of the floor of the nostril to reduce the width of the nasal sill; combined reduction of the alar base and nostril floor to decrease flare and reduce width (Fig. 4). The medial incision should be at the natural crease formed by the junction of the nasal sill and ala with the upper lip, and the lateral incision should be placed 1-2 mm above the alar-facial groove in order to avoid a visible scar. Incisions are closed with 6-0 prolene sutures, taking care to evert the edges of the skin. The sutures are removed on days 5-7 (Fig. 5).

Closure of incisions

Closure of midcolumellar incisions

If the technique is performed correctly, there will be no scar, whatever the type of skin. In dark-skinned patients, keloid formation is not seen in this area if treated properly. It is important to use 6-0 or 7-0 prolene and to evert the edges of the skin. The first suture is always placed in the midline, continuing with angled off-midline sutures. This helps to recruit skin medially and prevents lateral notching of columellar incision.[16] Suture removal is usually performed on days 4-6, with care being taken to tape the incision site afterwards.

Closure of intercartilaginous, transcartilaginous or marginal incisions, and septal mucosal incisions

These incisions are closed with one or two 5-0 or 6-0 absorbable (vicryl) sutures which are placed slightly laterally to the domes. Care should be taken not to distort the dome region or to produce notching of the nostril rim. Columellar extension of incisions should be closed with an additional

Table 4. Gradual approach to the nasal tip

Nasal tip procedures

A. Intact strip procedures
- cephalic trim of lateral crura
- transdomal suture narrowing technique
- double-dome unit technique
- lateral crural steal/new dome technique

B. Incomplete strip procedures
- lateral crural overlay
- vertical dome division
- medial crura division

C. Grafts
- shield graft
- shield graft with lateral crural steal
- shield graft + cap graft
- buttress graft
- alar batten grafts
- collumelar strut
- plumping pre-maxilla grafts

D. Septocolumellar suture

absorbable suture if the mucosal flaps of the vestibular skin have not been properly aligned.

Intranasal packs/closure of septal mucosal incisions

Closure of the mucoperichondrial flaps of the septum is performed using a continuous horizontal mattress absorbable suture. This prevents the formation of hematoma. Intranasal packing is not performed routinely, except when extensive septal surgery and reconstruction has been performed or when endoscopic sinus surgery procedures or turbinoplasty have been performed, and the risk of bleeding is high. In these cases, the objective of packing the nose is to provide some compression to the septal flaps and prevent hematoma formation, synechia, and decrease the risk of postoperative bleeding. Packing is usually left in place for 24-48 hours.

External nasal splints

Taping the nose and fixing a cast in place will help reduce dead space, edema and the formation of hematomas, will protect the nasal structures from external trauma and will prevent displacement of the newly aligned nasal structures. Tape should be placed over the dorsum and tip, and is immobilized with a nasal splint. This splint is removed on post-surgical day 7 and the nose is taped for an additional five to seven days. This will help lessen post-surgical edema, especially in the supratip region.

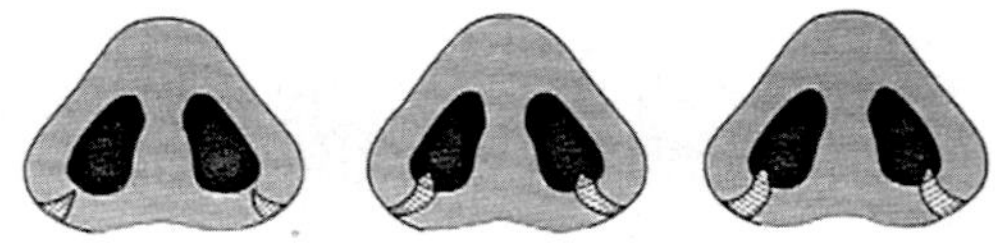

a b c

Fig. 4. Alar base resection. *a.* Reduction of alar flare can be performed in two ways without touching the nasal sill. 1. V-shaped reduction of the lateral alar base; 2. excision of tissue from the nostril floor without touching the nasal sill. *b.* Reduction of the width of the nasal floor with slight reduction of the alar flare. *c.* Combined reduction of the nasal floor width and alar flare.

Postoperative care

Patients should be given oral and written postoperative instructions to follow at home. This helps to prevent complications. Additionally, thick skinned patients should be warned that edema will be present for a longer period of time and that dark circles under the eyes can be accentuated for up to four to six months after surgery.

Persistent edema of the supratip region can be effectively treated with subdermal injections of 1-2 mg triamcinolone acetonide (Kenalog: 10 mg/ml) followed by taping of the nasal tip. These injections can be repeated every four weeks. In patients with a thick skin and greater risk of developing pollybeak deformity, injections can be started as early as the first week after surgery, but should not be used in excess and should not be placed intradermally as this can produce permanent cutaneous atrophy.[17]

Complications

Rhinoplasty in ethnic patients can be a very demanding and complicated operation

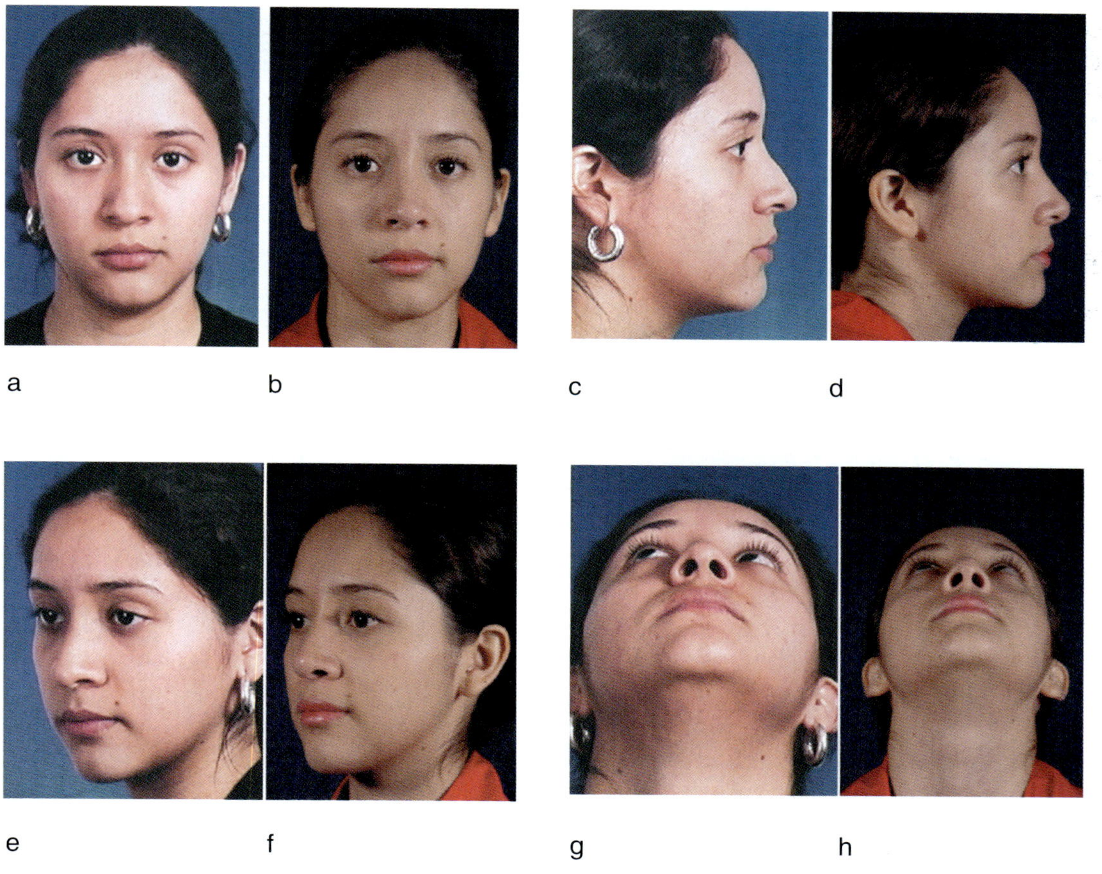

Fig. 5. Pre- (*a,c,e,g*) and post- (*b,d,f,h*) operative views of a female patient with a wide bulbous nasal tip with poor support, a wide nasal base with alar flaring, and a small osseo-cartilaginous hump. A conservative hump resection with lateral osteotomies was performed to narrow the nose. The tip and base were approached using a columellar strut, lateral crural steal and septo-columellar suture techniques, and alar base resection. The overall result was a narrower nose with a more defined and projected nasal tip.

where complex surgical maneuvers and placement of multiple grafts and sutures can be performed. The placement of grafts and performance of aggressive tip procedures will increase the chances dorsal and tip irregularities, fibrosis, and asymmetries. Sometimes, no matter what procedure is performed, there is a persistent fullness of the nasal tip. It is important for the surgeon to try to camouflage any grafts and implants as much as possible and to be meticulous with any tip procedures. Patients should be aware that these possible complications can occur, even in the best hands.

The best way to manage complications is to prevent them as much as possible. In reductive procedures, the surgeon should not forget that, to guarantee long-term results, support structures of the nose should be reconstituted and in many cases reinforced with the placement of sutures and grafts. In cases where support is a problem even before surgery, tip support must be obtained with the placement of sutures and very often with grafts, but it should always be borne in mind not to build up too much. The final result should be a balance, not only aesthetically, but also functionally.

In some cases, where the patient is dissatisfied, revision is needed when the final result does not blend in with the patient's ethnic features.[18] It is important for the surgeon not to over-resect a high dorsum or build up too much on a low one. The final goal of surgery should not be a 'perfect nose' but rather a harmonic nose that blends in with the individual patient's physical and facial characteristics (Fig. 6).

Conclusions

Rhinoplasty has always been one of the most popular facial plastic operations. Today, a large percentage of the world's

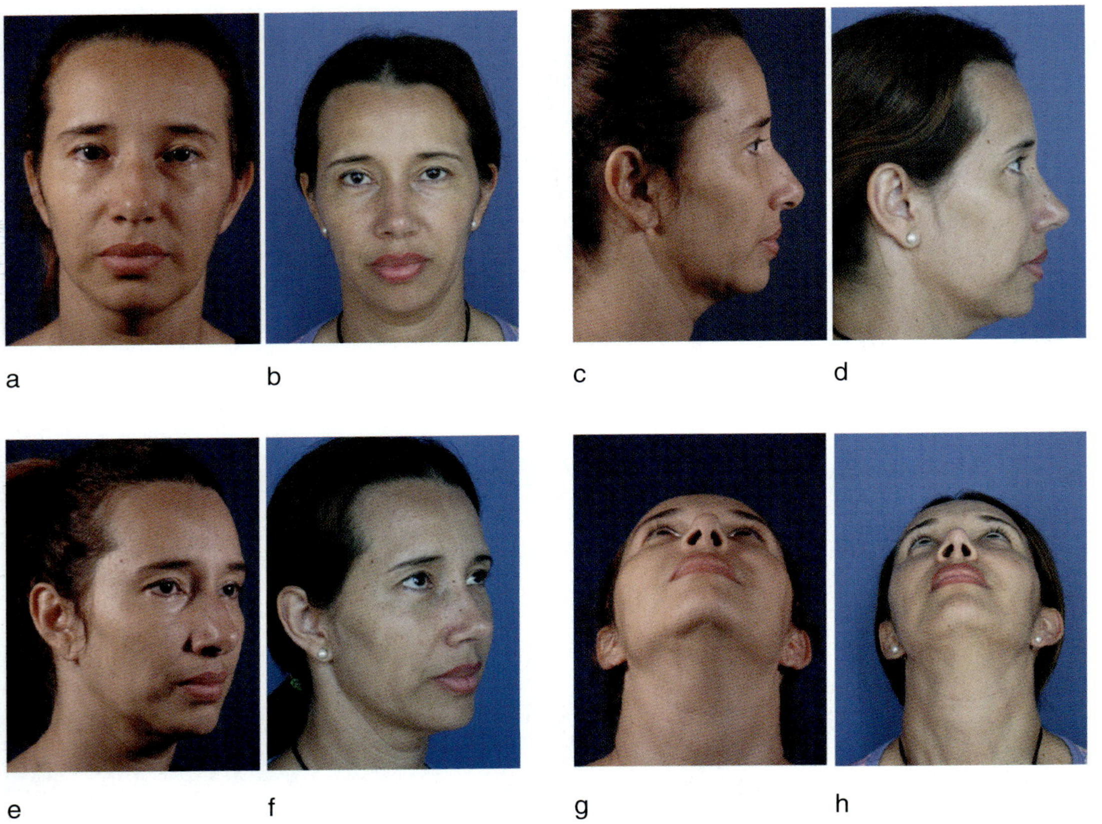

Fig. 6. Pre- (*a,c,e,g*) and post- (*b,d,f,h*) operative views of a female patient with a osseocartilaginous hump and wide dorsum, slightly boxy tip, and hanging columella. Lateral osteotomies with hump removal, the transdomal suture narrowing technique and conservative caudal excision of the septal cartilage give a more harmonious and balanced post-surgical result.

population is non-Caucasian, and it is very common to have ethnic patients requesting aesthetic nose surgery. Even though there is no special surgical technique that should be followed or standardized, the role of the surgeon is to have a clear understanding of the patient's ethnical background, and be able to define whether the patient can be provided with an effective solution that approaches what the patient considers to be 'beautiful' or 'aesthetically acceptable'. Finally, the surgeon should provide the patient with an insight into aesthetics, balance, and possible surgical options with their limitations and complications, and help point the patient towards realistic expectations.

28: BATTEN GRAFTS FOR NASAL VALVE COLLAPSE

W.J. Fokkens and G.J. Nolst Trenité

Introduction

The surgical treatment of nasal valve collapse aims to strengthen the anatomical structures in order to resist any negative pressure from the nasal sidewalls and/or to widen the valve in order to release negative pressure from the nasal airflow when this becomes too high. In severe cases, a combination of strengthening the sidewall and widening the internal and/or external valve is indicated.

In earlier literature and rhinology textbooks, the nasal valve is defined as being the narrowest part of the airway. An anatomical landmark bordered by the caudal margin of the upper lateral cartilage, the head of the inferior turbinate, the piriform aperture, and the nasal septum. In the more recent literature on rhinoplasty techniques, the distinction between the internal and external nasal valves becomes more prominent. The external nasal valve is the anatomical landmark determined by the nostril margin, formed by the alar rim, nostril sill and columella. A thin alar rim with a lack of skeletal support from the lower lateral cartilage, a broad columellar base, and an overprojected nasal tip can all result in slit-like nostrils, often displaying external valve collapse.

Diagnosis

For the adequate treatment of any nasal airway obstruction, a thorough medical history and physical examination are obligatory, if necessary, with the use of an endoscope. Any particular medical history data should be recorded, such as:

- nasal or sinus diseases (allergy, polyposis)
- medication (influencing the nasal mucosa and bleeding)
- nasal trauma
- previous septorhinoplasty
- facial palsy

Physical examination

It is important to determine between reversible (mucosa, hypertrophy of the inferior turbinate) and non-reversible obstructions (septal deviations, polyps, infractured nasal bone, scar tissue). The use of local decongestives and of an endoscope can be helpful in this. It is more difficult to assess the dynamic form of a nasal obstruction, which is influenced by the amount of negative pressure from the nasal airflow compared to the structural support of the lateral nasal sidewall. Finally, the site and amount of nasal valve collapse should be assessed in order to decide upon the most suitable surgical treatment.

Inspection

In certain cases, external inspection can reveal the etiology of the nasal airway obstruction, for example:

- narrow mid-nose
- inverted V syndrome
- pinched nose
- saddle nose
- overprojected tip with slit-like nostrils
- thin alar sidewalls
- broad columellar base
- facial palsy

The following pathologies, which cause nasal airway obstruction, can be found by means of internal inspection:

- inward protruding lateral crus
- septal deviation

- scar tissue
- too narrow and too wide a nasal valve angle
- hypertrophic head of the inferior turbinate
- narrowing of the piriform aperture
- mucosal pathology
- synecchiae
- polyps

The use of an endoscope and inspection after decongestion help to diagnose nasal airway pathology and to determine whether the obstruction is reversible. In order to diagnose the dynamic form of the obstruction and to determine the site of maximal collapse, inspection should be performed during rest as well as during more forceful inspiration through the nose, using a small probe to lateralize the collapsed segment.
A simple test for detecting any limitations in inhalation at the level of the ostium internum is by pulling the cheek laterally during gentle inspiration through the nose, the so-called Cottle test. The signs are positive when inhalation noticeably improves after this maneuver.

Treatment modalities for nasal valve collapse

Surgical treatment can be divided into various groups, depending on the underlying pathology, as follows:

- correction of a non-reversible obstructive component
  - deviated septum (see Chapter 24)
  - narrow piriform aperture
  - vestibular scarring (see Chapter 22)
  - broad columella
- widening the internal nasal valve (which is normally 10-15 degrees in the leptorrhine nose)
  - spreader grafts (see Chapter 9B)
  - modified-Z plasty (see Chapter 9A)
- remodelling of the nasal tip skeleton
- upward rotation of the lateral crus (see Chapter 8)
- deprojection of the overprojected tip
- strengthening of the nasal sidewall with autogenous graft material
  - alar battens

In many cases, more then one surgical procedure is necessary to correct alar collapse.

Surgical technique for alar batten grafting

In order to prevent nasal valve collapse, alar battens are indicated 'to strengthen the nasal side wall'. The graft material of choice is autogenous cartilage from the septum, auricle (concha) or rib. If available, septal cartilage is the first choice. In some cases the natural curvature of the concha is helpful, especially for restoring the curvature of the alar rim. In general, grafts measure 5-8 mm in width and 12-18 mm in length. They are sculpted in a rectangular shape. The batten should be of sufficient size to provide support, and it can be influenced by the stiffness of the cartilage, the thickness of the overlying skin, aesthetic appearance, and the severity of the nasal valve collapse.

The graft should be beveled in thin-skinned patients. A small inverted V-shaped cartilage resection at the base of the graft helps to prevent shifting after precise placement.

Depending on the further surgical procedures needing to be carried out, an endonasal or external approach can be indicated. The graft should be positioned at the margin of the piriform aperture and a mark made on the skin. The position of the batten depends on the site of maximum collapse: supra alar in internal valve collapse, and caudal to the cephalic position of the lateral crus in external valve collapse (Fig. 1a and b). The graft should extend laterally to the piriform aperture. There can be some

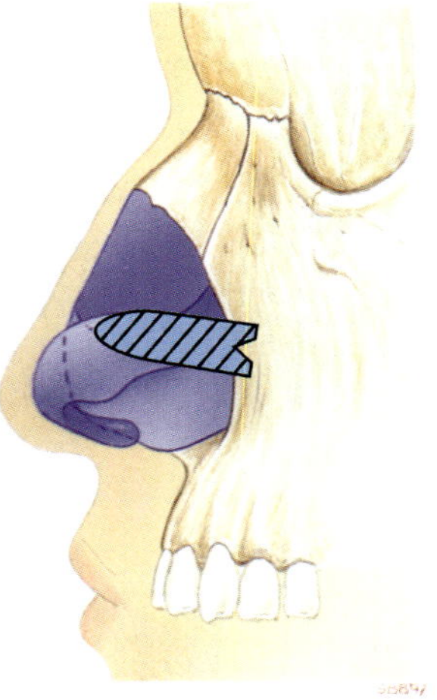

a

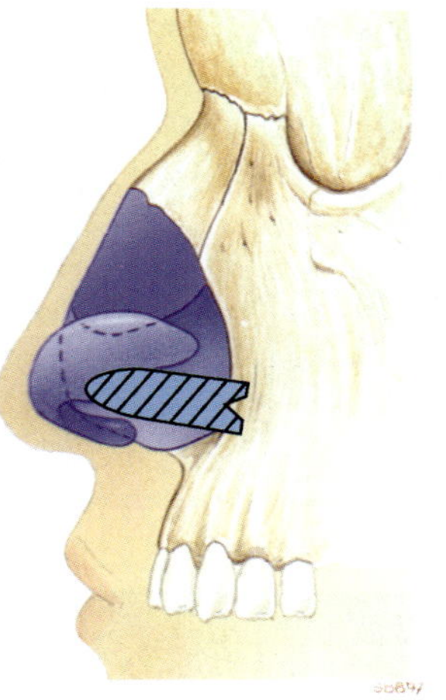

b

Fig. 1a. Position of the alar batten graft for correction of internal valve collapse.

Fig. 1b. Position of the alar batten graft for correction of external valve (alar) collapse.

overlap medially and cephalically with the upper and lower lateral cartilage.

In thin-skinned patients in particular, care should be taken to preserve the natural contours of the nasal side wall.

With the endonasal approach, a vestibular incision is made lateral to the determined pocket approximately 8-10 mm in length. A precise pocket is dissected subcutaneously up to the piriform aperture. Although no further fixation is needed if the graft fits well into the pocket, transcutaneous fixation over a button is helpful for preventing dead space and is obliqatory in cases of too wide a pocket.

Figures 2a-z show the surgical procedure by means of an endonasal approach in alar batten grafting in a patient with internal valve collapse, a slight polly beak, and deviation of the nasal dorsum and caudal septum to the left (Fig. 3a-f). When using the external approach, fixation of the graft to the nasal skeleton is often indicated.

Pitfalls during alar batten grafting

The following pitfalls are common during the surgical procedure for alar batten grafting:

- tears in the grafted material, which can weaken and distort the graft
- a batten that is too small in width (not strong enough) and in length (not extending to the piriform aperture)
- wrong positioning of the graft (not at the site of maximum collapse)
- too large a pocket with no fixation of the graft, resulting in postoperative shifting of the graft
- unaesthetic appearance due to visibility of the graft through the (thin) skin and/ or unnatural curvature of the nasal side wall or ala
- good structural support of the nasal side wall, but still too narrow an internal nasal valve angle in which combination with a spreader graft was indicated

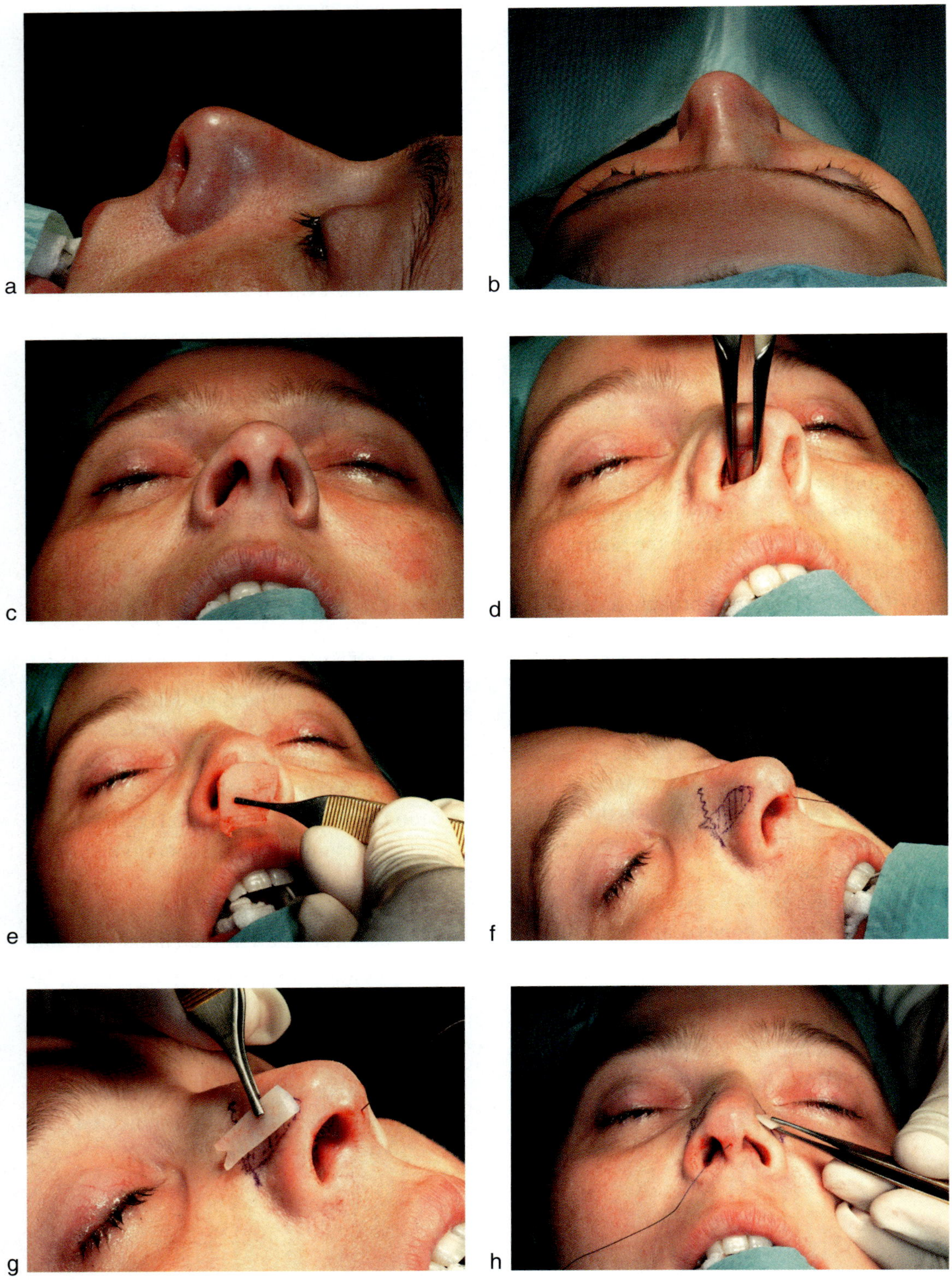

Fig. 2a-c. Preoperative lateral, bird's eye and basal views.

Fig. 2d,e. Harvesting septal cartilage through a hemitransfixion incision.

Fig. 2f. Lateral view after septoplasty with a midcolumellar guiding suture to secure the caudal septum in the midline. Lateral view shows the marking of the caudal rim of the bony pyramid and the position determined for the alar batten.

Fig. 2g,h. Sculpured alar batten for right and left sides.

Fig. 2i. Leftover crushed cartilage to fill the donor site in the cartilaginous septum.

Fig. 2j. View of the cartilaginous dorsum through an endonasal approach to correct a slight polly beak.

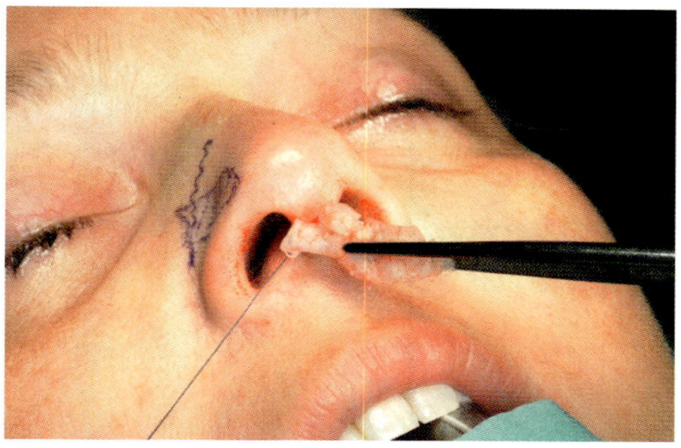

i

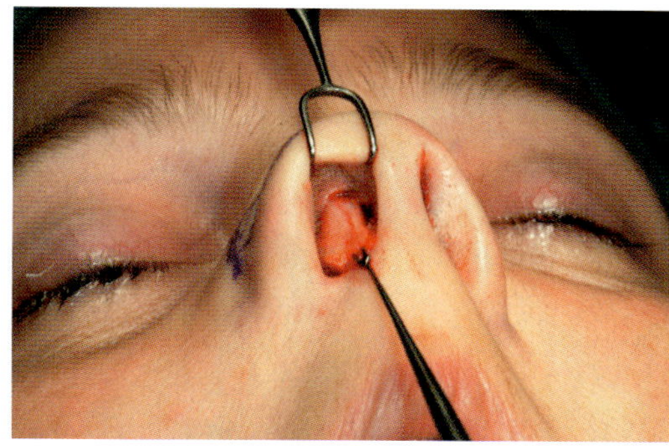

j

Fig. 2k,l. Marginal incision and blunt dissection to create a pocket for the alar batten.

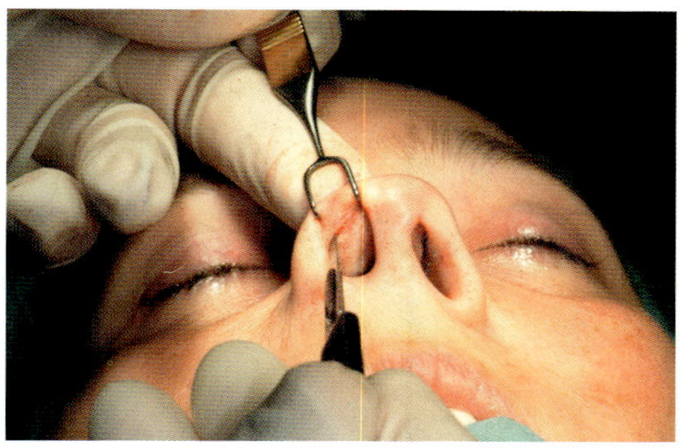

k

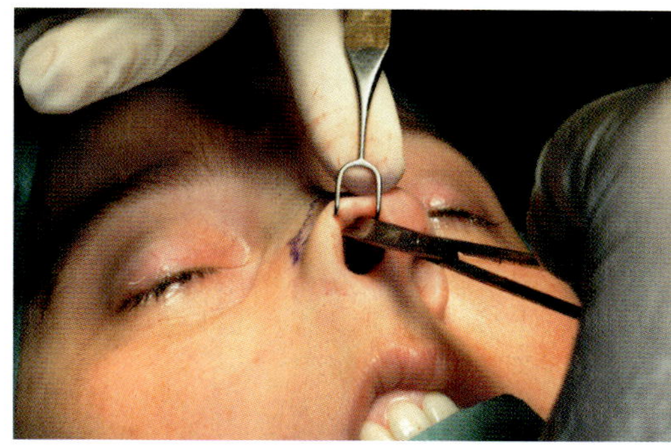

l

Fig. 2m,n. Guiding suture at the base of the alar batten and insertion of a straight needle with a guiding suture into the pocket.

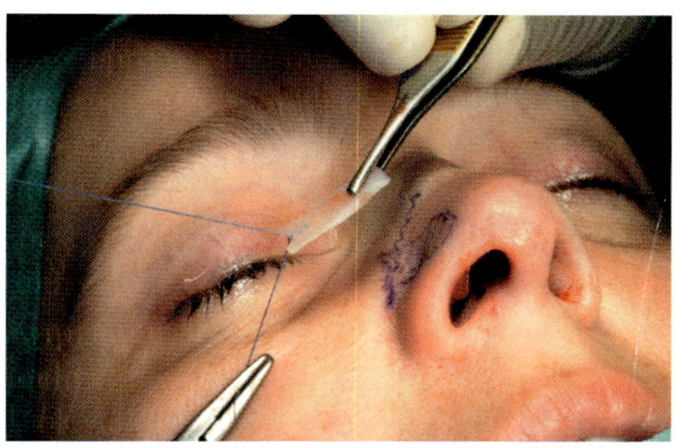

m

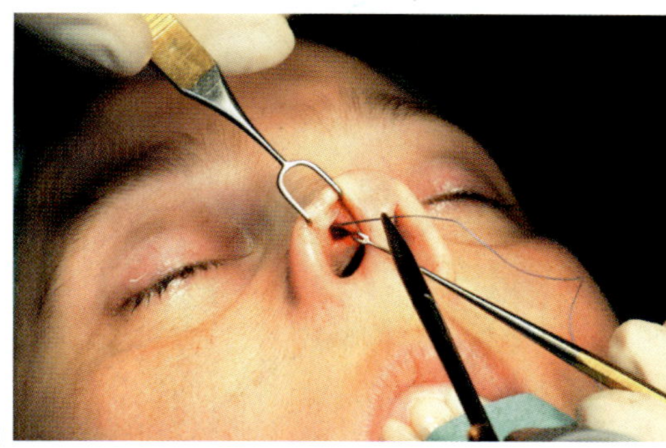

n

Fig. 2o,p. Positioning of the alar batten and closure of the marginal incision.

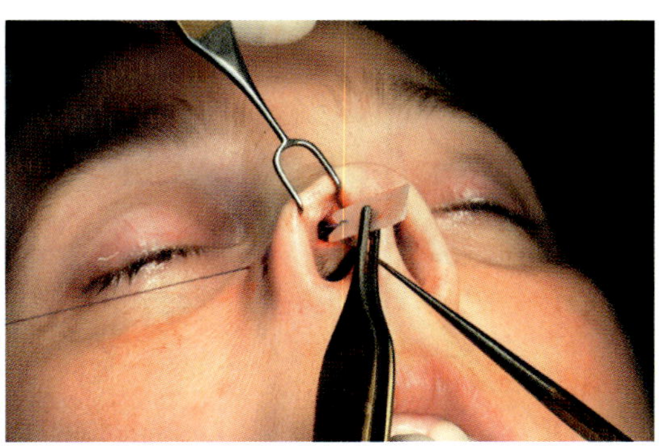

o

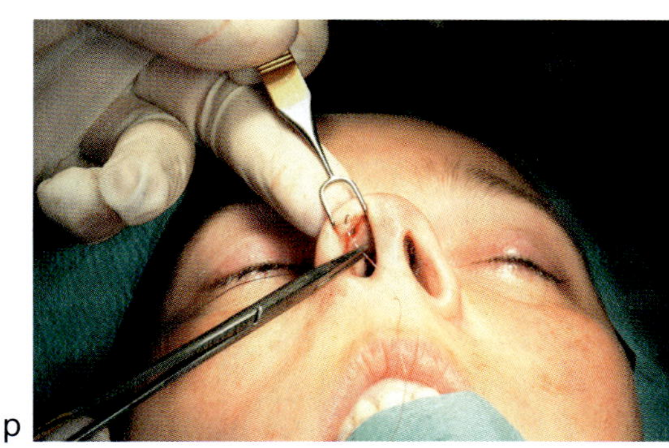

p

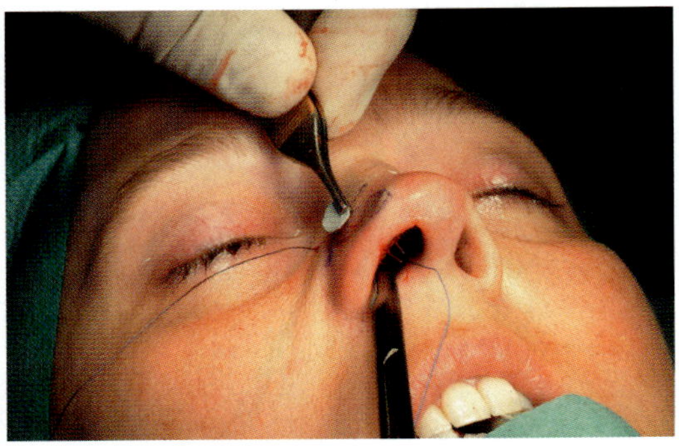

q

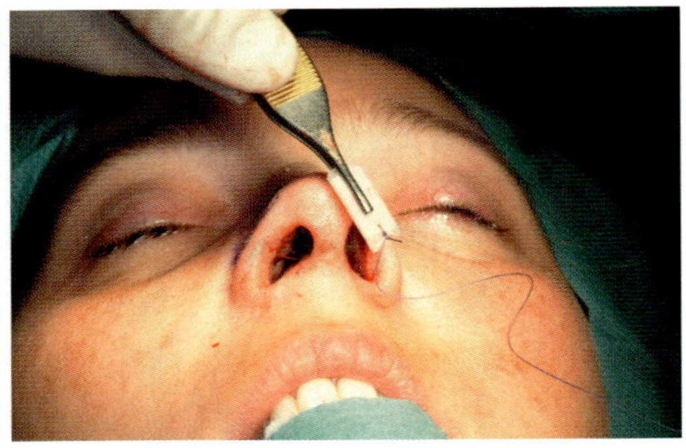

r

Fig. 2q. Transcutaneous suture over an aluminium button to fix the alar batten and to prevent a dead space.

Fig. 2r,s. Alar batten for the left side ready to be positioned in the pocket with a guiding suture.

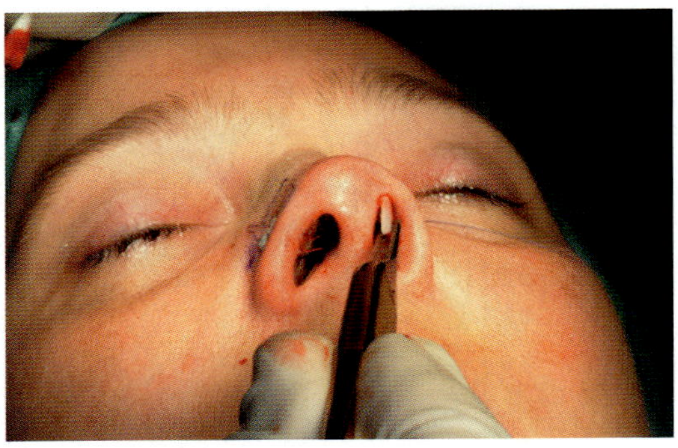

s

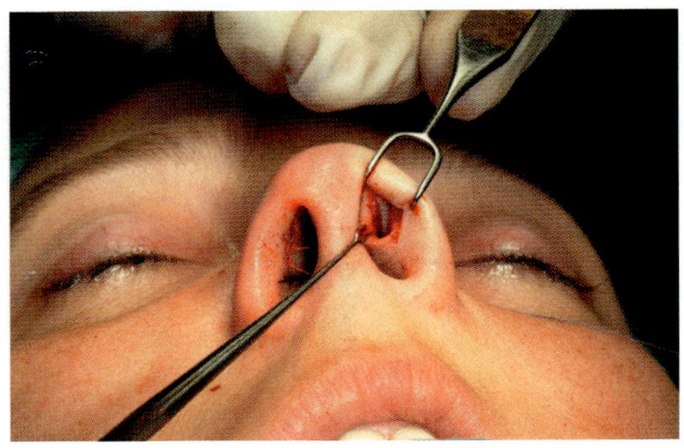

t

Fig. 2t. Alar batten *in situ* and fixed with a transcutanous suture over an aluminum button.

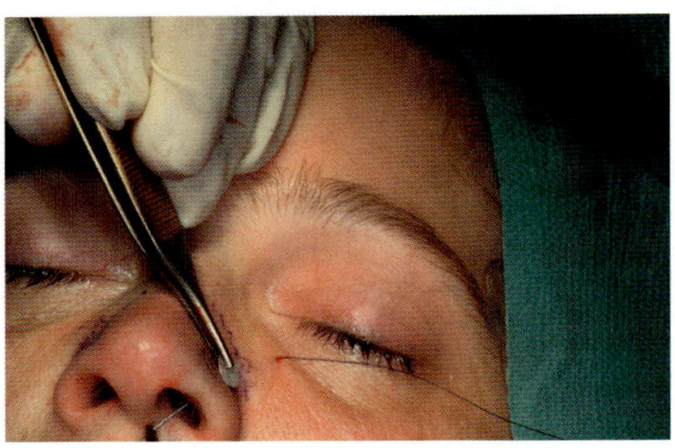

u

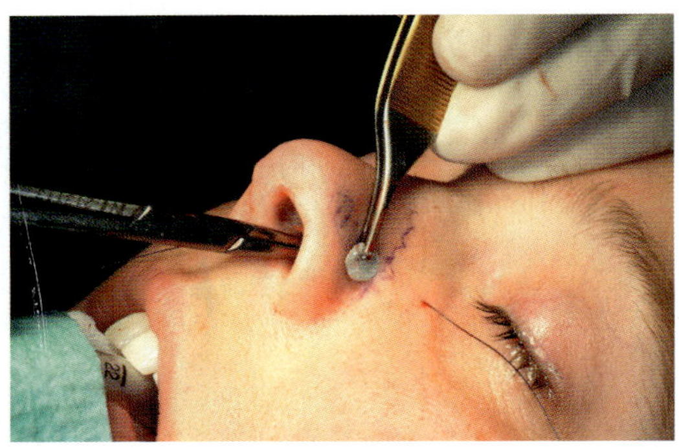

v

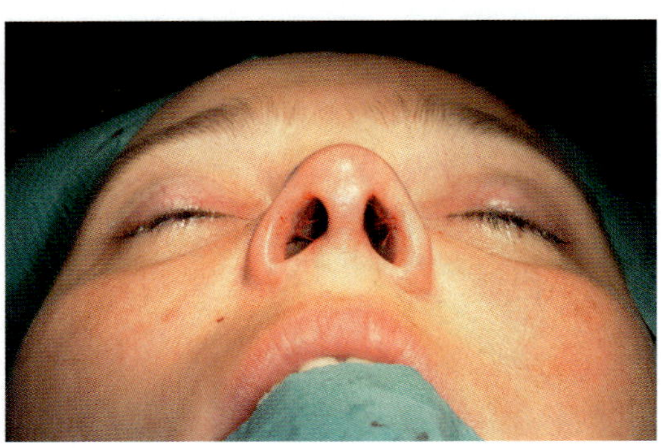

w

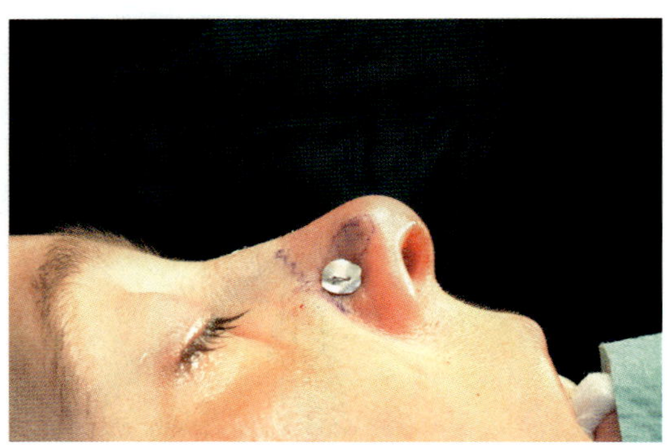

x

Fig. 2w-z. Direct postoperative basal and lateral views and after packing and dressing.

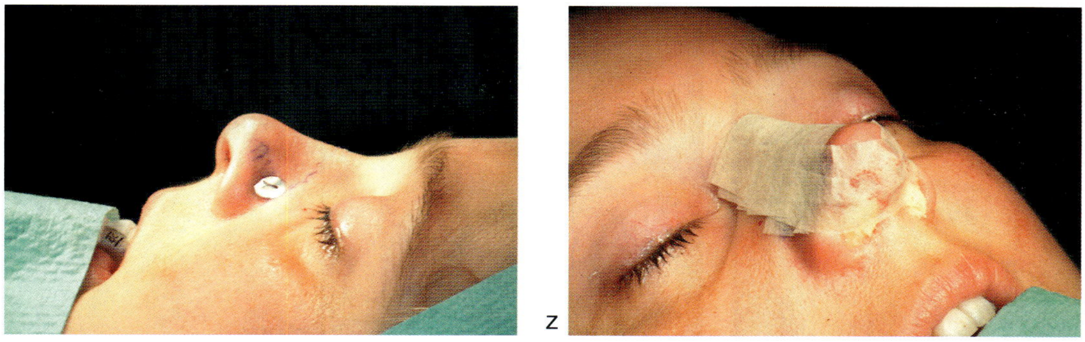

y z

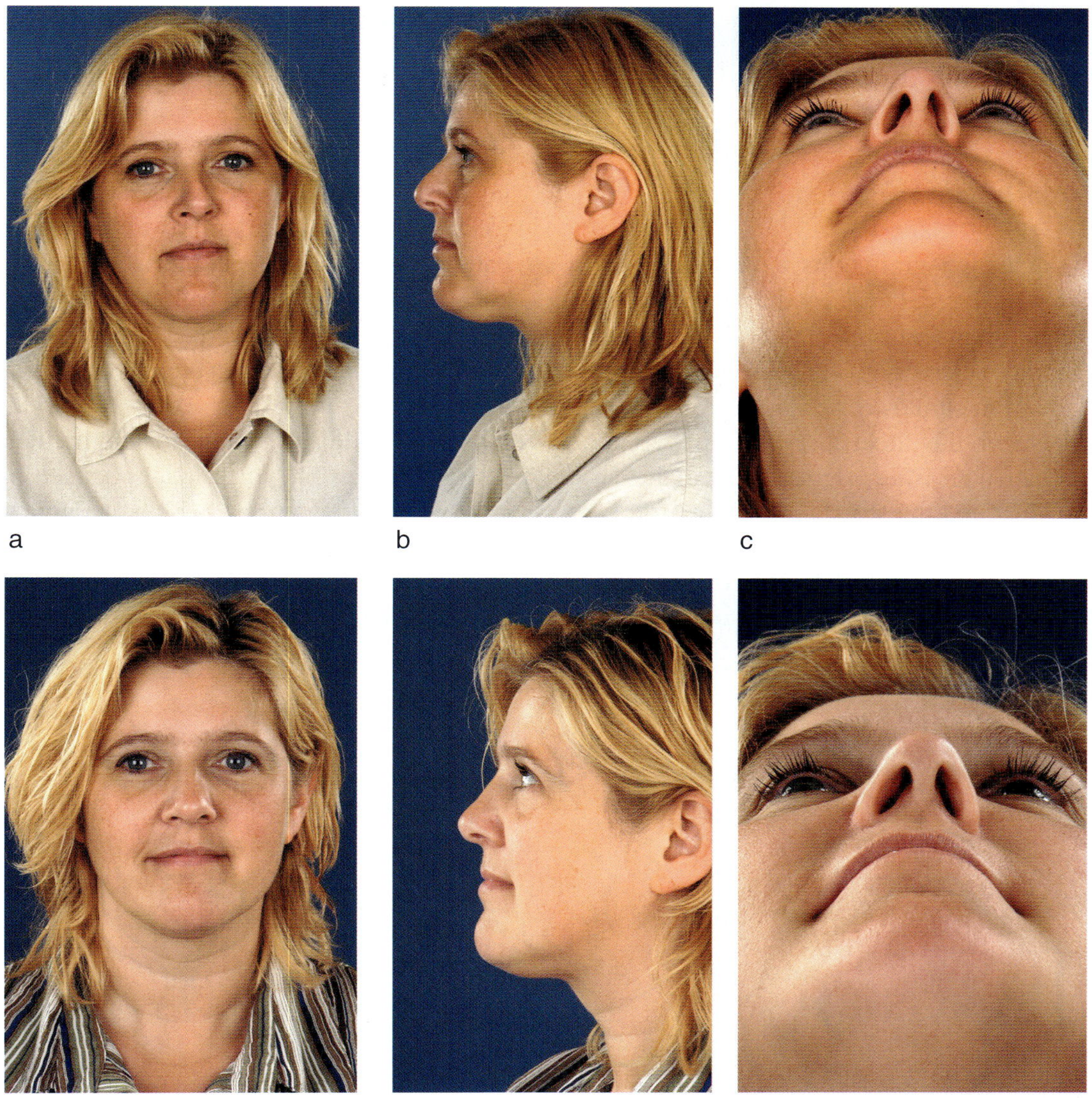

a b c d e f

Fig. 3a-f. Pre- and postoperative views of the patient with internal valve collapse, a slight polly beak, and deviation of the nasal dorsum and caudal septum to the left (surgical procedure shown in fig. 2a-z).

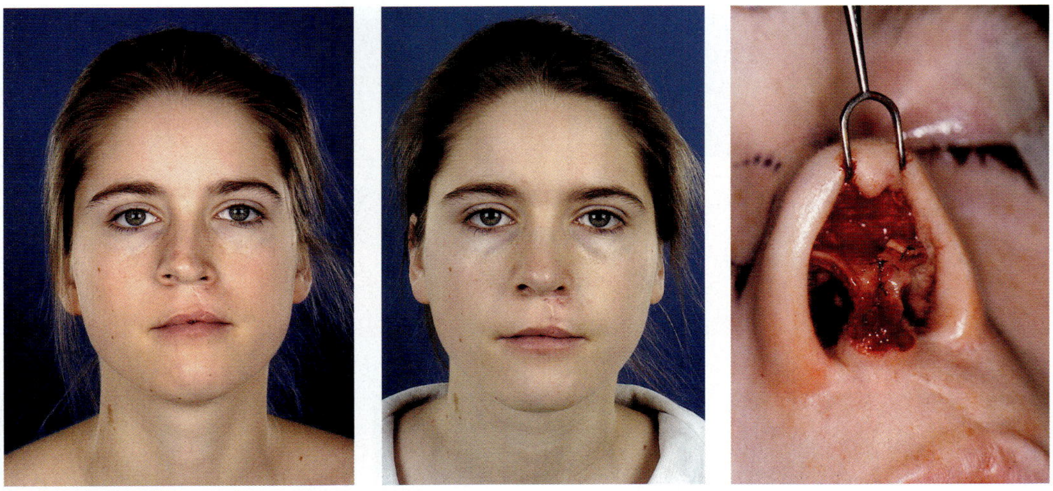

a b c

Fig. 4a,b. Pre- and postoperative frontal views of external rhinoplasty in a cleft lip patient with alar collapse at the left side.

Fig. 4c. Interoperative view of the same patient with an alar batten sutured to the repositioned lateral crus in order to correct external valve collapse and to improve the aesthetic appearance.

Conclusions

Alar batten grafting is a versatile tool in nasal valve collapse. A thorough examination for diagnosing other causes of nasal airway obstruction and for determining the site of maximal collapse is essential.

Due to the direct correlation between the negative pressure originating from the nasal airflow and the structural support from the nasal side wall, it can be difficult to choose the correct surgical procedure. Techniques to diminish the negative pressure by enlarging the nasal valve angle (spreader graft) or to strengthen the nasal side wall with alar battens can be performed. In specific cases, only a combination of both these procedures, batten graft and spreader graft placement, will be able to restore normal nasal airway.

Care should be taken to distinguish between reversible obstructions (mucosal swelling) and non-reversible anatomical obstructions, such as a deviated septum. Nasal valve collapse is a diagnostic and surgical challenge.

29: RECONSTRUCTION OF SKIN CANCER DEFECTS OF THE NOSE

Peter J.F.M. Lohuis, A.J.M. Balm and G.J. Nolst Trenité

Introduction

The nose has the highest incidence of skin cancer, and the management of a nasal defect following tumor removal is influenced by multiple factors. Tumor control is essential, since recurrence can lead to high patient morbidity and unnecessary donor site damage. Therefore, cosmetic considerations for compromising the margins of resection are indefensible. Excision by Mohs' micrographic surgery permits examination of the complete peripheral and deep resection margins in one plane. This technique is known for its high cure rate and, in most cases, permits primary reconstruction of the nasal defect.

The aim of reconstructive nasal surgery is not just to rebuild all or part of the nose, but rather to blend and tailor the new and old tissues in such a way as to create the best possible result. The challenge of reconstruction is related to the complexity of the defect in an organ where function, structural integrity, and contour should be maintained. Differences in color, texture, and thickness between the nasal remnants and the resources of skin available for the reconstruction pose aesthetic limits that are often difficult to overcome. Therefore, the decision on the possible use of a local flap is based on careful consideration of where tissue may be borrowed from, how it can be repositioned, what the immediate and long-term effects of moving that tissue will be, and how scars may be hidden. Age, general health, and the aesthetic goals of the patient should also be taken into account. In this chapter, we discuss the fundamentals of nasal reconstruction and describe various basic reconstructive options, depending on the size, depth, and location of the surgical wound.

Epidemiology

More than one-third of all cancers originate in the skin; 75% of these include basal cell carcinoma (BCC) and 20% squamous cell carcinoma (SCC).[1] Of the remaining 5%, melanoma is responsible for 4% of all skin cancers, and 1% comprises a group of relatively rare skin cancers (*e.g.*, Merkel cell carcinoma, sarcoma, malignant adnexal, and malignant lymphoid neoplasms of the skin).[2] Approximately 90% of all BCCs, 80% of all SCCs, and 15-20% of all melanomas are found in the head and neck. People with fair skin, fair hair, and blue eyes (Fitzpatrick's skin type I and II) are at greatest risk. Caucasian individuals residing closer to the equator have a higher risk of developing skin cancer, suggesting a direct correlation to exposure to sunlight or, more specifically, to the cumulative amount of ultraviolet radiation exposure.[3] Consequently, in the head and neck, skin cancers are predominantly found on sun-exposed sites such as the nose, and in particular the most projected lower two-thirds. In fact, cancer occurs more often on the skin of the nose than in any other organ of the body.[4] Although reports vary, the frequency of nasal BCC, SCC, and melanoma is (relative to each other) approximately 85%, 14%, and 1%, respectively.[5]

Tumor biology

The extent or aggressiveness of nasal skin cancer should not be underestimated. Inadequate treatment can lead to uncontrollable local recurrence, often resulting in (sub)total amputation and high patient morbidity. Proper treatment planning is essential for providing the patient with the best chance for cure and an optimal aesthetic

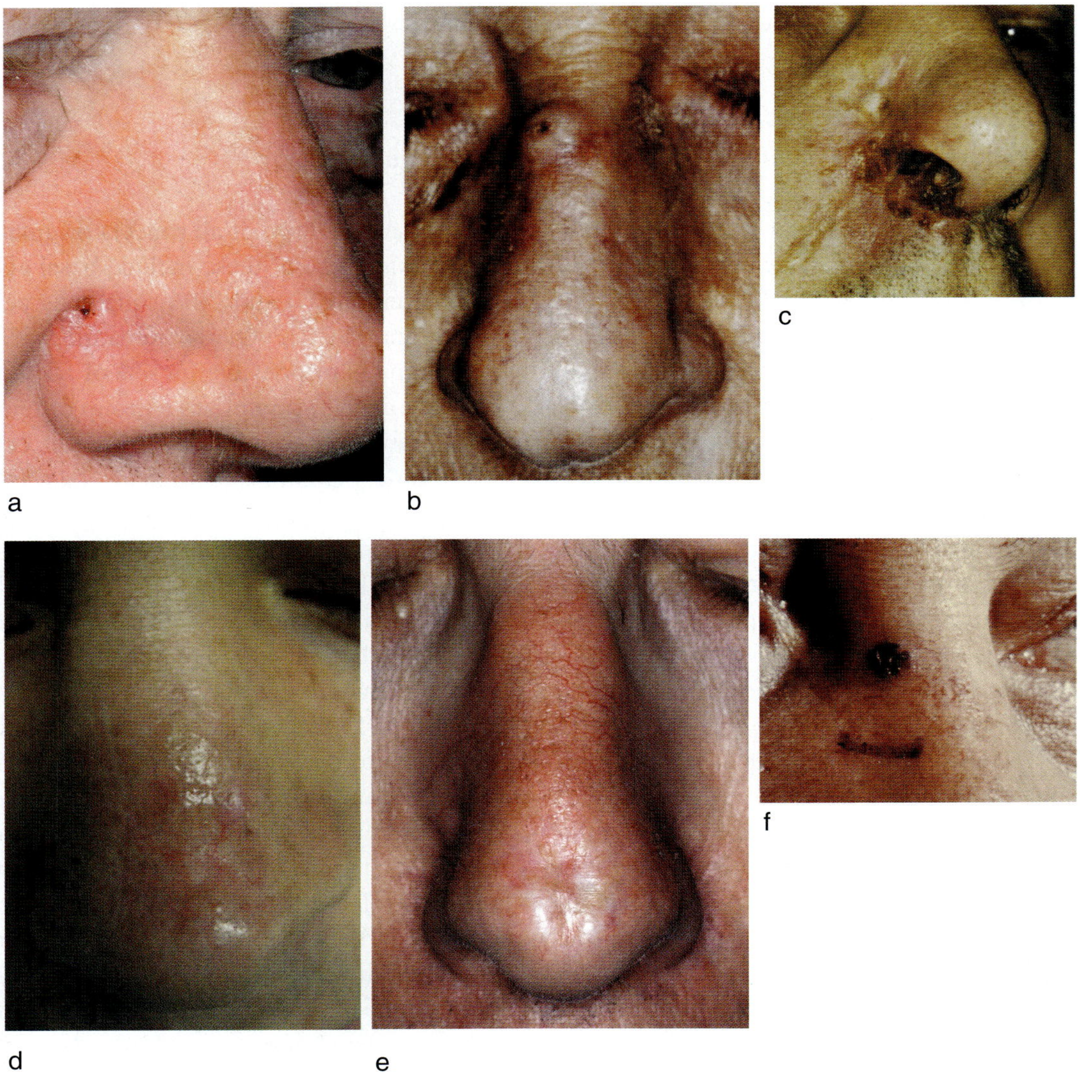

Fig. 1. BCC has man clinical manifestation The presentation of pearly teleangiectatic pa pule (*a,b*) is typical, bu BCC may also resembl an eczematous patch or a atrophic scar (*c,d,e*) wit indefinite borders. A pig mented BCC may resem ble a melanoma (f).

and functional result. Above all, the nasal reconstructive surgeon should be familiar with the tumor biology of the different types of skin cancer.[6] The biology of the three most frequently occurring nasal skin cancers (BCC, SCC, and melanoma) is briefly discussed in the following subsections.

Basal cell carcinoma

BCC is the most frequently occurring cutaneous malignancy in Caucasians, and has many clinical manifestations (Figs. 1a-f). The presentation of a pearly, teleangiectatic papule is typical, but BCC may also resemble an eczematous patch or an atrophic scar with indefinite borders.

In order to minimize the chance of recurrence after therapy, the clinician must be aware of the various clinical growth patterns and the multiple histopathological variations of BCC (Fig. 2a and b).[7,8] Histologically, five BCC subtypes can be discriminated, each with different clinical implications. These are, in order of increasing aggressiveness, superficial BCC (10%), nodular or solid BCC (50-70%), micronodular BCC, infiltrating BCC, and morpheaform BCC.[9] Combinations of different histologies (mixed-type) are also found. Micronodular, infiltrative, morpheaform,

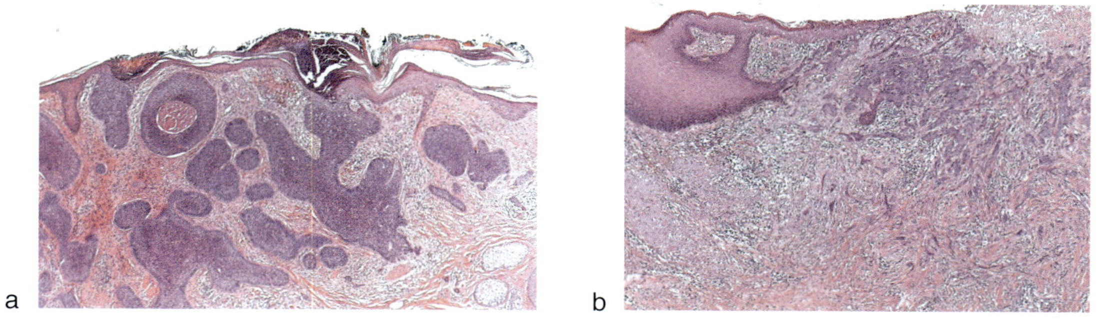

Fig. 2. Histological sections of a nodular (*a*) and an infiltrative (*b*) BCC. Infiltrative type BCCs tend to grow more invasively and often extend peripherally beyond the apparent clinical margin.

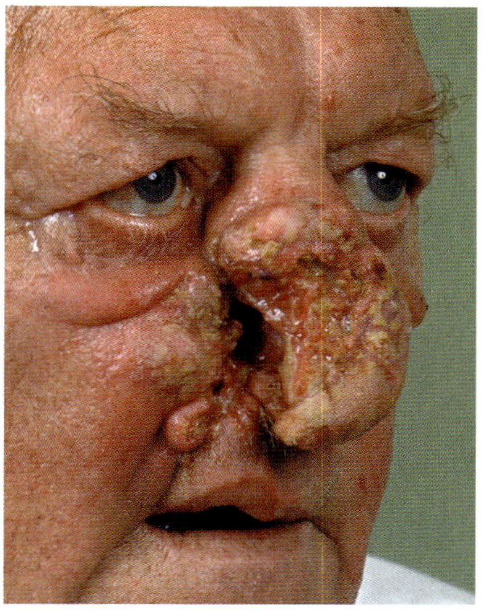

Fig. 3. Invasive ulcerating SCC with a granular, rolled margin of the nasal side wall, illustrating the sometimes aggressive tumor biology of SCCs.

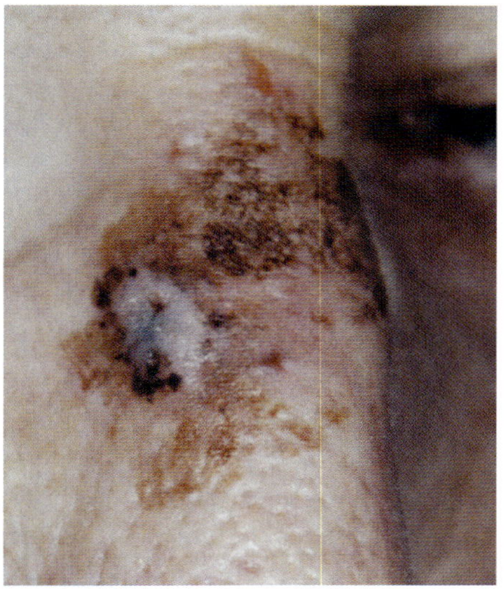

Fig. 4. Nodular malignant melanoma of the nasal dorsum arising in a patch of lentigo maligna (a precursor of malignant melanoma).

and mixed-type BCC tend to grow more invasively, and often extend peripherally beyond the apparent clinical margin.[10] Therefore, appropriate therapy should be tailored to the histopathology obtained by biopsy.

Squamous cell carcinoma

Invasive SCC demonstrates epidermal cells proliferating downwards in the direction of the dermis, often producing keratin pearls. Clinically, they present as a firm erythematous skin lesion (often covered with a crust), but an ulcerating, easily bleeding lesion is not exceptional (Fig. 3). Removal of a crust may reveal a granular, rolled margin. Increased tumor thickness and depth of invasion are the most consistent histopathological features of cutaneous SCC that recur and metastasize, but differentiation grade, perineural involvement, clinical size (diameter), immune status of the patient, and anatomical site may also be important.[11-13] At presentation, regional lymph node metastases are found in approximately 10% of cases;[12,14,15] their presence has a major influence on the final outcome of the disease. In these cases, local excision of the tumor is combined with therapeutic neck dissection and/or parotidectomy, followed by adjuvant postoperative radiotherapy when the prognostic signs are bad.[15,16] Distant metastases are very exceptional, but may occur in the lungs, bone, and liver in the event of extended regional disease.

Melanoma

Malignant melanoma is a malignancy arising from the melanocytes, the pigment-producing cells of the skin (Fig. 4). Three clinical types of malignant melanoma of the skin can be discriminated in the head and neck, as follows: superficial spreading malignant melanoma, lentigo maligna melanoma, and nodular malignant melanoma. The prognosis is strongly related to the depth of tumor invasion and the presence of regional lymph node metastases.[17] The depth of invasion is determined by Clark levels and, more precisely, by Breslow thickness. Breslow thickness measures the distance from the granular layer of the epidermis to the point of deepest invasion by tumor cells, and is ascertained by excisional biopsy. The definite treatment of melanoma of the skin includes wide re-excision of the initial biopsy site.

Although wide excision of melanoma is curative in some cases, all invasive melanomas carry some risk of metastases. In case of a regional nodal metastasis, tumor prognosis drops by more than 50%, depending on the number of positive lymph nodes.[18] Nevertheless, therapeutic lymph node dissection is still worth doing since it offers a potential chance of cure in melanoma patients with regional lymph node metastases.[18,19]

Tumor excision

Surgical excision of skin cancer provides a high cure rate and has the advantage of the histopathological control of complete tumor removal. Although important, cosmetic or functional concerns remain secondary to cure and should therefore not compromise safe and complete tumor removal. In order to pursue the safe excision of nasal skin cancer, the reconstructive surgeon should adhere to the following principles:

- apply proper surgical techniques and margins;
- screen for the presence of regional metastases; and
- delay reconstruction when radical excision is uncertain.

Apply proper surgical techniques and margins

Biopsy

Biopsies are used, not only for microscopic assessment or confirmation of the type of primary tumor, but also for establishing the level and depth of invasion as well as the presence of negative histological features.[20,21] For all nasal BCCs and SCCs, especially when large or aggressive, it is important first to make a diagnosis by incisional punch biopsy, in order to determine the proper margin and treatment strategy.

In case of a suspected melanoma, an excisional biopsy containing at least 2-3 mm of macroscopically normal skin around the lesion is performed to establish a diagnosis before more definite surgery can be planned.[6] Shave biopsies of suspected melanomas are never indicated. Histological evaluation of the entire tumor specimen is required in order to find the thickest and deepest part of the lesion, which determines the final Breslow thickness. The depth of invasion (Breslow thickness) in malignant melanomas forms a guide for the width of the margin of re-excision, and also represents the most important prognostic parameter.

Local anesthesia

When excising nasal skin cancer under local anesthesia, the visible tumor and resection margins should be outlined in ink before injecting the local anesthetic (Fig. 5). Local infiltration of the anesthetic directly under the tumor should be avoided, especially in SCCs and melanomas, since there is a theoretical chance of seeding tumor cells.[22] Instead, nerve blocks involving the infraorbital nerve, infratrochlear nerve, and/or external nasal branch of the anterior ethmoidal nerve are used, often in combination with field-block anesthesia around the tumor.

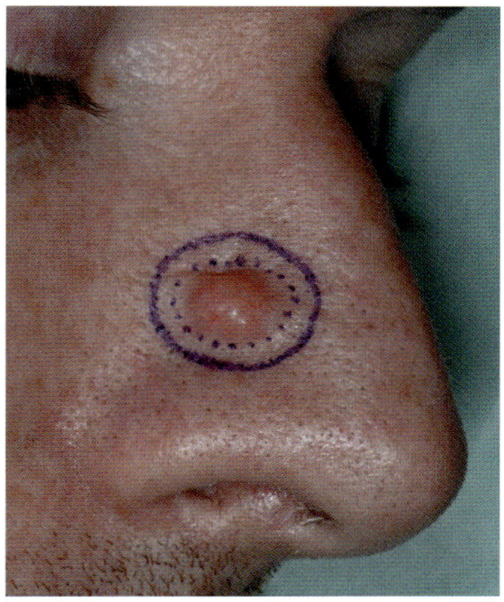

Fig. 5. Excision plan of a nodular BCC of the lateral nose. Biopsy was obtained to determine histology and subsequently to determine margin and treatment strategy. Clinical and resection margins (3 mm) are outlined before injecting local anesthesia.

Tumor excision

Biopsy is important for determining the margin and for making a treatment plan. For example, a small primary nodular BCC with a diameter of 10 mm or less requires a 3-mm margin in order to include all tumor extensions in 80% of cases (Fig. 5).[23-25] In contrast, morpheaform or infiltrating type BCCs are notoriously deceptive and can send out subclinical extensions of 7 mm or more beyond the clinically estimated borders (Fig. 2b).[23,26] Recurrent BCCs and SCCs also need notably larger excision margins. In general, a small SCC requires a therapeutic margin of at least 5 mm; this margin can be extended, depending on the size and estimated infiltration depth of the primary tumor.

Melanomas may contain satellites or in transit metastases and therefore needs wide excision. Table 1 shows the margin of excision that is required for the treatment of melanomas in relation to Breslow thickness, as determined by the excisional biopsy. Recently, there has been a trend towards narrower excision margins in the treatment of melanomas in the face. Generally, in the head and neck, a margin of at least 0.5 cm should be obtained for non-invasive or *in situ* melanomas, and a margin of at least 1 cm or more for invasive melanomas.[27] Patients with melanomas are best treated in a multidisciplinary center, because the biological behavior of these tumors is unpredictable.

Table 1. Breslow thickness and generally recommended margin of (re)excision

Breslow thickness	*Margin of excision*
In situ melanoma	0.5 cm
≤ 2.0 mm	1 cm
> 2.0 mm	2 cm (at least 1 cm in the face)

Of equal importance in planning the lateral margins is assessing the depth of the lesion prior to any reconstructive procedure. In particular in the lower third of the nose, there is an intimate attachment of skin and lower cartilages such that invasion of the cartilage occurs relatively early in the course of the disease.[28] Studies have shown that the highest percentage of recurrent BCCs are nasal, illustrating the difficulty of tumor control in this area. On the one hand, this may be due to a tendency towards narrow excision margins in an effort to simplify reconstruction in this aesthetically important area. On the other, skin cancer in the midface is known to show a local tumor spread, which appears to be related to the embryonic fusion planes at this site.[29] A tumor seems to prefer to invade in depth rather than to cross the borders of these fusion planes.

When BCCs or SCCs recur in a scar, flap, or graft, the entire scar, flap, or graft should be excised, since recurrent tumors tend to move in previously dissected planes. Similarly, in case of recurrence after radiotherapy, the entire field of irradiation should be excised. In particular with these difficult tumors, excision by Mohs' micrographic surgery (see next subsection) is applicable due to the high chance of cure using this technique.

Screen for the presence of regional metastases

The aggressiveness and potential regional metastatic spread of melanomas, and to a lesser extent of SCCs, are undisputed and strongly related to the invasion depth of the primary tumor. The midface and nose drain into lymphatics that follow the facial vessels to the facial, submental, and submandibular nodes (level I). However, the lymph nodes of the superficial lobe of the parotid gland are also known to play a filtering role for the lymph flow of the midface. For cutaneous nasal cancer, it is therefore important to palpate not only the cervical lymph nodes, but also the nodes of the parotid gland, buccal fat path, and nasolabial fold, since these locations may harbor the first-echelon lymph nodes (Fig. 6).[30,31] Ultrasound-guided fine-needle aspiration cytology (US-FNAC) has been shown to be of additional value in the detection of regional lymph node metastases.[32]

Delay reconstruction when radical excision is uncertain

Primary reconstruction of skin cancer defects is safe in most cases, under the conditions of proper patient selection and reliable histopathological examination techniques. Surgical delay in wound reconstruction should be considered, sometimes even after Mohs' surgery, if there is any doubt about the completeness of the tumor resection.[33,34] In particular in large, recurrent, or aggressive skin tumors (*e.g.*, perineural growth, deep invasion of the bony or cartilaginous framework of the nose), the timing of reconstruction should be postponed until more certainty has been obtained that no signs of tumor regrowth have occurred (Fig. 7).[11,35] Using a split- or full-thickness skin graft or secondary intention healing as an interim method for nasal reconstruction can offer surveillance of the operative site for recurrence.

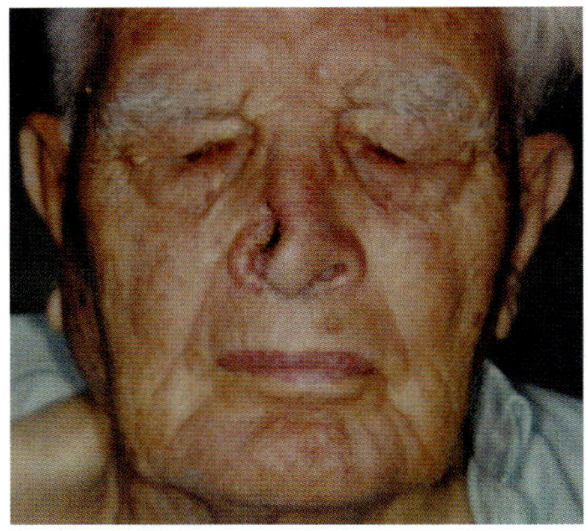

Fig. 6. Patient referred from another hospital after irradical excision of an SCC of the right ala, now presenting with a regional metastasis of the parotid gland requiring parotidectomy and radical modified neck dissection.

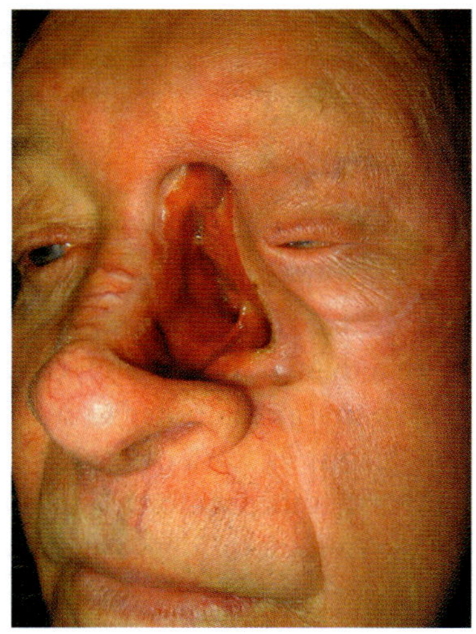

Fig. 7. Patient referred from another hospital with recurrent SCC of the upper nasal side wall after primary reconstruction with a cheek advancement flap (note the melolabial and infra-orbital incision lines), requiring subtotal amputation. Reconstruction was postponed until more certainty could be obtained that no signs of tumor regrowth had evolved.

Mohs' surgery

In order to establish high quality care in nasal reconstructive surgery, the methods used by the pathologist to examine tumor margins should be understood by the clinician. The more complete the examination of the surgical margin, the more accurately the chances of cure can be estimated. In case of a three-layer excision of the nasal ala, routine peripheral sectioning permits a complete check of the margins. However, in other cases, Mohs' micrographic surgery is ideal for controlling the complete peripheral and deep resection margins in one plane, permitting orientation, identification, mapping, and re-excision of microscopic tumor extensions (Fig. 8).[36-39] These extensions can be followed without having to sacrifice inappropriate amounts of normal tissue.

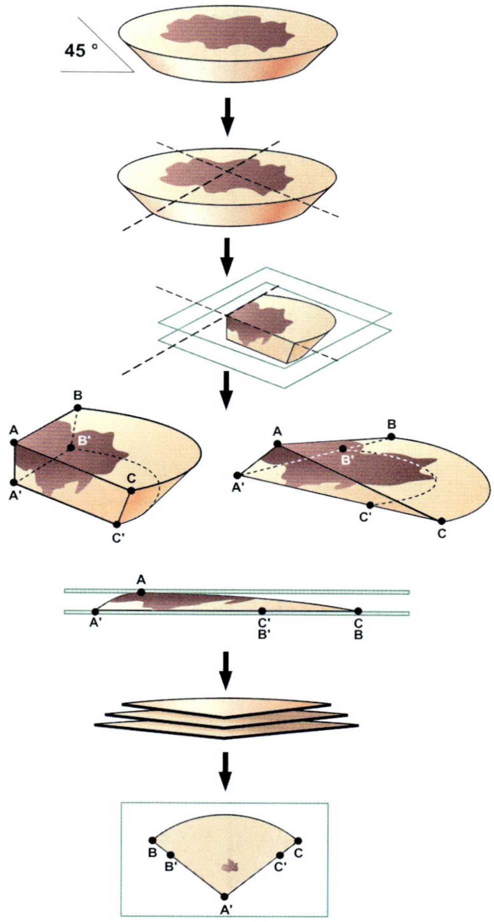

Fig. 8. Schematic drawing depicting the main principle of Mohs' micrographic surgery. Oblique peripheral sections are used to encompass peripheral and deep resection margins in one plane, theoretically allowing a 100% check of margins and mapping of possible microscopic tumor extensions.

Due to its high chances of cure, Mohs' surgery may be specifically indicated for SCCs and a subset of BCCs, including BCCs with an unfavorable histology or an unfavorable location, as well as large and recurrent BCCs (Table 2). In these cases, Mohs' surgery provides the best prospect for complete tumor removal and should therefore be considered compulsory when planning for primary reconstruction with local or regional transposition flaps (Table 3).[40]

Table 2. Indications for Mohs' micrographic surgery

– BCC
  – large
  – unfavorable histology (*e.g.*, infiltrating, morpheaform, micronodular)
  – recurrent
  – in functionally and aesthetically important areas (*e.g.*, nose, ear, eyelid)
– SCC

Table 3. Pros and cons of Mohs' micrographic surgery

Advantages:
– 100% check margins
– low percentage of recurrence (for a review: see Vuyk & Lohuis[37])
– saves valuable uninvolved skin (for reconstruction)
– primary reconstruction on the day of the excision

Disadvantages:
– time consuming

Key features of nasal reconstruction

Nasal units are covered by skin of a specific color, texture, and thickness. In addition, each unit has specific contours determined by soft and hard tissue. The decision-making process in the reconstruction of nasal defects should include careful consideration of where tissue may be borrowed from, how it can be repositioned, what the immediate and long-term effects of moving that tissue will be, and how scars may be hidden. In order to reach this goal, the nose must be restored as a major facial unit composed of each subunit. Three principles form the basis of this reconstructive process, as follows:[41-43]

– replace missing tissue with similar tissue;
– replace missing portions of the nasal skeleton with cartilage fashioned to precisely replicate the missing part; and
– divide the topography of the nose into aesthetic units and resurface the entire unit with a skin flap if the majority of the skin in the unit has been lost.

Replace missing tissue with similar tissue

Nasal skin varies in texture, color and appearance within the various areas of the nose (Fig. 9). The nasal dorsum, side walls, columella, alar margins and soft triangles are all covered with thin, smooth skin. The nasal tip and ala are covered with thick, pitted skin due to the presence of sebaceous

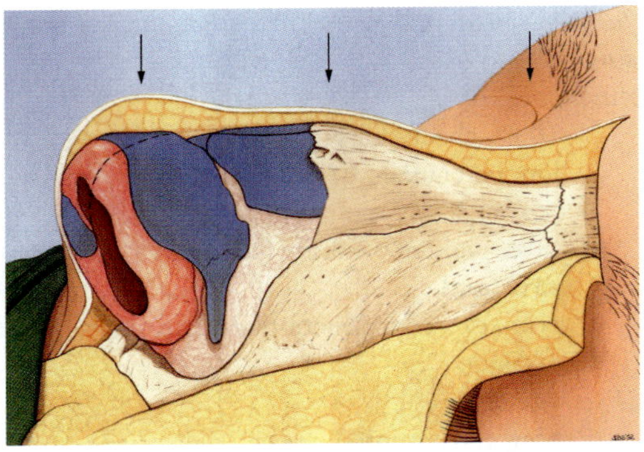

Fig. 9. Nasal skin varies in thickness and also in appearance between different areas of the nose.

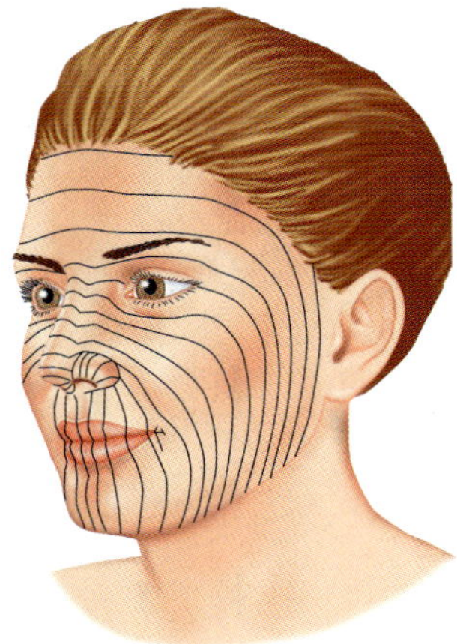

Fig. 10. The arrangement of the nasal relaxed skin tension lines (RSTL) is complex, since they are oriented transversely from the root to the tip, but change direction on the ala and columella, where they are oriented perpendicular to the nostril orifice.

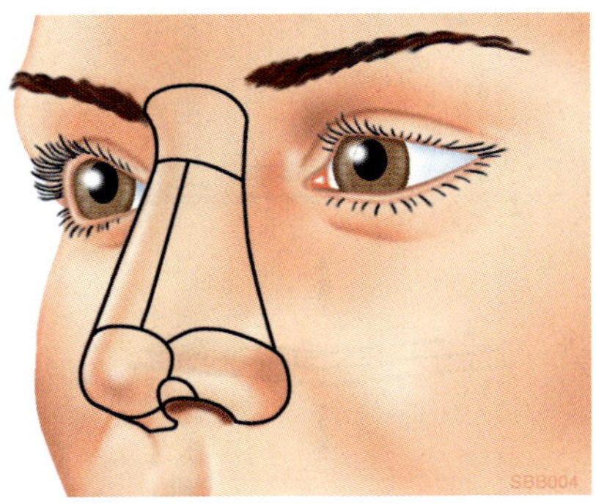

Fig. 11. The aesthetic unit theory is important in nasal reconstruction. Placing a scar between topographic units, where it follows the join of normal lighted ridges and shallow valleys, will make it less visible.

glands. The color of the skin may vary from pale with a matt texture on the side of the nose, to a shade of red-pink with a shiny appearance over the nasal tip.[44]

When replacing nasal skin with similar tissue, local flaps (unlike skin grafts) are especially useful in the thick-skinned zones because of their reliable color and texture. Regional flaps (especially the forehead flap) are used for larger, deeper defects, because their size, bulk, and vascularity permit the replacement of ideal skin cover and primary cartilage support and lining. Loss of nasal inner lining should be restored by septal mucosa or adjacent vestibular skin.

Replace missing portions of the nasal skeleton

Loss of primary cartilage support by removal of the upper and lower cartilages should be restored by replacing the missing portions of the nasal skeleton with septal or auricular cartilage. Defects extending to the alar margin may result in retraction or partial collapse of the nostril if the ala is not properly supported with a batten in the form of a cartilage graft. Structural alar grafts are usually obtained from the contralateral conchal cartilage. These grafts are positioned beneath the alar cartilages between the lateral crura and the vestibular skin, and are of sufficient length to extend from the crura to the alar base.

Alar batten grafts provide support for the nasal ala, but may also prevent constriction of the nasal valve in patients where two or more nasal aesthetic units have been resurfaced with a covering flap. For the same purpose, septal cartilage should replace the upper lateral (tri-angular) cartilage.

Aesthetic units

Strategic incision placement

Although we cannot control wound healing or prevent the development of scars, we can select the color, texture, and thickness of donor materials. We can also control the site, size, shape, and direction of incisions and excisions, and so manipulate the scars they produce.[45,46] Scars can be placed strategically so that they utilize relaxed skin tension lines (RSTL) (Fig. 10) or are camouflaged at the junction of subunits (Fig. 11). Border scars of skin flaps are best positioned so that they resemble the ridges and valleys of the nasal units.[47]

Fig. 12. Patient referred from another hospital after reconstruction of a dog bite with a superiorly based melolabial flap. Reconstruction of the entire alar subunit would probably have led to a better aesthetic result (*a*). Inproper use of a transposition flap in the supra-tip region, resulting in a conspicious scar and pincushing (*b*)

a

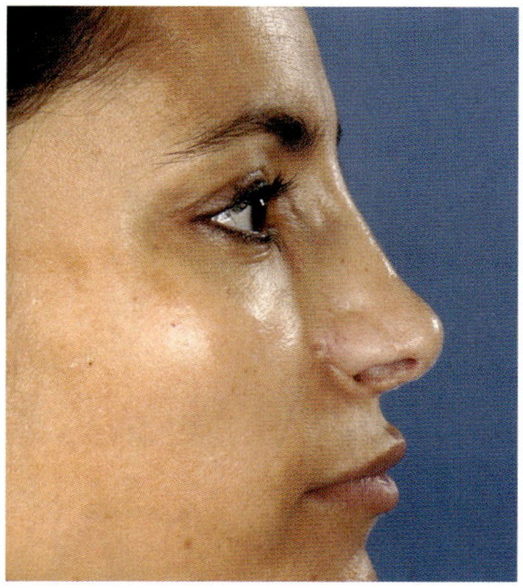

b

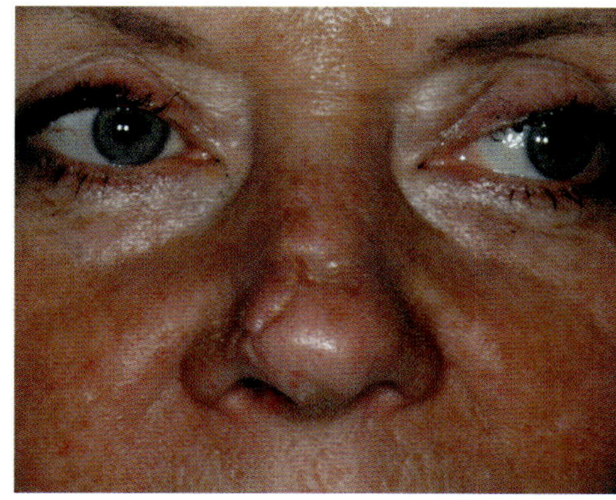

Figs. 13a and b. The subunit principle suggests that if a defect encompasses more than 50% of a subunit, excision of the residual normal tissue should be considered. In this patient with wide re-excision for a superficial spreading melanoma, the entire nasal dorsal subunit was reconstructed with a flap instead of only patching the original defect (same patient as in Fig. 39).

a

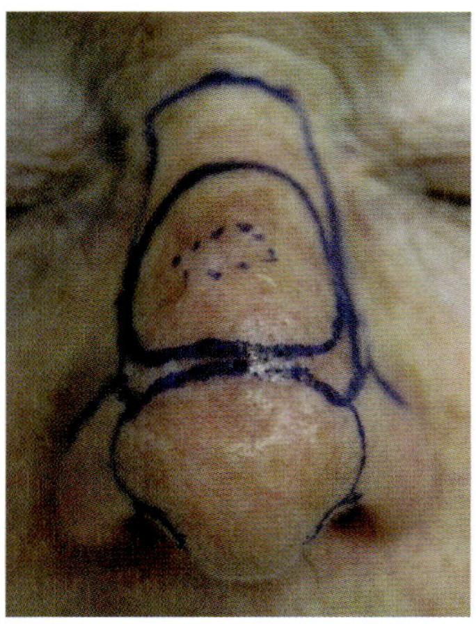

b

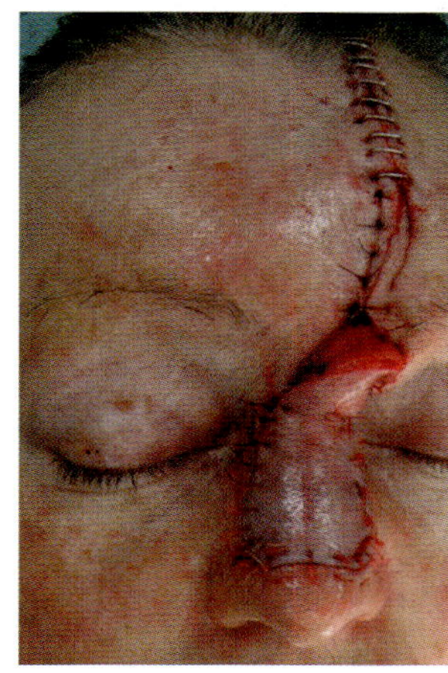

Fig. 14. Patient with excision of a recurrent infiltrative BCC after radiotherapy followed by reconstruction with a paramedian forehead flap. Although the texture and thickness of the donor site skin is quite different from the recipient site in this thin-skinned patient, resurfacing the entire subunit positioned the scars in joints between three-dimensional units.

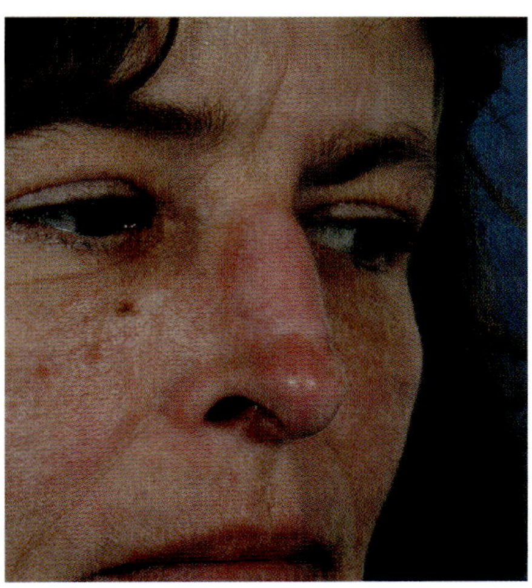

The subunit principle

The aesthetic unit theory is important in nasal reconstruction (Fig. 11). If a line of light or shadow (due to scarring) crosses a smooth surface where it is not expected, it will be noticed at a glance (Fig. 12). A 'good' scar remains hidden from view because it is visually perceived as a 'normal' facial fold or contour line. If a scar is placed between nasal topographic units, where it follows the join of normal lighted ridges and shallow valleys, it will also be taken as being normal. Equally importantly, the bulge of a flap caused by trapdoor contractions will mirror the normal contours of convex subunits.

The subunit principle suggests that if a defect encompasses more than 50% of a subunit, excision of the residual normal tissue should be considered (Fig. 13a).[48] In this way the entire subunit is reconstructed with a flap (Fig. 13b), instead of patching the original defect. Resurfacing a partial defect as an entire subunit may position scars in joints between three-dimensional units, where they may be hidden and less visible (Fig. 14). This maneuver is most effective in reconstruction of the tip and alar subunits, which are surrounded by fairly abrupt, distinct borders. In these locations, the subunit principle also makes use of the trapdoor effect to recreate a three-dimensional convexity, since many flaps have a tendency to pincushion and stand up as a bulge above the residual skin.[47]

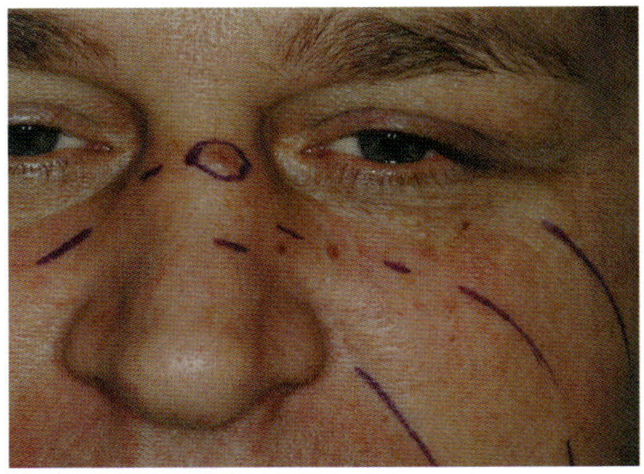

Fig. 15. Following the lines of relaxed skin tension (RSTL), small soft tissue wounds in the supra-tip region or in the thin mobile skin overlying the nasal bones and upper lateral cartilages can be primarily closed without appreciable deformity.

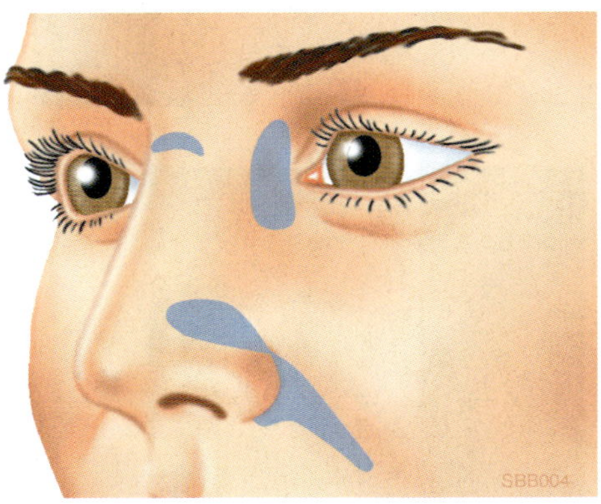

Fig. 16. Secondary intention healing is often ignored as a valuable alternative to immediate surgical reconstruction of a wound. Particularly wounds in concave areas such as the medial canthus, alar facial groove, and naso-alar crease, even though quite deep, often heal with excellent cosmetic results.

Nasal reconstruction techniques

A variety of reconstructive techniques are available for the reconstruction of skin cancer defects of the nose. The choice is based on the size, depth, and location of the surgical wound, as well as on the availability and condition of the surrounding tissue. Below we discuss some of the most important basic techniques, which have been the source of many small modifications.

Primary closure

Small soft tissue wounds of the supra-tip region or of the thin mobile skin overlying the nasal bones and upper lateral cartilages can be primarily closed without appreciable deformity. Incisions and lines of closure that follow the lines of relaxed skin tension (RSTL) should be used whenever possible (Fig. 15). Limited undermining may be necessary to ensure tension-free closure.

Scars from direct closure are usually minimal, particularly in the elderly population in whom skin tumors usually occur. In case of an unsightly non-depressed scar, dermabrasion six months postoperatively may help. The transverse primary closure of a large dorsal defect will result in upward rotation of the nasal tip, which may be an added bonus in case of a drooping nose in elderly patients.

Healing by secondary intention

Secondary intention healing is often ignored as a valuable alternative to immediate surgical reconstruction of a wound.[49,50] Due to a process of contraction and epithelialization, the cosmetic results of secondary intention healing are often equal to the results of more complex reconstructive surgery. In particular, wounds in concave areas such as the medial canthus, alar facial groove, and naso-alar crease, even though rather deep, often heal with excellent cosmetic results (Fig. 16). Upward retraction of the alar rim rarely occurs, unless the wound involves most of the alar surface or

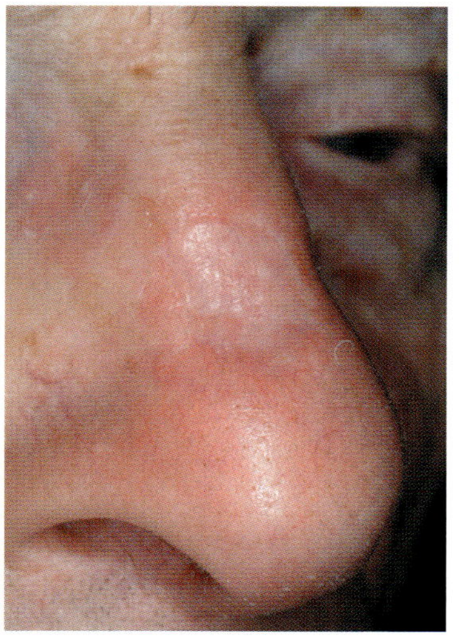

a

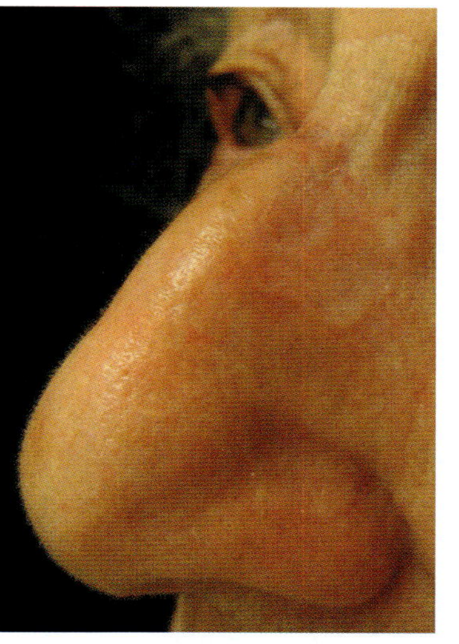

b

Fig. 17a. Preauricular FTSG of the dorsum of the middle nasal vault. Although a difference in thickness exists, the result of such a graft is acceptable in elderly patients with actinic skin.

Fig. 17b. FSTG from the upper eyelid over the left nasal bone and a preauricular FSTG in the naso-alar crease. Note that the texture of the preauricular skin matches the nasal skin better.

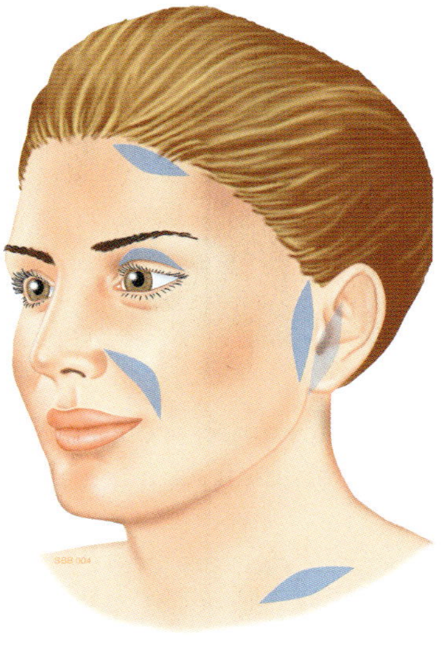

Fig. 18. Potential donor sites for FTSG.

is located within a few millimeters of the rim.[55] Secondary granulation of wounds on the nasal dorsum and tip is not indicated, since this invariably results in flattening of the nasal contour.

Grafts

Free skin grafts

Two factors critical to the success of any graft are the vascular capability of the recipient bed and the thickness of the tissue that is transposed. Split-thickness skin grafts (STSGs) are rarely employed in nasal reconstruction because they lose pigment during healing and because contraction of the underlying wound proceeds unchecked. This often leads to a pale, shiny irregular surface. However, full-thickness skin grafts (FTSGs) serve perfectly well for replacement of the upper two-thirds of the nose.[51] A prerequisite for skin grafting is a woundbed that allows vascular ingrowth, making avascular tissues such as exposed bone and cartilage generally inapplicable for supporting an FTSG. FTSGs in convex regions such as the nasal tip are often cosmetically inferior because of differences in thickness, texture, and color of the grafted skin (Fig. 17a and b).

The final choice of the donor area for FTSGs depends on the size, thickness, and pigmentation of the needed graft. Potential donor sites should be carefully examined under natural light in order to discover the best match. Skin from the postauricular, preauricular, and supraclavicular regions is frequently used, although in elderly people, the upper eyelid occasionally also serves as a potential donor site (Fig. 18). The postauricular skin is slightly redder and thinner than the nasal skin. The preauricular skin usually has a better color and texture match with the upper two-thirds of the nose, but is limited in size, particularly in hair-bearing male skin.[52,53] In contrast, the sebaceous skin of the melolabial fold provides an excellent color and texture match for small

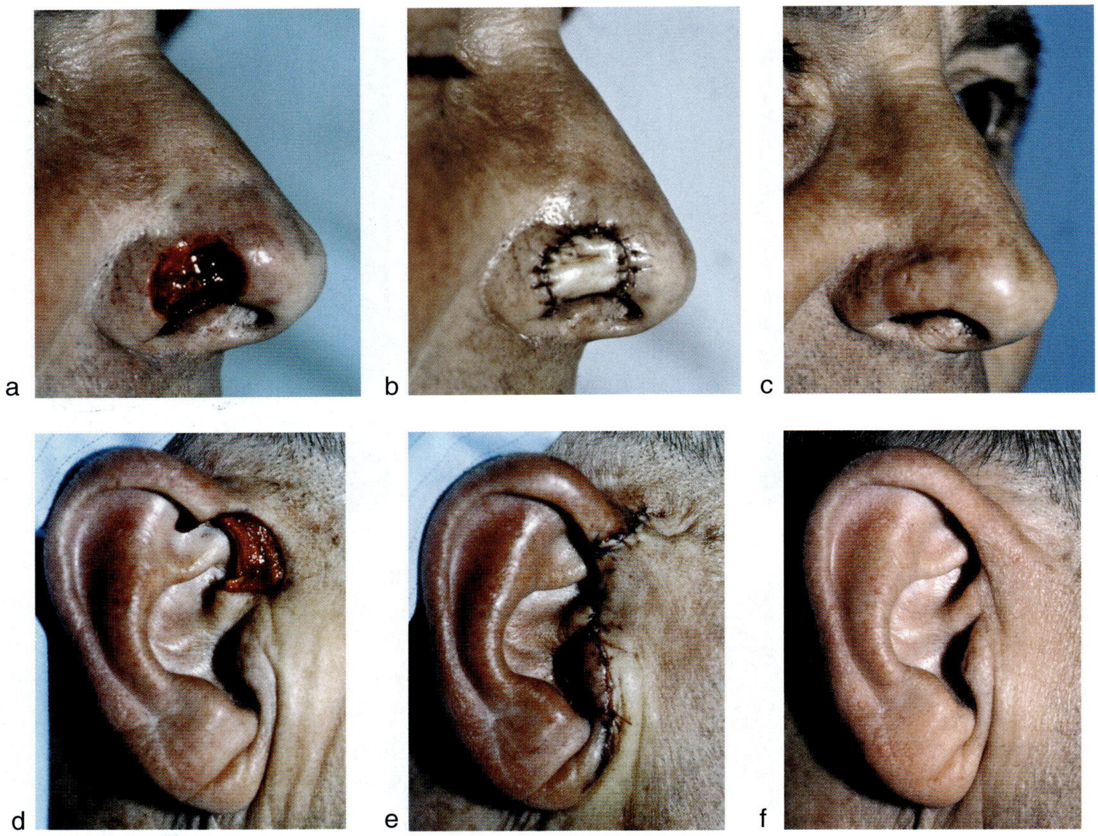

Fig. 19. Composite graft taken from the root of the helix to repair small defects of the alar rim. The donor site can be closed primarily with minimal cosmetic morbidity (courtesy of H.D. Vuyk).

defects in the nasal tip and infratip lobule.[54] Although relatively thick, the supraclavicular area can provide sufficient skin to reconstruct an entire lateral subunit of the nose.

Since the slightest amount of hematoma from the recipient site will result in the loss of the graft, hemostasis of the recipient site should be meticulous, and the graft should be held in place for four to five days using non-adhesive tape and a stent or (tie-over) bolster dressing.

Composite grafts

Composite grafts have the benefit of being relatively simple procedures, which can provide satisfactory results and minimal compromise if they do fail. Due to its thickness, a composite graft requires an almost ideal recipient bed. The use of epinephrine solutions for local anesthesia should be avoided. Allowing the recipient site to granulate for three days increases the probability of composite graft take. However, even in the best circumstances, complete survival is rare when the graft is more than 1.0 cm thick.

Composite grafts are best utilized for the repair of small defects of the alar rim (Fig. 19a-f) and columella, and are preferably taken from the root of the helix, where the donor site can be primarily closed with minimal cosmetic morbidity.[55] The occurrence of a notch on either side of the graft along the alar or columellar margin after healing is the rule rather than the exception. Correction of these notches should be delayed for approximately six months, and then performed under local anesthesia.[28]

Local skin flaps

Flaps are the only reliable way to transfer bulk tissue for reconstruction. Having its own source of nutrient blood makes the flap independent from the recipient bed for its survival. It may therefore be used to cover

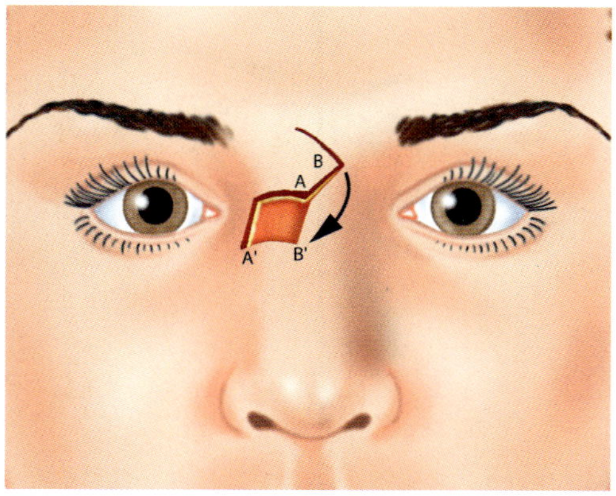

Fig. 20. Rhomboid flap from the glabellar root.

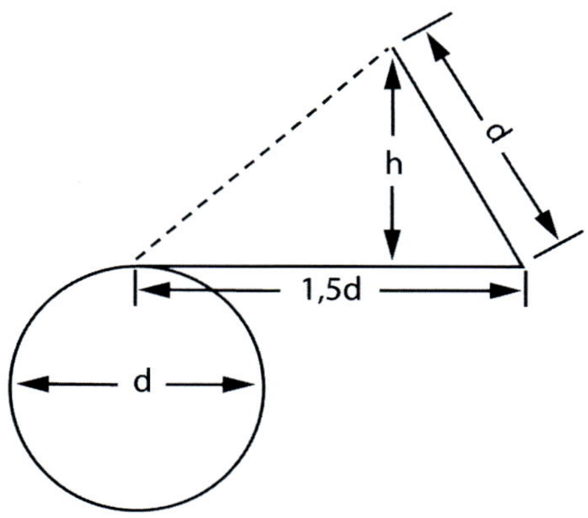

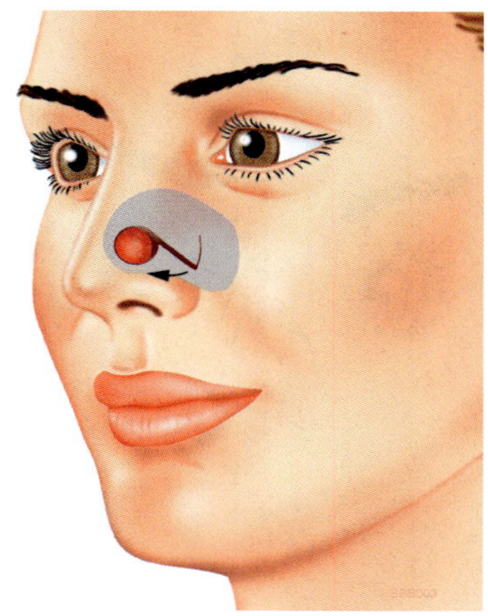

Fig. 21a,b. The note flap is an elegant alternative to the rhomboid flap. The principle is shown in a schematic drawing.

nonvascular structures such as bare bone and cartilage.[45] Local skin flaps, taken from within the aesthetic subunits of the nose, provide excellent aesthetic camouflage for small defects, largely because of skin match in terms of texture, color, and thickness.[56-58] Excess tissue, usually in the upper two-thirds of the nose, is moved into adjacent defects. The alar region is less suited for local transposition or rotation flaps, since the supra-alar crease is often lost.

Rhomboid flap

The rhomboid flap makes optimal use of tension distribution by orienting the flap design according to the lines of maximum extensibility (perpendicular to relaxed skin tension lines).[59] However, the geometric design of the rhomboid flap (with eight possible variations) onto the complicated RSTL pattern of the nose seldom fits to make optimal use of this concept. The possible exception to this is the lateral nasal side wall and the glabellar root (Fig. 20).

Note flap

An elegant alternative to the rhomboid flap is the note flap. This avoids having to sacrifice normal tissue at the edges of a circular defect in order to create the arbitrary geometric pattern which is required for the rhomboid flap. In essence, the note flap is a triangular transposition flap, which is capable of closing a circular defect with little donor site deformity. The simplest form of this flap is shown in Figure 21. It is extremely easy to design this flap in relation to the relaxed skin tension lines. For a circular defect, the surgeon draws two tangents approximately parallel to the relaxed skin tension lines of the nose. Four potential flaps are then designed and the surgeon chooses the best of four options. Ideally, the RSTL should parallel the final donor closure site. One of the disadvantages of the note flap is that there is frequently some dog-ear formation at the base of the triangular flap, although no tailoring is usually needed. A more important disadvantage is that it requires a fair amount of judgment based on experience. Since the flap is somewhat smaller than the defect, the surgeon must ensure that there is sufficient tissue laxity to allow closure.[60]

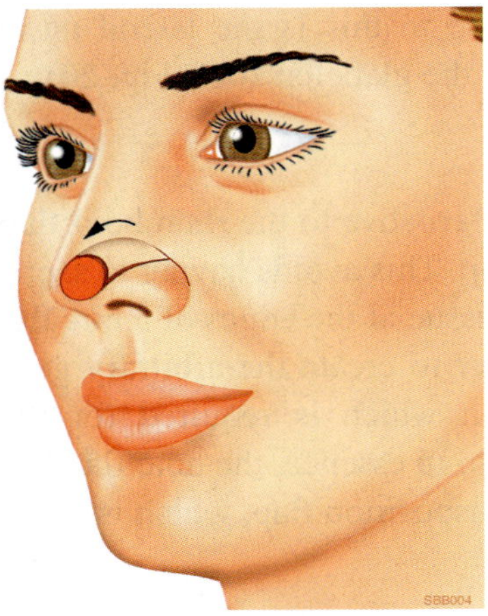

a

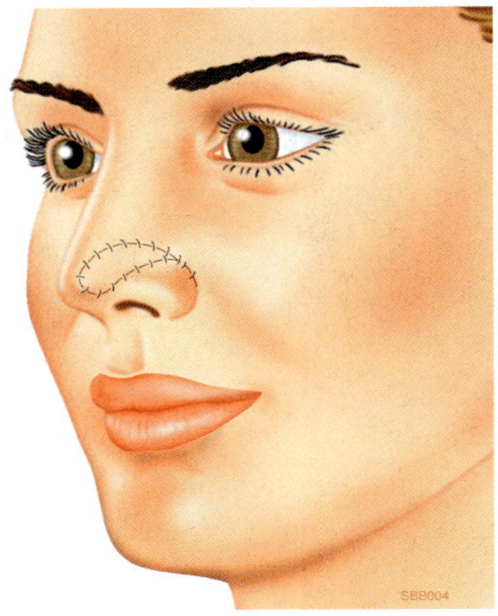

b

Fig. 22a,b. Locally applied V-to-Y island pedicle advancement flap, which can be used in the simple reconstruction of small defects located in the region of the anterior alar groove and lateral nasal tip, including the nasal facet.

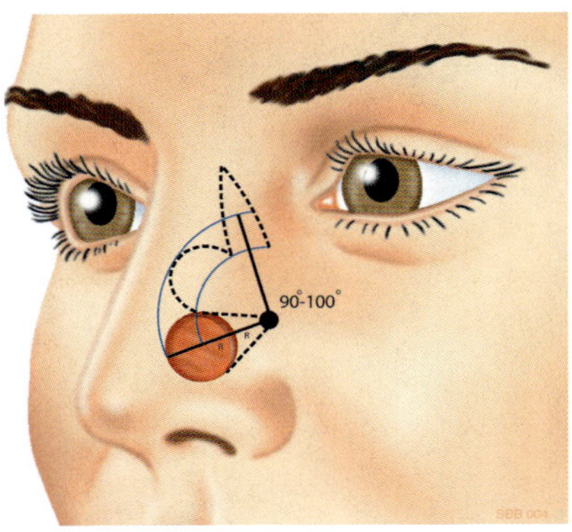

a

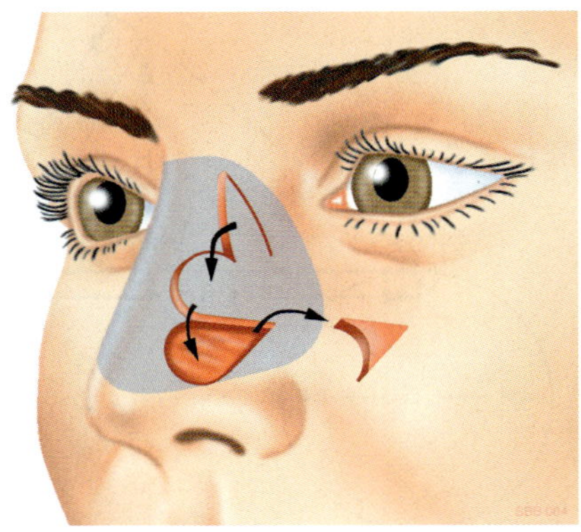

b

Fig. 23a,b. Bilobed double transposition flap.

V-to-Y island pedicle advancement flap

The V-to-Y island pedicle advancement flap is frequently used as a regional flap to replace soft tissue of the lower lateral nasal side wall in more extensive skin cancer defects. As a local flap, its use is limited. It is mentioned here because it might be helpful in the simple reconstruction of small defects located in the region of the anterior alar groove and lateral nasal tip, including the nasal facet (Fig. 22a and b).[43]

Bilobular transposition flap

By definition, the bilobed flap is a double transposition flap that allows movement of looser skin from the upper nose into small defects of the lateral lower nose and adjacent tip.[61] The defect should not exceed a diameter of 1.5 cm, and the pedicle is best based on the lateral aspect of the nose. The primary flap or lobe is used to repair the nasal defect, and a secondary lobe is created to repair the donor site of the primary lobe (Fig. 23a and b). The donor site of the secondary lobe is then primarily closed.[62,63] Wide undermining beneath the musculature is essential. In order to prevent excessive dog-ear deformity, the skin should not be transposed over more than 90 degrees.[64] A Burow's triangle is commonly excised adjacent to the defect.[65] The bilobed flap requires incisions that violate the boundaries of the subunits, but rotate skin of similar quality to cover the defect. However, with careful design, the bilobed flap may be individually designed to give excellent cosmetic results with minimal distortion.[63]

Regional flaps

If large areas of nasal skin are missing (more than 1.5 cm in diameter), or if the underlying nasal support is missing and the cartilage framework must be restored with

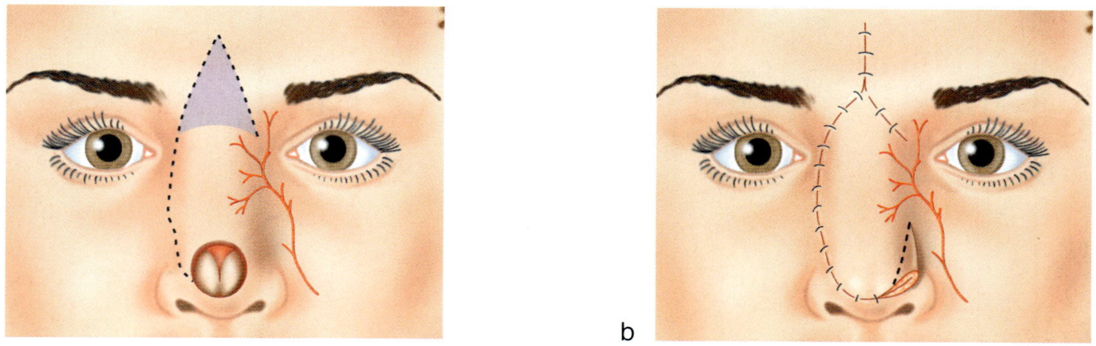

Fig. 24a,b. Nasal dorsal glabellar rotation flap. In the glabellar portion, the dissection is in the subcutaneous plane; in the nasal portion, it is beneath the musculature.

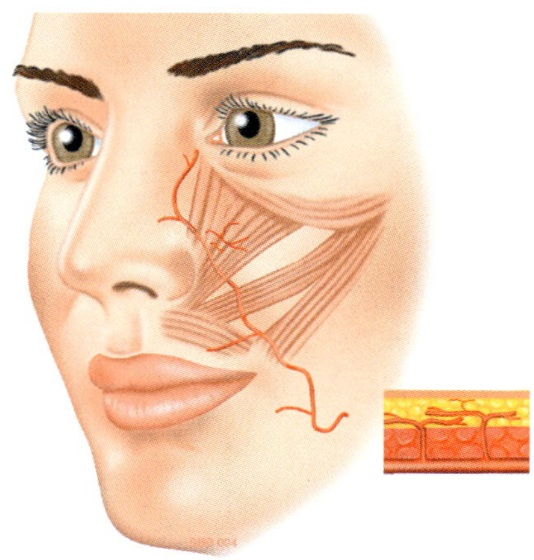

Fig. 25. The blood supply to the melolabial flap is not actually based on a specific vessel found in the flap. Rather, it is based on a directionally oriented subdermal plexus that courses parallel to the melolabial crease, thus making it a random pattern flap with a directional orientation to the blood flow of the angular artery.

primary cartilage grafts, a local flap is no longer applicable. These circumstances require a regional (distant) flap such as the nasal dorsal glabellar rotation, melolabial, or paramedian forehead flap. In case the defects extend to the paranasal region, regional flaps such as the cheek advancement flap and pedicled island advancement flap may serve to replace the soft tissue of the lower lateral nasal side wall and alar insertion.

Nasal dorsal glabellar rotation flap

The nasal dorsal glabellar rotation flap provides an excellent one-stage procedure for repairing medium-to-large distal surgical defects of the middle and distal part of the nose (1-2.5 cm in diameter).[66,67] The flap, which receives a versatile axial blood supply from the angular artery, takes tissue from the lax glabellar skin and may appear to be too aggressive for closure of a distal nasal or midnasal defect (Figs. 24a and b). However, because its design is primarily that of a rotation flap (with a back-cut in the glabella region), it must be larger than the primary defect in order to maximize tissue movement and decrease wound closure tension at the flap donor site. The effective length of the flap diminishes progressively as the flap rotates about its pivotal point, the medial canthus. Dissection in the subcutaneous plane in the glabellar portion of the flap is critical because the thicker glabellar skin of the flap is advanced to the medial canthus where the skin is thinner (Fig. 24a). The nasal portion is dissected beneath the musculature.[67]

The melolabial flap

Closure by tissue from the melolabial area not only allows a good color match at the recipient site, but also affords camouflage at the donor site defect, hidden in the often-present melolabial crease. The blood supply to the melolabial flap is not actually based on a specific vessel found in the flap. Rather, it is based on a directionally oriented subdermal plexus that courses parallel to the melolabial crease, thus making it a random pattern flap with a directional orientation to the blood flow of the angular artery (Fig. 25).[68]

Two variants are described below: the inferiorly based (two stage; interpolation) and superiorly based (one stage; transposition) melolabial flap.

Inferiorly based melolabial flap: this is a versatile flap for the reconstruction of a defect that remains within the aesthetic unit

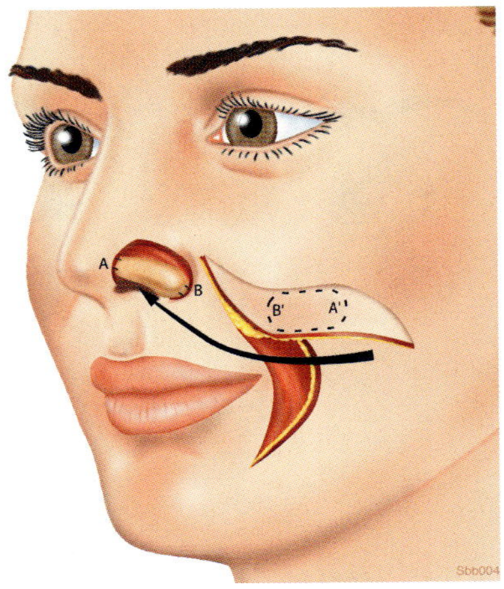

Fig. 26. Schematic figure of an inferiorly based melolabial flap.

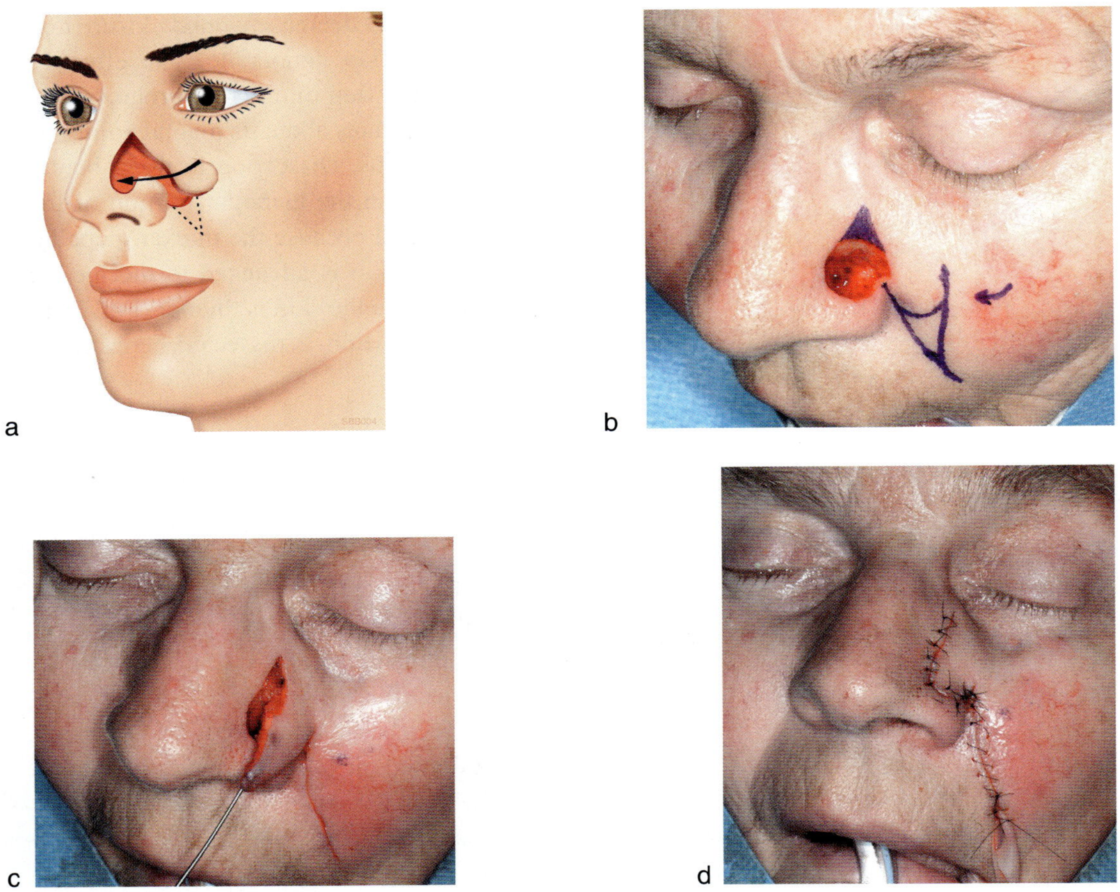

Fig. 27a-d. Schematic figure (*a*) and clinical example (*b,c,d*) of a superiorly based melolabial flap as a one-stage procedure.

of the ala or the columella. It is ideal for these sites because its soft fat contracts into a convexity that resembles normal contours.[43] However, if the defect exceeds this topographic unit to the nasal tip or the lateral nasal wall, the paramedian forehead flap is the flap of choice. The inferiorly based melolabial flap is designed as an interpolation flap in which the final scar of donor site closure will lie exactly in the melolabial sulcus (Fig. 26). For safe melolabial flap elevation, the depth of dissection is limited medially by identification of the orbicularis muscle and laterally by SMAS

Fig. 28. Example of a scalp flap. The indications for the scalp flap, the forerunner of the paramedian forehead flap, have largely been replaced by the more delicate paramedian forehead flap.

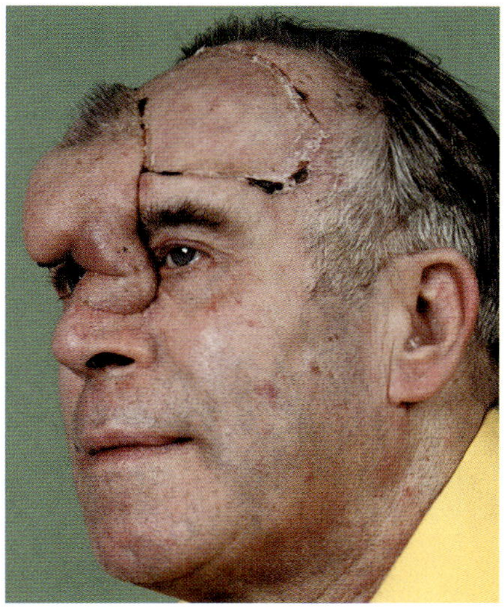

Fig. 29. The blood supply to the forehead is depicted schematically. The supratrochlear and ipsilateral supraorbital arteries, both terminal branches of the ophthalmic artery in the internal carotid artery system, demonstrate rich collateral circulation and anastomosis. The supratrochlear artery also richly anastomoses with the terminal branches of the angular artery supplied by the external carotid artery system.

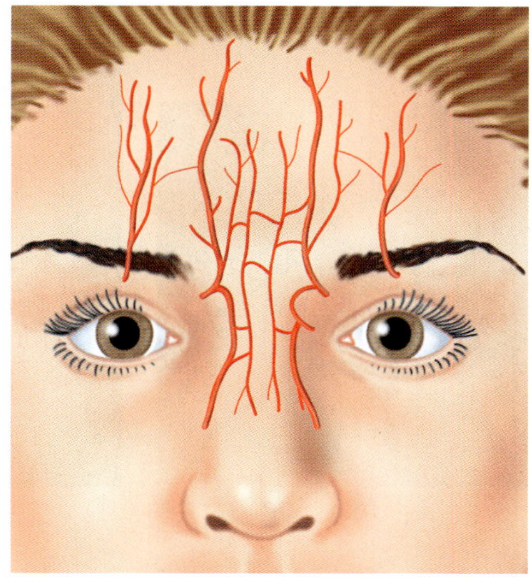

fibers coursing to meet the former. The donor site is closed by undermining adjacent cheek skin and advancing it inferiorly and medially. More than three weeks later, the pedicle is divided in a second-stage procedure, which also allows for debulking and contouring at the recipient site.

Superiorly based melolabial flap: defects of the ala can usually also be handled well with a superiorly based melolabial flap (Fig. 27a). If the defect does not involve the alar base and if the flap is thinned appropriately at the time of initial transfer, the procedure can be completed in one stage (Fig. 27b-d).[69,70] These flaps can remain edematous for a significant period of time. However, with the injection of steroids (Kenacort, 10 mg/ml) and occasional defatting, reasonable results can be achieved, particularly in elderly patients with large melolabial folds.

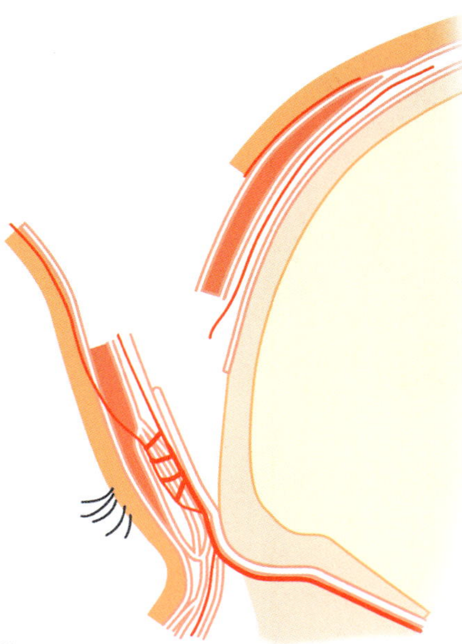

a

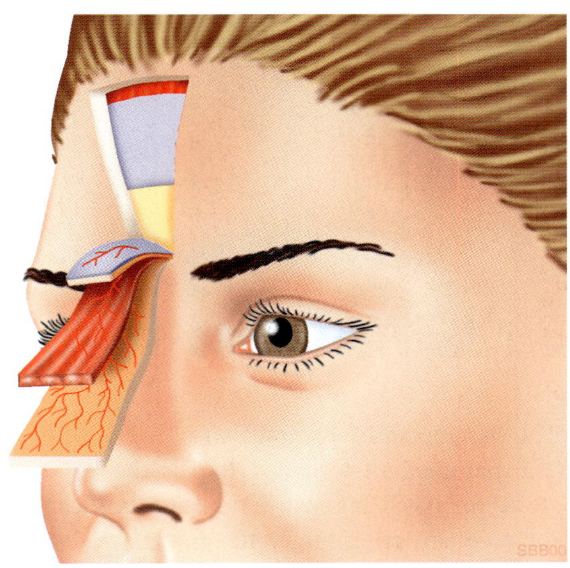

b

Fig. 30a,b. It is important to be familiar with the progressive change in plane taken by the supratrochlear artery, which forms the major blood supply to the paramedian forehead flap, as it ascends the forehead. This artery runs from the orbit over the periosteum, through the frontalis muscle towards the subcutaneous tissue of the distal flap.

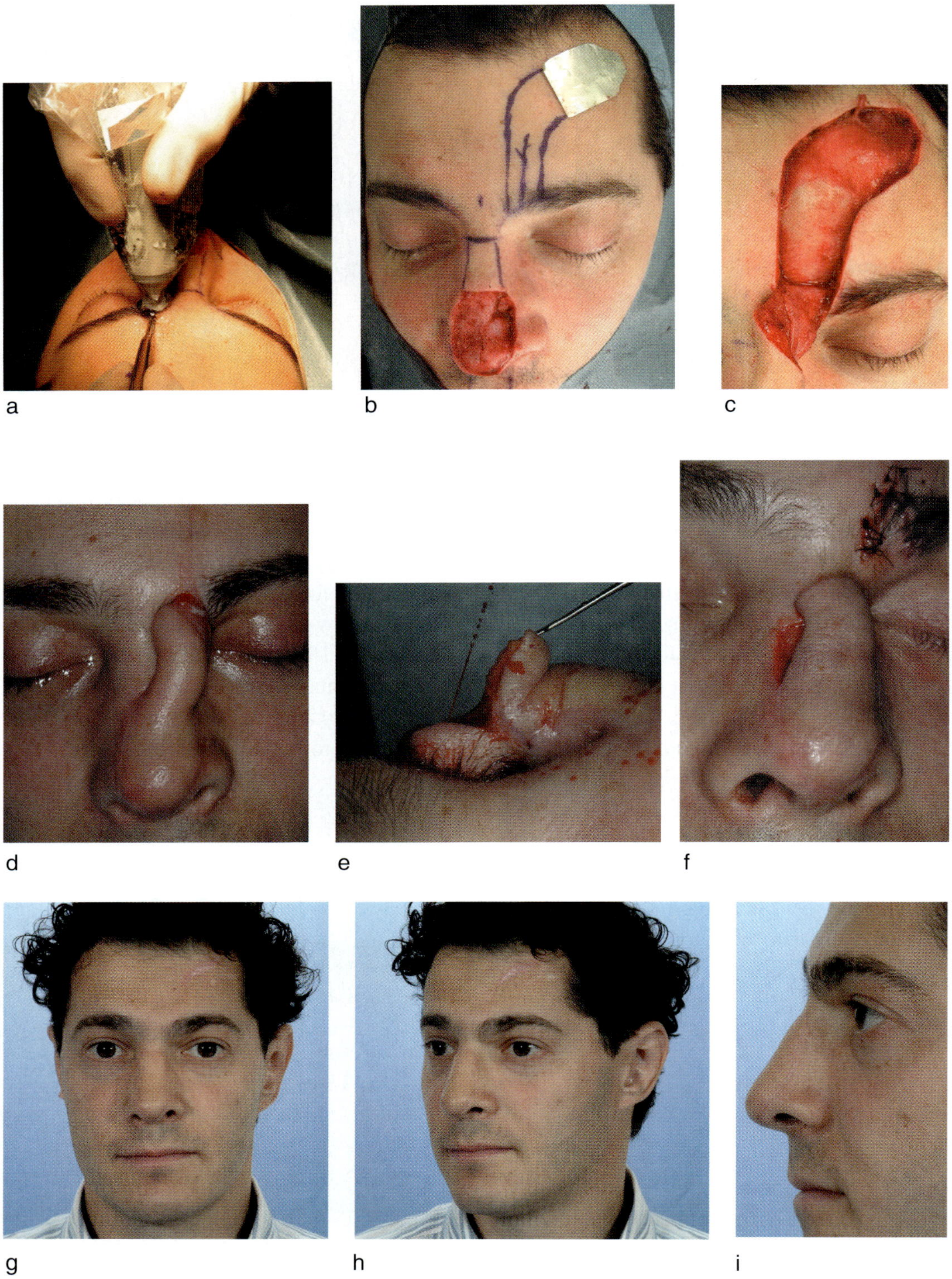

Fig. 31a-i. A young patient with a defect of the nasal tip after removal of an infiltrating BCC. The supratrochlear artery is identified by a Doppler (*a*). The paramedian forehead flap is directed laterally because of the shape and low position of the hairline in this particular patient, but was still closed primarily (*b*). About 2 cm above the supra-orbital rim, the periosteum is incised and the dissection carried inferiorly in a subperiosteal plan (*c*). Pedicled flap in place (*d*). The flow pressure in the supratrochlear artery is clearly visible when the pedicle is divided after three weeks (*e*). The nasal dorsal aesthetic unit is further excised and the brow reconstructed (*f*). Postoperative result after three months, no additional contouring was required (*g-i*). The broadened frontal scar is ideally re-excised six months after the initial procedure (*h*).

The paramedian forehead flap

The paramedian forehead flap is the keystone for nasal reconstruction and is ideal for reconstructing large, full-thickness defects of the lower two-thirds of the nose, including the nasal tip, ala, columella, dorsum, and nasal side wall.[55,71-73] It is a far more delicate lap than its forerunner, the scalp flap, which is now more or less obsolete (Fig. 28). The color and texture of the forehead skin provides an excellent match for nasal reconstruction, whereas the blood supply to the flap is extremely reliable. The major blood supply comes from the supratrochlear artery (Fig. 29 and 30a and b), which demonstrates collateral circulation and anastomosis with the ipsilateral supraorbital artery. Both arteries are terminal branches of the ophthalmic artery in the internal carotid artery system. The supratrochlear artery also richly anastomoses with the terminal branches of the angular artery supplied by the external carotid artery system. Therefore, the flap has two blood supplies: an axial pattern supply from the supratrochlear artery and a random pattern supply from branches of the facial and angular arteries.[55,74]

Since the paramedian forehead flap is the workhorse for nasal reconstruction, it is described in detailed steps below as a two-stage procedure (Fig. 31a-i). The first stage is the development of the flap as well as closure of the defect and the donor site. The second stage is the division of the pedicle, appropriate debulking and contouring at the recipient site, as well as closure of the brow region.

First stage

Developing the flap

- Care should be taken to design the flap over the supratrochlear vessels. The supratrochlear artery crosses the superomedial orbit vertically approximately 1.7-2.2 cm lateral to the midline[74].
- It is helpful to identify the artery with a Doppler (Fig. 31a) since this allows a narrow base to be planned (7 mm of tissue is taken on each side of the vessel), thus improving the arc of flap rotation and effective flap length.
- A pattern is cut from the foil of a suture pack to match the exact size of the defect or aesthetic unit.
- If the hairline of a patient is low or if the flap is required for columellar reconstruction, the orientation of the flap can be bent laterally to avoid the transplantation of hair-bearing skin (Fig. 31b). However, the design may also be extended into the hairline, because in a second-stage procedure the hair follicles can be carefully pulled out from the distal end of the flap via its deep surface.
- The greatest part of the flap is in a supraperiosteal plane. About 2 cm above the supra-orbital rim, the periosteum is incised and the dissection carried inferiorly in a subperiosteal plan. This is done to safeguard the supratrochlear artery and to allow the flap to be rotated from a much lower position in the orbit without tension (Fig. 31c).
- The excellent blood supply of the flap allows thinning of the distal portion of the flap, enhancing pliability and final contouring, especially in case of a defect of the nasal tip.
- After limited undermining, closure of the defect should take place with eversion of wound edges.

Closure of the donor site

- Closure of the forehead with staples (Fig. 13b) decreases wound tension and, in most cases, allows primary closure of the donor site with minimal scarring.
- A Burow's triangle is usually cut out in the hairline, in order to prevent dog-ear formation.
- Occasionally, particularly if part of the wound has been allowed to heal by secondary intention, it may be necessary to revise the forehead scar at a later date, most commonly after a period of six months (Fig. 31h).

Second stage

Dividing the pedicle and thinning of the flap

- The pedicle of the flap is divided approximately three weeks after the primary procedure (Fig. 31d-f). As far as vascularity permits, this is also the time for appropriate debulking and contouring of the transplanted skin flap. Alternatively, an intermediate stage before final pedicle division allows for

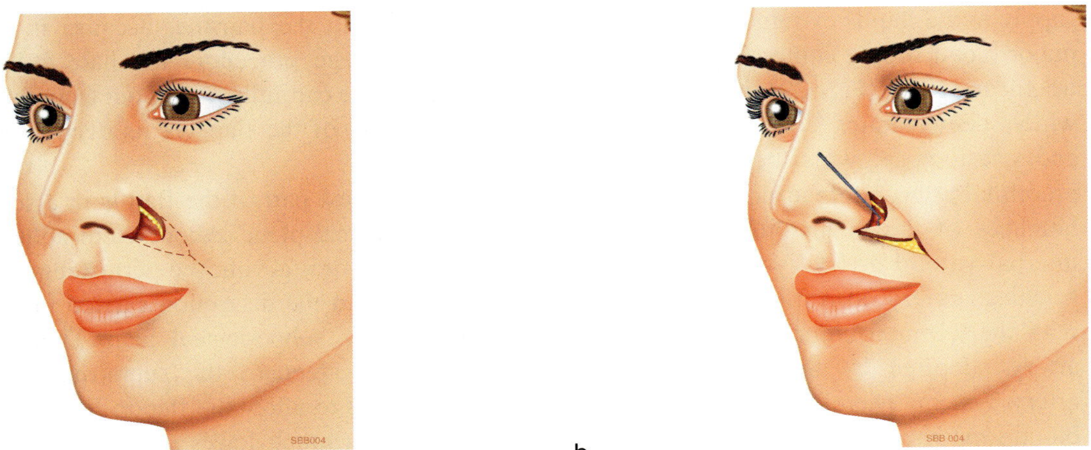

a b

Fig. 32a,b. Subcutaneously based V-to-Y flaps are most commonly used for soft-tissue replacement of the lower lateral nasal side wall. The flap is incised and freed from the adjacent cheek fat but remains attached in the deep plane.

more aggressive sculpturing and contouring at three weeks, the pedicle division being delayed until week six.

- The unused portion of the forehead flap is amputated and discarded, except for a small triangle of hair-bearing skin for closing the brow.
- Closure of the brow region is performed with wide undermining and meticulous suturing in order to avoid a trapdoor deformity (Fig. 31f). The pedicle should never be replaced higher than the level of the eyebrow, because it will show up as a finger-like deformity on an otherwise smooth forehead.

Cheek and cervicofacial flaps

For larger wounds of the lateral nose, lateral upper lip, and cheek, the upper cervical and cheek areas can provide ample amounts of well vascularized tissue for reconstruction. A variety of flap designs has been described in these areas and is primarily discussed in terms of the location or mode of transfer of donor tissue. Four basic designs are described below:

V-to-Y island pedicle advancement flap
Subcutaneously based V-to-Y flaps are most commonly used for soft tissue replacement of the lower lateral nasal side wall, but they may also be used to repair small and deep skin defects of the ala.[75,76]

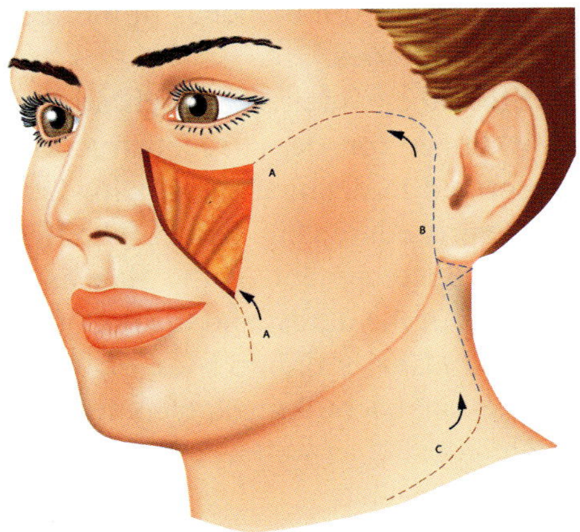

Fig. 33a-c. Schematic example of the use of a cheek advancement flap (*a*), which can be extended to a cheek rotation flap (*b*), and a cervicofacial flap (*c*). For larger wounds of the lateral nose, lateral upper lip, and cheek, the upper cervical and cheek areas can provide ample amounts of well vascularized tissue for reconstruction.

The flap is incised and freed from the adjacent cheek fat, but it remains attached in the deep plane (Fig. 32a and b). If the pedicle causes excessive fullness adjacent to the ala, a secondary procedure to contour this region is planned two to three months after the flap transfer.

Cheek advancement flap
The cheek advancement flap is used for closure of defects involving the lateral nose and adjacent cheek. Elevation of this flap should be performed in the mid-subcutaneous plane as far laterally as is needed to advance the flap to fill the nasal and/or cheek wound. The superior limb of this flap should be placed at the lower orbital rim or in a natural lower eyelid crease and carried to a more superior location at the lateral canthus in order to avoid postoperative ectropion. The inferior limb is usually

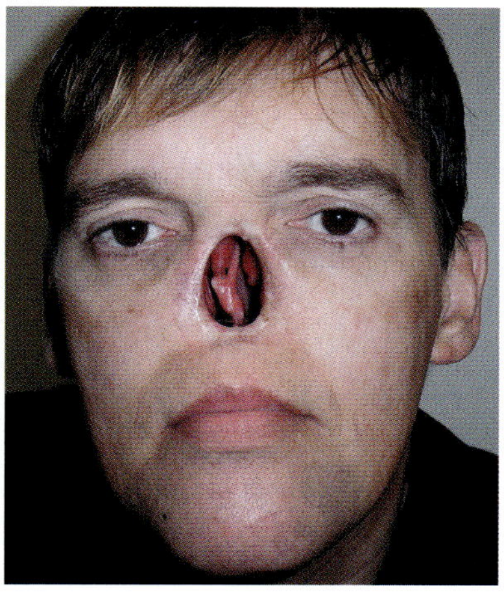
a

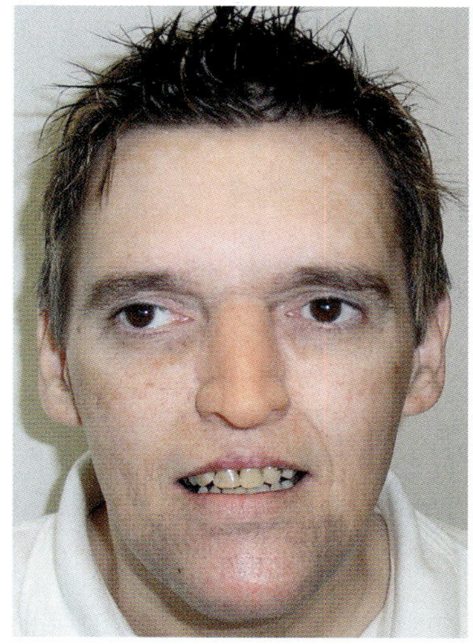
b

Fig. 34a,b. Young male patient after total nasal amputation because of a recurrent SCC (*a*). Situation after reconstruction with a silicone prosthesis (*b*).

placed in the nasolabial cheek fold (Fig. 33).[55,77]

Cheek rotation flap

The cheek advancement-rotation flap has been proven to be useful in the repair of larger and more complex cheek defects of the lateral nose, cheek, and lateral upper lip. This flap is extremely vital and its scars can be well concealed, especially in elderly patients. The design follows the classic outline of Mustardé's flap (Fig. 33). If the superior edge of the flap is located in the area of the infraorbital rim, the posterior extension of this limb must be carried a little higher to the level of the lateral canthus, and then back and anterior to the ear. After incision of the superficial musculoaponeurotic system (SMAS), undermining is continued below the plane of the SMAS level, above the facial nerve branches. In its superior location, it is imperative to secure the dermis of the flap to the periosteum of the lateral orbital rim in order to avoid postoperative ectropion. Incising back along the base of the flap or removing a Burow's triangle of skin along the outer side of the donor site helps to distribute the lines of closure equally.

Cervicofacial flap

This rotation-advancement flap is basically an extension of the inferiorly based cheek rotation flap into the neck in order to obtain additional cervical skin to increase the size of the wound that can be closed (Fig. 33).[55] Defects of as large as 6 x 10 cm can be closed in one stage with this flap. Cervicofacial flaps are random in that they rely entirely on the circulation of the subdermal plexus coming from the branches of the facial vessels. The blood supply and reliability can be significantly improved by dissecting the flap in the deep plane (*i.e.*, below the superficial musculoaponeurotic system). In the cervical region, undermining is performed beneath the platysma, which is transected transversely in the lower cervical region to allow good upward mobility and satisfactory transposition of the flap.[77] The cervicofacial flap offers excellent exposure for concomitant dissection of the parotid gland and cervical lymph node chains if skin cancer has metastasized to the parotid gland or neck.

Near-total nasal reconstruction

A description of the reconstructive techniques used in patients with near-total nasal amputation is beyond the scope of this chapter. In these cases, prosthetic rehabilitation using osseo-integrated implants should be borne in mind as an excellent alternative (Fig. 34a and b).

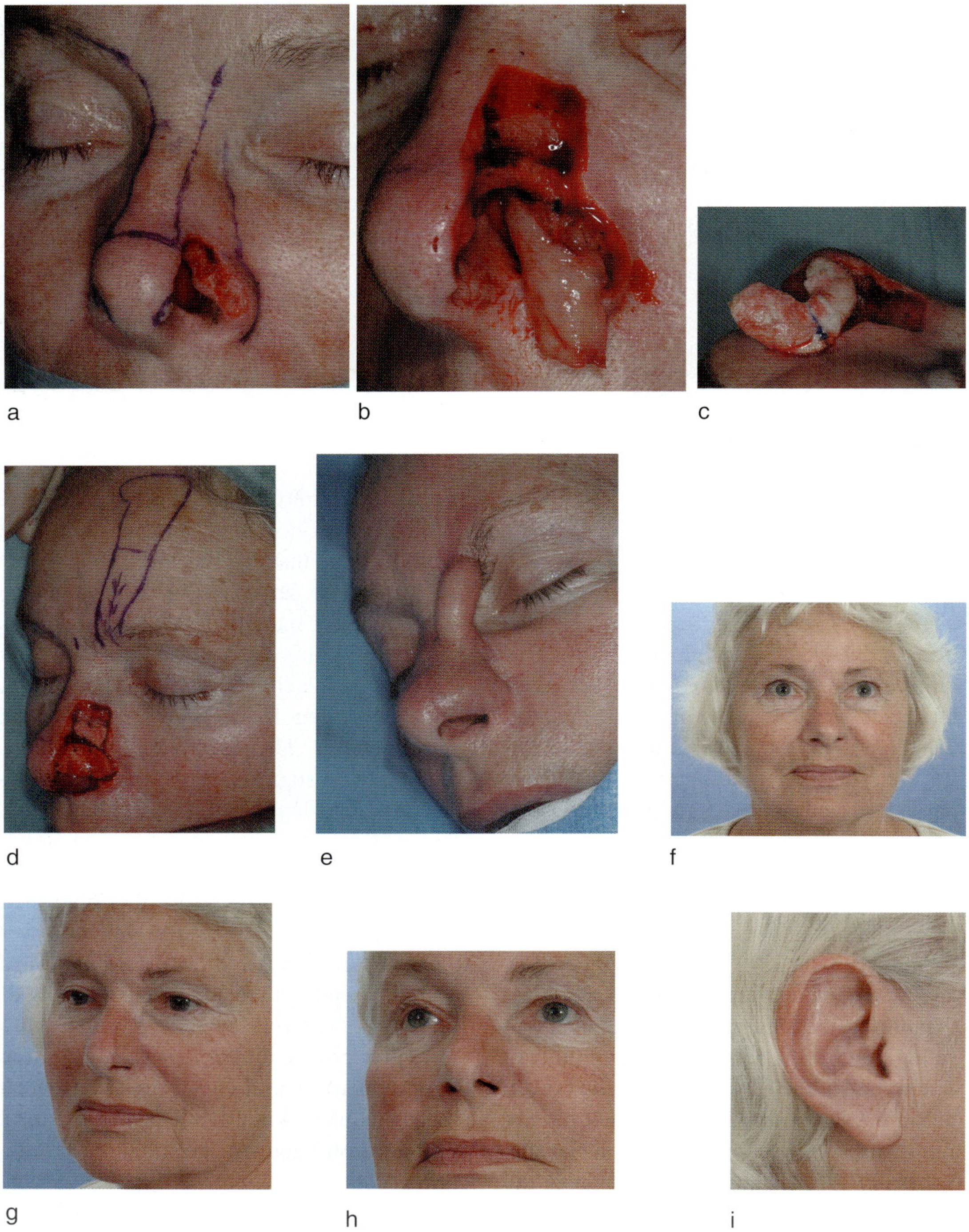

Fig. 35a-i. Patient with a full thickness defect of the nasal ala after removal of an infiltrating BCC (*a*). A caudally based ipsilateral septal mucoperichondrial hinge flap was used for the inner lining (*b*). Contralateral auricular cartilage is used as a graft to restore contour and to avoid retraction of the alar rim (*c,d*). Flap in place, situation after three weeks (*e*). Postoperative result after three months. Some extra contouring of the alar groove may still be required (*f-h*). The position and shape of the donor auricle from which conchal cartilage was grafted remains unchanged (*i*).

Nasal lining

The importance of ensuring adequate osseo-cartilaginous support and internal nasal lining cannot be overemphasized. It can prevent scar formation and retractions resulting in a deformity worse than the one to be concealed.[78] Reconstruction of a full-thickness defect should thus involve three-layers: the outer lining, nasal skeleton, and inner lining (Fig. 35a-i). Cartilage grafting to reconstruct the nasal skeleton is essential in preventing retraction of the alar margin, in order to avoid collapse of the nasal valve,

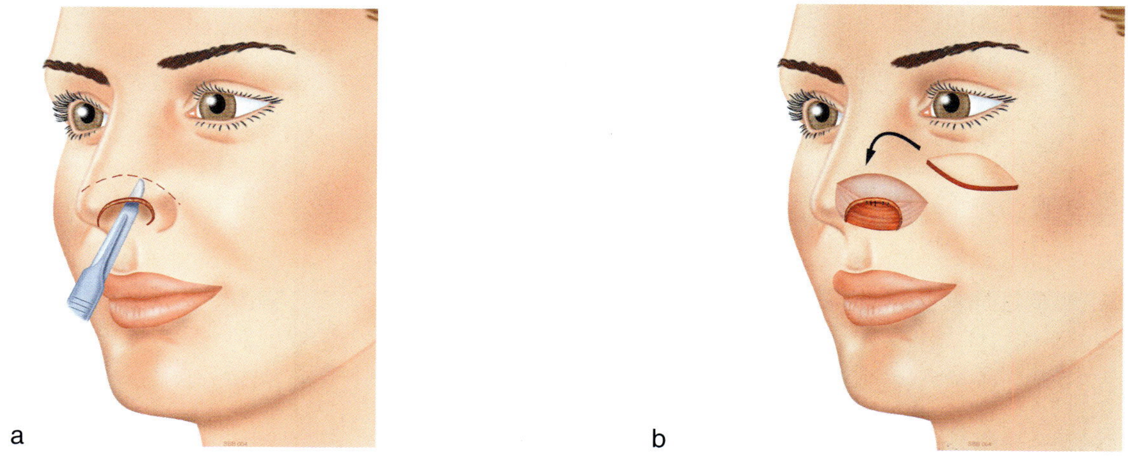

Fig. 36a,b. The bi-pedicled vestibular skin advancement flap is a flap of residual vestibular skin based medially on the nasal septum and laterally on the nasal floor.

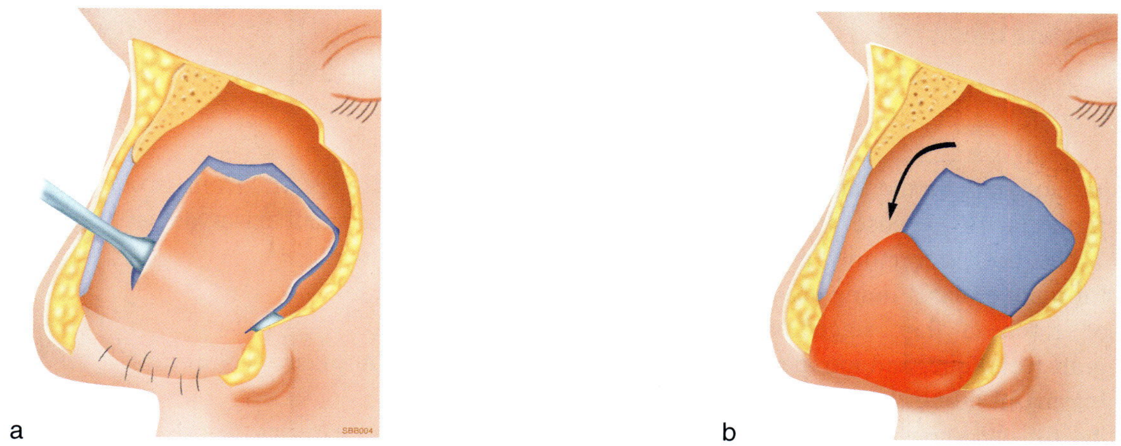

Fig. 37a,b. The septomucoperichondrial hinge flap is based on a 1.5-2-cm pedicle located in the area of the nasal spine and supplied by the ipsilateral septal branch of the superior labial artery.

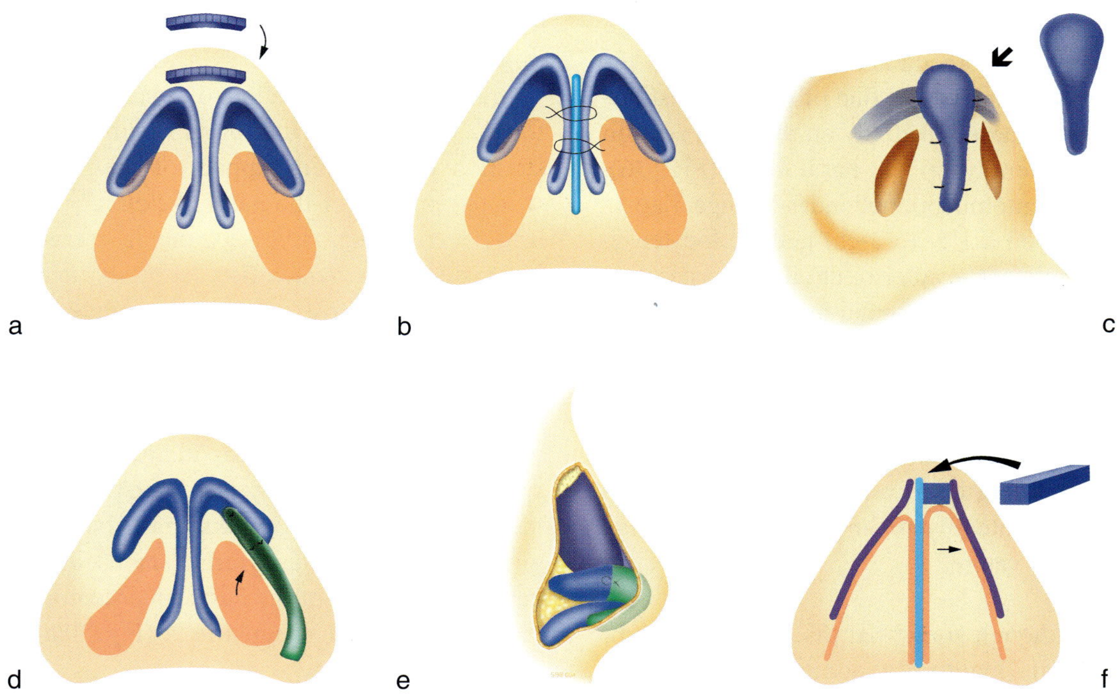

Fig. 38a-f. Grafts play an essential role in nasal reconstruction since they form the basis to provide sufficient strength for maintaining support of the underlying bony-cartilaginous nasal skeleton. Onlay graft (*a*), columellar strut (*b*), shield graft (*c*), alar batten graft (*d*), contour/rim graft from conchal cartilage (*e*), spreader graft (*f*).

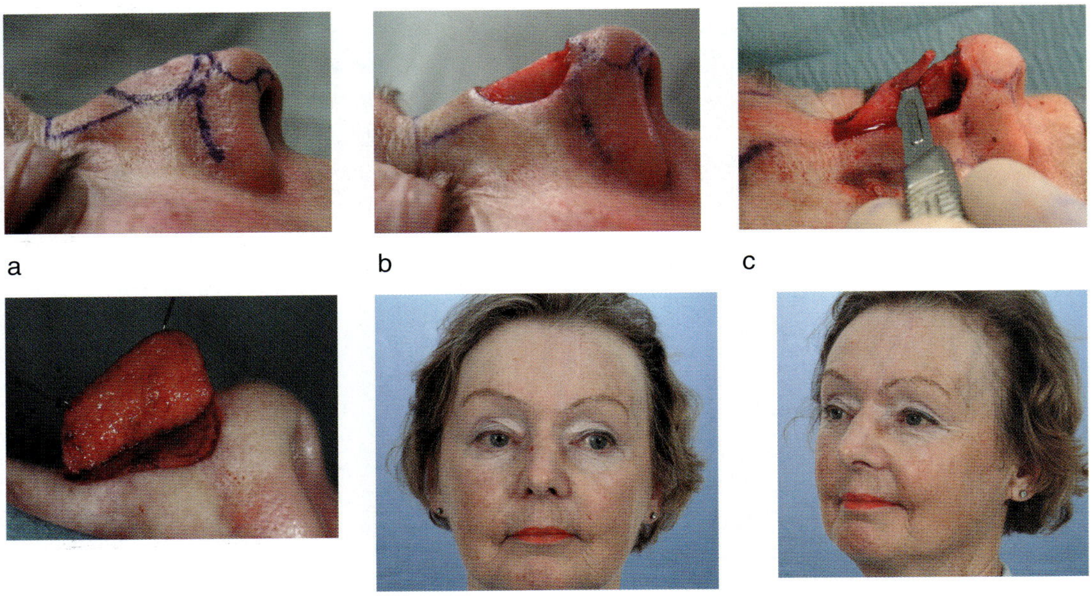

a b c d e f

Fig. 39a-f. Patient after a wide excision of a superficial spreading melanoma with an underlying cartilaginous hump (*a,b*), which was resected (*c*). Third-phase contouring by defatting of the transplanted forehead skin after four weeks (*d*). Final result (*e,f*) after three months (Same patient as in Fig. 13).

and to maintain the three-dimensional configuration of the nose (Fig. 35c and d).[79]

The most commonly described choices for internal nasal lining are the prefabricated forehead flap, staged sequential skin graft technique, and intranasal lining flaps. Intranasal lining flaps are preferred for lining full-thickness nasal defects and include the bipedicled vestibular skin advancement flap and septal mucoperichondrial hinge flap. The bipedicled vestibular skin advancement flap is a flap of residual vestibular skin based medially on the nasal septum and laterally on the nasal floor (Fig. 36). The septomucoperichondrial hinge flap is based on a 1.5- to 2-cm pedicle located in the area of the anterior nasal spine, supplied by the ipsilateral septal branch of the superior labial artery (Fig. 35b and 37a and b). For larger defects, a contralateral septomucoperichondrium flap, based on the dorsum of the septum and supplied by the anterior ethmoid artery, can also be used. It is hinged laterally to line the side walls and middle vault.[80]

Although somewhat thick, stiff, and limited in length, in some cases adjacent turnover flaps based on a scar (secondary granulation/skin graft) from around the periphery of a small nasal defect can be very useful as well.[80,81]

Adjuvant rhinoplasty techniques

In addition to external nasal lining, the nasal skeleton can be entirely recreated using technical experience gained from rhinoplasty surgery.

Grafts play an essential role, since they form a basis on which to provide sufficient strength to maintain support of the constructed portion of the nasal skeleton.[82] In nasal reconstruction, grafts mainly serve three functions: restoration, support, and contour. Restorative grafts replace defects of the nasal skeleton and may be constructed of bone or cartilage, depending on the missing framework. Support grafts (columellar strut, lateral alar batten graft, spreader grafts) provide reinforcement to the existing skeleton. Contour grafts (shield graft, cap graft, onlay grafts) are used to enhance the shape of the nasal tip or to correct topographical irregularities (Fig. 38a-f).[43]

Auricular cartilage grafts are mostly used

to replace missing segments of alar cartilages and to support the ala. A columellar strut is fashioned from septal cartilage to provide structural support to the central tip and columella. By changing the angle of its placement in the inferior columella, the strut can also be used to augment the nasolabial angle or to increase columellar prominence. Lateral alar batten from septal or auricular cartilage produces slight lateral flaring of the alar cartilage in the region of the internal and external nasal valves, increasing the nasal aperture. Spreader grafts are used to lateralize upper lateral cartilage and to increase the aperture of the internal nasal valve. Shield grafts of septal or auricular cartilage are used to enhance tip definition, projection, and rotation. However, adjusting the amount of replaced nasal dorsal skin can also influence tip rotation. A cap graft of cartilage is used in single or double layers to enhance tip definition, projection, and rotation. Septal or auricular cartilage is also used to correct areas of contour depression on the surface of the nose.

Other modifications of the nasal skeleton include tip sutures to narrow the domes, hump resection to lower the nasal dorsum, and osteotomies to medialize the bony side walls. Second- or third-phase contouring procedures, which involve sculpting the subcutaneous tissues of the covering flap, are usually necessary and can be performed under local anesthesia (Fig. 39a-f).

Despite efforts to assemble a delicate nostril, the resultant ala may also be too thick. Secondary defatting is then best carried out by means of rim incisions. When the defect extends cephalically to the alar groove, a specific contouring procedure is necessary to create a new alar groove, which is often obliterated by the base of the reconstructive flap. A template of the contralateral normal ala is made, reversed, placed over the reconstructed ala, and carefully traced with a marking pen.[43] Excision of soft tissue and cartilage is performed by accessing the upper cephalic incision of the flap or by creating a new incision in the flap along the superior border of the tracing. Dermabrasion of the incisional scars may help to smooth out any minor discrepancies in contour and texture. The thick skin of the nose and face lends itself well to dermabrasion.

Postoperative care

Written instructions for the postoperative care of the wound should be provided to the patient and must be specific for each procedure. In general, after 24 hours, the patients can remove their dressings and take a shower. Any crusts should be gently removed. Subsequently, suture lines should be cleaned with soap or diluted hydrogen peroxide twice daily, after which a thin layer of antibiotic ointment should be applied to the wound. Bolster dressings for skin grafts should remain in place for approximately four days. In case of an interpolation flap, the pedicle should be kept moist by means of fatty gauze and antibiotic ointment to improve epithelialization.

Follow-up

Patients with a high risk of recurrence or metastatic spread should be followed closely for long periods of time. SCCs, melanomas, and Merkel cell carcinomas have definite metastatic potential. It is important to stress that, unlike many malignancies, melanomas have a tendency to recur many years after the primary tumor has been removed. According to a consensus of the Dutch Melanoma Working Party, a follow-up period of five years is sufficient for patients with a melanoma of > 1-2 mm Breslow thickness (provided there are no histological signs of regression) and of ten years when the Breslow thickness is > 2 mm.[27]

Following treatment of BCC, the patient should be clinically examined for recurrent tumors once every six months for the first two years and then once a year for the following three, according to the Dutch guidelines for the treatment of BCC. Thereafter, the patient should be examined for new primary tumors at yearly intervals by a dermatologist. Prospectively, it has been found that 36% of patients who develop a BCC will develop a second primary within the ensuing five years, usually in the sun-exposed head and neck region.[83] Early diagnosis and treatment of recurrent BCCs or another primary BCC is desirable, since treatment of the disease in its earliest stages results in less patient morbidity.

30: INSTRUMENTS

G.J. Nolst Trenité

Apart from knowledge, skill and experience, the use of appropriate instruments is a prerequisite for performing a reliable operation.

The main goal in modern rhinoplasty is to perform the operation as atraumatically as possible, to prevent unpredictable scar formation and to ensure good long-term postoperative results. The use of delicate, sharp and high quality instruments is fundamental in lessening surgical trauma and entering the right surgical planes, resulting in less bleeding, shorter duration of the operative procedure and, ultimately, better postoperative results.

During my frequent visits to international authorities on rhinoplasty, I noted that they were using delicate rhinoplasty instruments that were not available in the Netherlands. While doing rhinoplasties as a 'guest surgeon', I noticed that an ENT surgeon taking his first steps in aesthetic rhinoplasty will do this with instruments which were readily available for functional rhinoplastic surgery (but not always state-of-the-art). This inspired me to design some specific rhinoplasty instruments

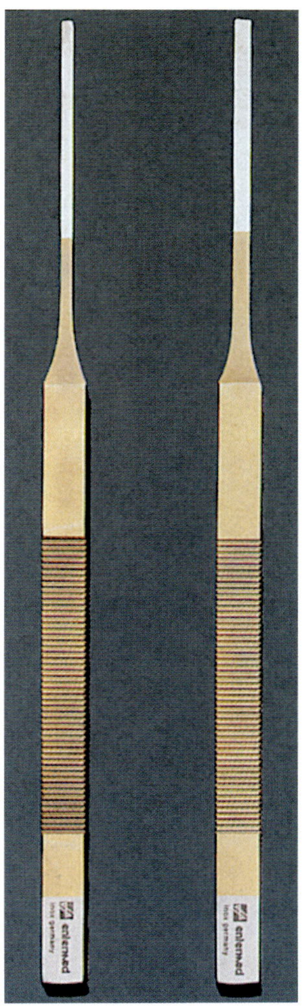

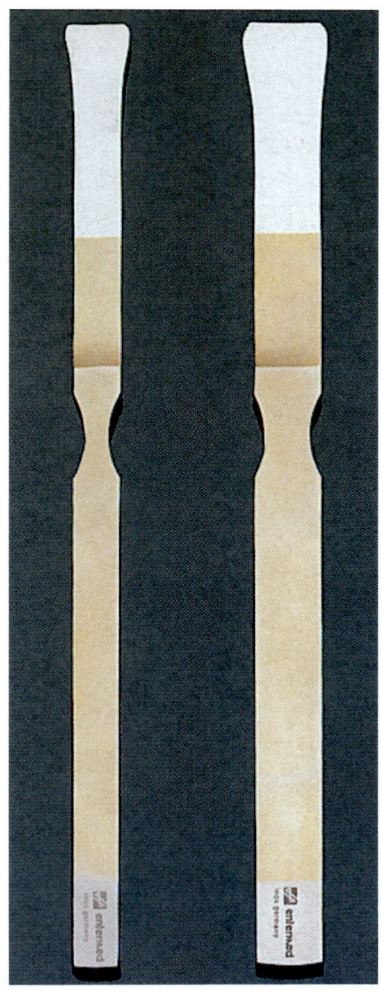

Fig. 1. Micro-osteotomes (2 mm and 3 mm blades).

Fig. 2. Hump osteotomes (10 mm and 14 mm blades).

(Figs. 1–3). This was finally realized with the help of John Vos of Entermed bv, Woerden, the Netherlands, and the instruments were manufactured by Max and Katharina Müller of Explorent GmbH, Tuttlingen, Germany. Combined with specially selected instruments (Figs. 4–7), these form a supplementary rhinoplasty set to be used with instruments already available for functional rhinoplastic surgery. This complete set of very delicate, high quality instruments has a special gold finish for easy recognition on the operating table.

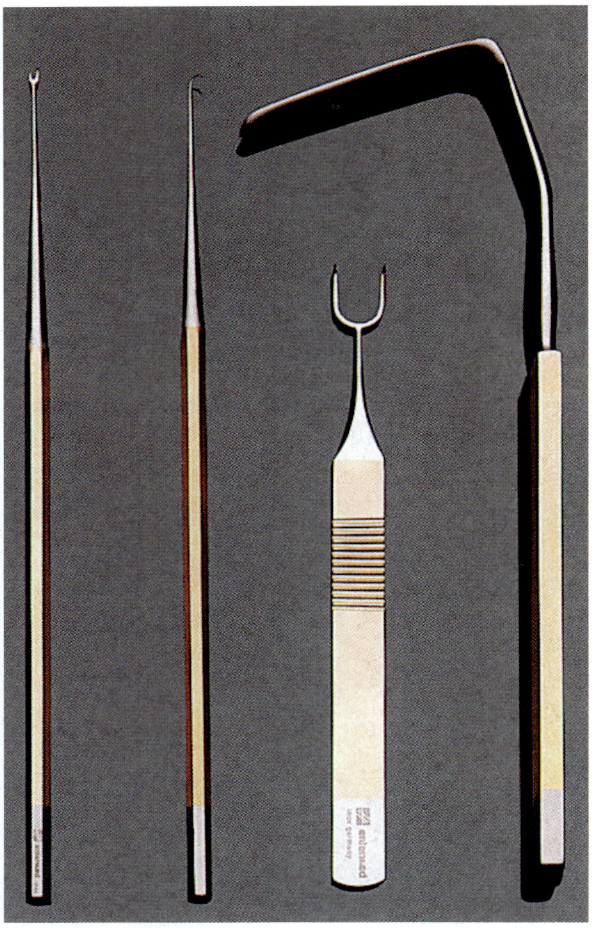

Fig. 3. Skin hooks:
1 prong
2 prong (2 mm)
2 prong (10 mm)
Nasal retractor.

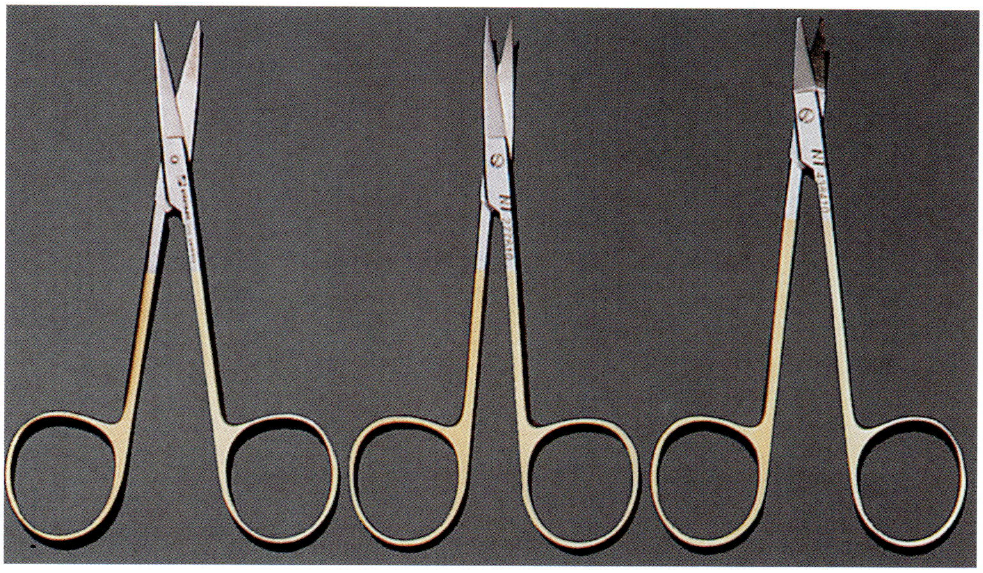

Fig. 4. Rhinoplasty scissors:
straight, sharp (10 cm)
curved, sharp (10 cm)
angled, Walter type (10 cm).

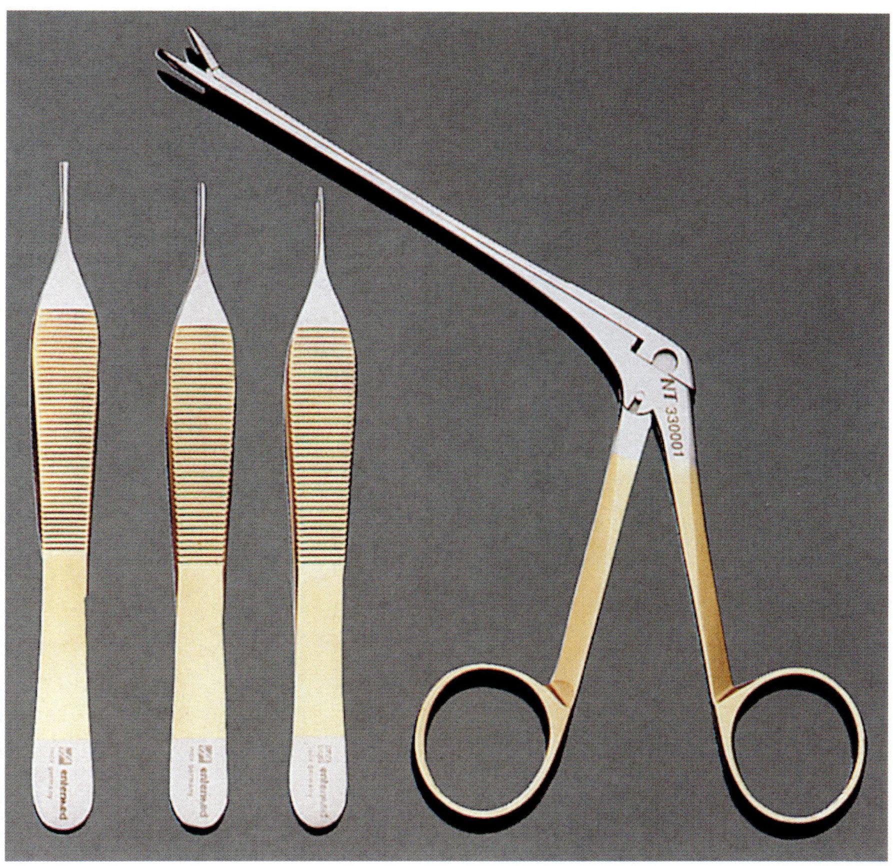

Fig. 5. Tissue forceps with side-grasping teeth, Adson-Brown type (12 cm)
Dressing forceps, Adson type (12 cm)
Tissue forceps, Adson type (12 cm)
Nasal forceps, Blackesley type (small).

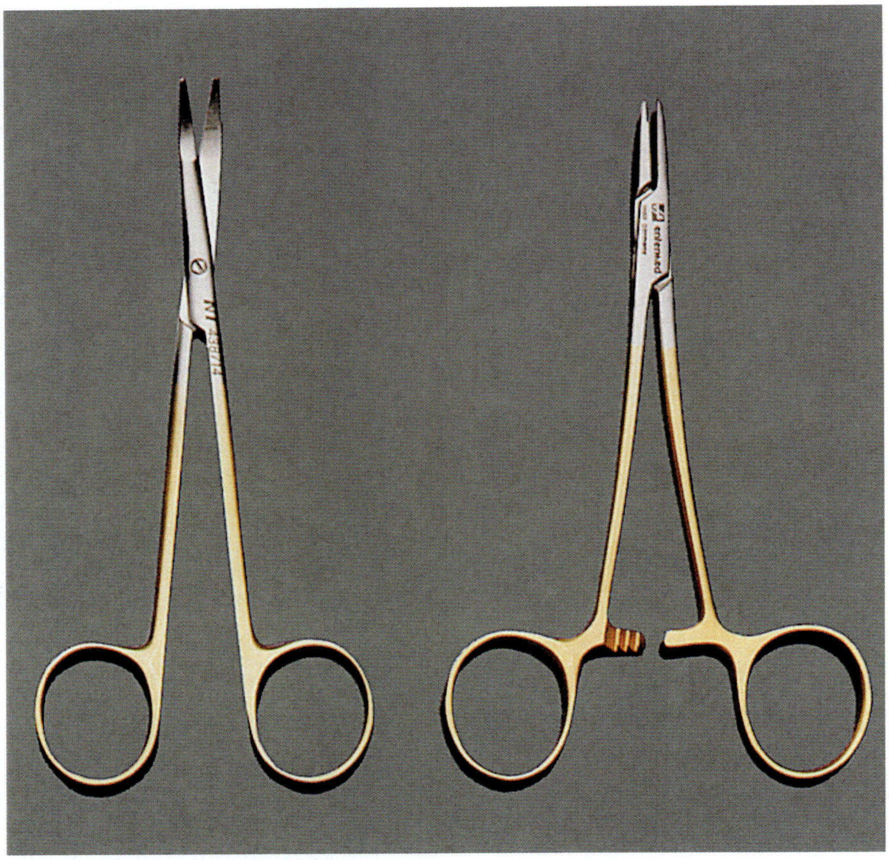

Fig. 6. Dissection scissors, Killner type (14 cm) Needle holder, Halsey type, tungsten carbide inserts (13 cm).

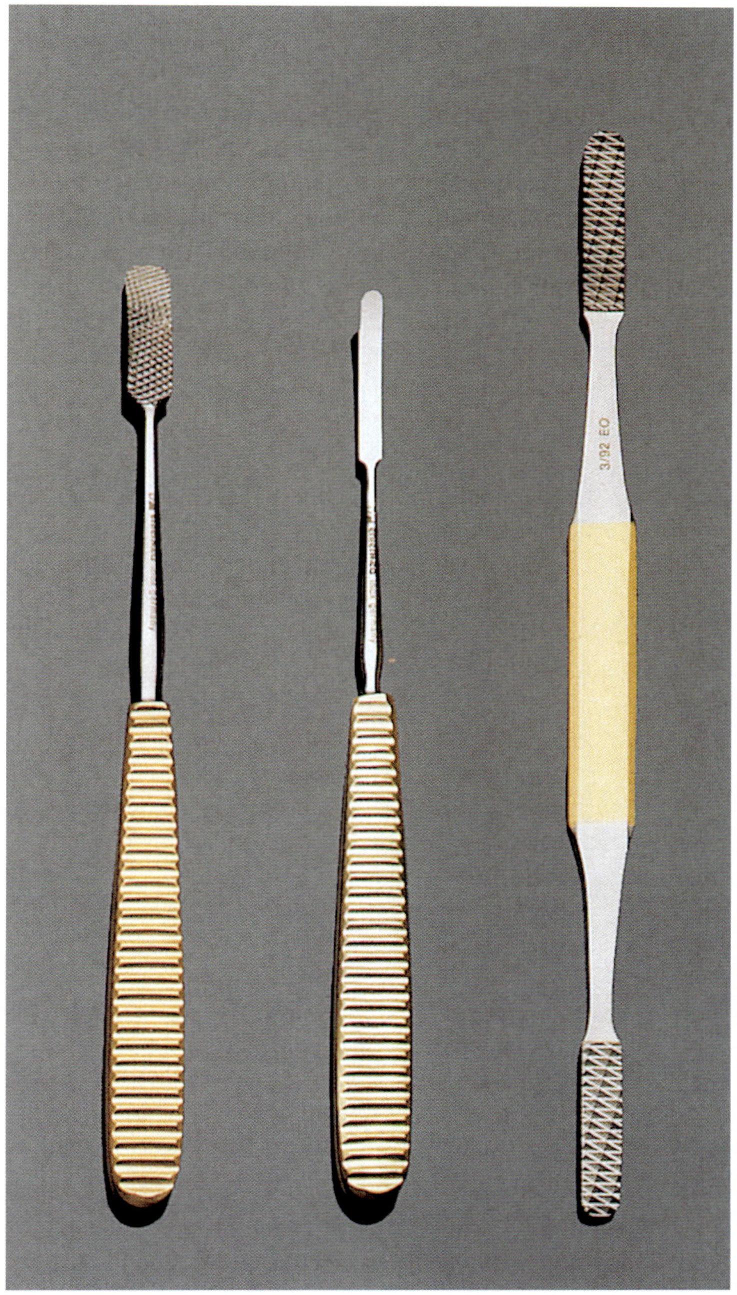

Fig. 7. Glabella rasp
Periosteal elevator, Joseph type (3 mm blade)
Nasal rasp, double blade, tungsten carbide inserts 5/6 (7/8 not shown).

These instruments are available through Entermed bv, Woerden, the Netherlands and Explorent GmbH, Tuttlingen/Germany.

ABOUT THE EDITOR

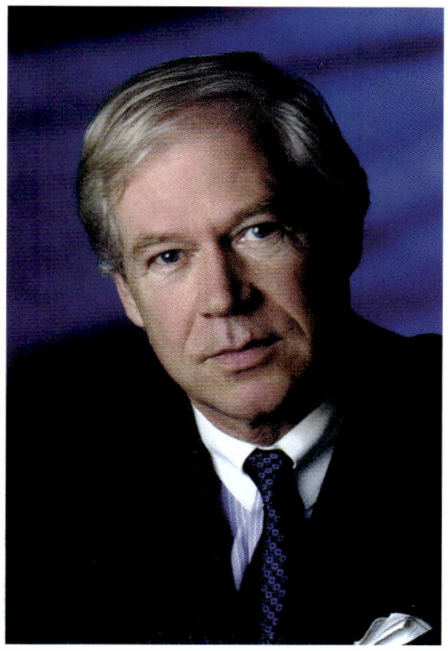

Gilbert Nolst Trenité's special interest in surgery of the nose started during his ENT residency, when he was carrying out experimental work on implants in a growing nasal septum. His frequent visits abroad to experts on rhinoplasty (Bull, Mackay, Masing, Tardy, Walter, etc.) greatly stimulated him to improve his knowledge and technique. As vice president of the Dutch ENT society, he was one of the initiators of *Rhinoplasty, a practical guide to functional and aesthetic surgery of the nose*. The enlarged second edition was a world first with an active CD ROM containing live surgery video clips. Enlarged even more, the third edition is combined with an interactive DVD ROM, containing more than four hours of live surgery.

In his enthusiasm for facial plastic surgery, and in particular for rhinoplasty, Nolst Trenité has given many lectures and live surgery demonstrations on this subject all over the world, and has designed various specific instruments for rhinoplasty, including a custom-made vestibulum device.

As former head of the Rotterdam cleft palate center, he became deeply involved in the highly challenging secondary rhinoplasty for cleft-lip patients. Since the early 1990s, he has been one of the Dutch vice presidents of the European Academy of Facial Plastic Surgery, and he also joined the editorial board of Facial Plastic Surgery International Quarterly Monographs. He has worked in private practice as an ENT surgeon for nearly thirteen years.

Since 1994 he has been second-in-command of and associate professor at the ENT Department of the Academic Medical Center, the University Hospital of the University of Amsterdam (former head Professor P.F. Schouwenburg, present head Professor Wytske Fokkens). Moreover, he is consultant surgeon for facial plastic surgery at Professor Amiri's clinic in Bad Wiessee, Germany.

He established the annual International Course on Modern Rhinoplasty Techniques in Amsterdam, and started a research group on chondroneogenesis in collagenous matrices with tissue growth factors, as well as a further research project with the Rotterdam cleft palate center on the influence of orthodontic treatment (the Weil method) on facial growth in cleft-lip patients. He also established a mid-European course at the University of Pécs, (director, Professor Joseph Pytel) in Hungary, for which he received the Gold Medal from the University, and was appointed guest professor. Moreover, he initiated a 'promising' research project in cartilage healing in the growing septum at Pécs and became honorary member of the Hungarian ENT Society. He has also been appointed guest professor at the University of Ghent, Belgium (head of the ENT Department, Professor Van Couwenberge). He is an honorary member of the South African ENT Society, was an honorary visiting professor at the Rhinofest at the Mayo Clinics in the USA in 2003 and, in 2004, became honorary member of the Polish Rhinologic Society.

Professor Nolst Trenité is president of the European Academy of Facial Plastic Surgery. For many years, he represented the Dutch ENT Society at the Union Européenne Médicins Spécialistes (UEMS) and he is president of the international Lazarus Leprosy Society, through which he has become involved in facial rehabilitation surgery in leprosy patients. He is also president of the board of the Rotterdam cleft palate center. As a member of the executive board of the International Federation of Facial Plastic Surgery Society (in 2004 he became vice president), he developed an international certification process for use in facial plastic surgery, in collaboration with Dr Roxana Cobo from Colombia. He is one of the editors in chief of *Facial Plastic Surgery Monographs* (Thieme, New York, Stuttgart) and a member of the editorial board of *Archives of Facial Plastic Surgery* (AMA Journal). He has also contributed to many international textbooks and peer-reviewed medical journals.

ACKNOWLEDGEMENTS

I would like to extend my grateful thanks to all those who helped make the third enlarged edition of *Rhinoplasty, a Practical Guide to Functional and Aesthetic Surgery of the Nose* with interactive DVD possible. Special thanks go to the following people:

- To all the contributors for their enthusiastic cooperation in the preparation of their manuscripts, which have given this book such special dimensions;
- To Eugene Tardy for his willingness to review the first, second, and third editions, and for this encouraging and positive foreword;
- To Jan Keet, Cor de Ruyter, Cees Hersbach, and my son Gilean (third year medical student) for their high quality photography;
- To Bas Blankenvoort for his expert and beautiful illustrations;
- To the late Willem van Asperen, Tineke Wierenga, and the video crew for filming and editing the live surgery videos;
- To Yvonne Steenvoorden-Wijnveld, Els Tjong Joe Wai (my former secretary) and Margalith van Huiden-ten Brink (my present secretary) for their efficient help and for typing the manuscript;
- To Werner Degger, Gerard van Groningen, Bob van Gijzel, and Jaap Tuyp at the Audio Visual Center of the Academic Medical Center for their excellent developmental work on the Rhinoplasty DVD;
- To Peter Bakker and his son Simon at Kugler Publications for their efforts in bringing the manuscripts into line, and for liaising the entire production process;
- To my wife Bregtje and our children Sanne, Tessa, and Gilean for their unfailing support.

Gilbert J. Nolst Trenité

LITERATURE

Chapter 1

1. Bosma JF: Anatomy of the Infant Head. Johns Hopkins University Press, Baltimore, MD 1986
2. Dehneke HJ, Meyer R: Plastic Surgery of Head and Neck: Corrective and Reconstructive Rhinoplasty, Vol I. New York, NY: Springer Verlag 1967
3. Hafferl A: Lehrbuch der topografischen Anatomie. Dritte Auflage. Berlin: Springer Verlag 1969
4. Lam SM, Williams EF: Anatomic considerations in aesthetic rhinoplasty. Facial Plast Surg 14(4):209, 2002
5. Lang J: Klinische Anatomie der Nase, Nasenhöhle und Nebenhöhlen. Stuttgart: George Thieme Verlag 1988
6. Papel ID: Anatomy and physiology of the skin. In: Papel ID et al (eds): Facial Plastic and Reconstructive Surgery, 2nd Edn, pp 3-14. New York, NY: Thieme Medical Publishers Inc 2002
7. Perkins SW: Anatomy and physiology. In: Krause ChJ (ed): Aesthetic Facial Surgery. Philadelphia, PA: Lippincott Company 1991
8. Poublon RML: The cartilaginous nasal dorsum and the postnatal growth of the nose. Thesis, Rotterdam 1987
9. Straatsma BR, Straatsma CR: The anatomical relationship of the lateral nasal cartilage to the nasal bone and the cartilaginous nasal septum. Plast Reconstr Surg 8:443-455, 1951
10. Tardy ME: Misadventures in nasal tip surgery. Otolaryngol Clin N Am 20(4):797-823, 1987
11. Tardy ME: Surgical Anatomy of the Nose. New York, NY: Raven Press 1990
12. Tardy ME: Practical surgical anatomy. In: Tardy ME (ed): Rhinoplasty, the Art and the Science, Vol 1, pp 2-125. Philadelphia, PA: WB Saunders Co 1997

Chapter 2

1. Anderson JR, Ries WR: Rhinoplasty: Emphasizing the External Approach, pp 34-110. New York, NY: Thieme Inc 1986
2. Becker OJ: Rhinoplasty: cultural, esthetic and psychological aspects. Chicago Med 64:230-235, 1961
3. Bernstein L: Esthetics in rhinoplasty. Otolaryngol Clin N Am 8:705-715, 1975
4. Denecke HJ, Meyer R: Plastic Surgery of the Head and Neck. New York, NY: Springer Verlag 1967
5. Goode RL: Personal communication 1983
6. Krugman ME: Photoanalysis of the rhinoplasty patient. J Ear Nose Throat 60:56-59, 1981
7. Papel ID: Aesthetic facial analysis. In: Papel ID et al (eds): Facial Plastic and Reconstructive Surgery, 2nd Edn, pp 135-144. New York, NY: Thieme Medical Publishers Inc 2002
8. Peck H, Peck S: A concept of facial esthetic angles. Orthod 40:284-317, 1970
9. Powell N, Humphreys B: Proportions of the Aesthetic Face. New York, NY: Thieme-Stratton Inc 1984
10. Ricketts RM: Divine proportions in facial aesthetics. Clin Plast Surg 9:401-422, 1982

11. Sheen JH: Aesthetic Rhinoplasty, Vol 1, pp 68-127. St Louis, MO: CV Mosby Co 1987
12. Tardy ME: Practical surgical anatomy. In: Tardy ME (ed): Rhinoplasty, the Art and the Science, Vol 1, pp 8-36. Philadelphia, PA: WB Saunders Co 1997

Chapter 3

1. Anderson J: On the selection of patients for rhinoplasty. Otolaryngol Clin N Am 8:685, 1960
2. Berman WE: Rhinoplastic Surgery, p 156. St Louis, MO: CV Mosby Co 1989
3. Gorney M: Patient selection criteria: an ounce of prevention. In: Kaye BL, Gradinger GP (eds): Symposium on problems and complications in aesthetic plastic surgery of the face, Vol 23, ASPRS. St Louis, MO: CV Mosby Co 1984
4. Heinberg CE, Kern EB: The Cottle sign: an aid in the physical diagnosis of nasal airflow disturbance. Int Rhinol 11:89-94, 1973
5. Janeke JB, Wright WK: Studies on the support of the nasal tip. Arch Otolaryngol 93:458, 1971
6. Micheli-Pellegrini V, Manfrida GM: Rhinoplasty and its psychological implications: applied psychology observations in aesthetic surgery. Aesthetic Plast Surg 3:229, 1979
7. Papel ID: Computer imaging for facial plastic surgery. In: Papel ID et al (eds): Facial Plastic and Reconstructive Surgery, 2nd Edn, pp 110-115. New York, NY: Thieme Medical Publishers Inc 2002
8. Papel ID: Photography in facial plastic surgery. In: Papel ID et al (eds): Facial Plastic and Reconstructive Surgery, 2nd Edn, pp 116-124. New York, NY: Thieme Medical Publishers Inc 2002
9. Rees TD: Aesthetic Plastic Surgery, Vol I, p 99. Philadelphia, PA: WB Saunders Co 1980
10. Sheen JH: Aesthetic Rhinoplasty, Vol I, p 131. St Louis, MO: CV Mosby Co 1987
11. Tardy ME: Rhinoplasty in Otolaryngology – Head and Neck Surgery, p 699. St Louis, MO: CV Mosby Co 1986
12. Tardy ME: Principles of photography in facial plastic surgery. New York, NY: Thieme-Stratton, 1992

Chapter 4

1. Cook WW, Johnson CM, Quatela VC, Torinmi DM: Anaesthesia. In: Open Reconstructive Rhinoplasty, p 33. Philadelphia, PA: WB Saunders Co 1990
2. De Jong RH: Toxicity of local anaesthetics. Reg Anaesth 8, 1977
3. Kattz RM, Matteo RS, Papper EM: Injection of epinephrine during general anesthesia with halogenated hydrocarbons and by cyclopropane in man. Anaesthesiology 23:597, 1962
4. Lynch S: Anaesthesia. In: Aesthetic Plastic Surgery, Vol I, p 40. Philadelphia, PA: WB Saunders Co 1980
5. Papel ID: Anesthesia in facial plastic surgery. In: Papel ID et al (eds): Facial Plastic and Reconstructive Surgery, 2nd Edn, pp 145-152. New York, NY: Thieme Medical Publishers Inc 2002
6. Perlow M: Anaesthesia for facial plastic surgery. In: Facial Plastic and Reconstructive Surgery, p 24. St Louis, MO: CV Mosby Co 1992
7. Schmidt KF: Evaluation of candidates for outpatient anaesthesia and surgery. Int Anaesthesiol Clin 14:9, 1976
8. Tom L, Tardy ME: Anaesthesia in rhinoplasty. Facial Plast Surg 1:2, 1984

Chapter 5

1. Beekhuis GJ: Nasal obstruction after rhinoplasty: etiology and techniques for correction. Laryngoscope 86:540, 1976
2. Bull TR: Stigmata of rhinoplasty. In: Bernstein L (ed): Plastic and Reconstructive Surgery, Vol 1, p 66. Aesth Surg 1981
3. Fairbanks DNF, Fairbanks GR: Nasal septal perforation: prevention and management. Ann Plast Surg 5:452, 1980
4. Huizing EH: The management of septal abscesses. Facial Plast Surg 3:4, 1986
5. Huizing EH: Long term results of reconstruction of the septum in the acute phase of a septal abscess in children. Rhinology 22:55, 1984
6. Masing H: Zur plastisch-operativen Versorgung von Septumhämatomen und Abscessen. HNO Wegweiser 13:235, 1965
7. Nolst Trenité GJ, Verwoerd CDA, Verwoerd-Verhoef HL: The influence of resection and reimplantation of septal cartilage upon nasal growth: an experimental study in rabbits. Rhinoplasty 25:225, 1987
8. Nolst Trenité GJ: Revision Surgery. Abstractbook Basic and Advanced Course in Modern Rhinoplasty Techniques. Amsterdam 1995
9. Reiter D, Alfor E, Jabourian Z: Alternatives to packing in septorhinoplasty. Arch Otolaryngol Head Neck Surg 115:1203, 1989
10. Rettinger G, Masing H, Heinl W: Surgical closure of septal perforations with a septal mucosa rotation flap. HNO 34:461, 1986
11. Sclafani AP, Romo T 3rd, Barnett JG, Barnett CR: Adjustment of subtle postoperative nasal defects: managing the 'near-miss' rhinoplasty. Facial Plast Surg 19(4):349-361, 2003
12. Tardy ME: Rhinoplasty tip ptosis: etiology and prevention. Laryngoscope 83:923, 1973
13. Thomas JR, Tardy ME: Complications of rhinoplasty. In: Complications of Head and Neck Surgery. Philadelphia, PA: BC Decker, 1986
14. Walter C: Komplikationen bei rhinoplastischen Eingriffen. In: Handbuch der plastische Chirurgie, Bd II. Beitrag p 34. Berlin: Walter de Gruyter 1966
15. Webster RC: Revisional rhinoplasty. Otolaryngol Clin N Am 8:753, 1975

Chapter 6

1. Bönisch M, Mink A: Septum reconstruction with PDS implant. HNO 47(6):546-550, 1999 (in German)
2. Cottle MH: Nasal surgery in children: effect of early nasal injury. EENT Monthly 30:32, 1951
3. Cottle MH, Loring RM, Fischer GC, Gaynon IE: The maxilla-premaxilla approach to extensive nasal septum surgery. Arch Otolaryngol 68:303, 1958
4. Courtiss EH, Goldwyn RM: Resection of obstructing inferior turbinates: a 6-year follow-up. Plast Reconstr Surg 72:913, 1983
5. Fry HJH: Interlocked stress in human septal cartilage. Br J Plast Surg 18:276, 1966
6. Hinderer KH: Fundamentals of Anatomy and Surgery of the Nose. Birmingham, AL: Aesculapius Publ Co 1971
7. Jeppesen F: Septo- and Rhinoplasty: a Step-by-Step Instruction. Copenhagen: Munksgaard 1986
8. Kilian G: The submucous window resection of the nasal septum. Ann Otol Rhinol Laryngol 14:363, 1905
9. Murakami W, Wong L, Davidson J: Application of the biomedical behaviour of cartilage to nasal septoplastic surgery. Laryngoscope 92:300, 1982

10. Van Delden MR, Cook PR, Davis WE: Endoscopic partial inferior turbinoplasty. Otolaryngol Head Neck Surg 121(4):406-409, 1999

Chapter 7

1. Becker DG, Becker SS, Saad AA: Auricular cartilage in revision rhinoplasty. Facial Plast Surg 19(1):41-52, 2003
2. Bönisch M, Mink A: Healing process of cartilage attached to a polydioxanone implant. HNO 48(10):745-746, 2000 (in German)
3. Escobar Sanz-Dranguet P, Marquez Dorsch F, Villacampa Auba JM, Sanabria Brassart J, Gutierrez Fonseca R, Pastormerlo Botegia G, Cenjor Espanol C: Cartilaginous grafts in rhinoplasty. Acta Otorrinolaringol Esp 53(10):736-740, 2002 (in Spanish)
4. Gurley JM, Pilgram T, Perlyn CA, Marsh JL: Long-term outcome of autogenous rib graft nasal reconstruction. Plast Reconstr Surg 108(7):1895-1905, 2001
5. Helder AH, Huizing EH: Transplantation terminology in nasal surgery. Rhinology 24:235, 1986
6. Hellmich S: Nasal grafts. Proceedings Int Meet Joseph Soc London. Birmingham: R Evans 1981
7. Hellmich S: Cartilage implants in rhinoplasty – problems and prospects. Rhinology 10:1, 1972
8. Huizing EH: Implantation and transplantation in reconstructive nasal surgery. Rhinology 12:106, 1974
9. Kamer FM, Churukian MM: Shield graft for the nasal tip. Arch Otolaryngol 110:608, 1984
10. Kim YO, Park BY, Lee WJ: Aesthetic reconstruction of the nasal tip using a folded composite graft from the ear. Br J Plast Surg 57(3):238-244, 2004
11. Micheli-Pellegrini V: Passato, presente e futuro dei materiali alloplastici in chirurgia estetica. Minerva Chir 38:871, 1983
12. Millard DR: Congenital nasal tip retrusion and three little composite ear grafts. Case report. Plast Reconstr Surg 48:501, 1972
13. Nolst Trenité GJ: Cartilage autografts in nasal surgery. FACE 1:1-7, 1994
14. Nolst Trenité GJ: Autogenous grafts in rhinoplastic surgery. Russian Rhinol 1:26-33, 1996
15. Ortiz-Monasterio F, Olmedo A, Ortiz-Oscoy L: The use of cartilage grafts in primary aesthetic rhinoplasty. Plast Reconstr Surg 67:597, 1981
16. Peck GC: The onlay graft for nasal tip projection. Plast Reconstr Surg 71:27, 1983
17. Tardy ME, Denneny JC, Fritsch MH: The versatile cartilage autograft in reconstruction of the nose and face. Laryngoscope 95(5):523, 1985
18. Tardy ME, Schwartz MS, Parras G: Saddle nose deformity: autogenous graft repair. Facial Plast Surg 6:2, 1989
19. Van Lange JW, de Roo K, Middelkoop E, Van den Bos T, Everts V, Nolst Trenité GJ: Perichondrium-wrapped collagenous matrices to induce chondroneogenesis: an in vitro study. Arch Facial Plast Surg 3(2): 22-126, 2001
20. Walter C: Composite grafts in nasal surgery. Arch Otolaryngol 90:6, 1969

Chapter 8

1. Becker DG, Becker SS: Treatment of nasal obstruction from nasal valve collapse with alar batten grafts. J Long Term Eff Med Implants 13(3):259-269, 2003
2. Bull TR, Mackay IS: Alar collapse. Facial Plast Surg 3(4):268, 1986
3. Cinelli JA: Physiologic rhinoplasty principles. In: Maloney WH (ed): Otolaryngology, New York, NY: Harper & Row Publishers Inc 1971

4. Cottle MH: The structure and function of the nasal vestibule. Arch Otolaryngol 62:173, 1955
5. Masing H: Experimentelle Untersuchungen über die Stromung im Nasenmodell. Arch Klin Exp Ohren Nasen Kehlkopfheilkd 189:59, 1967
6. Meyer R: Nasenflügelkollaps. In: Denecke HJ, Meyer R (eds) Korrigierende und rekonstruktive Nasenplastik, p 105. Berlin: Springer Verlag 1964
7. Meyer R, Jovanovic B, Derder S: All about nasal valve collapse. Aesthetic Plast Surg 20(2):141-151, 1996
8. Rettinger G, Masing H: Rotation of the air cartilage in collapsed ala. Int Rhinol 19:81, 1981
9. Rettinger G, Masing H: Behinderte Nasenatmung durch altersbedingte Veränderungen der Flügelknorpel. In: Neubauer H (ed) Plastische und Wiederherstellungschirurgie des Alters. Berlin/Heidelberg: Springer Verlag 1986
10. Toriumi DM, Josen J, Weinberger M, Tardy ME Jr: Use of alar batten grafts for correction of nasal valve collapse. Arch Otolaryngol Head Neck Surg 123(8):802-808, 1997
11. Walter C: Zum Thema: Nasenflügelkollaps. Laryngol Rhinol Otol (Stuttgart) 55:447, 1976
12. De Wit G, Kapteyn TS, Van Bochove W: Some remarks on the physiology, the anatomy and the radiology of the vestibulum and the isthmus nasi. Int Rhinol 3:37, 1965

Chapter 9A

1. Andre RF, Paun SH, Vuyk HD: Endonasal spreader graft placement as treatment for internal nasal valve insufficiency: no need to divide the upper lateral cartilages from the septum. Arch Facial Plast Surg 6(1):36-40, 2004
2. Goode RL: Surgery of the incompetent nasal valve. Laryngoscope 95:546, 1985
3. Haight JSJ, Cole P: The site and function of the nasal valve. Laryngoscope 93:49, 1983
4. Hinderer KH: Surgery of the nasal valve. Int Rhinol 8:60, 1970
5. Kern EB: Surgery of the nasal valve. In: Sisson GA, Tardy ME (eds) Plastic and Reconstructive Surgery of the Face and Neck. Stuttgart: Georg Thieme Verlag 1975
6. McCaffrey TV, Kern EB: Clinical evaluation of nasal obstruction: a study of 1,000 patients. Arch Otolaryngol 105:542, 1979
7. Ozturan O: Techniques for the improvement of the internal nasal valve in functional-cosmetic nasal surgery. Acta Otolaryngol 120(2):312-315, 2000
8. Rohrich RJ, Hollier LH: Use of spreader grafts in the external approach to rhinoplasty. Clin Plast Surg 23(2):256-262, 1996
9. Van Dishoeck HAE: The part of the valve and the turbinates in total nasal resistance. Int Rhinol 3:19, 1965
10. Walter C: Surgical approaches to problems of the nasal valve area and the extra mucosal rhinoplasty. In: Rees ThD (ed): Rhinoplasty, Problems and Controversies. A Discussion with the Experts, Ch. 24, p 204. St Louis, MO: CV Mosby Co 1988

Chapter 9B

1. Adamson PA: Open rhinoplasty. Otolaryngol Clin N Am 20(4):837-852, 1987
2. Converse JM: In: Reconstructive Plastic Surgery, 2nd Edn, p 1086. Philadelphia, PA: WB Saunders Co 1977
3. Courtiss E, Gargan T, Courtiss G: Nasal physiology. Ann Plast Surg 13:214, 1984
4. Goode RL: Surgery of the incompetent nasal valve. Laryngoscope 95:546-555, 1985

5. Johnson CM Jr, Toriumi DM: Open Structure Rhinoplasty, Ch 8, pp 179-205. Philadelphia, PA: WB Saunders Co 1990
6. Kern EB: Surgical approaches to abnormalities of the nasal valve. Laryngoscope 93:49-55, 1983
7. Peck GC: Techniques in Aesthetic Rhinoplasty, p xiii. New York, NY: Thieme-Stratton Inc 1984
8. Sheen JH: Secondary rhinoplasty. Plast Reconstr Surg 56:137, 1975
9. Sheen JH: Aesthetic Rhinoplasty, p 26. St Louis, MO: CV Mosby Co 1978
10. Sheen JH: Spreader graft: A method of reconstruction of the roof of the middle nasal vault following rhinoplasty. Plast Reconstr Surg 73(2):230-237, 1984
11. Sheen JH: In: Rees ThD (ed) Rhinoplasty: Problems and Controversies. A Discussion with the Experts, Ch 19, pp 155-162. St Louis, MO: CV Mosby Co 1988
12. Sulsenti G, Palma P: A new technique for functional surgery of the nasal valve area. Rhinology Suppl no 10, 1989
13. Tardy ME: Surgical Anatomy of the Nose, Ch 4, pp 55-97. New York, NY: Raven Press 1990
14. Vinayak BC, Nolst Trenité GJ: External rhinoplasty. Exploiting the benefits. FACE 5(2):77-92, 1997

Chapter 10

1. Aiach G: External transcolumnellar approach and cartilage grafting: a very complementary association. Rev Stomatol Chir Maxillofac 104(4):215-222, 2003 (in French)
2. Adamson PA: Refinement of the nasal tip. Facial Plast Surg 5:115, 1988
3. Berman WE: Surgery of the nasal tip. Otolaryngol Clin N Am 10:563, 1975
4. Bloom DC, Cupp CL: The percutaneous columnellar strut. Am J Rhinol 17(6):357-361, 2003
5. Bull TR: The tip. In: Rees ThD (ed): Rhinoplasty, Problems and Controversies. A Discussion with the Experts, Ch 5, p 35. St Louis, MO: CV Mosby Co 1988
6. Denecke HG, Meyer R: Plastische Operationen an Kopf und Hals, Vol I. In: Nasen Plastik, p. 82. Berlin: Springer Verlag 1964
7. Foda HM: Management of the droopy tip: a comparison of three alar cartilage-modifying techniques. Plast Reconstr Surg 112(5):1408-1417, discussion 1418-1421, 2003
8. Goodman WS: External approach to rhinoplasty. Can J Otolaryngol 2:207, 1973
9. Kridel RWH, Konior RJ: The under projected tip. In: Krause CHK (ed): Aesthetic Facial Surgery, Vol 12, p 191. Philadelphia, PA: JB Lippincott Co 1991
10. Mahe E, Gambling J: La voie transcartilagineuse dans la chirurgie de la pointe du nez. Ann Chir Plast 27:147, 1982
11. Nolst Trenité GJ: The surgical approach to the nasal tip. Clin Otolaryngol 16(1):109, 1991
12. Nolst Trenité GJ: Surgical correction of nasal tip deformities. In: Proceedings of the XVI World Congress of Otorhinolaryngology Head and Neck Surgery, Sydney, pp 138-144. Bologna: Monduzzi Editore SpA, 1997
13. Parell GJ, Becker GD: The “tensin nose”. Facial Plast Surg 1:2-81, 1984
14. Ponti L: Aesthetic problems in surgical technique of the nasal tip. In: Plastic and Reconstructive Surgery of the Face and Neck, Proceedings of the Second International Symposium, Vol 1. New York, NY: Grune & Stratton 1977

15. Tardy ME, Hewell TS: Nasal tip refinement – reliable approaches and sculpture techniques. Facial Plast Surg 1(2):87, 1984
16. Tardy ME, Younger R, Key M, et al: The overprojecting tip – anatomic variation and targeted solutions. Facial Plast Surg 4:4, 1987
17. Tardy ME: Transdomal suture refinement of the nasal tip. Facial Plast Surg 4:4, 1987
18. Tardy ME, Toriumi DM: Philosophy and principles of rhinoplasty. In: Papel ID, Nachlas NE (eds): Facial Plastic and Reconstructive Surgery, Ch 31, p 278. St Louis, MO: CV Mosby Co 1991
19. Tardy ME: Rhinoplasty. The Art and the Science, Vol II. Philadelphia, PA: WB Saunders Company, 1997
20. Webster RC: Advances in surgery of the tip: intact rim cartilage techniques and the tip-columella-lip esthetic complex. Otolaryngol Clin N Am 8:615, 1975

Chapter 11

1. Acarturk S, Gencel E: The spreader-splay graft combination: a treatment approach for the osseocartilaginous vault deformities following rhinoplasty. Aesthetic Plast Surg 27(4):275-280, 2003
2. Becker DG, Toriumi DM, Gross CW, Tardy ME Jr: Powered instrumentation for dorsal reduction. Facial Plast Surg 13(4):291-297, 1997
3. Berman WE: Rhinoplastic Surgery, p 156. St Louis, MO: CV Mosby Co 1989
4. Courtiss EH: Objectives in aesthetic surgery. In: Courtiss EH (ed): Male Aesthetic Surgery. St Louis, MO: Mosby Co 1982
5. Huizing EH: Push-down of the external nasal pyramid by resection of wedges. Rhinology 13:185, 1975
6. Jeppesen F: Septo- and Rhinoplasty, p 96. Copenhagen: Munksgaard 1986
7. Johnson CM, Toriumi DM: Open Structure Rhinoplasty, Ch 8, p 179. Philadelphia, PA: WB Saunders Co 1990
8. Mckinney P: In: Cunningham BL (ed): Rhinoplasty, Ch 9, p 131. New York, NY: Churchill Livingstone 1989
9. Mackay IS: Percutaneous osteotomies. In: Symposium on Rhinology, Odense, Denmark 1984
10. Meyer R: Secondary and Functional Rhinoplasty: The Difficult Nose, Ch 26, p 77. Orlando, FL: Grune & Stratton Inc 1988
11. Nolst Trenité GJ: Micro-osteotomies. Clin Otolaryngol 15(6):563, 1990
12. Nolst Trenité GJ: Trauma reduction in rhinoplastic surgery. Rhinology 29:111, 1991
13. Nolst Trenité GJ: Rhinoplasty: modern techniques. Russian Rhinol 1:17-25, 1996
14. Peck GC: Technique in Aesthetic Rhinoplasty, p 80. New York, NY: Gower Med Publ 1984
15. Pirsig W, Konings D: Wedge resection in rhinosurgery. A review of the literature and long-term results in a hundred cases. Rhinology 26:77, 1988
16. Rees TD: Aesthetic Plastic Surgery, Vol I, p 153. Philadelphia, PA: WB Saunders Co 1980
17. Rohrich RJ, Minoli JJ, Adams WP, Hollier LH: The lateral nasal osteotomy in rhinoplasty: an anatomic endoscopic comparison of the external versus the internal approach. Plast Reconstr Surg 99(5):1309-1312, discussion 1313, 1997
18. Skoog T: A method of hump reduction in rhinoplasty. Arch Otolaryngol 83:283, 1966

19. Tardy ME, Denneny JC: Micro-osteotomies in rhinoplasty. Facial Plast Surg 1(2), 1984
20. Tardy ME, Kron TK, Younger R, et al.: The cartilaginous pollybeak: etiology, prevention and treatment Facial Plast Surg 6:2, 1989
21. Tardy ME: Rhinoplasty. The Art and the Science, Vol I. Philadelphia, PA: WB Saunders Company, 1997
22. Walter C: Komplikationen bei rhinoplastische Eingriffen. In: Handbuch der plastische Chirurgie, Bd II. Beitrag 34. Berlin: Walter de Gruyter 1966
23. Webster RC, Davidson TM, Smith RC: Curved lateral osteotomy for airway protection in rhinoplasty. Arch Otolaryngol 103:454, 1977

Chapter 12

1. Adamson PA: Open rhinoplasty. Otolaryngol Clin N Am 20:837-852, 1987
2. Adamson PA: Refinement of the nasal tip. Facial Plast Surg 5:115-134, 1988
3. Adamson PA, Zylker TD, Vuyk HD: Open approach for septo-rhinoplasty. Video Dept, Dept Otolaryngol-Head Neck Surg, Maastricht Univ 1989
4. Adamson PA, Smith O, Tropper GJ: Incision and scar analysis in open (external) rhinoplasty. Arch Otolaryngol Head Neck Surg 116:671-675, 1990
5. Anderson JR: New approach to rhinoplasty: a five-year reappraisal. Arch Otolaryngol Head Neck Surg 93:284-291, 1971
6. Constantian MB: Grafting the projecting nasal tip. Ann Plast Surg 14:5, 1985
7. Johnson CM, Quatela VC: Nasal tip grafting via the open approach. Facial Plast Surg 4:301-316, 1987
8. Johnson CM, Toriumi DM: Open Structure Rhinoplasty. Philadelphia, PA: WB Saunders Co 1990
9. Kamer FM, Churukian MM: Shield graft for the nasal tip. Arch Otolaryngol Head Neck Surg 110:608-610, 1984
10. Ortiz-Monastero F, Olmedo A, Ortiz Oscoy L: The use of cartilage grafts in primary aesthetic rhinoplasty. Plast Reconstr Surg 5:597-605, 1981
11. Sheen JH: Achieving more nasal tip projection by the use of a small autogenous vomer or septal cartilage graft. Plast Reconstr Surg 56:35-40, 1975
12. Sheen JH: Aesthetic Rhinoplasty. St Louis, MO: CV Mosby Co 1978
13. Tardy ME, Schwartz M, Parras G: Saddle nose deformity: autogenous graft repair. Facial Plast Surg 6:121-134, 1990
14. Thomas C, Mishra P: Open tip rhinoplasty along with the repair of cleft lip in cleft lip and palate cases. Br J Plast Surg 53(1):1-6, 2000
15. Wright WK, Kridel RWH: External rhinoplasty: a tool for teaching and for improved results. Laryngoscope 91:945-951, 1981
16. Zylker TD, Vuyk HD: The open septo-rhinoplasty: experience with 80 patients. Ned T Geneesk (Dutch Med J) 27:1303-1308, 1990

Chapter 13

1. Gillies H: Plastic Surgery of the Face. London: H Frowde, Hodder and Stoughton Co 1920
2. Rethi A: Operation to shorten an excessively long nose. Rev Chir Plast 2:85, 1934
3. Sercer A, Mundnich K: Plastische Operationen an der Nase und an der Ohrmuschel. Stuttgart: Georg Thieme Verlag 1962
4. Goodman WS, Charbonneau PA: External approach to rhinoplasty. Laryngoscope 84:2195-2201, 1974

5. Anderson JR: The dynamics of rhinoplasty. In: Int Congress Series No 206: Proceedings of the Ninth International Congress in Otolaryngology, Mexico, August 1969, pp 708-710. Amsterdam: Excerpta Medica 1969
6. Anderson JR: New approach to rhinoplasty: a five year appraisal. Arch Otolaryngol Head Neck Surg 93:284-291, 1971
7. Johnson CM Jr, Toriumi DM: Open Structure Rhinoplasty. Philadelphia, PA: WB Saunders 1990
8. Snell D: History of external rhinoplasty. J Otolaryngol 7:1, 1978
9. Rogers, Blair O: John Orlando Roe – not Jacques Joseph – the father of aesthetic rhinoplasty. Aesth Plast Surg 10(2):63-88, 1986
10. Aufricht G: Joseph's rhinoplasty with some modifications. Surg Clin N Am 51(2):299-316, 1971
11. Tardy ME: Sculpturing of the nasal tip. In: Tardy ME (ed) Rhinoplasty, the Art and the Science. Vol 2, pp 374-571. Philadelphia, PA: WB Saunders Co, 1997
12. Tardy ME, Denneny J, Fritsch MH: The versatile cartilage autograft in reconstruction of the nose and face. Laryngoscope 95:523, 1985
13. Goodman WS, Charles DA: Technique of external rhinoplasty. Can J Otolaryngol 7:13-18, 1978
14. Goodman WS, Charles DA: Why external rhinoplasty? J Otolaryngol 7:9-12, 1978
15. Wright WK, Kridel RWH: External septorhinoplasty: a tool for teaching and for improved results. Laryngoscope 91:945-951, 1981
16. Adamson PA, Smith O, Tropper GJ: Incision and scar analysis in open (external) rhinoplasty. Arch Otolaryngol Head Neck Surg 116:671-675, 1990
17. Farrior RT: Modifications in rhinoplasty: where and when. Trans Am Acad Ophthalmol Otolaryngol 78:341, 1974
18. Danial RK: The nasal tip; anatomy and aesthetics. Plast Reconstruct Surg 89:216, 1992
19. Sheen JH, Sheen AP: Aesthetic Rhinoplasty, 2nd Edn. St Louis, MO: CV Mosby 1987
20. Larrabee WF: Open rhinoplasty and the upper third of the nose. Facial Plast Surg Clin N Am 1(1):23-38, 1993
21. Kern EB: Surgical approaches to abnormalities of the nasal valve. Laryngoscope 93:49-55, 1983
22. Sheen JH: Spreader graft: a method of reconstructing the roof of the middle nasal vault following rhinoplasty. Plast Reconstruct Surg 73(2):230-239, 1984
23. Rohrich RJ, Hollier LH: Use of spreader grafts in the external approach to rhinoplasty. Clin Plast Surg 23(2):255-262, 1996
24. Webster RC, Smith RC: Lateral crural retrodisplacement for superior rotation of the tip in rhinoplasty. Aesth Plast Surg 3:65-78, 1979
25. Kridel RWH, Konior RJ: Controlled nasal tip rotation via the lateral crural overlay technique. Arch Otolaryngol Head Neck Surg 117:411-415, 1991
26. Kridel RWH, Konior RJ, Shumrick K et al: Advances in nasal tip surgery: the lateral crural steal. Arch Otolaryngol Head Neck Surg 115:1206, 1989
27. Sheen JH: Achieving more nasal tip projection by the use of a small autogenous vomer or septal cartilage: a preliminary report. Plast Reconstruct Surg 56(1):35-40, 1975
28. Kamer FM, McQuown SA: Revision rhinoplasty: analysis and treatment. Arch Otolaryngol Head Neck Surg 114:257, 1988

29. Webster RC: Revision rhinoplasty. Otolaryngol Clin N Am 8:753, 1975
30. Skoog T: A method of hump reduction in rhinoplasty: a technique for preservation of the nasal roof. Arch Otolaryngol 83:283-287, 1966
31. Tardy ME: Cartilage autografts reconstruction of the nose. In: Rhinoplasty, the Art and the Science, Vol 2, pp 648-724. Philadelphia, PA: WB Saunders Co, 1997
32. Kridel R, Appling D, Wright W: Closure of septal perforation: a simplified method via the external septorhinoplasty approach. In: Plastic and Reconstructive Surgery of the Head and Neck: Proceedings of the Fourth International Symposium, Vol 1. St Louis, MO: CV Mosby Co 1984
33. Kridel R, Appling D, Wright W: Septal perforation closure utilizing the external septorhinoplasty approach. Arch Otolaryngol Head Neck Surg 112:168, 1986
34. Arnstein DP: Surgical considerations in the open rhinoplasty approach to septal perforations. Arch Otolaryngol Head Neck Surg 115:435-438, 1989
35. Fairbanks DNF, Chen SCA: Closure of large nasal septal perforations. Arch Otolaryngol Head Neck Surg 91:403-406, 1970
36. Fairbanks DNF, Fairbanks GR: Surgical management of large nasal septal perforations. Br J Plast Surg 24:382, 1971
37. Rettinger G, Masing H, Heinl W: Management of septal perforation by rotation plasty of the septal mucosa. HNO 34:461-466, 1986
38. Cottle MH: The Cottle nasal syndromes. In: Rhinology: The Collected Writings of Maurice H Cottle, pp 189-190, 1987
39. Johnson CM Jr, Godin MS: The tension nose: open structure rhinoplasty approach. Plast Reconstruct Surg 95(1): 43-51, 1995
40. Nolst Trenité GJ: Secondary surgery of the cleft lip nose. In: Nolst Trenité GJ (ed): Rhinoplasty: A Practical Guide to Functional and Aesthetic Surgery of the Nose, 1st Edn. Amsterdam/New York: Kugler Publ 1993
41. Sykes JM, Senders CW: Surgery of the cleft lip nasal deformity. Operat Tech Otolaryngol Head Neck Surg 1:2119-224, 1990
42. Gorney M: Reconstruction of the postcleft nasal deformity. In: Rees TD (ed) Rhinoplasty: Problems and Controversies, Ch 46, p 410. St Louis, MO: CV Mosby Co, 1988
43. Nolst Trenité GJ: Rhinoplasty: the cleft lip patient. Cleft Palate J 34(1):1-6, 1997
44. Nolst Trenité GJ: Secondary rhinoplasty in the bilateral cleft lip patient. FACE 4(1):15-23, 199?
45. Sykes JM, Senders CW, Wang TD, Cook TA: Use of the open approach for repair of secondary cleft-lip nasal deformities. Facial Plast Surg Clin N Am 1(1):111-126, 1993
46. Guyuron B, Varghai A: Lengthening the nose with a tongue-and-groove technique. Plast Reconstr Surg 111(4):1533-1539, discussion 1540-1541, 2003
47. Foda HM: External rhinoplasty: a critical analysis of 500 cases. J Laryngol Otol 117(6):473-477, 2003
48. Werther JR: External rhinoplasty approach for repair of posttraumatic nasal deformity. J Craniomaxillofac Trauma 2(4):12-19, 1996

Chapter 14

1. Denecke HJ, Meyer R: Plastische Operationen an Kopf und Hals, Vol I, Nasenplastik, p 108. Berlin: Springer Verlag 1964
2. Foda HM: Alar setback technique: a controlled method of nasal tip deprojection. Arch Otolaryngol Head Neck Surg 127(11):1341-1346, 2001

3. Fuleihan NS, Webster RC, Smith RC: Deformity of the nasal base. In: Kranse CHJ (ed): Aesthetic Facial Surgery, Ch 17, p 289. Philadelphia, PA: JB Lippincott Co 1991
4. Hinderer KH: Correction of deformities of the base of the nose. In: Sission GA (ed): Plastic and Reconstructive Surgery of the Face and Neck. New York, NY: Grune & Stratton 1977
5. Meyer R: Residual deformities of the ala. In: Meyer R (ed) Secondary and Functional Rhinoplasty: The Difficult Nose. New York, NY: Grune & Stratton 1988
6. Peck GC: Alar rim sculpturing. In: Peck GC (ed) Techniques in Aesthetic Rhinoplasty. New York, NY: Thieme-Stratton Inc 1984
7. Rees TD: The tip columella complex and the alar base. In: Rees TD (ed): Aesthetic Plastic Surgery. Philadelphia, PA: WB Saunders Co 1980
8. Sheen JH: Aesthetic Rhinoplasty, Vol I, p 252. St Louis, MO: CV Mosby Co 1987

Chapter 15

1. Ahuja RB: Radical correction of secondary nasal deformity in unilateral cleft lip patients presenting late. Plast Reconstr Surg 108(5):1127-1135, 2001
2. Cho BC, Park JW, Baik BS: Correction of severe secondary cleft lip nasal deformity using a composite graft: current approach and review. Ann Plast Surg 48(2):131-137, 2002
3. Clark JM, Skoner JM, Wang TD: Repair of the unilateral cleft lip/nose deformity. Facial Plast Surg 19(1):29-40, 2003
4. Cronin TD: Lengthening columella by use of skin from nasal floor and alae. Plast Reconstr Surg 21:417, 1958
5. Denecke HJ, Meyer R: Plastische Operationen an Kopf und Hals. Vol I. Nasenplastik, Ch XIV p 230. Berlin: Springer Verlag 1964
6. Farrior RT: The problem of the unilateral cleft lip nose. A composite operation for revision of secondary deformity. Laryngoscope 72:289, 1962
7. Farrior RT: The cleft-lip nose septo-rhinoplasty and combined lip repair. In: Sission GA, Tardy ME (eds): Plastic and Reconstructive Surgery of the Face and Neck. New York, NY: Grune & Stratton 1977
8. Gorney M: Reconstruction of the postcleft nasal deformity. In: Rees ThD (ed): Rhinoplasty "Problems and Controversies", Ch 46, p 410. St Louis, MO: CV Mosby Co 1988
9. Han S, Choi MS: Three-dimensional Z-plasty in the correction of the unilateral cleft lip nasal deformity. Cleft Palate Craniofac J 38(3):264-267, 2001
10. Matsuya T, Iida S, Kogo M: Secondary rhinoplasty using flying-bird and vestibular tornado incisions for unilateral cleft lip patients. Plast Reconstr Surg 112(2):390-395, 2003
11. Meyer R: Hare-lip nose. In: Meyer R (ed): Secondary and Functional Rhinoplasty in the Difficult Nose, Ch 20, p 335. New York, NY: Grune & Stratton Inc 1988
12. Millard DR: Columella lengthening by a forked flap. Plast Reconstr Surg 22:454, 1958
13. Millard DR: Rotation advancement in the repair of unilateral cleft lip. In: Gralib WC, Rosenstein SW, Bzoch KR (eds): Cleft Lip and Palate-Surgical, Dental and Speech Aspects. Boston, MA: Little, Brown & Co 1971
14. Nolst Trenité GJ, Weil J, De Roos P: Observation: A comment on "a discussion of presurgical orthodontics in patients with clefts". Cleft Palate I, 27(4):419, 1990

15. Nolst Trenité GJ: Neuschirurgie bij de schisispatient. Ned T Geneesk 136, no 16, 1992
16. Nolst Trenité GJ: Cleft-lip nose surgery. Abstractbook Vth European Craniofacial Congress, Copenhagen 1995
17. Nolst Trenité GJ: Secondary rhinoplasty in the bilateral cleft lip patient. FACE 4(1):15-23, 1995
18. Nolst Trenité GJ, Paping RHL, Trenning AH: Rhinoplasty in the cleft lip patient. Cleft Palate Craniofacial Journal. 34(1):63-68, 1997
19. Nolst Trenité GJ: Secondary rhinoplasty in the bilateral cleft. Facial Plast Surg 18(3):179-186, 2002
20. Nolst Trenité GJ: Secondary rhinoplasty in the bilateral cleft. Facial Plast Surg 18(3):179-186, 2002
21. Ortiz-Monasterio F, Olmedo A: Cleft lip nose. In: Rees ThD (ed): Rhinoplasty: Problems and Controversies, Ch 45, p 397. St Louis, MO: CV Mosby Co 1988
22. Romo T 3rd, Choe KS, Sclafani AP: Secondary cleft-lip rhinoplasty utilizing porous high-density polyethylene. Facial Plast Surg 19(4):369-377, 2003
23. Smith HW: Cosmetic rhinoplasty on the cleft lip patient. In: Berman WE (ed): Rhinoplastic Surgery, Ch 25, p 300. St Louis, MO: CV Mosby Co 1989
24. Verwoerd CDA, Mladina R, Nolst Trenité GJ, Pigott RW: The nose in children with unilateral cleft-lip and palate. Int J Ped Otorhinolaryngol, 32(Suppl):45-52, 1995
25. Weil J: Orthopaedic growth guidance and stimulation for patients with cleft lip and palate. Scand J Plast Reconstr Surg 21:57-63, 1987

Chapter 16

1. Bull TR: Rhinoplasty: problems and controversies. In: Rees TD, Baker DC (eds): The Nasal Tip, Ch 5, p 41. St. Louis, MO: CV Mosby Co 1988
2. Lipsett EM: A new approach to surgery of the lower cartilagenous vault. Arch Otolaryngol 70:52–57, 1959
3. Meyer HJ, Denecke R: Plastic Surgery of Head-Neck: Corrective and Reconstructive Rhinoplasty. Berlin: Springer Verlag 1967
4. Pedroza F: A 20-year review of the 'new domes' technique for refining the drooping nasal tip. Arch Facial Plast Surg 4(3):157-163, 2002

Chapter 17

1. Converse J: Reconstructive Plastic Surgery, 2nd Edn, Vol 2, p 1141. Philadelphia, PA: WB Saunders 1977
2. De Jong JH: Rib grafts in the treatment of saddle deformity. Presented at the European Academy of Facial Surgery, London, May 1983
3. Elahi MM, Jackson IT, Moreira-Gonzalez A, Yamini D: Nasal augmentation with Surgicel-wrapped diced cartilage: a review of 67 consecutive cases. Plast Reconstr Surg 111(3):1309-1318, discussion 1319-1321, 2003
4. Gibson T, Davis B: The fate of preserved bovine cartilage implants in man. Br J Plast Surg 6:4-25, 1953
5. Gibson T, Davis B: The long-term survival of cartilage homografts in man. Br J Plast Surg 2:177-187, 1977
6. Mackay IS, Bull TR: The fate of Silastic in the management of saddle deformity of the nose. J Laryngol Otol 97:43-47, 1983
7. Marvin JA: The application of cantilever bridge principle to Silastic nasal support. Br J Plast Surg 33:404-406, 1980

8. Milward TM: The fate of Silastic and vitrathene nasal implants. Br J Plast Surg 25: 1276-1278, 1972
9. Muhlbauer WD: Long-term behaviour of preserved homologous rib cartilage in the correction of saddle nose deformity. Br J Plast Surg 124:325-383, 1971
10. Reicht J: The application of dermis grafts in deformities of the nose. Plast Reconstr Surg 71:772-780, 1983
11. Riechelmann H, Rettinger G: Three-step reconstruction of complex saddle nose deformities. Arch Otolaryngol Head Neck Surg 130(3):334-338, 2004
12. Romo T 3rd, Sclafani AP, Sabini P: Reconstruction of the major saddle nose deformity using composite allo-implants. Facial Plast Surg 14(2):151-157, 1998
13. Rozner L: Augmentation rhinoplasty. Br J Plast Surg 33:377-382, 1980
14. Stucker FJ: Technical aspects of facial contouring using polyamide mesh. Otolaryngol Clin N Am 15:123-131, 1982
15. Tardy EM, Schwartz M, Parras G: Saddle nose deformity: autogenous graft repair. Facial Plast Surg 6:2: 1989
16. Thompson N: The subcutaneous dermis graft. Plast Reconstr Surg 26:1-22, 1960
17. Wallace AF: The Progress of Plastic Surgery. Oxford: WA Meeuws 1980

Chapter 18

1. Cottle MH, Loring RM: Corrective surgery of the external nasal pyramid and the nasal septum for restoration of normal physiology. Eye Ear Nose Throat Monthly 26:207, 1947
2. Dirlewanger A, Meyer R: Plastik und Rekonstruktion des Nasenseptums. Schweiz ORL Congress Délémont 1968
3. Akyildiz AM: Septoplasty in perforations of the nasal septum. Int Rhinol 7:1, 1993
4. Hertig P, Meyer R: Closure of septal defects and septocolumellar reconstruction. In: Int Congress Series No. 206: Proceedings of the Ninth International Congress, Mexico, August 1969, p 714. Amsterdam: Excerpta Medica 1969
5. Meyer R: Total nasal reconstruction. In: Conley J, Dickinson JT (eds): Plastic and Reconstructive Surgery of the Face and Neck. New York, NY: Grune and Stratton 1972
6. Schmid RE, Widmajer WI: Ueber die Hautknorpel-Transplantationen aus der Ohrmuschel und ihre funktionelle und ästhetische Bedeutung bei der Deckung von Gesichtsdefekten. Fortschr Kiefer Gesichtschir 7:48, 1961
7. Jacobs KF: Angeborene Aplasie von Nasensteg und knorpeligem Septum. Laryngol Rhinol Otol 63:344, 1984
8. Ellis DAF, Le Liever WC: The nose-check flap in total columellar reconstruction. In: Bernstein L (ed): Plastic and Reconstructive Surgery of the Head and Neck. Third International Symposium, Vol 2, p 26. 1981
9. Matton G, Beck H: Closure of a large nasal septal perforation with a lined nasolabial flap. Chir Plast 93:61, 1985
10. Meyer R: Die partielle Ersatzplastik der Nase. Aesth Med Heft 1:1, 1963
11. Meyer R: Verschluss von Septumperforationen. In: Denecke HJ, Meyer R (eds), Plastische Operationen an Kopf und Hals: korrigierende Nasenplastik. Berlin: Springer-Verlag 1964
12. Meyer R: Complications tardives en rhinoplasties. Med Hyg 39:742, 1981
13. Meyer R: Secondary and Functional Rhinoplasty: The Difficult Nose. Orlando, FL: Grune & Stratton Inc. Harcourt Brace Jovanovich Publ 1988

14. Meyer R, Kesselring UK: Reconstructive surgery of the nose. Clin Plast Surg 8:435, 1981

Chapter 19

1. Adamson PA: Refinement of the nasal tip. Facial Plast Surg 5:115-134, 1988
2. Anderson JR, Ries WR: Rhinoplasty: Emphasizing the External Approach. New York, NY: Thieme Inc 1986
3. Bull TR, Mackay JS: Augmentation rhinoplasty. Facial Plast Surg 1:125-136, 1984
4. Denecke HJ, Ey W: Die Operationen an der Nase und im Nasopharynx. Berlin: Springer Verlag 1984
5. Early MJ, Lendrum J: The alar swing technique in the correction of the saddle nose deformity. Br J Plast Surg 37:307-312, 1984
6. Erdem T, Ozturan O: Graft materials used in the reconstruction of saddle nose. Kulak Burun Bogaz Ihtis Derg 9(6):435-440, 2002 (Review in Turkish)
7. Gunther JP, Rohrich RJ: Augmentation rhinoplasty: dorsal onlay grafting using shaped autogenous septal cartilage. Plast Reconstr Surg 86:39-45, 1990
8. Johnson CM, Toriumi DM: Open Structure Rhinoplasty. Philadelphia/London/ Toronto: WB Saunders Co 1990
9. Masing H, Rettinger G: Eingriffe an der Nase. In: Theissing J (ed): Mund-, Hals- und Nasenoperationen. Stuttgart/New York: Georg Thieme Verlag 1988
10. Masing H, Lehmann W, Stadler J: Über Sekundäroperationen nach submuköser Septumresektion. Laryngol Rhinol Otol 57:931, 1978
11. Mayer TG, Fleming RW: The nasal dorsum: open approach. Facial Plast Surg 5:143-159, 1988
12. Meyer R: Secondary and Functional Rhinoplasty: The Difficult Nose. New York, NY: Grune & Stratton Inc 1988
13. Nagel F: Wichtige Gesichtspunkte bei der Korrektur der Sattelnase. Laryngol Rhinol Otol 62:356-358, 1983
14. Riechelmann H, Rettinger G: Three-step reconstruction of complex saddle nose deformities. Arch Otolaryngol Head Neck Surg 130(3):334-338, 2004
15. Romo T 3rd, Sclafani AP, Sabini P: Reconstruction of the major saddle nose deformity using composite allo-implants. Facial Plast Surg 14(2):151-157, 1998
16. Staindl O: Zur Therapie der Sattelnase. Laryngol Rhinol Otol 62:348-355, 1983
17. Thibault J, Sevigny B: Use of isografts and homografts in reconstruction of the nasal pyramid. J Otolaryngol 11:9-13, 1982
18. Thomassin JM, Paris J, Richard-Vitton T: Management and aesthetic results of support grafts in saddle nose surgery. Aesth Plast Surg 25(5):332-337, 2001

Chapter 20

1. Cottle MH: An introduction to conservative septum-pyramid surgery. Int Rhinol 2:11, 1964
2. Crysdale WS, Tatham B: External septorhinoplasty in children. Laryngoscope 95:12, 1985
3. Huizing EH: Septum surgery in children: indications, surgical technique and long-term results. Rhinology 17:91, 1979
4. Van Loosen J, Verwoerd-Verhoef HL, Verwoerd CDA: The nasal septal cartilage in the newborn. Rhinology 26:161, 1988
5. Van Loosen J, Juong Yiang, Howard CV, Van Zanten GA, Verwoerd-Verhoef HL, Verwoerd CDA, Van Velzen D: Nasal cartilage maturation assessed by automated

computer-assisted image analysis. Otolaryngology in ASEAN Countries. Adv Otorhinolaryngol 51:51-60, 1997

6. Mladina R: The role of maxillary morphology in the development of pathological septal deformities. Rhinology 25:199, 1987
7. Metzenbaum M: Replacement of the lower end of the dislocated septal cartilage versus submucous resection of the dislocated end of the septal cartilage. Arch Otolaryngol 9:282, 1929
8. Nolst Trenité GJ, Verwoerd CDA, Verwoerd-Verhoef HL: Reimplantation of autologous septal cartilage in the growing nasal septum. I. The influence of resection and reimplantation of septal cartilage upon nasal growth: an experimental study in rabbits. Rhinology 25:225, 1987
9. Nolst Trenité GJ, Verwoerd CDA, Verwoerd-Verhoef HL: Reimplantation of autologous septal cartilage in the growing nasal septum. II. The influence of reimplantation of rotated or crushed autologous septal cartilage on nasal growth: an experimental study in growing rabbits. Rhinology 26:25, 1988
10. Pirsig W: Rhinoplasty and the airway in children. Facial Plast Surg 3:225, 1988
11. Pirsig W, Bean JK, Lenders H, Verwoerd CDA, Verwoerd-Verhoef HL: Cartilage transformation in a composite graft of demineralized bovine bone matrix and ear perichondrium used in a child for the reconstruction of the nasal septum. Int J Pediat Otorhinolaryngol 32:171-181, 1995
12. Poublon RML, Verwoerd CDA, Verwoerd-Verhoef HL: Anatomy of the upper lateral cartilages in the human newborn. Rhinology 28:41, 1990
13. Subaric M, Mladina R: Nasal septum deformaties in children and adolescents: a cross sectional study of children from Zagreb, Croatia. Int J Pediat ORL 63:41, 2002
14. Stucker FJ, Bryarly RC, Shockley WW: Management of nasal trauma in children. Arch Otolaryngol 110:190, 1984
15. Takahashi R: The evolution of the nasal septum and the formation of septal deformity. Rhinology (Suppl):6, 1988
16. Tardy ME, Broadway D: Septorhinoplasty in the preadolescent. In: Healy G (ed) Common Problems in Pediatric Otolaryngology. Chicago, IL: Yearbook Medical Publ 1990
17. Van Velzen D, Van Loosen J, Verwoerd CDA, Verwoerd-Verhoef HL: Persistent pattern of variations in thickness of the human nasal septum: implications for stress and trauma as illustrated by a complex fracture in a 4-year-old boy. Otolaryngology in ASEAN countries. Adv Otorhinolaryngol 51:46-50, 1997
18. Verwoerd CDA, Van Loosen J, Schütte HE, Verwoerd-Verhoef HL, Van Velzen D: Surgical aspects of the anatomy of the vomer in children and adults. Rhinology (Suppl) 9:87, 1989
19. Verwoerd CDA, Verwoerd-Verhoef HLV, Meeuwis CA: Stress and wound healing of the cartilaginous nasal septum. Acta Otolaryngol (Stockh) 107:441-445, 1989
20. Verwoerd CDA, Verwoerd-Verhoef HL: Developmental aspects of the deviated nose. Facial Plast Surg 6:2, 1989
21. Verwoerd CDA, Verwoerd-Verhoef HL, Meeuwis CA, Van der Heul RO: Wound healing of the nasal septal perichondrium in young rabbits. ORL 52:180-186, 1990
22. Verwoerd CDA, Verwoerd-Verhoef HL, Meeuwis CA, Van der Heul RO: Wound healing of autologous implants in the nasal septal cartilage. ORL 53:310, 1991

23. Verwoerd-Verhoef HL, Meeuwis CA, Van der Heul RO, Verwoerd CDA: Histologic evaluation of crushed cartilage grafts in the growing nasal septum of young rabbits. ORL 53:305, 1991
24. White P, Forte V: Surgical management of nasal airway obstruction in children. J Otolaryngol 18:155, 1989

Chapter 21

1. Aiach G: Intéret d'une direction extraunquese dans le traitement de certaines sténoses. Ann Chir Plast 19:273-276, 1974
2. Bagal AA, Adamson PA: Revision rhinoplasty. Facial Plast Surg 18(4):233-244, 2002
3. Becker DG, Becker SS, Saad AA: Auricular cartilage in revision rhinoplasty. Facial Plast Surg 19(1):41-52, 2003
4. Rees TD, Krupp S, Wood-Smith D: Secondary rhinoplasty. Plast Reconstr Surg 46:332-340, 1970
5. Rees TD, Wood-Smith D: Cosmetic Facial Surgery
6. Romo T 3rd, Sonne J, Choe KS, Sclafani AP: Revision rhinoplasty. Facial Plast Surg 19(4):299-307, 2003
7. Sclafani AP, Romo T 3rd, Barnett JG, Barnett CR: Adjustment of subtle postoperative nasal defects: managing the 'near-miss' rhinoplasty. Facial Plast Surg 19(4):349-361, 2003
8. Sheen JH: Aesthetic Rhinoplasty, p 600. St Louis, MO: CV Mosby 1978
9. Walter C: Composite grafts in nasal surgery. Arch Otolaryngol 90:622-630, 1969
10. Walter C: Survey of the use of composite grafts in the head and neck region. Otolaryngol Clin N Am 5:571-602, 1972
11. Walter C: Secondary nasal revisions after rhinoplasties. Trans Am Acad Ophthalmol 519:519-526, 1974
12. Walter C: Aesthetische Nasenchirurgie. Arch Oto-Rhino-Laryngol 216:251-350, 1977
13. Walter C: The use of composite grafts in the head and neck region. In: English GM (ed) Otolaryngology, pp 1-31. Philadelphia, PA: JB Lippincott 1988
14. Walter C: Plastisch-chirurgische Eingriffe im Kopf-Hals-Bereich. Stuttgart/New York, NY: Thieme Verlag 1997
15. Wong BJ, Giammanco PF: The use of preserved autogenous septal cartilage in 'touch-up' rhinoplasty. Arch Facial Plast Surg 5(4):349-353, 2003

Chapter 22

1. Kern AP: Surgery of the nasal valve. In: Sisson GA, Tardy ME (eds) Plastic and Reconstructive Surgery of the Face and Neck. Stuttgart: George Thieme Verlag 1970
2. Teichgraber DF, Wainwright DJ: Treatment of nasal valve obstruction. Plast Reconstr Surg 93(6):1174-1182, 1994
3. Constantian MB: The incompetent external nasal valve: pathophysiology and treatment in primary and secondary rhinoplasty. Plast Reconst Surg. 93(5):919-931, 1994
4. Naasen A, Page RE: The double cross plasty: a new technique for nasal stenoses. Br J Plast Surg 45:165-168, 1992
5. Blandini D et al: Iatrogenic nostril stenosis: aesthetic correction using a vestibular mucosa flap. Aesthet Reconstr Surg 95(3):569-571, 1994
6. Verwoerd CDA, Mladina R, Nolst Trenité GJ, Pigott RW: The nose in children with

unilateral cleft lip and palate. Int J Pediatr Otorhinolaryngol 32(Suppl):S45-S52, 1995

7. Nolst Trenité GJ: Secondary rhinoplasty in the bilateral cleft-lip patient. FACE 4(1):15-23, 1995
8. Nolst Trenité GJ: Treatment of congenital and iatrogenic stenoses of vestibulum nasi. Clin Otolaryngol 21(5):467-468, 1996
9. Nolst Trenité GJ, Paping RHL, Trenning AH: Rhinoplasty in the cleft-lip patient. Cleft Palate J 34(1):63-78, 1997
10. Nakajima T, Yoshimuri Y, Sakalihara H: Augmentation of the nostril splint for retaining the correct contour of the cleft lip nose. Plast Reconstr Surg 182-186, 1992

Chapter 23

1. Nolst Trenité GJ: Coursebook 4th International Course in Modern Rhinoplasty Techniques, 1997

Chapter 24

1. Rees ThD: Aesthetic Plastic Surgery, Vol 1, Part 2: Rhinoplasty. Philadelphia, PA: WB Saunders Company 1980
2. Tardy ME, Thomas JR, Roeder J, Fitzpatrick ME: Reconstructive Surgery of the Deviated Septum and Nose. Richards Manufactoring Co, Inc 1-19, 1982
3. Kern EB: Nasal septal reconstruction. In: Rees ThD, Baker DC, Tabbel N (eds) Rhinoplasty: Problems and Controversies, Ch 28, pp 242-257. St. Louis, MO: CV Mosby Company 1988
4. Gorney M: The septum in rhinoplasty. In: Rees Thd, Baker DC, Tabbel N (eds) Rhinoplasty: Problems and Controversies, Ch 31, pp 269-277. St. Louis, MO: CV Mosby Company 1988
5. Bull TR, Tardy ME: The damaged nose. Facial Plast Surg 6:2, 1989
6. Wustrow ThPU: Challenges in rhinoplasty. Facial Plast Surg 11:3, 1995
7. Rettinger G: Complications of septo-rhinoplasty. Facial Plast Surg 13:1, 1997
8. Farrior EH: Contemporary rhinoplasty in facial plastic surgery. Facial Plast Surg 13:3, 1997
9. Park SS, Holt GR: Rhinoplasty and septoplasty. Part 1. Otolaryngol Clin N Am, February 1999
10. Park SS, Holt GR: Rhinoplasty and septoplasty. Part 2. Otolaryngol Clin N Am, August 1999

Chapter 25

1. Tardy ME Jr: Rhinoplasty: The Art and the Science. Philadelphia, PA: WB Saunders 1997
2. Rees TD: Surgical correction of the severely deviated nose by extramucosal excision and replacement as a free graft. Plast Reconstr Surg 78:320-330, 1986
3. Toriumi DM, Mueller RA, Grosch T, Bhattacharyya TK, Larrabee WF: Vascular anatomy of the nose and the external rhinoplasty approach. Arch Otolaryngol Head Neck Surg 122:22-34, 1996
4. Jugo SB: Total septal reconstruction through decortication (external) approach in children. Arch Otolaryngol Head Neck Surg 113:173-178, 1987
5. M. Bönisch, A. Mink: Septal reconstruction with a polydioxanon plate (PDS®). FACE 6:149-154, 1999
6. Merten HA, Luhr HG: Resorbierbare PDS-Folien zur Orbitadefektüberbrückung im tierexperimentellen Vergleich. Dtsch Z Mund Kiefer Gesichtschir 18:100-104, 1994

7. Bönisch M, Mink A: Heilungsprozess des Knorpels in Verbindung mit PDS-Folie. HNO 48:743-746, 2000
8. Bönisch M, Hajas T, Nolst Trenité GJ: Influence of polydioxanone foil on growing septal cartilage after surgery in an animal model. Arch Facial Plast Surg 5:316-319, 2003
9. Nolst Trenité GJ, Verwoerd CDA, Verwoerd-Verhoef HL: Reimplantation of autologous septal cartilage in the growing nasal septum. I. Rhinology 25:225-236, 1987
10. Nolst Trenité GJ, Verwoerd CDA, Verwoerd-Verhoef, HL: Reimplantation of autologous septal cartilage in the growing nasal septum. II. Rhinology 26:25-32, 1988.
11. Verwoerd CDA, Verwoerd-Verhoef HL, Meeuwis CA et al: Wound healing of autologous implants in the nasal septal cartilage. ORL 53:310-314, 1991
12. Bönisch M, Mink A: Clinical and histological results of septoplasty with a resorbable implant. Arch Otolaryngol Head Neck Surg 126:1373-1377, 2000

Chapter 26

1. Snell D: History of external rhinoplasty. J Otolaryngol 7:1,1978
2. Aufricht G: Joseph's rhinoplasty with some modifications. Surg Clin N Am 51(2):299-316, 1971
3. Gillies H: Plastic Surgery of the Face. London: H Frowde, Hodder and Stoughton Co 1920
4. Rethi A: Operation to shorten an excessively long nose. Rev Chir Plast 2:85, 1934
5. Sercer A: Dekortication der Nose. Chir Maxillofac Plast (Zagreb) 1:49, 1958
6. Padovan T: External approach in rhinoplasty (decortication). Symp ORL 4:354, 1966
7. Goodman WS, Charbonneau PA: External approach to rhinoplasty. Laryngoscope 84: 2195-2201, 1974
8. Goodman WS: The external approach to rhinoplasty. Can J Otolaryngol 2(3):207, 1973
9. Anderson JR: New approach to rhinoplasty: a five year appraisal. Arch Otolarynol Head Neck Surg 93:284-291, 1971
10. Toriumi DM, Johnson CM Jr: Open structure rhinoplasty. Facial Plast Surg Clin N Am 1:1-22, 1993
11. Whitaker EG, Johnson CM Jr: The evolution of open structure rhinoplasty. Arch Facial Plast Surg 5:291-300, 2003
12. Johnson CM Jr, Toriumi DM: Open Structure Rhinoplasty, pp 47-98. Philadelphia, PA: WB Saunders Co 1990
13. Nolst Trenité GJ: Basic approaches and techniques in nasal tip surgery. In: Rhinoplasty: A Practical Guide to Functional and Aesthetic Surgery of the Nose. 1st edition. Amsterdam/New York: Kugler Publ 1993
14. Adamson PA, Smith O, Tropper GJ: Incision and scar analysis in open (external) rhinoplasty. Arch Otolaryngol Head Neck Surg 116(6): 671-675, 1990
15. Hanasono MM, Kridel RWH, Pastorek NJ et al: Correction of the soft tissue pollybeak using triamcinolone injection. Arch Facial Plast Surg 4:26-30, 2002
16. Toriumi DM, Becker DG. Rhinoplasty Dissection Manual. Philadelphia, PA: Lippincott Williams and Wilkins 1999
17. Johnson CM Jr, Godin MS: The tension nose: open structure rhinoplasty approach. Plast Reconstr Surg 95:43-51, 1995
18. Kridel RWH: Combined septal perforation repair with revision rhinoplasty. Facial Plast Surg Clin N Am 3(4):459-470, 1995
19. Adamson PA, Huang H: Open rhinoplasty. In: Papel ID (ed) Facial Plastic and Reconstructive Surgery, 2nd Edn, pp 390-401. New York, NY: Georg Thieme 2002

20. Larrabee WF: Open rhinoplasty and the upper third of the nose. Facial Plast Surg Clin N Am 1:23-38, 1993
21. Toriumi DM: Management of the middle nasal vault in rhinoplasty. Operat Tech Plast Reconstr Surg 2:16-30, 1995
22. Toriumi DM, Ries WR: Innovative surgical management of the crooked nose. Facial Plast Surg Clin N Am 1:63-78, 1993
23. McCollough EG, English JL: A new twist in nasal tip surgery: an alternative to the Goldman tip for the wide or bulbous lobule. Arch Otolaryngol Head Neck Surg 111:524-529, 1985
24. Tardy ME, Cheng E: Transdomal suture refinement of the nasal tip. Facial Plast Surg 4:317-326, 1987
25. Konior RS, Kridel R: Controlled nasal tip positioning via the open rhinoplasty approach. Facial Plast Surg Clin N Am 1:53-62, 1993

Chapter 27

1. Hoefflin S: Ethnic Rhinoplasty. New York, NY: Springer/Verlag Inc 1997
2. Powell N, Humphreys B: Proportions of the Aesthetic Face. New York, NY: Thieme-Stratton Inc 1984
3. Matory WE Jr: Ethnic Considerations in Facial Aesthetic Surgery. New York, NY: Lippincott-Raven 1997
4. Nolst Trenité GJ: Preoperative management. In: Nolst Trenité GJ (ed) Rhinoplasty, a Practical Guide to Functional and Aesthetic Surgery of the Nose, pp 18-24, 2nd edition. The Hague: Kugler Publications 1998
5. Palma P, Bignami M et al: Rhinoplasty for the Mediterranean nose. Facial Plast Surg 19(3): 279-294, 2003
6. Cobo R: Mestizo rhinoplasty. Facial Plast Surg 19(3):257-268, 2003
7. Tardy ME Jr: Rhinoplasty: The Art and the Science. Philadelphia, PA: WB Saunders Co 1997
8. Nolst Trenité GJ: Basic approaches and techniques in nasal tip surgery. In: Nolst Trenité GJ (ed) Rhinoplasty: A Practical Guide to Functional and Aesthetic Surgery of the Nose, 2nd edition. The Hague: Kugler Publications 1998
9. Godin MS, Waldman SR, Johnson CM Jr: The use of expanded polytetrafluoroethylene (Gore-Tex) in rhinoplasty: a six-year experience. Arch Otolaryngol Head Neck Surg 121:1131-1136, 1995
10. McCurdy: The Asian nose: augmentation rhinoplasty with L-shaped silicone implants. Facial Plast Surg Monographs 18: 245-252, 2002
11. Romo T III, Abraham MT: The ethnic nose. Facial Plast Surg 19(3):269-277, 2003
12. Murakami GS, Cook T, Guida RA: Nasal reconstruction with articulated irradiated rib cartilage. Arch Otolaryngol Head Neck Surg 117:327-330, 1991
13. Kridel RWH, Kraus W: Grafts and implants in revision rhinoplasty. Facial Plast Surg Clin N Am 3(4):473-486, 1995
14. Wang TD: Non-Caucasian rhinoplasty. Facial Plast Surg 19(3):247-255, 2003
15. Whitaker EG, Johnson CM: The evolution of open structure rhinoplasty. Arch Facial Plast Surg 5:291-300, 2003
16. Toriumi DM, Johnson CM Jr: Open structure rhinoplasty: featured technical points and long-term follow-up. Facial Plast Surg Clin N Am 1(1):1-22, 1993
17. Hanasono MM, Kridel RWH, Pastorek NJ, Galsgold MJ, Koch RJ: Correction of the soft tissue pollybeak using triamcinolone injection. Arch Facial Plast Surg 4:26-30, 2002

18. Nolst Trenité GJ: Considerations in ethnic rhinoplasty. Facial Plast Surg 19(3):239-245, 2003

Chapter 28

1. Beekhuis GJ: Nasal obstruction after rhinoplasty: etiology and techniques for correction. Laryngoscope 86:540-548, 1976
2. Bull TR, Mackay IS: Alar collapse. Facial Plast Surg 3(4):268, 1986
3. Constantian MB, Clardy RB: The relative importance of septal and nasal valvular surgery in correcting airway obstruction in primary and secondary rhinoplasty. Plast Reconstr Surg 98:38-54, 1996
4. Constantian MB: The incompetent external nasal valve: pathophysiology and treatment in primary and secondary rhinoplasty. Plast Reconstr Surg 93:919-931, 1994
5. Courtiss E, Gargan T, Courtiss G: Nasal physiology. Ann Plast Surg 13:214, 1984
6. Fuleihan NS, Webster RC, Smith RC: Deformity of the nasal base. In: Kranse CHJ (ed) Aesthetic Facial Surgery, Ch 17, p 289. Philadelphia, PA: JB Lippincott Co 1991
7. Goode RL: Surgery of the incompetent nasal valve. Laryngoscope 95:446, 1985
8. Haight JSJ, Cole P: The site and function of the nasal valve. Laryngoscope 93:49, 1983
9. Heinberg CE, Kern EB. The Cottle sign: an aid in the physical diagnosis of nasal airflow disturbance. Int Rhinol 1(11):89-94, 1973
10. Johnson CM, Toriumi DM: Open Structure Rhinoplasty. Philadelphia, PA: WB Saunders Co 1980
11. Kaspenbauer JL, Kern EB: Nasal valve physiology: implications in nasal surgery. Otolaryngol Clin N Am 20:699-719, 1987
12. Kern EB: Surgery of the nasal valve. In: Rees (ed) Rhinoplasty: Discussion with the Experts, pp 209-222. St Louis, MO: Mosby Year Book Inc 1995
13. Kern EB: Surgery of the nasal valve. In: Sisson GA, Tardy ME (eds) Plastic and Reconstructive Surgery of the Face and Neck. Stuttgart: Georg Thieme Verlag 1975
14. Kern EB: Surgical approaches to abnormalities of the nasal valve. Laryngoscope 93:49-55, 1983
15. Khosh MM, Jen A, Honrado C, Pearlman SJ: Nasal valve reconstruction. Arch Facial Plast Surg 6(31):167-171, 2004
16. Meyer R: Residual deformities of the ala. In: Meyer R (ed) Secondary and Functional Rhinoplasty: The Difficult Nose. New York, NY: Grune & Stratton 1988
17. Nolst Trenité GJ: Alar insufficiency. In: Nolst Trenité GJ (ed) Rhinoplasty: A Practical Guide to Functional and Aesthetic Surgery of the Nose, Ch 8, pp 45-57, 2nd edition. The Hague: Kugler Publ 1998
18. Peck GC: Alar rim sculpturing. In: Opeck GC (ed) Techniques in Aesthetic Rhinoplasty. New York, NY: Thieme-Stratton Inc 1984
19. Rees TD: The tip columella complex and the alar base. In: Rees TD (ed) Aesthetic Plastic Surgery. Philadelphia, PA: WB Saunders Co 1980
20. Sheen JH: Spreader graft: a method of reconstructing the roof of the middle nasal vault following rhinoplasty. Plast Reconstr Surg 73:230-237, 1984
21. Sheen JH, Shean AP: Aesthetic Rhinoplasty. St Louis, MO: Mosby Year Book Inc 1987
22. Stucker FJ, Hoasjoe DK: Nasal reconstruction with conchal cartilage: correcting valve and lateral nasal collapse. Arch Otolaryngol Head Neck Surg 120:653-658, 1994
23. Sulsenti G, Palma P: A new technique for functional surgery of the nasal valve area. Rhinology (Suppl 10), 1989
24. Tardy ME: Surgical Anatomy of the Nose, Ch 4, pp 55-97. New York, NY: Raven Press 1990

25. Tardy ME, Garner ET: Inspiratory nasal obstruction secondary to alar and nasal valve collapse: technique for repair using autologous cartilage. Oper Tech Otolaryngol Head Neck Surg 1:215-218, 1980
26. Toriumi DM: Management of the middle nasal vault in rhinoplasty. Oper Tech Plast Reconstr Surg 2:16-30, 1995
27. Toriumi DM, Josen J, Weinberger M, Tardy ME: Use of alar batten grafts for correction of nasal valve collapse. Arch Otolaryngol 123:802-808, 1997
28. Walter C: Zum Thema: Nasenflügelkollaps. Laryngol Rhinol Otol 55:447, 1976
29. Walter C: Surgical approaches to problems of the nasal valve area and the extra mucosal rhinoplasty. In: Rees TD (ed): Rhinoplasty, Problems and Controversies: A Discussion with the Experts, Ch 24, p 204. St Louis, MO: CV Mosby Co 1988
30. Zijlker TD, Vuyk HD: In: Nolst Trenité GJ (ed) Rhinoplasty: A Practical Guide to Functional and Aesthetic Surgery of the Nose, Ch 9b, pp 67-75, 2nd edition. The Hague: Kugler Publ 1998

Chapter 29

1. Preston DS, Stern RS: Nonmelanoma cancers of the skin. N Engl J Med 327:1649-1662, 1992
2. Gloster AM, Brodland JG: The epidemiology of skin cancer. Dermatol Surg 22:217-226, 1996
3. Urbach F: Ultraviolet radiation and skin cancer of humans. J Photochem Photobiol B 40:3-7, 1997
4. Bennett JE, Moore TS, Vellios F, Hugo NE: Surgical treatment of skin cancer of the nose. Am J Surg 117:382-387, 1969
5. Conley J: Cancer of the skin of the nose. Ann Otol Rhinol Laryngol 83:2, 1974
6. Lohuis PJFM, De Rie MA, Balm AJM: Cutaneous malignancies of the head and neck. In: Vuyk HD, Lohuis PJFM (eds) Facial Plastic Reconstructive Surgery. London: Hodder 2005 in press
7. Sexton M, Jones DB, Maloney ME: Histologic pattern analysis of basal cell carcinoma: study of a series of 1039 consecutive neoplasms. J Am Acad Dermatol 23:1118-1126, 1990
8. Emmett AJ: Surgical analysis and biological behaviour of 2277 basal cell carcinomas. Aust NZ J Surg 60:855, 1990
9. Verhaegh MEJM: Growth Characteristics of Basal Cell Carcinoma. Thesis, University of Maastricht 1998
10. Orengo IF, Salasche SJ, Fewkes J et al: Correlation of histologic subtypes of primary basal cell carcinoma and number of Mohs stages required to achieve a tumor-free plane. J Am Acad Dermatol 37:395-397, 1997
11. Goepfert H et al: Perineural invasion of squamous cell skin carcinoma of the head and neck. Am J Surg 148:542, 198
12. Rowe DE, Carroll RJ, Day CL: Prognostic factors for local recurrence, metastasis, and survival rates in squamous cell carcinoma of the skin, ear, and lip: implications for treatment modality selection. J Am Acad Dermatol 26:976, 1992
13. Hendrix JD, Slingluff CL: Cutaneous malignancies: diagnosis and treatment. In: Papel ID (ed) Facial Plastic and Reconstructive Surgery, pp 485-511. New York, NY: Thieme 2002
14. Breuninger H, Black B, Rassner G: Microstaging of squamous cell carcinomas. Am J Clin Pathol 94:624-627, 1990
15. Jol JAD, Van Velthuysen MLF, Hilgers FJM et al: Treatment results of regional metas-

tasis from cutaneous head and neck squamous cell carcinoma. Eur J Surg Oncol 29:81-86, 2002
16. Lay SY, Weinstein GS, Chalian AA et al: Parotidectomy in the treatment of aggressive cutaneous malignancies. Arch Otolaryngol Head Neck Surg 128(5):521-526, 2002
17. Jonk A, Strobbe LJ, Kroon BB, Mooi WJ, Hart AA, Nieweg OE, Balm AJ: Cervical lymp node metastases from cutaneous melanoma of the head and neck: a search for prognostic factors. Eur J Surg Oncol 24(4):298-302, 1998
18. White RR, Stanley WE, Johnson JL et al: Long-term survival in 2,505 patients with melanoma with regional lymph node metastasis. Ann Surg 235:879-887, 2002
19. Meyer T, Merkel S, Gohl J, Hohenberger W: Lymph node dissection for clinically evident lymph node metastasis of malignant melanoma. Eur J Surg Oncol 28:424-430, 2002
20. Petter G, Haustein UF: Squamous cell carcinoma of the skin: histopathological features and their significance for clinical outcome. J Eur Acad Dermatol Venereol 11:37-44, 1998
21. Breuninger H, Black B, Rassner G: Microstaging of squamous cell carcinoma. Am J Clin Pathol 94:624-627, 1990
22. Fortner JG: Inadvertent spread of cancer at surgery. J Surg Oncol 53(3):191-196, 1993
23. Breuninger H, Dietz K: Prediction of subclinical tumour infiltration in basal cell carcinoma. J Dermatol Surg Oncol 17:74-578, 1991
24. Brodland DG, Zitelli JA: Surgical margins for excision of primary cutaneous squamous cell carcinoma. J Am Acad Dermatol 27:241-248, 1992
25. Wolff DJ, Zitelli JA: Surgical margins of basal cell carcinoma. Arch Dermatol 123:340-344, 1987
26. Salache SJ, Amonett RA: Morpheaform basal cell epitheliomas: a study of subclinical extension in a series of 51 cases. J. Dermatol Surg Oncol 56:387-394, 1981
27. Kroon BBR, Bergman W, Coebergh JWW, Ruiter DJ: Consensus on the management of malignant melanoma of the skin in the Netherlands. Dutch Melanoma Working Party. Melanoma Res 9(3):207-212, 1999
28. Argenta LC: The nose. In: Soutar DS, Tiwari RM (eds). Excision and Reconstruction in Head and Neck Cancer, p 239. London: Churchill Livingstone 1994
29. Panje W, Ceilley R: The influence of embryology of the mid-face on the spread of epithelial malignancies. Laryngoscope 89:1914-1920, 1979
30. Pathak I, O'Brien CJ, Petersen-Schaeffer K et al: Do nodal metastases from cutaneous melanoma of the head and neck follow a clinically predictable pattern? Head Neck 23:785-790, 2001
31. Shah JP, Kraus DH, Dubner S, Sarkar S: Patterns of regional lymph node metastases from cutaneous melanomas of the head and neck. Am J Surg 162:320-323, 1999
32. Van den Brekel MW, Castelijns JA: Imaging of lymph nodes in the neck. Semin Roentgenol 35(1):42-53, 2000
33. Thomas RJ, Frost TW: Immediate versus delayed repair of skin defects following resection of carcinoma. Otolaryngol Clin N Am 26:203-213, 1993
34. Evans GR, Williams JZ, Ainslie NB: Cutaneous nasal malignancies: is primary reconstruction safe? Head Neck 19(3):182-187, 1997
35. Levine H: Cutaneous carcinoma of the head and neck: management of massive and previously uncontrolled lesions. Laryngoscope 93:87, 1983
36. Lohuis PJFM, Vuyk HD: Micrografische chirurgie volgens Mohs voor de behandeling van non-melanoma huidkanker in het aangezicht. NTV Dermatol Venereol 11:12-16, 2001

37. Vuyk HD, Lohuis PJFM: Mohs micrographic surgery for facial skin cancer: a review. Clin Otolaryngol 26:265-273, 2001
38. Rowe DE, Carroll RJ, Day CL Jr: Mohs surgery is the treatment of choice for recurrent (previously treated) basal cell carcinoma. J Dermatol Surg Oncol 15:424-431, 1989
39. Snow SN, Madjar DD Jr: Mohs surgery in the management of cutaneous malignancies. Clin Dermatol 19(3):339-347, 2001
40. Baker RA, Swanson NA, Grekin RC: Mohs' surgical treatment and reconstruction of cutaneous malignancies of the nose. Facial Plast Surg 1987; 5: 1, 29-47, 1987
41. Menick FJ: Artistry in aesthetic surgery: aesthetic perception and the subunit principle. Clin Plast Surg 14(4):723-734, 1987
42. Burgett GC, Menick FJ: Aesthetic Reconstruction of the Nose. St Louis, MO: CV Mosby 1994
43. Baker SR, Naficy S: Principles of Nasal Rconstruction. St Louis, MO: CV Mosby 2002
44. Watts S, Vuyk HD, Kirkland P: Nasal reconstruction. In: Vuyk HD, Lohuis PJFM (eds) Facial Plastic Reconstructive Surgery. London: Hodder 2005
45. Barton FE: Aesthetic aspects of nasal reconstruction. Clin Plast Surg 15(1):155-166, 1988
46. Singh DJ, Bartlett SP: Aesthetic consideration in nasal reconstruction and the role of modified nasal subunits. Plast Reconstr Surg 111:639-651, 2003
47. Menick FJ: A 10-year experience in nasal reconstruction with the three-stage forehead flap. Plast Reconstr Surg 109(6):1839-1855; discussion 1856-1861, 2002
48. Burgett GC, Menick FJ: The subunit principle for nasal reconstruction. Plast Reconstr Surg 76:239-247, 1985
49. Zitelli JA: Secondary intention healing: an alternative to surgical repair. Clin Dermatol 2:92-106, 1984
50. Gosler JB, Pollack SV: Healing by secondary intention. In: Thomas RJ, Roller J (eds) Cutaneous Facial Surgery. Stuttgart: Thieme Med Publ 1992
51. Johnson TM, Radner D, Nelson BR: Soft tissue reconstruction with skin grafting. J Am Acad Dermatol 27(2):151-162, 1992
52. Breach HM: Preauricular full-thickness skin grafts. Br J Plast Surg 71:124-126, 1978
53. Field LM: The preauricular site for donor grafts of skin. J Dermatol Surg Oncol 6:40-44, 1980
54. Booth SA, Zalla MJ, Roenigk RK, Phillips PK: The nasolabial fold donor site for full-thickness skin grafts of nasal tip defects. J Dermatol Surg Oncol 19:553-559, 1993
55. Becker FF, Hillstrom RP: Reconstruction of the nose and midface. In: Papel IA, Nachlas NE (eds) Facial Plastic and Reconstructive Surgery. St Louis, MO: CV Mosby 1992
56. Zitelli JA, Fasio MJ: Reconstruction of the nose with local flaps. J Dermatol Surg Oncol 17:184-189, 1991
57. Becker FF: Local flaps in facial plastic surgery. J Dermatol Surg Oncol 14:635-647, 1988
58. Becker FF, Langford FP: Local flaps in nasal reconstruction. Facial Plast Surg Clin N Am 4:505-515, 1996
59. Larrabee WF, Trachy R, Sutton D: Rhomboid flap dynamics. Arch Otolaryngol 107:755-757, 1981
60. Walike JW, Larrabee WF: The nose flap. Arch Otolaryngol 111:430-433, 1985
61. Flint ID, Siegle RJ: The bipedicled flap revisited. J Dermatol Surg Oncol 20:394-400, 1994

62. Tardy ME, Tenta LT, Azem K: The bilobed flap in nasal repair. Arch Otolaryngol 95:1-5, 1992
63. Moy RL, Grossfeld JS, Baum M, Rivlin D, Eremia S: Reconstruction of the nose utilizing a bilobed flap. Int J Dermatol 33:657-660, 1994
64. Zitelli JA: The bilobed flap for nasal reconstruction. Arch Dermatol 125:957-559, 1990
65. Murakami CS, Odland PD: Bilobed flap variations. Oper Tech Otolaryngol Head Neck Surg 4:76-79, 1993
66. Dzubow LM: Nasal dorsal flaps. In: Baker SR, Swanson NA (eds) Local Flaps in Facial Reconstruction. St Louis, MO: CV Mosby 1995
67. Johnson TM, Swanson NA, Baker SR, Brown MD, Nelson BR: The Rieger flap for nasal reconstruction. Arch Otolaryngol Head Neck Surg 121:634-637, 1995
68. Younger RAL: The versatile melolabial flap. Otolaryngol Head Neck Surg 107:721-726, 1992
69. Field LM: The nasolabial flap: a defensive reappraisal. J Dermatol Surg Oncol 16:429-436, 1990
70. Zitelli JA: The nasolabial flap as a single-stage procedure. Arch Dermatol 126:1445-1448, 1990
71. Park SS: Reconstruction of nasal defects larger than 1.5 cm in diameter. Laryngoscope 110:1241-1250, 2000
72. Quatela GC, Sherris DA, Rounds MF: Aesthetic refinements of forehead reconstruction. Arch Otolaryngol Head Neck Surg 121:1106-1113, 1995
73. Alfort EL, Baker SR, Shumrick KA: Midforehead flaps. In: Baker SR, Swanson NA (eds) Local Flaps in Facial Reconstruction. St Louis, MO: CV Mosby 1995
74. Shumrick KA, Smith TL: The anatomic basis for the design of forehead flaps in nasal reconstruction. Arch Otolaryngol Head Neck Surg 118:373-379, 1992
75. Fosko SW, Dzubow LM: Nasal reconstruction with the cheek island pedicle flap. J Am Acad Dermatol 35:580-587, 1996
76. Johnson TM, Baker SR, Brown MD et al: Utility of the subcutaneous hinge flap in nasal reconstruction. Dermatol Surg 30:459, 1994
77. Kroll SS, Reece GP, Robb G, Black J: Deep-plane cervicofacial rotation-advancement flap for reconstruction of large cheek defects. Plast Reconstr Surg 94:88-93, 1994
78. Burgett GC, Menick FJ: Nasal support and lining: the marriage of beauty and blood supply. Plast Reconstruc Surg 84:189-203, 1989
79. Robinson JA, Burgett GC: Nasal valve malfunction resulting from resection of cancer. Arch Otolaryngol Head Neck Surg 116:1419-1424, 1990
80. Menick FJ: Lining options in nasal reconstruction. Oper Tech Plast Reconstr Surg 5:65-75, 1998
81. Park SS, Cook TA, Wang TD: The epithelial 'turn-in' flap in nasal reconstruction. Arch Otolaryngol Head Neck Surg 121:1122-1127, 1995
82. Lohuis PJFM, Vuyk HD: Shaping and positioning of the nasal tip. In: Vuyk HD, Lohuis PJFM (eds) Facial Plastic and Reconstructive Surgery. London: Hodder 2005
83. Robinson JK: Risk of developing another basal cell carcinoma: a 5 year prospective study. Cancer 60:118, 1987

SUBJECT INDEX

N

Q